CARDIOPULMONARY CRITICAL CARE

CARDIOPULMONARY CRITICAL CARE

Thomas L. Higgins

Chief, Critical Care Division
Baystate Medical Center, Springfield, MA, USA
Associate Professor of Medicine and Anesthesiology,
Tufts University, School of Medicine, Boston, MA, USA

Jay S. Steingrub

Director, Medical Intensive Care Unit
Baystate Medical Center, Springfield, MA, USA
Associate Professor of Medicine,
Tufts University, School of Medicine, Boston, MA, USA

Robert M. Kacmarek

Director, Respiratory Care
Massachusetts General Hospital, Boston, MA, USA
Associate Professor of Anesthesiology,
Harvard Medical School, Boston, MA, USA

James K. Stoller

Head, Section on Respiratory Therapy
Department of Pulmonary/Critical Care Medicine, The Cleveland Clinic Foundation, Cleveland, OH, USA
Vice Chairman, Division of Medicine Associate Chief of Staff
The Cleveland Clinic Foundation, Cleveland, OH, USA
Professor of Medicine,
CCF Health Science Center of Ohio State University, Columbus, OH, USA

BIOS Scientific Publishers Ltd
9 Newtec Place, Magdalen Road, Oxford OX4 1RE, UK
Tel. 144 (0) 1865 726286. Fax 144 (0) 1865 246823
World Wide Web home page: http://www.bios.co.uk/

Distributed exclusively in the United States of America, its dependent territories, Canada, Mexico, Central and South America, and the Carribean by Springer-Verlag New York Inc., 175 Fifth Avenue, New York, USA, by arrangement with BIOS Scientific Publishers Ltd., 9 Newtec Place, Magdalen Road, Oxford OX4 1RE, UK

Important Note from the Publisher

The information contained within this book was obtained by BIOS Scientific Publishers Ltd from sources believed by us to be reliable. However, while every effort has been made to ensure its accuracy, no responsibility for loss or injury whatsoever occasioned to any person acting or refraining from action as a result of information contained herein can be accepted by the authors or publishers.

The reader should remember that medicine is a constantly evolving science and while the authors and publishers have ensured that all dosages, applications and practices are based on current indications, there may be specific practices that differ between communities. You should always follow the guidelines laid down by the manufacturers of specific products and the relevant authorities in the country in which you are practising.

Production Editor: Aimie Haylings
Designed and typeset by J&L Composition Ltd, Filey, North Yorkshire, UK
Printed by Cromwell Press, Trowbridge, UK

Contents

Contents

Abbreviations

ABG	arterial blood gas		BUN	blood urea nitrogen
A/C	assist/control		CABG	coronary artery bypass grafting
ACE	angiotensin converting enzyme		CAD	coronary artery disease
ACEI	angiotensin-converting enzyme inhibitor		cAMP	3′,5′-cyclic adenosine monophosphate
ACLS	advanced cardiac life support		CAP	community-acquired pneumonia
ACT	activated clotting time		CAVH	continuous arteriovenous hemofiltration
ADH	antidiuretic hormone			
AF	atrial fibrillation		CHF	congestive heart failure
AFl	atrial flutter		CI	cardiac index
AG	anion gap		CNS	central nervous system
ALI	acute lung injury		CO	cardiac output
ALV	adaptive lung ventilation		COMT	catecholamine-o-methyl transferase
AMI	acute myocardial infarction			
AP	accessory pathway		COP	colloid osmotic pressure
APACHE	Acute Physiology and Chronic Health Evaluation		COPD	chronic obstructive pulmonary disease
APD	atrial premature depolarization		CPAP	continuous positive airway pressure
APRV	airway pressure release ventilation		CPB	cardiopulmonary bypass
APS	adaptive pressure support		CPK	creatine phosphokinase
aPTT	activated partial thromboplastin time		CPR	cardiopulmonary resuscitation
			CRRT	continuous renal replacement therapy
AR	adrenergic receptor			
AR	aortic regurgitation		CSM	carotid sinus massage
ARDS	adult/acute respiratory distress syndrome		CT	computer tomography
			CVC	central venous catheter
ARF	acute respiratory failure		CVP	central venous pressure
AS	aortic stenosis		CVVHD	continuous veno-venous hemofiltration with dialysis
ATC	automatic tube compensation			
AV	atrio-ventricular		CXR	chest radiograph
a-vDO$_2$	arteriovenous O$_2$ content difference		DAG	diacylglycerol
			DCA	dichloroacetate
AVNRT	atrioventricular nodal re-entrant tachycardia		DIC	disseminated intravascular coagulation
AVRT	atrioventricular re-entrant tachycardia		DOPA	dihydroxyphenylethylamine
BAL	broncho-alveolar lavage		2,3-DPG	2,3-diphosphoglycerate
BiPAP	bi-level positive airway pressure		DVT	deep venous thrombosis
BOOP	bronchiolitis obliterans organizing pneumonia		ECCO$_2$R	extracorporeal membrane carbon dioxide removal

ECG	electrocardiogram/ electrocardigraphy		LA	left atrial
ECMO	extracorporeal membrane oxygenation		LAP	left atrial pressure
			LBBB	left bundle branch block
EDV	end-diastolic blood volume		LDUH	low-dose unfractionated heparin
EKG	electrocardiograph		LMWH	low molecular weight heparin
ELISA	enzyme-linked immune serum assay		LPVS	lung-protective ventilatory strategy
EMG	electromyogram		LR	lactated Ringer's solution
ERV	expiratory reserve volume		LV	left ventricle/ ventricular
ESBL	extended spectrum β-lactamase		LVEDP	left ventricular end-diastolic pressure
ESV	end-systolic blood volume		LVEDV	left ventricular end-diastolic blood volume
ETA	endotracheal aspirate			
FAST	focused abdominal sonogram for trauma		LVSWI	left ventricular stroke work index
			MAO	monoamine oxidase
FEV$_1$	forced expiratory volume in 1 s		MAP	mean arterial pressure
FFP	fresh frozen plasma		MAT	multifocal atrial tachycardia
FiO$_2$	fraction of inspired oxygen		MCT	medium-chain triglyceride
FOB	fiberoptic bronchoscopy		MI	myocardial infarction
FRC	functional residual capacity		MIC	minimal inhibitory concentration
FVC	forced vital capacity		MICU	medical intensive care unit
GI	gastrointestinal		MIP	maximal inspiratory pressure
Gi	G-inhibitory (protein)		MMV	mandatory minute ventilation
Gs	G-stimulatory (protein)		MODS	multiple organ dysfunction syndrome
HAP	hospital-acquired pneumonia			
HALF	hypertonic albuminated fluid		MPAP	mean pulmonary arterial pressure
HFJV	high-frequency jet ventilation		MPM	Mortality Probability Model
Hgb	hemoglobin		MR	mitral regurgitation
HSS	hypertonic saline solution		MRI	magnetic resonance imaging
5-HT	5-hydroxytryptamine		MRSA	methicillin-resistant *Staphylococcus aureus*
HTN	hypertension			
IABC	intraaortic balloon counterpulsation		MS	mitral stenosis
			MSOF	multiple system organ failure
IABP	intraaortic balloon pump		MV	mechanical ventilator
IC	inspiratory capacity		MVV	maximal voluntary ventilation
ICD	internal cardiac defibrillator		MW	molecular weight
ICU	intensive care unit		NE	norepinephrine
IL	interleukins		NG	nasogastric
IJV	internal jugular vein		NIF	negative inspiratory force
IMV	intermittent mandatory ventilation		NIPPV	noninvasive positive pressure ventilation
INR	international normalized ratio		NPV	negative predictive value
IP3	inositol 1,4,5-triphosphate		NS	normal saline solution
IPC	intermittent pneumatic compression		NSTEMI	non-ST elevation myocardial infarction
IPG	impedance plethysmograpy		OHS	open-heart surgery
IRV	inspiratory reserve volume		OR	operating room

PA	pulmonary artery		SB	sinus bradycardia
PA/C	pressure assist/control		SCM	sternocleidomastoid muscle
PAC	pulmonary artery catheterization/catheter		SDD	selective digestive decontamination
$PaCO_2$	arterial CO_2 tension		SI	stroke index
PACU	post-anesthesia care units		SILV	synchronous independent lung ventilation
PAI-1	plasminogen activator inhibitor I			
PAO	pulmonary artery occlusion		SIMV	synchronized intermittent mandatory ventilation
PaO_2	mixed venous O_2 tension			
PAOP	pulmonary artery occlusion pressure		SIRS	systemic inflammatory response syndrome
PAP	pulmonary artery pressure		SR	sinus rhythm
PAWP	pulmonary artery wedge pressure		ST	sinus tachycardia
PBS	protected brush specimens		ST	surface tension
PCIRV	pressure control inverse ratio ventilation		STEMI	ST elevation myocardial infarction
PCWP	pulmonary capillary wedge pressure		SV	stroke volume
			SVC	superior vena cava
PDI	phosphodiesterase inhibitor		SVR	systemic vascular resistance
PE	pulmonary embolism		SVT	supraventricular tachycardia
PEA	pulseless electrical activity		TBW	total body water
PEEP	positive end-expiratory pressure		TCO	thermodilution cardiac output
PLV	partial liquid ventilation		TdP	Torsades de Pointes
PMC	point of maximum compliance change		TEE	transesophageal echocardiogram
			TFPI	tissue factor protein inhibitor
Ppl	intrathoracic/intrapleural pressure		THAM	tromethamine
PPV	positive predictive value		TLC	total lung capacity
PRVC	pressure-regulated volume control		TNF	tumor necrosis factor
PS	pressure support		TV	tidal volume
PSV	pressure support ventilation		UAG	urinary anion gap
PVC	premature ventricular contraction		UIP	upper inflection point
PVR	pulmonary vascular resistance		US	compression ultrasonography
q	every		VAP	ventilator-associated pneumonia
RBBB	right bundle branch block		VAPS	volume-assured pressure support
RBC	red blood cells		VC	vital capacity
rhAPC	recombinant activated protein C		VILI	ventilator-induced lung injury
RIJV	right internal jugular vein		VIP	vasoactive infusion port
RPF	renal plasma flow		VO_2	O_2 consumption
RPP	rate pressure product		VQ	ventilation-perfusion (ratio)
RTA	renal tubular acidosis		VRE	vancomycin-resistant enterococci
rtPA	recombinant tissue type plasminogen activator		VS	volume support
			VT	ventricular tachycardia
RV	residual volume		VTE	venous thromboembolism
RV	right ventricle/ventricular		WCT	wide complex tachycardias
RVSWI	right ventricular stroke work index		WOB	work of breathing
SaO_2	arterial O_2 saturation		WPW	Wolfe-Parkinson-White (pattern)

Contributors

Ali Al-Khafaji MD
Critical Care Medicine, Dartmouth-Hitchcock
Medical Center, Lebanon, New Hampshire,
USA

C. Allen Bashour MD FACS FCCP
Department of Cardiothoracic Anesthesiology,
Division of Anesthesiology and Critical Care
Medicine, The Cleveland Clinic Foundation,
Cleveland, Ohio, USA

Howard L. Corwin MD FCCM FACP
Critical Care Medicine, Dartmouth-Hitchcock
Medical Center, Lebanon, New Hampshire,
USA

Marcus J. Hampers MD
Critical Care Medicine, Dartmouth-Hitchcock
Medical Center, Lebanon, New Hampshire,
USA

Thomas L. Higgins MD MBA FACP FCCM
FACC
Critical Care Division, Baystate Medical
Center, Springfield, Massachusetts, USA

Paul Jodka MD
Critical Care Division, Baystate Medical
Center, Springfield, Massachusetts, USA

Robert M. Kacmarek RRT PhD
Respiratory Therapy Department,
Massachusetts General Hospital, Boston,
Massachusetts, USA

Laurie A. Loiacono MD
Critical Care Division, Baystate Medical
Center, Springfield, Massachusetts, USA

William T. McGee MD MHA
Critical Care Division, Baystate Medical
Center, Springfield, Massachusetts, USA

Magdy Migeed MD
New York Heart Center, 1000 East Genesse St,
Syracuse, New York, USA

Imtiaz A. Munshi MD
Trauma Division, Baystate Medical Center,
Springfield, Massachusetts, USA

Lawrence S. Rosenthal MD PhD FACC
Division of Cardiology, University of
Massachusetts Memorial Medical Center,
Worcester, Massachusetts, USA

Marc Schweiger MD FACC
Division of Cardiology, Baystate Medical
Center, Springfield, Massachusetts, USA

Jay S. Steingrub MD FACP FCCM
Medical Intensive Care Unit, Baystate
Medical Center, Springfield, Massachusetts,
USA

James K. Stoller MD FACP FCCM FCCP
Respiratory Therapy Department, Cleveland
Clinic Foundation, Cleveland, Ohio, USA

Introduction

Does the world need another critical care textbook? As I look around my office, I count four hefty, comprehensive critical care tomes, five ICU handbooks, and more than two dozen related texts on mechanical ventilation, nutritional support, arrhythmia management, monitoring and pharmacotherapy. My handheld organizer provides me with instant antibiotic and drug-dosage recommendations, and I can easily search the literature on computers in my office, at home, and at every nursing station. With all of this information readily at hand, why would anyone want another critical care text?

The answer may be found in the concept of the evolutionary 'niche'. The audience for this book is not necessarily the expert in critical care, who presumably also has a well-stocked bookshelf in his or her office. This book is intended for clinicians with intermittent responsibilities for critically ill patients in a world of competing demands. Our target audience includes the medical student on a final-year elective, the house officer on a one-month rotation in the ICU, the nurse or respiratory therapist seeking more information, and the general internist, surgeon or anesthesiologist who occasionally cares for critically ill patients. Hospitalists (hospital-based doctors) may find this book to be particularly useful, especially if their hospital does not support full-time critical care staff. Our goal was to create a work with more depth than the typical pocket reference, while avoiding the bulk and expense of a more encyclopedic work. In order to achieve this goal, we have concentrated this volume on cardiac and pulmonary issues in the ICU. While the intent is for this book to be part of a larger family of books that would, in

total, approximate a standard text this volume also stands on its own. The hope is that it will provide a logical approach and best-practice suggestions for a variety of common critical care issues, while remaining small enough to be read cover-to-cover. The authors recognize that controversy exists in many treatment decisions, but have chosen to present a consensus approach, buttressed by essential references. My feeling is that questions raised at 3 in the morning should be answered succinctly. I'm happier to engage in a spirited discussion supported by 200 conflicting references when the patient has been stabilized.

Where possible, chapters have been arranged to present a brief overview of the disease process and epidemiology, diagnostic criteria, important differential diagnostic considerations, and practical, evidence-based advice on patient management. We have only touched on prognostic information, enough to use in discussions with family members. Tables have been used to facilitate quick reference, and the figures are similar to what we would hand-draw on morning rounds to illuminate a concept. Some chapters are intended to expose background information (Respiratory and Cardiac Physiology, Oxygen Delivery and Utilization, Clinical Shock States, Respiratory Muscle Function, ARDS) while others are more practically oriented (Pressors and Inotropes, Hypertensive Emergencies, Cardiac Rhythm Disturbances, Nosocomial Pneumonia, Weaning from Mechanical Ventilation, and Postoperative Care). In looking through other textbooks, we felt that the mechanics of line placement were seldom detailed, and have included a richly illustrated chapter on Line Placement Techniques.

In order to keep the book to a reasonable size, we have deliberately omitted important aspects of critical care – specifically neurologic and neurosurgical management, gastrointestinal bleeding, toxicity and poisoning, hematalogic and oncologic management, renal issues including dialysis, and infectious/immunologic issues. Plans are in the works for companion volumes to address these topics.

Just as the practice of critical care is a multidisciplinary, team effort, so to is the process of bringing a textbook to life. The authors would like to recognize the efforts of a number of individuals whose contributions were essential to this book. First and foremost, Ms. Suzanne Allen, administrative assistant for Baystate Medical Center's Critical Care Division, spent countless hours typing and retyping manuscripts, chased down letters of permission to reprint figures and tables, and kept the project moving and organized. Mr. Jonathan Gregory initiated the project for BIOS Scientific Publishers Ltd, helped formulate the style of the book and provided much-needed encouragement during the battle to complete the manuscripts. Ms. Victoria Oddie and Dr. Katie Deaton, of the Editorial Department at BIOS, helped tidy up the manuscript and fix the many overlooked details as the book wound its way to production. Aimie Haylings, our Production Editor, gracefully pushed the book through its final months, and managed to turn indecipherable scrawls and eighth-generation photocopies into art.

Special thanks is also due to our colleagues: attending physicians, nurses, respiratory therapists, fellows, residents and medical students who asked the right questions at the right times, and who generously read manuscript drafts and offered valuable suggestions. Our spouses and families deserve thanks for their unconditional love, patience, wit and support when another impossible deadline loomed. Above all, we thank our patients and their families, from whom we have learned so much to be applied in the future.

Thomas L. Higgins MD

Acknowledgements

'To Louis and Mary Higgins, who started me on this journey, and to Suzanne, my traveling companion during the best years' – TLH

'To Milagros and my son, Oron, who define love and happiness as not a destination, but rather, a method of life' – JSS

'To my wife, Jan, who has consistently encouraged my academic pursuits and to my children Robert, Julia, Katie, and Callie who make it all worthwhile' – RMK

'To Terry, for her abiding support and love, and to Jake, who gives purpose, grounding, and love.' – JKS

Chapter 1

Respiratory physiology/pulmonary gas exchange

Robert M. Kacmarek, PhD, RRT

Contents

1.1 Introduction

Managing respiratory dysfunction is a fundamental aspect of critical care medicine. Although respiratory failure is a rare cause of death in the intensive care unit (ICU)[1], the vast majority of patients admitted to the ICU experience respiratory dysfunction[2]. This introductory chapter focuses on pulmonary mechanics as related to critical care and pulmonary gas exchange, V/Q relationships, dead space, shunting, and evaluation of hypoxemia and hypercarbia. Such knowledge provides a framework that clarifies the rationale behind the various approaches to mechanical ventilatory support.

1.2 Lung mechanics

The maximum gas-containing capacity of the lungs (total lung capacity, TLC) is divided into four basic volumes and four capacities comprising the four basic volumes (*Table 1.1* and *Figure 1.1*). Of these, the two that have the most relevance to critical care are the functional residual capacity (FRC) and the vital capacity (VC). The FRC is critical to gas exchange; it is an established gas reservoir allowing exchange of oxygen and carbon dioxide on a continual basis during both inspiration and expiration[3]. Loss of FRC results in intrapulmonary shunting and oxygenation

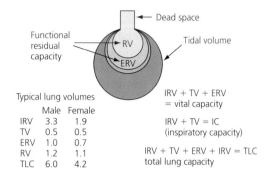

Typical lung volumes

	Male	Female
IRV	3.3	1.9
TV	0.5	0.5
ERV	1.0	0.7
RV	1.2	1.1
TLC	6.0	4.2

IRV + TV + ERV = vital capacity

IRV + TV = IC (inspiratory capacity)

IRV + TV + ERV + IRV = TLC total lung capacity

Figure 1.1 The normal spirogram with all four lung volumes and capacities illustrated. See *Table 1.1* for definitions.

deficits. Much of the management of the critically ill mechanically ventilated patients is focused on restoring and maintaining the FRC (Chapter 15).

Vital capacity is critical because it defines the ventilatory reserve of a patient[3,4]. The closer a patient's TV is to his or her VC, the less capable the patient is of responding to ventilatory stress and sustaining spontaneous ventilation. VC is decreased postoperatively, as a result of the prolonged effects of anesthesia. Neuromuscular/neurologic insult, and changes in the elastic recoil of the lungs and thorax as well as a result of pneumonia, atelectasis or edema also cause decreases in VC. Restoration of the VC is an essential aspect of recovery from ventilatory failure[3].

Table 1.1 Volume subdivisions and capacities of the lung

Residual volume	RV	Gas remaining in the lung after maximum exhalation
Expiratory reserve volume	ERV	Gas that can be forcefully exhaled after passive exhalation
Tidal volume	V_T or TV	Gas inspired and expired each breath
Inspiratory reserve volume	IRV	Gas that can be forcefully inhaled above normal V_T
Functional residual capacity	FRC	RV + ERV
Inspiratory capacity	IC	V_T + IRV
Vital capacity	VC	ERV + V_T + IRV
Total lung capacity	TLC	RV + ERV + V_T + IRV

1.2.1 Pulmonary mechanics

Anatomically the lung and the thorax are configured to move in opposite directions (*Figure 1.2*). The normal elastic recoil of the lungs favors the smallest unstressed volume while the rib cage and chest wall tend to expand to a volume of about 60–70% of total lung capacity after which the chest wall tends to contract[5,6]. Movement of the lungs and thorax is controlled by the muscles of ventilation. Opposing this movement are the elastic properties of the lung and thorax and the resistance of gas flow into the lung.

1.2.2 Elastic properties of the respiratory system

The lung and thorax (chest wall) can be viewed in terms of a set of springs. The recoil tendency of a spring can be expressed in terms of an unstressed or resting length and a length–tension relationship. Similarly, the relevant properties of expandable volumetric structures are the unstressed volume and the relationship between volume and the transmural pressure required to achieve that volume[7]. Transmural pressure is expressed as the difference between the pressure inside and that outside the structure, or distending pressure. For the respiratory system the transmural pressure is equal to alveolar pressure (P_{alv}) minus body surface pressure (P_{BS}). During spontaneous breathing a negative transmural pressure ($P_{alv} - P_{BS}$) causes lung volume to become larger (distending pressure), whereas a positive transmural pressure (recoil pressure) causes lung volume to become smaller. If lung volume is plotted against transmural pressure the classic sigmoid compliance curve of the respiratory system is established (*Figure 1.3*). The slope of the linear section of this pressure–volume relationship (*P–V* curve) is compliance of the total respiratory system (C_{RS}):

$$C_{RS} = \Delta V/\Delta P. \qquad (1.1)$$

1.2.3 Compliance

Compliance is the inverse of elastance and used to estimate the ease of distensibility of the respiratory system. In *Figure 1.3*, the point where the *P–V* curve crosses the volume line represents FRC; to the left of zero on the horizontal axis the transmural pressure is positive, and to the right negative[8]. It should be noted also that as the elastic limits of the system are reached (TLC and RV) a greater pressure change is required for any volume change, whereas,

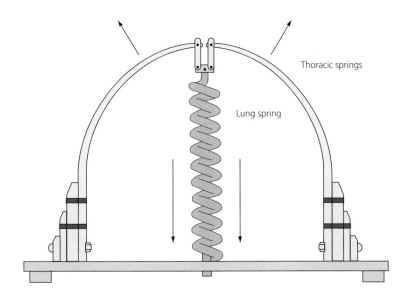

Thoracic springs

Lung spring

Figure 1.2 The lung and thorax may be conceptualized as two springs opposing the movement of each other, the thorax expanding to 60–70% of TLC and the lung contracting. Reproduced with permission from: Scanlan, C.L., Wilkins, R.L. and Stoller, J.K. (1999) *Egan's Fundamentals of Respiratory Care,* 7th Edn. St. Louis: Mosby-Yearbook

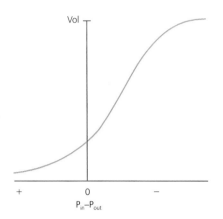

Figure 1.3 The normal pressure–volume relationship for the total respiratory system. As noted beyond FRC (to the right of the vertical volume line) the P–V relationship is linear until TLC (maximum volume) is approached.

between FRC and roughly 60–70% of TLC, the P–V relationship is generally linear[5]. Compliance is usually measured on this linear aspect of the curve and is expressed in 1 cm^{-1} H$_2$O; however, in mechanically ventilated patients it is frequently expressed as ml cm^{-1} H$_2$O. Compliance is dependent on size: the greater the size of the lungs the greater the compliance. However, compliance divided by lung volume is volume independent and referred to as non-dimensional specific compliance[5].

At FRC the transmural pressure is zero. It is at this level that the opposing forces of the lung and thorax are equal and opposite. The elastic properties of the lung and thorax can be independently determined by measuring esophageal pressure (a reflection of pleural pressure, P_{PL}) and comparing it with alveolar pressure[8]. During spontaneous breathing esophageal pressure is reflective of the elastic recoil of the lungs and is used to calculate lung compliance (C_L):

$$C_L = \Delta V/P_{alv} - P_{PL}. \tag{1.2}$$

To calculate thoracic compliance (C_{Th}) the effect of the ventilatory muscles must be eliminated (using paralysis or heavy sedation) and lung volume provided by mechanical

ventilation. In this setting esophageal pressure represents the elastic recoil of the thorax:

$$C_{Th} = \Delta V/P_{alv} - P_{PL}. \tag{1.3}$$

Change in bladder pressure can be used as a substitute for esophageal pressure for the calculation of thoracic compliance[9]. Bladder pressure has been clearly shown to be reflective of abdominal/thoracic recoil pressure in critically ill patients receiving controlled mechanical ventilation. Compliance of the total respiratory system, the lungs and the thorax are related by the following equation:

$$1/C_{RS} = 1/C_L + 1/C_{Th}. \tag{1.4}$$

Figure 1.4 plots the compliance curves of the respiratory system, the lungs, and the thorax. As indicated, the thoracic and lung compliance curves cross the zero recoil pressure line at different lung volume levels. Any change in either lung or thoracic compliance affects the compliance of the total respiratory system.

1.2.4 Surfactant and effect of surface tension

At the surface of any liquid the intermolecular attraction of the molecules in the liquid establishes a barrier or force, surface tension (ST), preventing disruption at the surface. Surface tension established at the air–liquid interface

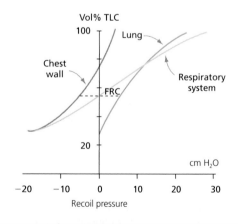

Figure 1.4 The compliance curves of the thorax, lungs, and total respiratory system.

within the alveoli is an important component of the elastic properties of lung. As noted in *Figure 1.5* the pressure–volume relationship of the lung during inspiration and expiration is different dependent upon whether the lung is fluid or air filled[10]. The fluid-filled lung can be distended with much less pressure than an air-filled lung. The air-filled lung also demonstrates a marked hysteresis, that is, the inflation and deflation *P*–*V* relationship is different[5,10]. The reason for this difference is the presence of surfactant, the phospholipid secreted by type 2 alveolar cells. Surfactant reduces surface tension and stabilizes lung volume. Without the presence of surfactant at end exhalation the alveoli would collapse. The relationship between ST and the pressure within a sphere is defined by LaPlace's Law:

$$P = 2\,ST/r \qquad (1.5)$$

where the relationship of the pressure (*P*) within a fluid sphere to the tension (*ST*) created at the surface of the sphere is dependent upon the radius (*r*) of the sphere[5]. The overall

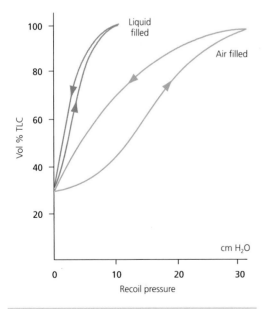

Figure 1.5 Inflation and deflation pressure–volume curves of the normal air-filled lung and a fluid-filled lung. See text for discussion.

quantity of surfactant within the lung during health is constant, decreasing surface tension during exhalation and increasing surface tension during inspiration. As a result, any disruption in surfactant production results in an increase in elastic recoil of the lung or a decrease in lung compliance, decreasing the compliance of the total respiratory system and increasing the likelihood of atelectasis.

1.2.5 Flow resistance

Airflow between atmosphere and the distal lung is dependent upon driving pressure and the resistance to gas flow. Resistance (*R*) to flow in any system is dependent upon the structure of the system and is determined by the pressure gradient (ΔP) needed to maintain flow and the flow rate ($\dot{V}$):

$$R = \Delta P/\dot{V}. \qquad (1.6)$$

Resistance is specifically affected by a number of physical factors of the fluid and system: density (*D*) and viscosity (*n*) of the gas flowing, and radius (*r*) and length (*l*) of the airway[5]. These factors relationship to resistance are illustrated in a modification of Poiseuille's Law[11]:

$$R = \Delta P/\dot{V} = nl8/\pi r4 \qquad (1.7)$$

where *B* is a constant, and by the Reynold's Number (RN)[5]:

$$RN = (\text{Diameter})(\text{Velocity}) \\ (\text{Density})/\text{Viscosity}. \qquad (1.8)$$

Specifically, as the radius of the airway decreases by 50% the resistance to flow increases 16-fold and the less dense and more viscous a gas the more likely it is to flow in a laminar manner[11]. Laminar and turbulent flow are very different. Laminar flow is smooth and uniform flow with the molecules in the center of the gas column proceeding more rapidly than those at the periphery because they do not encounter the resistance of the sides of the vessel. Turbulent flow is rough and tumbling flow where all molecules in the system encounter the sides of the container. The concern between these different flow patterns is the pressure to maintain flow. During laminar flow, R is directly related to the flow, whereas with turbulent flow R is directly related to the flow rate squared. As a result, a much greater pressure gradient is required to maintain turbulent than laminar flow. The use of helium–oxygen mixtures is directly based on these physical properties. The lower-density, higher-viscosity helium generally results in less driving pressure to maintain the same flow[12].

1.2.6 Normal and abnormal values
Table 1.2 lists normal values in adults for resistance and compliance[5] and levels generally present during different clinical settings in the ICU. However, these are estimates and are affected by the size of the patient. A 5 ft tall, 95 pound woman and 6 ft 6 in tall, 220 pound man will have very different normal compliance and resistance.

1.2.7 Measurements during mechanical ventilation
Bedside estimations of both compliance and resistance in mechanically ventilated patients are possible. However, precision in these measurements is generally lacking. The specific instrumentation available in the Pulmonary Function Laboratory is generally not available in the ICU. Ideally, calculation of compliance requires a precise measurement of the static volume of gas maintained in the lung and the pressure required to maintain it. With most ventilators, the tidal volume displayed does not take into consideration volume lost to gas compression in the ventilator tubing and humidifier[13]. As a result, delivered tidal volume must be corrected for system specific compressed volume (CV), which with most ventilating circuits equals about 1–2 ml cm^{-1} H$_2$O (P_{PLAT})[14]. This correction can be avoided if actual exhaled tidal volume (V_{et}) is measured at the artificial airway. Static inspiratory plateau pressure P_{PLAT} must be corrected for total positive end-expiratory pressure (PEEP) (applied plus auto PEEP) to determine the actual pressure maintaining the static lung volume. Thus

an estimate of static total respiratory system compliance (C_{RS}) can be made using the following equation:

$$C_{RS} = V_{et}/P_{PLAT} - PEEP_A - PEEP_I \quad (1.9)$$

where $PEEP_A$ is applied PEEP and $PEEP_I$ is auto-PEEP.

Compliance of the thorax can be determined in a similar manner except that static end expiratory esophageal (eso) or bladder pressure replaces airway pressure:

$$C_T = V_{et}/P_{PLAT} \text{ (eso)} - PEEP_A - PEEP_I. \quad (1.10)$$

To estimate airway resistance the pressure required to establish a constant flow is generally determined. This requires volume ventilation with a square wave flow be delivered. As noted in *Figure 1.6* the difference between peak and plateau pressure when V_T is delivered with a constant gas flow $\dot{V}$ establishes the pressure gradient required to maintain flow:

$$R = P_IP - P_{PLAT}/\dot{V}. \quad (1.11)$$

1.3 The law of motion

From the previous discussion it becomes apparent that the pressure required to ventilate either spontaneously or mechanically is affected by compliance, resistance, volume and flow. These variables are related by the law of motion, which states that the pressure needed to ventilate a patient is equal to volume (V) divided by compliance plus resistance times flow:

$$P = V/C + R\dot{V}. \quad (1.12)$$

Peak ventilating pressure is a result of the combined effects of resistance and compliance whereas P_{PLAT} is solely a reflection of the pressure to overcome compliance and the difference between P_IP and P_{PLAT} the pressure to overcome airways resistance. A change in compliance would change the slope of the airway pressure curve from zero pressure to point A (*Figure 1.6*) and the magnitude of both A and B, whereas a change in resistance would

Table 1.2 Normal and abnormal compliance and airway resistance levels

Total respiratory system[a] (RS)	0.08–0.1 l cm^{-1} H$_2$O
Lung[a]	0.16–0.2 l cm^{-1} H$_2$O
Thorax[a]	0.16–0.2 l cm^{-1} H$_2$O
Specific compliance[a]	0.08 (no units)
RS medically ventilated	60–80 ml cm^{-1} H$_2$O
RS ARDS	<40 ml cm^{-1} H$_2$O
Airway resistance[a] (R)	0.6–2.4 cm H$_2$O l^{-1} s^{-1} at a flow of 0.5 l s^{-1}
R—mechanically ventilated normal	<5 cm H$_2$O difference P$_I$P – P$_{PLAT}$, constant flow
R—mechanically ventilated marked obstruction	>10 cm H$_2$O difference P$_I$P – P$_{PLAT}$, constant flow

[a]Normal values from Comroe, J.H. (1974) *Physiology of Respiration*, 2nd Edn. Year Book Medical Publishers, Chicago, IL.

P$_I$P, peak inspiratory pressure; P$_{PLAT}$, end inspiratory plateau pressure.

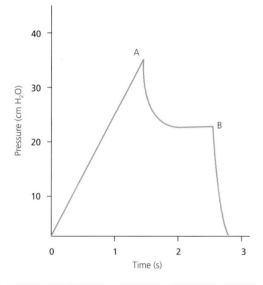

Figure 1.6 An inspiratory positive pressure waveform with an end inspiratory pause. Gas flow is delivered with a constant flow. A, peak airway pressure; B, end inspiratory plateau pressure.

to ventilate the system. In controlled ventilation the ventilator provides all of the effort (pressure) to ventilate; during spontaneous ventilation the patient provides all of the effort. During all forms of assisted ventilation the effort is shared between the patient and the ventilator. A frequent observation during the transition from assisted to controlled ventilation is an increase in airway pressure. The reason for this increase is that the negative intra-thoracic pressure established during assisted ventilation must now be provided by the mechanical ventilator. The actual pressure required to ventilate has not increased, it simply has shifted from the patient to the ventilator.

1.4 Auto-PEEP

Auto-PEEP, also referred to as intrinsic PEEP, is a result of incomplete emptying of the lung at end expiration or air trapping. The term unidentified PEEP is also used to refer to auto-PEEP because auto-PEEP is not identified on the pressure manometer of the ventilator unless an end expiratory hold is imposed[15]. Auto-PEEP is established as a result of the intrinsic properties of the lung, not as a result of setting PEEP on the ventilator. As illustrated in *Figure 1.7*, at normal end exhalation alveolar pressure is greater than central airway pressure when auto-PEEP is present as a result of dynamic flow limitation. But when an end expiratory hold is established, alveolar, central airway and ventilator circuit pressures equilibrate, indicating the average 'system' end

change the magnitude of the difference between A and B and the magnitude of A. Similarly, a change in volume or flow would alter this relationship. It is essential to realize that the pressure generated during ventilation is solely affected by these factors regardless of whether pressure or volume ventilation is used or assisted or controlled ventilation is provided. The greater the volume, flow or airway resistance and the lower the compliance of the system the greater the transmural pressure required

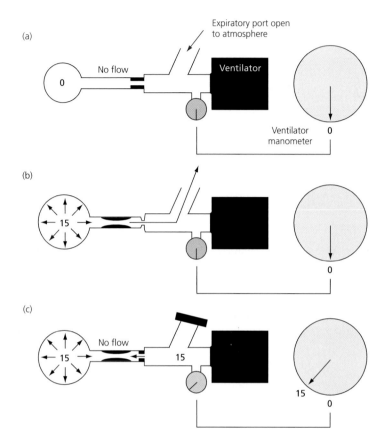

Figure 1.7 Relationship between alveolar, central airway and ventilator circuit pressure during (a) normal conditions and in the presence of severe dynamic airway obstruction, (b) with the expiratory port open, and (c) with the expiratory port occluded. Auto-PEEP level during occlusion can be read on the pressure manometer. From: Pepe, P.E. and Marini, J.J. (1982) Occult positive end expiratory pressure in mechanically ventilated patients with airflow obstruction: the auto-PEEP effect. Reproduced with permission from the *American Review of Respiratory Disease*.

expiratory pressure. In addition to dynamic airflow limitation, large minute ventilation and inadequate expiratory time can cause auto-PEEP.

As already illustrated, auto-PEEP does affect ventilatory mechanics and must be considered during all measurements. Failure to do so results in a misleading interpretation of P–V relationships (lower compliance). During assisted ventilation, auto-PEEP also increases patient effort/work of breathing.

1.5 $\dot{V}/\dot{Q}$ relationships

Ventilation ($\dot{V}$) and perfusion ($\dot{Q}$) distribute throughout the respiratory system in a manner to establish the normal overall $\dot{V}/\dot{Q}$ relationship of 0.8. Maintenance of the $\dot{V}/\dot{Q}$ relationship insures arterial blood gases do not deviate from normal. However, any alteration

in the overall normal $\dot{V}/\dot{Q}$ relationship can result in hypoxemia or hypercarbia.

1.5.1 Ventilation
Distribution of ventilation is gravity dependent, a greater percentage of tidal volume is distributed to gravity dependent lung than non-gravity dependent lung (*Figure 1.8*)[16]. As the lung is contained within the visceral pleural and separated from the parietal pleural by a thin layer of fluid, gravity can dramatically affect local pleural pressure and as a result local FRC and distribution of V_T. In general, lung units that are non-gravity dependent have a more negative pleural pressure, greater FRC and lower compliance than gravity dependent units. A lower percentage of tidal volume distributes to non-gravity dependent than to gravity dependent units. That is, the majority of the tidal volume distributes to gravity,

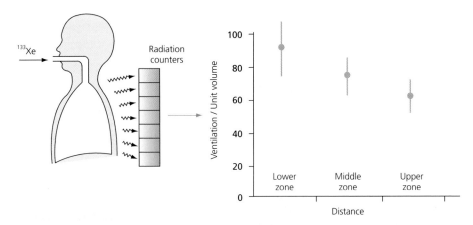

Figure 1.8 Measurement of regional differences in ventilation with radioactive xenon. Ventilation decreases from the apex to the base of the lung in the standing position. From: West, J. (1990) *Respiratory Physiology: The Essentials*, 4th Edn. Reproduced with permission from Lippincott, Williams & Wilkins.

whereas the majority of FRC is distributed to non-gravity dependent lung. The largest proportion of ventilation is distributed to gravity regardless of position.

1.5.2 Perfusion

Distribution of perfusion is similar to that of ventilation, although at the extremes of the lung (base and apex) the differences are greater than those observed with ventilation[17]. John West has proposed a three-zone model of pulmonary perfusion (*Figure 1.9*)[17].

In zone 1, the apex of the lung, alveolar pressure is generally greater than arterial, which is greater than venous pressure. This results in essentially no pulmonary capillary flow during rest. In zone 2, the middle portion of the lung, perfusion is intermittent during rest, as arterial pressure is greater than alveolar but alveolar pressure is greater than venous. In zone 3, perfusion is continuous (during inspiration and expiration), as arterial pressure and venous pressure are greater than alveolar pressure.

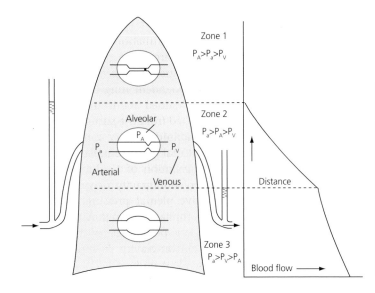

Figure 1.9 John West's model of uneven distribution of blood flow. Pulmonary blood flow is based on vascular and alveolar pressures affecting actual blood flow to capillaries. From: West, J.B., Dollery, C.T. and Naimark, A. (1964) Distribution of blood flow in isolated lung: relation to vascular and alveolar pressure. Reproduced with permission from *The Journal of Applied Physiology*.

West's model also dictates that the gravitational distribution of perfusion is maintained regardless of position. However, recent animal data[18,19] cast some doubt on redistribution of ventilation based on gravity in other than the erect or supine position. However, no data are currently available on patients to contradict West's theory of $\dot{V}/\dot{Q}$ matching. In addition, recent data demonstrating the efficacy of prone positioning on oxygenation in about 70% of adult respiratory distress syndrome (ARDS) patients studied would lend support to West's model[20,21].

From the above discussion, it is understood that there are specific relationships in health between $\dot{V}$ and $\dot{Q}$ that establish the normal variability between $\dot{V}/\dot{Q}$ relationships from the apex to the base of the lungs. The base is normally better perfused than the apex and the apex is normally better ventilated. At the apex $\dot{V}/\dot{Q}$ approaches infinity because of the lack of perfusion, whereas the $\dot{V}/\dot{Q}$ is greater than about 3.0 in the base, with the overall $\dot{V}/\dot{Q}$ maintained in health at 0.8[22].

1.5.3 Shunting and dead space

A $\dot{V}/\dot{Q}$ other than 1.0 indicates a maldistribution of either ventilation or perfusion. Numerous pathophysiologic conditions can alter $\dot{V}/\dot{Q}$ relationships (*Table 1.3*). If the $\dot{V}/\dot{Q}$ is greater than 1.0 dead space is present, whereas a $\dot{V}/\dot{Q}$ less than 1.0 indicates the presence of intrapulmonary shunting. *Figure 1.10* illustrates the extremes of $\dot{V}/\dot{Q}$ relationships[23]. A normal unit is one in which ventilation and perfusion are perfectly matched, whereas a silent unit has complete absence of either ventilation or perfusion. A dead space unit occurs if ventilation is present but perfusion is absent, and a shunt unit occurs when ventilation is absent but perfusion is present. In addition to these extreme conditions, a dead space effect is established whenever ventilation is in excess of perfusion or whenever the $\dot{V}/\dot{Q}$ relationship exceeds 1.0. A shunt effect occurs whenever the $\dot{V}/\dot{Q}$ relationship is less than 1.0.

Table 1.3 Cause of altered $\dot{V}/\dot{Q}$ relationships

Decreased $\dot{V}/\dot{Q}$ (shunt)
- Anatomic distribution of venous blood to the left heart
- Arterial or ventricular septal defects
- Arteriovenous anastomosis
- Severe liver disease
- Vascular pulmonary tumors
- Congenital cardiac anomalies
- Atelectasis
- Consolidating pneumonia
- Pneumothorax
- Pleural effusion
- Retained secretions
- Bronchospasm
- Partial or complete airway obstruction
- Regional increases in fibrotic lung tissue
- Decreased tidal volume
- Mucosal edema
- Any condition in which ventilation is less than perfusion

Increased $\dot{V}/\dot{Q}$ (dead space)
- Positive pressure ventilation
- PEEP/continuous positive airway pressure (CPAP)
- Mechanical dead space
- Pulmonary emboli
- Emphysema
- ARDS
- Rapid shallow breathing
- Decreased cardiac output
- Alveolar septal wall destruction
- Any condition in which ventilation is greater than perfusion

1.6 Evaluation of hypoxemia

Hypoxemia can be caused by a number of pathophysiologic abnormalities, most commonly alveolar hypoventilation, $\dot{V}/\dot{Q}$ mismatch (low $\dot{V}/\dot{Q}$) and true shunting. Diffusion abnormalities do cause hypoxemia as a result of delays in passage of O_2 molecules across the alveolar capillary membrane. However, as noted in *Figure 1.11*, hemoglobin molecules become fully saturated with oxygen in about 0.25 s whereas the normal transit time for hemoglobin through the pulmonary capillaries is about 1.0 s[16]. As a result, the impact of a diffusion abnormality is usually limited. In

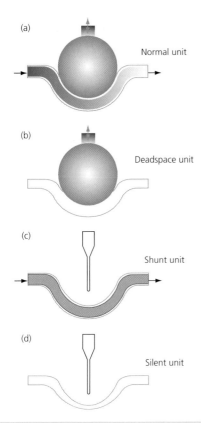

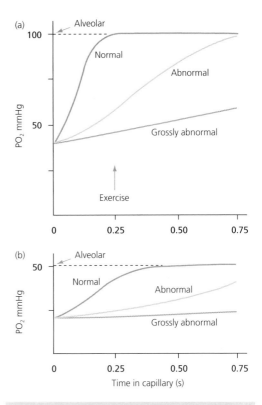

Figure 1.10 The theoretical respiratory unit (a) normal ventilation, normal perfusion; (b) normal ventilation, no perfusion; (c) no ventilation, normal perfusion; (d) no ventilation, no perfusion. From: Shapiro, B.A., Harrison, R.A. and Walton, Jr. (1982) *Clinical Application of Arterial Blood Gases,* 3rd Edn. Year Book Medical Publishers.

Figure 1.11 Oxygen equilibration time across the alveolar–capillary membrane. (a) Time course when alveolar PO_2 is normal. (b) Time course when alveolar PO_2 is markedly decreased. From: West, J. (1990) *Respiratory Physiology: The Essentials,* 4th Edn. Reproduced with permission from Lippincott, Williams & Wilkins.

patients with severe interstitial edema or gross pulmonary edema diffusion defects do contribute to hypoxemia but the precise level of contribution is difficult to establish.

Alveolar hypoventilation always results in hypoxemia if severe. As noted from the alveolar gas equation,

$$P_AO_2 = \frac{(P_B - P_{H_2O})(F_IO_2) - (P_ACO_2)}{(F_IO_2 + 1 - F_IO_2/R)} \quad (1.13)$$

where P_B is the barometric pressure and R is the respiratory quotient and increases in alveolar PCO_2 result in a decrease in alveolar PO_2.

The last part of Equation (1.13) is frequently simplified to

$$(P_ACO_2)(F_IO_2 + 1 - F_IO_2/R) \approx P_ACO_2/R. \quad (1.14)$$

In other words, for approximately every 1 mmHg P_ACO_2 increase the alveolar PO_2 decreases by 1.25 mmHg (R = 0.8). Alveolar hypo- or hyperventilation can markedly alter the alveolar PO_2 and thus the arterial PO_2 (P_aO_2). Of all of the causes of hypoxemia this is the easiest to correct. Reestablishment of normal alveolar ventilation returns P_aO_2 to its normal range.

1.6.1 $\dot{V}/\dot{Q}$ mismatch

A $\dot{V}/\dot{Q}$ mismatch results in hypoxemia when a reduction in ventilation is out of proportion to the change in perfusion. Although low $\dot{V}/\dot{Q}$ areas result in the same level of hypoxemia as observed in a similar level of true shunting,

differentiation between the two is important because of their varied response to hypoxemia[24]. As illustrated in *Figure 1.12*, the hypoxemia as a result of low $\dot{V}/\dot{Q}$ areas responds well to a small increase in the F_IO_2 whereas true shunting (*Figure 1.13*) does not. With low $\dot{V}/\dot{Q}$ areas,

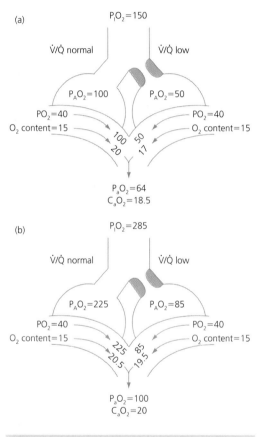

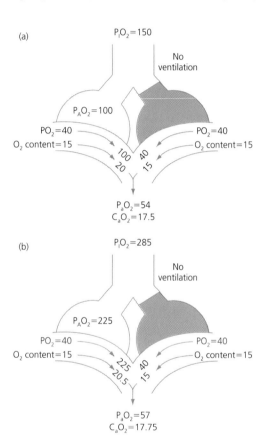

Figure 1.12 Hypoxemia as a result of low $\dot{V}/\dot{Q}$ mismatch and the effect of supplemental oxygen. (a) With room air, insufficient O_2 reaches the poorly ventilated alveolus to fully saturate its capillary blood. (b) With 40% O_2, P_AO_2 in the low $\dot{V}/\dot{Q}$ alveolus is raised enough to make its capillary PO_2 nearly normal. Note that the average P_aO_2 of the mixture of blood from both capillaries is a result of the average of the two O_2 contents, not PO_2s. From: Pierson, D.J. (1992) Respiratory failure: introduction and overview. In: *Foundations of Respiratory Care* (eds D.J. Pierson and R.M. Kacmarek). Reproduced with permission from Churchill Livingstone.

Figure 1.13 Hypoxemia as a result of true shunting and the effect of supplemental oxygen. (a) Blood leaving the normal alveoli is fully saturated; however, no oxygen enters the blood of the capillary associated with the unventilated alveoli. (b) The addition of 40% oxygen has essentially no effect on oxygenation, as little O_2 can be added to the blood perfusing the normal alveolus and no oxygen can be added to the blood passing the unventilated alveolus. From: Pierson, D.J. (1992) Respiratory failure: introduction and overview. In: *Foundations of Respiratory Care* (eds D.J. Pierson and R.M. Kacmarek). Reproduced with permission from Churchill Livingstone.

the airway is partially open even though the alveoli are grossly underventilated. As a result, the administration of an increased F_iO_2 allows the alveolar PO_2 in the low $\dot{V}/\dot{Q}$ area to increase sufficiently to reverse the hypoxemic effect. It is for this reason that the hypoxemia in many chronic obstructive pulmonary disease (COPD) patients can be easily reversed by low flow oxygen via a nasal cannula. The administration of oxygen confirms the cause of hypoxemia, for small increases in F_iO_2 generally do not improve P_aO_2 if true shunting is the cause of hypoxemia.

Frequently the blood flow to an area of low $\dot{V}/\dot{Q}$ is also reduced as a result of hypoxic vasoconstriction. However, the reduction in blood flow often is inadequate to match the reduction in ventilation. Certain vasoactive drugs reduce hypoxic vasoconstriction and cause significant worsening of arterial oxygenation. Inhaled nitric oxide in COPD patients has been shown to increase hypoxemia, as have other systemic vasodilators (nitroprusside).

When low $\dot{V}/\dot{Q}$ mismatch is the cause of hypoxemia, the administration of high F_iO_2s (>60%) can result in increased true shunting because of nitrogen washout atelectasis. As the extraction of oxygen by blood in a low $\dot{V}/\dot{Q}$ area may be greater than the replenishment of oxygen by ventilation, the absence of nitrogen can lead to instability. If the size of the alveoli continually decreases and nitrogen is absent, closing volume will eventually be reached and atelectasis develops.

In critically ill patients, low $\dot{V}/\dot{Q}$ areas are generally considered the primary cause of hypoxemia.

1.6.2 True shunting

An intrapulmonary shunt is referred to as a right to left shunt, because essentially blood leaving the right heart enters the left heart without participating in gas exchange, or as defined above, an area of lung perfused but without ventilation. As noted in *Figure 1.13* this results in venous blood mixing with oxygenated blood and a dramatic decrease in the

P_aO_2 because the amount of oxygen carried by hemoglobin (1.34 ml O_2 g^{-1} Hb at 100% saturation) is much larger than that dissolved in the plasma (0.003 ml O_2 ml^{-1} blood per mmHg PO_2). Additional O_2 can be added to plasma only in well-ventilated lung, as hemoglobin is usually saturated or near saturated in normal lung units. As a result, little O_2 is available to increase O_2 content in blood from shunted areas.

The majority of shunting is a result of unventilated lung units but high pulmonary artery pressure can cause the foramen ovale to open directly, shunting blood from the right to left heart. In addition, congenital cardiac anomalies and the emptying of a few veins (pleural, bronchial, thebesian veins) into the left heart and the development of A–V anastomoses from severe liver disease also increase the shunt fraction. As illustrated in *Figure 1.13*, simple oxygen therapy is not effective in reversing the hypoxemia associated with true shunting. To reverse the hypoxemic effect of true shunting the cause must be reversed, by the resolution of pneumonia, the expansion atelectasis areas or the closing of a patent foramen ovale. The specific ventilator therapy designed to address true shunting is PEEP. As discussed in Chapter 15, PEEP keeps unstable lung units open and improves oxygenation.

1.6.3 Dead space

Dead space is caused by a ventilation/perfusion mismatch greater than 1.0. Anatomically, as the conducting airways and the upper respiratory tract do not participate in gas exchange, the volume of gas in these areas is considered dead space. In the healthy adult, this volume equals about 1 ml kg^{-1} of ideal body weight. About 25–40% of the tidal volume normally does not participate in gas exchange. Any pathophysiologic condition that results in increased ventilation as compared with perfusion causes an increase in dead space (*Table 1.3*). The most obvious cause of an increase in dead space is pulmonary emboli, preventing

13

all blood flow to an area. However, the common disease states seen in the ICU (i.e. COPD, ARDS) also result in increased dead space (COPD as a result of the loss of the overall pulmonary capillary bed and ARDS because of occlusion of pulmonary capillaries). In addition, any time cardiac output decreases, dead space increases. Of primary concern in the ICU is application of positive pressure ventilation and PEEP to patients with inadequate vascular tone or volume, or inadequate cardiac output.

An often overlooked cause of increased dead space and as a result increased P_aCO_2 is auto-PEEP. Frequently, auto-PEEP is not recognized because it is not observed on the ventilator unless an end expiratory pause is activated. However, simple observation of the expiratory flow waveforms can identify the presence but not the magnitude of auto-PEEP (*Figure 1.14*). Whenever end expiratory flow does not return to zero auto-PEEP is present. A common reason for CO_2 elevation in the asthmatic, the post (or during) cardiac arrest patient, the postoperative patient, or the patient with COPD is overly aggressive delivery of mechanical ventilation. In these settings a decrease in minute ventilation resulting in a decrease in auto-PEEP may improve P_aCO_2 especially if cardiac output is depressed by the auto-PEEP. In all settings an increase in dead space results in an increase in P_aCO_2 if the minute ventilation remains constant.

1.6.4 Estimation of shunt and dead space

The classic method of measuring total shunt effect is the shunt equation:

$$Q_S/Q_T = (C_aO_2 - C_cO_2)/(C_{\bar{v}}O_2 - C_cO_2) \quad (1.15)$$

where Q_S/Q_T is total shunt per cent, C_aO_2 arterial O_2 content, mixed venous O_2 content and C_cO_2 capillary $C_{\bar{v}}O_2$ content in well-ventilated and perfused lung units. However, to use this equation, the P_aO_2 must be greater than 150 mmHg to insure 100% saturation of hemoglobin in capillary blood, and access to blood from the pulmonary artery must be available to calculate mixed venous O_2 content. As a result, clinically this approach is rarely used. As noted in *Table 1.4*, three other 'estimates' of shunting are widely used. Of these, the P_aO_2/P_AO_2 ratio is the least affected by anything but oxygenation status. However, clinically and experimentally the P_aO_2/F_IO_2 is the most commonly used index.

Estimation of dead space to tidal volume ratio (V_D/V_T) uses a modification of the Bohr equation:

$$V_D/V_T = P_aCO_2 - PECO_2/P_aCO_2 \quad (1.16)$$

where $PECO_2$ is equal to the mixed exhaled PCO_2. However, as noted above, whenever the minute ventilation is increased without an associated decrease in P_aCO_2, dead space must be elevated.

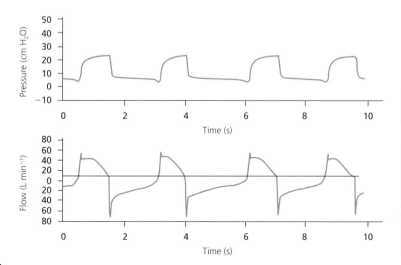

Figure 1.14 Pressure and flow curves from a COPD patient with auto-PEEP. Note the expiratory flow, an initial spike then marked decrease and expiration ended before flow reached zero. Whenever flow fails to return to zero auto-PEEP is present.

Table 1.4 Estimation of intrapulmonary shunting and dead space

Index	Normal value	Abnormal value	Limitation
Q_s/Q_T	2–5%	>10%	Invasive
$P_AO_2 - P_aO_2$	7–14 mmHg room air 31–56 mmHg 100% O_2	100–150 at F_IO_2 1.0	Varies with F_IO_2
PaO_2/P_AO_2	>0.75	<0.75	–
PaO_2/F_IO_2	450–500	<300–350	Varies with $PaCO_2$ and F_IO_2
V_D/V_T	25–40%	>40%	–

References

1. Montgomery, A.B., Stager, M.A., Carrico, C.J. and Hudson, L.D. (1985) Causes of mortality in patients with adult respiratory distress syndrome. *Am. Rev. Respir. Dis.* **132**: 485–489.
2. Knaus, W.A., Draper, E.A., Wagner, D.P. and Zimmerman, J.E. (1985) Prognosis in acute organ-system failure. *Ann. Surg.* **202**: 685–693.
3. Alex, C.G. and Tobin, M.J. (1995) Assessment of pulmonary function in critically ill patients. In: *Textbook of Critical Care*, 3rd Edn (eds S.M. Shoemaker, A. Grenvik, P.R. Holbrook and W.C. Shoemaker). W.B. Saunders, Philadelphia, PA, pp. 649–658.
4. Chevrolet, J.-C. and Deleamont, P. (1991) Repeated vital capacity measurements as predictive parameters for mechanical ventilation need and weaning success in the Guillain–Barré syndrome. *Am. Rev. Respir. Dis.* **144**: 814–819.
5. Comroe, J.H. (1974) Mechanical factors in breathing. *Physiology of Respiration*, 2nd Edn. Yearbook Medical Publishers, Chicago, IL, pp. 94–141.
6. Scanlan, C.L., Wilkins, R.L. and Stoller, J.K. (1999) *Egan's Fundamentals of Respiratory Care*, 7th Edn. St. Louis: Mosby-Yearbook.
7. Culver, B.H. (1992) Mechanics of ventilation. In: *Foundations of Respiratory Care* (eds D.J. Pierson and R.M. Kacmarek). Churchill Livingstone, New York, pp. 83–92.
8. Murry, J.F. (1974) Ventilation. *The Normal Lung: The Basis for Diagnosis and Treatment of Pulmonary Disease*. W.B. Saunders, New York, pp. 77–112.
9. Gattinoni, L., Pelosi, P., Suter, P.M., Pedoto, A., Vercesi, P. and Lissoni, A. (1998) Acute respiratory distress syndrome caused by pulmonary and extrapulmonary disease: different syndromes? *Am. J. Respir. Crit. Care Med.* **158**: 3–11.
10. Clements, J.A. and Tierney, D.F. (1964) Alveolar instability associated with altered surface tension. In: *Handbook of Physiology, Section 3, Respiration, Vol. II* (eds W.O. Fenn and H. Rahr). American Physiological Society, Washington, DC, pp. 1565–1583.
11. Slonim, N.B. and Hamilton, L.H. (1971) Resistance to breathing. *Respiratory Physiology*. C.V. Mosby, St. Louis, MO, pp. 16–65.
12. Manthous, C.A., Morgan, S., Pohlman, A. and Hall, J.B. (1997) Heliox in the treatment of airflow obstruction: a critical review of the literature. *Respir. Care* **42**: 1034–1042.
13. Kacmarek, R.M. and Hess, D. (1994) Basic principles of ventilator machinery. In: *Principles and Practice of Mechanical Ventilation* (ed. M.J. Tobin). McGraw–Hill, New York, pp. 65–110.
14. Kacmarek, R.M., Hess, D. and Stroller, J.K. (1993) Airway pressure, flow and volume waveforms and long mechanisms during mechanical ventilation. *Monitoring in Respiratory Care*. Mosby Year Book, St. Louis, MO, pp. 497–544.
15. Pepe, P.E. and Marini, J.J. (1982) Occult positive end expiratory pressure in mechanically ventilated patients with airflow obstruction: the auto-PEEP effect. *Am. Rev. Respir. Dis.* **126**: 166–170.
16. West, J. (1990) Ventilation. *Respiratory Physiology: The Essentials*, 4th Edn. Williams and Wilkins, Baltimore, MD, pp. 11–20.
17. West, J.B., Dollery, C.T. and Naimark, A. (1964) Distribution of blood flow in isolated lung: relation to vascular and alveolar pressure. *J. Appl. Physiol.* **19**: 713–724.
18. Glenny, R.W., Lamm, W.J., Albert, R.K. and Robertson, H.T. (1991) Gravity is a minor

determinant of pulmonary blood flow distribution. *J. Appl. Phys.* **71**: 620–629.

19. **Glenny, R.W., Bernard, S., Robertson, H.T. and Hlastala, M.P.** (1999) Gravity is an important but secondary determinant of regional pulmonary blood flow in upright primates. *J. Appl. Phys.* **86**: 623–632.

20. **Jolliet, P., Bulpa, P., Ritz, M., Riccou, B., Lopez, J. and Chevrolet, J.C.** (1997) Additive beneficial effects of the prone position, nitric oxide, and almitrive bismesylate on gas exchange and oxygen transport in ARDS. *Crit. Care Med.* **25**: 786–794.

21. **Chatte, G., Sab, J.M., Dubois, J.M., Sirodot, M., Gaussorgues, P. and Robert, D.** (1997) Prone position in mechanically ventilated patients with severe acute respiratory failure. *Am. J. Respir. Crit. Care* **155**: 473–480.

22. **West, J.B.** (1985) *Ventilation/Blood Flow and Gas Exchange*, 4th Edn. Blackwell, Oxford.

23. **Shapiro, B.A., Harrison, R.A. and Walton, J.R.** (1982) The Physiology of external respiration. *Clinical Application of Arterial Blood Gases*, 3rd Edn. Year Book Medical Publishers, Chicago, IL, pp. 55–64.

24. **Pierson, D.J.** (1992) Respiratory failure: introduction and overview. In: *Foundations of Respiratory Care* (eds D.J. Pierson and R.M. Kacmarek). Churchill Livingstone, New York, pp. 295–302.

Chapter 2

Cardiac physiology

Jay S. Steingrub, MD

Contents

2.1 Cardiac function

Cardiac performance is regulated by the integration of four major determinants:

- preload: an estimate of ventricular end-diastolic volume, highly predictive of systolic function;
- afterload: the degree of ventricular wall tension;
- inotropy: the contractility of the ventricular muscle;
- heart rate.

Cardiac muscle has the inherent ability to adapt to varying demands and conditions. This adaptation to alterations and length of resting myocardial muscle fibers is known as the Frank–Starling's mechanism or Starling's law[1]. Ventricular contraction is facilitated by increasing fiber length during diastole, thereby permitting the ventricle to increase, up to a limit, the quantity of blood ejected from the ventricle with each beat (stroke volume). However, beyond the limits of optimal fiber length, contraction is impaired. The pressure in the atria is directly related to the filling of the ventricle in diastole. With normal hearts, as atrial pressure increases in response to venous return, cardiac output increases. The calculation of cardiac output can be determined by multiplying the stroke volume by the heart rate. The term 'cardiac index' is used, and refers to cardiac output divided by body surface area expressed in square meters (m²). Indexing cardiac output permits us to compare values between large and small patients.

2.2 Preload

Preload refers to the initial muscle fiber length or stretch on the cardiac muscle before ventricular contraction. Increases in preload are associated with increases in both the extent and velocity of muscle fiber shortening, which combine to produce an increase in stroke volume. In the normal heart, preload corresponds to end-diastolic blood volume (EDV) in the ventricles, just before ventricular systole, and

is directly related to venous return to the heart during diastole. As pressure is directly related to blood volume, diastolic pressure is a surrogate measure of diastolic volume. There is a direct relationship between preload and the force of myocardial contraction and stroke volume. Preload may be described by both right and left ventricular end-diastolic ventricular filling pressures and is clinically assessed by measurements of both right and left atrial pressure or pulmonary capillary wedge pressure (PCWP). The terms generally referring to left ventricular preload include: left ventricular end-diastolic blood volume (LVEDV), left ventricular end-diastolic pressure (LVEDP), left atrial pressure (LAP), pulmonary capillary wedge pressure/pulmonary artery wedge pressure (PAWP), or pulmonary artery occlusion pressure (PAOP).

2.2.1 Frank–Starling curve

The relationship between preload and left ventricle (LV) function during systole is graphically depicted by the Frank–Starling curve (*Figure 2.1*). This curve plots preload (end-

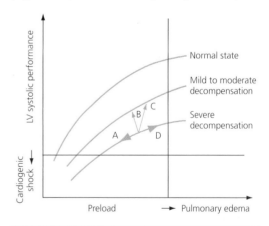

Figure 2.1 The Frank–Starling curve plots preload (end-diastolic volume) against an indicator of left ventricular (LV) performance (such as stroke volume or cardiac output) at a given level of contractility (inotropic state) and impedance. The three curves shown here represent a normal state as well as mild to moderate and severe decompensation.
Reproduced with permission from: *The Journal of Critical Illness* (1996) **11**: 86–87.

diastolic volume) against an indicator of LV systolic performance (cardiac output (CO), stroke volume, stroke work) at a given level of contractility (inotropic state) and impedance (any load acting against LV contraction).

The Starling curve fosters our understanding of how the heart responds to acute injury and chronic decompensation, and how different disease states can cause acute decompensation. The three curves in *Figure 2.1* represent three clinical states. In the presence of systolic dysfunction or increased impedance, the LV performs on a lower curve. Cardiogenic shock can develop when cardiac index falls below 2.2 l min^{-1} m^{-2} [2]. Pulmonary edema generally occurs when LVEDV rises to greater than or equal to 25 mmHg. Left ventricular performance moves to a higher curve when contractility increases or impedance decreases. Diuretics will decrease LVEDV and LV filling pressure, but may also decrease systolic performance (*Figure 2.1*, A), without shifting the curve. Vasodilators or inotropes increase stroke volume at any preload level so that ventricular function shifts to a higher curve (*Figure 2.1*, B). Inotropes plus volume infusion increase both preload and stroke volume (*Figure 2.1*, C). With severe LV dysfunction, fluids may increase systolic performance, but at the risk of pulmonary edema (*Figure 2.1*, D).

2.2.2 Pressure–volume relationships

The relationship between ventricular end-diastolic pressure and stroke work (the ventricular function curve) can be altered by pharmacologic or neurohumoral influences[3]. A nonlinear relationship exists between stroke volume and end-diastolic pressure, and hearts with diminished contractility are less responsive to increases in end-diastolic pressure or preload. In the failing heart, the ventricular function curve is shifted to the right because as atrial pressure rises, cardiac output does not increase proportionately to the same level as it does in the normal heart, and levels off at a lower magnitude of cardiac output. For the same work (LV systolic performance), the normal heart performs at a lower filling pressure than the failing heart.

2.2.3 Alterations of preload

Alterations of preload greatly alter the cardiac output in both the normal and failing hearts. Reduction of preload resulting in a decrease in cardiac output or stroke work may be observed with hypovolemia, displacement of blood from the thorax (positive pressure ventilation) or cardiac compression (tamponade). Furthermore, impairment of right ventricular contractility such as in right heart failure may lead to a decrease in left ventricular filling. Any alteration in contractility or preload may be manifested by tachycardia as a compensation for a decrease in stroke volume.

Clinically, with chronic systolic dysfunction, the LV dilates to maintain a normal stroke volume (SV). At rest, a dilated LV usually performs near the peak of the Starling curve, such that further increases in preload will have little effect on stroke volume. Therefore, heart rate will often increase to maintain cardiac output in patients with LV dilatation. Any conditions that increase venous return and thus increase preload (end-diastolic volume) will increase heart rate and inotropy to compensate for elevation in LVEDV.

2.2.4 Ventricular interdependence and LV preload

Ventricular interdependence describes the process by which alterations in ventricular contraction and volume modify the function of the other ventricle. This interaction is the result of the close anatomic association between the ventricles, which are encircled by common muscle fibers, share a septal wall, and are enclosed within the pericardium.

As right ventricular (RV) volume and pressure increase, the left ventricular pressure–volume curve shifts to the left and becomes steeper (*Figure 2.2*). Conversely, as left ventricular volume and pressure increases, the right ventricular pressure–volume curve shifts to the left and becomes steeper. The mechanism for this interaction is diastolic alteration in

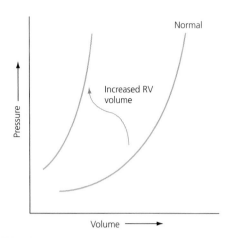

Figure 2.2 Increases in RV volume can cause a septal shift and changes in the pressure–volume relationship of the left ventricle as a result of ventricular interdependence. Reproduced with permission from Blackwell Science, *The Journal of Intensive Care Medicine* (1989) **4**: 86.

ventricular configuration caused by contra-lateral ventricular volume changes. Acute distention of one ventricle causes septal displacement and the distensibility of each ventricle is altered. The greater the right ventricular volume, the less compliant is the left ventricle. Therefore, for the same left ventricular filling pressure, right ventricular dilatation will decrease LVEDV and cardiac output.

Increases in lung volume and increases in alveolar pressure (*Table 2.1*) impede right ventricular outflow by increasing pulmonary vasculature resistance, which in the volume resuscitated patient will cause the right ventricle to dilate, pushing the intraventricular septum into the left ventricle and further

Table 2.1 Ventricular interdependence

Right ventricular pressure overload state
- Acute pulmonary hypertension
- Pulmonary embolism
- Chronic pulmonary disease
- Mitral stenosis

Right ventricular volume overload states
- Atrial septal defect
- Tricuspid insufficiency
- Pulmonary insufficiency

decreasing left ventricular diastolic compliance. Clinically, this reduction in left ventricular stroke volume for a given pulmonary artery wedge pressure may be misinterpreted as left ventricular failure when it merely represents a mechanically induced reduction of left ventricular diastolic compliance.

The reduction in venous return during positive pressure ventilation is amplified in the settings of hypovolemia and vasodilatory states, such as in shock, sepsis, and adrenal insufficiency. Management consists of intra-vascular volume replacement, use of vasopressors, and perhaps smaller tidal volume ventilation.

2.3 Afterload

Although stroke volume reduction can result in arterial hypotension, arterial blood pressure can also be maintained with a compensatory increase in peripheral systemic vascular resistance. Afterload is the tension created in the walls of the left ventricle as the muscle fibers shorten during contraction. Its determinants include the peripheral vascular resistance and the resistance against which the ventricle contracts (the impedance of aortic wall and valve). Hypertension (increased peripheral resistance), arteriosclerosis (stiff arterial walls) or aortic stenosis increase afterload. Both aortic pressure and systemic vascular resistance are critical determinants of the amount of blood pumped by the ventricle. The total sum of the forces resisting left ventricular ejection is referred to as impedance, which includes the resistance of the small arteries and arterioles, the compliance of the large arteries, blood viscosity, and the forces of inertia. The arterioles are the main resistant vessels and most resistance to flow occurs in the peripheral region. Pulmonary vascular resistance (PVR) and systemic vascular resistance (SVR) reflect the afterload of the right and left side of the heart, respectively. Afterload alterations can increase or decrease systolic LV performance when the inotropic state remains constant (*Figure 2.3*). Drugs that decrease

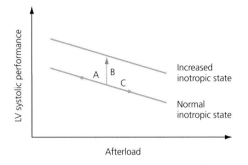

Figure 2.3 Changes in afterload (primarily those resulting from impedance) can increase or decrease systolic left ventricular performance if the inotropic state remains constant. Reproduced with permission from *The Journal of Critical Illness*, (1996) **11**: 86–87.

peripheral vascular resistance (decrease afterload) increase systolic performance without altering the inotropic state (A). Inotropic agents that increase contractility increase systolic performance but do not affect impedance (B). Vasoconstrictors decrease systolic performance by increasing peripheral vascular resistance (impedance) (C).

2.3.1 Stroke work

Stroke work is a measure of the work required of the left ventricle to develop blood pressure and eject blood with each heartbeat. Stroke work can be calculated for either side of the heart and is commonly indexed and presented in hemodynamic profiles as LVSWI and RVSWI (stroke work index).

All of these myocardial and vascular factors are interdependent and alterations of one physiological parameter will affect the others. An increase in afterload via elevation in blood pressure or systemic vascular resistance will lead to a compensatory increase in preload to maintain stroke volume in the normal functioning heart. However, in the presence of heart dysfunction, an increase in afterload frequently decreases stroke volume and cardiac output. Conversely, the reduction in afterload causes the impedance to ventricular ejection to decrease (decrease wall tension) with subsequent stroke volume increase.

2.4 **Contractility**

Contractility or the inotropic state of the heart is defined by the force and velocity of ventricular contraction, and is independent of preload, afterload and heart rate. The term refers to the strength of the contraction and the amount of cardiac muscle shortening that occurs with a given fiber length (preload) against a given afterload. An increase in fiber length signifies an increase in the stretch or preload. With normal contractility, increasing end-diastolic fiber length increases stroke volume. If contractility increases, stroke volume increases for the same fiber length (preload). At any given level of end-diastolic volume and degree of peripheral vascular resistance, as the inotropic state increases so does the stroke volume and, as a result, the ejection fraction also increases. As shown in *Figure 2.1*, there is a shift in the ventricular function curve to the right with decreased contractility. Left ventricular stroke work does not increase to the same level as occurs with normal contractility as end-diastolic fiber length increases (preload). In the presence of a reduction of contractility, preload must increase to maintain stroke volume. Ejection fraction, the ratio of stroke volume to the LVEDV, is used as a clinical measure of contractility. With a normal contractile state, cardiac output is dependent more on preload and afterload than on the inotropic state of the myocardium. Thus in normal subjects, augmentation of contractility does not necessarily elevate cardiac output. In contrast, when the myocardial contractile state is depressed, augmentation of the contractile state will increase cardiac output. In the perioperative period, several factors may predispose to myocardial depression, including anesthetic drugs, hypoxia, hypercapnia, acid–base disturbance, electrolyte abnormalities, surgical manipulation, drugs, and pre-existing heart disease. The terms contractility and myocardial performance often contribute to confusion when reviewing cardiac physiology. Myocardial performance is a summation of preload, afterload, contractility and heart rate, and is usually measured as cardiac output. Contractility is only one component of myocardial performance, much as the engine is only one component of a sports car's performance. Although contractility may not be measurable directly, it is important conceptually because of its ability to be enhanced by inotropic agents. Although it may be reasoned that increasing the inotropic state improves LV function, agents that increase contractility may also increase heart rate and myocardial oxygen consumption, causing life-threatening ventricular arrhythmias. Chapter 8 more fully discusses inotropic agents and their effect on myocardial performance.

2.5 Heart rate

Heart rate is a major determinant of cardiac output, one that is subject to extrinsic autonomic modulation. Alterations in heart rate within the physiologic range may produce significant changes in cardiac output. Such changes may be important when cardiac dysfunction is impaired or stroke volume is limited. Tachycardia often serves as a compensatory response when stroke volume decreases. A reduction in diastolic filling time and possibly reduction in cardiac output may occur with heart rates above 160 beats min^{-1}. An increase in heart rate raises myocardial oxygen consumption and may affect the management of patients with congestive heart failure (CHF).

2.5.1 Pacemakers

Temporary pacing is indicated for actual or threatened bradycardia caused by acute myocardial infarction, conduction system disease, procedures associated with important bradycardia or overdrive suppression of tachy-arrhythmias[4]. There are no categorical rules regarding the necessity of temporary pacing. *Table 2.2* classifies situations in which temporary pacing may be useful or effective.

2.5.2 Transcutaneous temporary cardiac pacing

Transcutaneous pacing can be used as an alternative to transvenous pacing and avoids some of the possible complications of central venous cannulation[5]. The application of electrical stimuli of long duration and high current can cause skeletal muscle stimulation and severe pain. Transcutaneous ventricular pacing can be employed as an alternative to transvenous pacing for Class I, Class IIA, and IIB indications as noted above. When the patient is dependent on pacing to maintain an appropriate heart rate or when it is anticipated that temporary pacing will be needed for greater than 24 h, insertion of a transvenous pacemaker is usually preferred. Transcutaneous ventricular pacing can be useful in acute settings such as cardiac arrest to avoid delays and complications from central venous cannulation.

2.6 Diastolic function

Intrinsic LV compliance is defined as the change in intrachamber pressure that occurs as a volume of blood enters the left ventricle. In a compliant ventricle, as blood volume in the chamber increases, the wall distends. This will allow accommodation of large volumes of blood, normally with minimal changes in diastolic pressure. However, in a noncompliant ventricle, small changes in volume result in marked changes in pressure. *Figure 2.4* demonstrates the relationship between left ventricular pressure and volume during increases and decreases in LV compliance. The points on the curve reflect the volume of blood remaining in the LV at end-systole and the amount entering the ventricle during diastole. Pulmonary edema can develop in the presence of decreased, normal, or increased compliance as depicted by the pressure–volume curve. With decreased left ventricular compliance, a normal left ventricular volume may increase diastolic pressure enough to cause pulmonary edema (A); with lower volume, pressure increases, but to a lesser extent (B). Volume overload states can cause pulmonary edema even with normal LV compliance (C). Chronic valvular regurgitation (D) and LV dilatation (E) increase compliance, allowing large volumes of blood to be accommodated with small

Table 2.2 Indications for transvenous temporary pacings

Class I – usually indicated and considered useful/effective
1. Bradycardia owing to conduction system disease (permanent pacing not immediately available)
   A. Complete heart block with:
      1. symptomatic bradycardia
      2. congestive heart failure
   B. Second-degree atrio-ventricular (AV) block with symptomatic bradycardia
   C. Atrial fibrillation or flutter with periods of symptomatic bradycardia or congestive heart failure attributable to bradycardia
   D. Symptomatic bradycardia in the setting of electrolyte abnormalities or drug toxicity
   E. Torsades de point
   F. Heart rate <30 beats min^{-1} persisting for ≥10 min
2. Acute myocardial infarction:
   A. Asystole
   B. Complete heart block
   C. Right bundle branch block with left anterior or left posterior hemiblock with acute anterior myocardial infarction
   D. Type II second-degree AV block with acute anterior myocardial infarction
   E. Symptomatic bradycardia unresponsive to atropine
3. Procedures that may be associated with significant bradycardia
   A. General anesthesia with complete heart block or Type II second-degree AV block
4. Overdrive suppression of tachyarrhythmias
   A. Symptomatic recurrent ventricular tachycardia refractory to drug therapy
   B. Symptomatic recurrent supraventricular tachycardia refractory to drug therapy

Class II – acceptable, of uncertain efficacy, may be controversial
   A. Weight of evidence in favor of usefulness
   B. Not well-established evidence, possibly helpful but not harmful

Class IIA
1. Acute myocardial infarction
   A. Left bundle branch block with an acute infarction
   B. Right bundle branch block with left anterior or left posterior hemiblock with an acute inferior infarction
   C. Type II second-degree AV block within acute inferior infarction
   D. Sinus bradycardia with hypotension, unresponsive to atropine
   E. Recurrent sinus pauses unresponsive to atropine
   F. Atrial or ventricular overdrive pacing for incessant ventricular tachycardia

Class IIB
1. Bradycardia owing to conduction system disease (permanent pacing not immediately available)
   A. Asymptomatic complete heart block
   B. Asymptomatic type II second-degree AV block
2. Acute myocardial infarction
   A. Bradycardia with acute inferior infarction responding to atropine
   B. Left bundle branch block with first-degree heart block of unknown duration
   C. Bifascicular block of unknown duration
3. Procedures associated with important bradycardia
   A. General anesthesia with right bundle branch block with left anterior or left posterior hemiblock
   B. Right heart catheterization in the presence of left bundle branch block

Class III – not indicated, may be harmful
1. Bradycardia owing to conduction system disease
   A. First-degree AV block
   B. Asymptomatic type I second-degree AV block
   C. Congenital third-degree heart block without symptoms
   D. Intermittent AV dissociation without bradycardia or heart block
2. Acute myocardial infarction
   A. New right bundle branch block
   B. Pre-existing bundle branch block
   C. Asymptomatic type I second-degree AV block or first-degree AV block
   D. Accelerated idioventricular rhythm causing AV dissociation

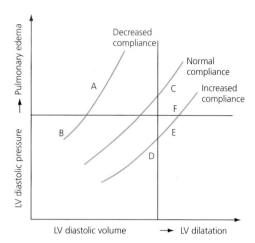

Figure 2.4 Pulmonary edema may develop whether left ventricular (LV) compliance is decreased, normal or increased—as indicated by the pressure–volume curves depicted here. With decreased LV compliance, even a normal LV volume may increase diastolic pressure enough to cause pulmonary edema (A); when the volume is low, pressure also increases, but to a lesser extent (B). Volume overload states may lead to pulmonary edema even if LV compliance is normal (C). Chronic valvular regurgitation (D) and LV dilatation (E) increase compliance; this allows large volumes of blood to be accommodated with only small changes in pressure. However, eventually the diastolic volume rises enough to increase the diastolic pressure above the threshold level for pulmonary edema (F). Reproduced with permission from *The Journal of Critical Illness*, (1996) **11**: 86–87.

changes in pressure. Ultimately, diastolic volume rises enough to increase the diastolic pressure above the threshold level for pulmonary edema (F). Conditions such as LV hypertrophy, myocardial ischemia, hypertrophic cardiomyopathy, and restrictive ventricular disease decrease compliance. With decreased compliance, diastolic pressure increases at all volume levels.

For example, in hypertensive patients with concentric LV hypertrophy, LV compliance may decrease during diastole despite the ventricle's small size and strong contractions. Hence, small changes in LV filling may generate a marked increase in diastolic pressures and lead to pulmonary edema. Up to 40% of

patients with congestive heart failure have isolated diastolic LV dysfunction[6]. Clinically, one needs to evaluate for LV diastolic dysfunction so as to determine whether therapeutic interventions that increase or decrease filling volume should be employed. With decreased diastolic compliance, volume reduction can lead to a significant decrease in systolic performance, according to the Frank–Starling mechanism. Volume support can quickly lead to pulmonary edema as a result of this increase in both diastolic pressure and PAWP.

Conversely, chronic volume overload states (aortic or mitral regurgitation) and dilated cardiomyopathy can increase compliance. Hence, the diastolic volume may be high enough to increase the diastolic pressure above the threshold level for pulmonary edema (commonly 25–30 mmHg) to develop.

Coronary artery disease, including ischemia and/or acute myocardial infarction, can alter chamber stiffness resulting in a change in compliance shifting the diastolic pressure–volume relationship up and to the left, so that small changes in end-diastolic volume are translated into much larger increments in end-diastolic pressure. Diastolic dysfunction is commonly a diagnosis of exclusion. The primary treatment of heart failure with normal systolic function but abnormal diastolic function is diuretics. ACE-inhibitors are useful. However, in the presence of heart failure, beta-blockers and calcium channel blockers must be added cautiously, although they improve diastolic compliance.

2.7 Diagnosis and therapy of acute congestive heart failure

In the diagnosis of acute heart failure in ICU patients, either the systolic and/or the diastolic performance may be affected. In those situations where the diastolic function of the ventricle in impaired, both diastolic and pulmonary venous pressure increase, leading to pulmonary edema. When systolic function is present, cardiac output decreases and may result in only fatigue as the initial presentation. The patient's medical history and physical examination may provide the only clues that point to possible left ventricular dysfunction[7].

Physical findings are associated with varying degrees of diagnostic or prognostic significance, and must be interpreted within the specific clinical setting. Although laboratory testing is required to support the diagnoses of LV dysfunction, the following should be considered:

- In patients with moderate to severe dysfunction, an S_3 gallop reflects poor LV diastolic compliance.
- Pulsus alternans is found in patients with severe LV dysfunction, and reflects a poor prognosis.
- Marked pulmonary edema suggests severe LV dysfunction and is a poor prognostic sign, particularly in the setting of acute aortic or mitral regurgitation.
- Evidence of right ventricular dysfunction is common in patients with moderate or severe LV dysfunction. Its prognostic significance depends on the degree of the dysfunction in both the right and left ventricles.
- Mild LV dysfunction in patients who have myocardial infarctions may signify poor prognosis if chronic and life-threatening arrhythmias develop.

2.7.1 Pathophysiology of congestive heart failure

Although CHF is a constellation of clinical symptoms, the underlying pathophysiology is characterized by impaired cardiac function, with the failing myocardium unable to adequately perfuse tissues to meet the metabolic demands. The fundamental defect leading to CHF is impaired myocardial contractility. Virtually any form of cardiac disease can cause heart failure (*Table 2.3*).

With progressive LV failure, increased filling pressure leads to pulmonary vascular congestion and eventually pulmonary edema and respiratory failure. The failing myocardium's inability to meet the body's metabolic needs

Table 2.3 Causes of heart failure
• Acute myocardial infarction
• Acute myocardial ischemia
• Uncontrolled hypertension
• Valvular disease
• Pulmonary embolism
• Pericardial disease
• Pregnancy
• Anemia
• Adverse drug effects
• Hyperthyroidism or hypothyroidism
• Nutritional disorders (vitamin deficiency)
• Severe sepsis

leads to increased neurohumeral tone, with elevated circulatory levels of catecholamines. Normally, low cardiac output causes both cardiac and aortic baroreceptor dysfunction, which will exert an inhibitory effect on sympathetic tone. Instead, there is increasing release of circulatory catecholamines, activation of the renin–angiotensin axis, leading to sodium and water retention, volume overload and progressive cardiac failure[8]. Elevated adrenergic tone causes vasoconstriction, and with subsequent increase in myocardial work leads to both cardiac irritability and potentially fatal arrhythmias. With left ventricular failure present, right ventricular failure can develop from increased pulmonary vascular resistance.

2.7.2 Compensatory mechanisms

In chronic congestive heart failure, three principal compensatory mechanisms are activated to maintain the heart's normal function as a pump. Initially, the Frank–Starling mechanism operates to increase preload (end-diastolic volume), which maintains stroke volume. The heart dilates to maintain a near-normal or normal stroke volume despite a markedly reduced ejection fraction. Myocardial hypertrophy also occurs secondarily, which maintains wall stress as the heart dilates. The amount of contractile tissue also increases during hypertrophy. Finally, augmentation of the sympathetic nervous system will occur, which increases heart rate and contractile function while maintaining perfusion pressure to vital organs. These compensatory mechanisms augment cardiac function in the early phases of heart failure. However, elevated venous pressure causes pulmonary and circulatory congestion. Cardiac dilatation causes high wall stress, which reduces performance. Increasing peripheral resistance may worsen afterload stress on an already poorly contracting heart. The net result is the full expression of CHF, and at this point the patient may benefit from more aggressive management in an ICU setting.

2.7.3 Diagnosis of CHF (*Table 2.4*)

If LV dysfunction is suspected, the next steps are to define the extent of any diastolic or systolic impairment, diagnose any structural or functional abnormalities, identify the underly-

ing cause of the dysfunction, and determine the prognosis. Systolic as well as diastolic dysfunction must be evaluated. In the absence of systolic LV dysfunction, abnormalities in diastolic performance, except possibly for infiltrative myocardial disease, carry a more favorable prognosis. It is important to remember that CHF and LV dysfunction are clinical syndromes, not laboratory diagnoses. The severity or extent of the impairment cannot be determined by one measurement.

2.7.4 Electrocardiography

Specific electrocardiographic patterns associated with left ventricular hypertrophy, previous myocardial infarction and ventricular branch block suggest left ventricular disease. A biphasic

Table 2.4 Etiology of left ventricular hemodynamic dysfunction

Condition	Hemodynamic profile
Myocardial disease • Myocardial infarction • Myocardial ischemia • Myocarditis • Dilated cardiomyopathy	Decreased contractility
Extracardiac disorder • Hypovolemia • Cardiac tamponade • Pulmonary embolism • Mitral stenosis	Increased/decreased atrial preload
Infiltrative disease • Restrictive cardiomyopathy	Decreased compliance
Pressure overload • Hypertension • Aortic stenosis • Aortic sclerosis • Aortic coarctation	Increased afterload
Volume overload states • Renal failure • Ventral septal defect • Anemia • Arteriovenous fistula	Increased preload, high output states
Aortic regurgitation • Acute • Chronic	Increased preload, increased impedance Increased preload, normal impedance
Mitral regurgitation • Acute • Chronic	Increased preload, very low impedance Increased preload, low impedance

P wave (P-mitrale) marks discoordinate atrial contraction, often a marker of valvular disease. Atrial fibrillation results in the loss of atrial 'kick', which assumes increasing importance in determining preload as ventricular compliance decreases. However, electrocardiography alone cannot be used to assess LV function.

2.7.5 Echocardiography
Echocardiography can comprehensively evaluate LV structure and function. Doppler echocardiography assesses valvular stenosis or regurgitation, estimates the left to right shunt ratios at the atrial or ventricular level, and measures the peak tricuspid Doppler velocity and thereby the pulmonary artery pressure[9]. Studies of global LV function and regional wall motion can provide important prognostic information. Stroke volume is derived by subtracting the end-systolic volume (ESV) from end-diastolic volume (EDV), and ejection fraction calculated by dividing stroke volume by EDV. Substantial regional wall motion abnormalities, however, introduce inaccuracy into these calculations. In patients with chronic mitral and aortic regurgitation, determinations of LV dimensions at end-systole can guide decisions regarding the need for surgical intervention.

2.7.6 Radiologic evaluation
Roentgenography can provide supporting evidence for LV dysfunction. Venous markings in the upper lung field and Kerley B-lines both suggest increased pulmonary venous pressure. Assessment of the size of the left ventricle can also provide additional clues.

2.7.7 Hemodynamic evaluation
Pulmonary capillary wedge pressure recordings and cardiac output may be measured with a pulmonary artery catheter. Further discussions of hemodynamic monitoring are found in Chapter 5.

2.8 Therapy

Current management techniques for heart failure include preventing volume overload, reducing myocardial work via afterload reduction though vasodilator use, and augmentation of cardiac output by administration of positive inotropic agents that act directly on the myocardium to improve cardiac performance (see Chapter 8). Titration of inotropic or vasodilator therapy for heart failure in the ICU setting depends on establishing clear therapeutic end-points. Inotropic agents are normally used to augment cardiac output, improve urine output and lower pulmonary capillary wedge pressure while avoiding sinus tachycardia or ventricular ectopy. Bedside hemodynamic measurements via pulmonary artery catheterizations are sometimes important in titrating inotropic therapy. However, in the setting of acute pulmonary edema, appropriate treatment (see below) often provides rapid resolution of this hemodynamic disorder and obviates the need for invasive monitoring. Pulmonary artery catheters are most useful when there is uncertainty regarding left ventricular filling pressure or cardiac output.

2.8.1 Diuretics
Diuretic-induced reduction in right-sided pressures may improve LV compliance, thereby improving cardiac output and renal perfusion. A decrease in ventricular filling pressures with diuretics will enhance cardiac performance in both tricuspid and mitral regurgitation. For those patients not previously receiving diuretics, low-dose furosemide (20–40 mg) is initially recommended. The dose is increased by 50% to 100% when there is no response within 1 h after administration. Short-acting loop diuretics (Bumetanide 1–5 mg IV) may also be employed for acute heart failure. Rarely larger doses (furosemide 250–500 mg; bumetanide ≥10 mg) are needed for patients with reduced renal function. Continuous furosemide infusion (5–10 mg h^{-1}) is effective to improve diuresis in critically ill patients who require a controllable diuretic or who demonstrate diuretic resistance. Furosemide may not be well absorbed orally in patients with decompensated heart failure. Diuretics will often dramatically relieve symptoms by lowering right

and left atrial filling pressures. Improved diuretic efficacy (synergism) exists between various classes of diuretics. Loop diuretics are often used in conjunction with thiazides, potassium sparing diuretics or metolazone in patients exhibiting resistance to initial therapy. The potassium sparing diuretic, spironolactone, has unique properties that are beneficial in congestive heart failure, and has been shown to reduce morbidity and mortality for class III or IV heart failure[10].

2.8.2 Digoxin

Clinical investigations have substantiated the efficacy of digoxin in the treatment of heart failure. Hemodynamic studies in both animals and humans have shown that digoxin increases cardiac index and decreases left filling pressure, right atrial pressure and heart rate. Digoxin improves heart inotropy by inhibiting sodium–potassium ATPase, leading to an increase in intracellular calcium levels and improved inotropy. Digoxin produces a modest improvement in cardiac output in patients with right heart failure secondary to pulmonary hypertension. Clinical trials support a long-term benefit of digoxin in preventing recurrent hospitalization, improving symptoms and functional capacity in patients with CHF, but not in reducing mortality[11]. Although there is no strong evidence for the benefit of digoxin in the acute setting of CHF, the drug is still recommended in the absence of abnormal atrioventricular conduction. A loading dose is not necessary in the treatment of heart failure. Treatment can begin with a dose of 0.25 mg day^{-1}. As a result of changes in lean body mass and renal function, the therapeutic range of digoxin in the elderly is lower. In patients over 70 years of age, digoxin concentrations from 0.5 to 1.3 mg ml^{-1} can be associated with higher toxicity. There are no data supporting the use of serum levels to guide dosing. It remains uncertain whether high doses are more effective than lower ones in the management of CHF.

In critically ill patients, a loading dose of digoxin is generally applied for the treatment of acute atrial arrhythmias associated with a rapid ventricular response rate. Rapid digitalization, independent of renal function, can be accomplished by giving 10–15 µg kg^{-1} ideal body weight (IBW) in divided doses. Typically, a regimen would include 50% of the total loading dose administered immediately, followed by 25% 6 h later, and the final 25% 6 h after that. A typical regimen when initiating digoxin for CHF may include a maintenance oral or parenteral therapy without a loading dose (0.125–0.25 mg day^{-1}), depending on the extent of renal dysfunction.

2.8.3 Beta agonists and phosphodiesterase inhibitors

Beta adrenergic agonists and phosphodiesterase inhibitors are mainstays of treatment for heart failure in the ICU, and are discussed in detail in Chapter 8.

2.8.4 Multimodal therapy

In the presence of acute heart failure, diuresis should be initially attempted. In the presence of renal dysfunction or hypoperfusion, inotropes and vasodilators (nitroglycerin, nitroprusside, ACE-inhibitors) are frequently required. Diuresis-induced reductions in right-sided pressures improve LV compliance, increasing both cardiac output and renal perfusion.

Inotropes and vasodilators may be used in the presence of a low-output state or when diuretics are found to be ineffective or exacerbate renal dysfunction. Concomitantly, efforts should be attempted to initiate long-term pharmacologic management, which should include a diuretic, an angiotensin converting enzyme inhibitor, a vasodilator, digoxin and beta-blockers[10]. ACE-inhibitor administration is associated with a decrease in end-diastolic and end-systolic volume, an increase in chamber stiffness, and perhaps a decrease in LV mass. In the setting of acute exacerbation of heart failure, shorter-acting vasodilators such as nitrates rather than ACE-inhibitors are more appropriate initially. Although high levels of norepinephrine in

CHF are linked with poor prognoses, beta-blockade is helpful. However, beta-blockers have no documented short-term benefit and can be harmful during acute exacerbation. Synergism between beta-agonists and the phosphodiesterase inhibitors has been documented, and varying combinations can be utilized to achieve desired amounts of inotropy and vasodilation.

2.9 Patient subsets

2.9.1 Right ventricular failure

Right ventricular (RV) failure is often a consequence of LV failure. Other mechanisms of RV failure include right ventricular myocardial infarction, and dilated cardiomyopathy. RV pressure overload may be secondary to chronic LV failure, chronic mitral valve disease or 'cor pulmonale' from COPD or pulmonary emboli. RV volume overload may be secondary to pulmonic or tricuspid regurgitation or a left to right intracardiac shunt.

Patients with acute right ventricular (RV) failure secondary to an RV infarction or acute pulmonary embolism may manifest signs of low cardiac output and elevated jugular venous pressure, a murmur of tricuspid regurgitation, right-sided S_3 gallop, and Kussmaul's sign. Patients with chronic RV pressure overload have signs of pulmonary hypertension including an RV S_4 gallop, RV heave and an accentuated pulmonic component to the second heart sound. Patients with chronic RV failure frequently present with edema, ascites, and pleural effusions. Diuretics are useful in decreasing the central venous pressure elevation and edema seen in RV failure. Loop diuretics can improve cardiac output by decreasing the degree of tricuspid regurgitation, decreasing RV distention and thereby reducing a ventricular-interdependent restraint on LV filling. In addition, spironolactone can reduce edema from RV failure because activation of the renin–angiotensin–aldosterone system is involved in sodium retention in these patients. Systemic arteriolar vasodilators used in LV failure therapies act as pulmonary vasodilators (i.e.

ACE-inhibitors, nitrates, nitroprusside) and improve RV output by reducing RV afterload[12].

Supplemental oxygen may also decrease pulmonary hypertension in these patients and should be employed acutely. Bronchodilators can improve RV function and symptoms in cor pulmonale exacerbation as a result of its bronchodilatory, pulmonary vasodilatory, and inotropic effects.

2.9.2 Valvular heart disease

Several valvular lesions can lead to symptoms of heart failure. Although medical management can provide short-term benefit, timing of surgical intervention is of essential importance (*Table 2.5*).

2.9.3 Mitral regurgitation

The most common causes of acute mitral regurgitation (MR) requiring ICU admission are acute infective endocarditis, chordal rupture in patients with myxomatous valves, papillary muscle rupture or dysfunction in the setting of inferior ischemia, and blunt or perforating chest trauma resulting in leaflet tear or chorda rupture.

Acute MR presents with signs of left atrial pressure overload and resulting pulmonary venous hypertension. High-pressure regurgitant flow from the left ventricle into the non-compliant left atrium produces left atrial systolic 'v' waves that are transmitted through the pulmonary venous system into the pulmonary capillaries, resulting in pulmonary edema. Left ventricular ejection into the 'low-pressure' left atrium can lead to an acute reduction in cardiac output with subsequent hypotension and cardiogenic shock. In chronic MR, chronic LV volume overload results in progressive dilation. As the LV may decompress itself into the low-pressure left atrium, afterload is reduced and ejection fraction is maintained in the presence of impaired intrinsic contractility.

In patients with pulmonary edema and hemodynamic collapse, clinical features that are suggestive of the diagnosis of acute MR include:

Table 2.5 Valvular surgery indications

Mitral regurgitation	Onset of symptoms with moderate or severe MR Or Asymptomatic LV systolic dysfunction (LVESD* ≥4.5 cm)
Mitral stenosis	Symptoms (heart failure, thromboembolism, fatigue) refractory to medical therapy with moderate or severe MS
Aortic regurgitation	Symptoms with moderate or severe AR Or Asymptomatic LV systolic dysfunction (LVESD ≥5.5 cm)
Aortic stenosis	Symptoms (angina, syncope or heart failure) with moderate or severe AS

*LVESD, left ventricular end-systolic dimension.

- a hyperdynamic apical impulse, possibly along with an RV heave;
- a loud P_2 caused by pulmonary hypertension;
- a holosystolic murmur heard best at the apex and radiating into the axilla;
- a third heart sound; with severe MR the murmur can be soft.

Electrocardiogram can show only sinus tachycardia although patients with ischemic MR may show evidence of inferior wall infarction. The chest X-ray demonstrates pulmonary edema.

Doppler echocardiography is essential for accurate and rapid evaluation of the cause and pathophysiology of MR in the hemodynamically unstable ICU patient. Chordal disruption, valvular abnormalities including flail leaflets and vegetations caused by endocarditis and papillary muscle dysfunction and rupture can be diagnosed. Color Doppler can be used to confirm the presence of MR to evaluate severity, and to identify eccentric regurgitant jets. The severity of left atrial pressure overload can be inferred from the characteristics of the regurgitant jet.

In the unstable population, pulmonary artery catheterization may be helpful in confirming the significance of mitral regurgitant lesions. With severe acute MR, the pulmonary capillary 'v' wave to mean pressure ratio is usually greater than two. In addition, serial cardiac output measurements assist in the selection of medical therapy.

Therapy for acute MR and pulmonary edema includes left ventricular afterload reduction, best achieved using parenteral vasodilator therapy, usually with nitroprusside and/or angiotensin-converting enzyme inhibitors[13]. Nitrates are helpful in the presence of myocardial ischemia leading to papillary muscle dysfunction. Diuretics may be necessary for the treatment of pulmonary edema. Intra-aortic balloon pumping is particularly useful to reduce left ventricular afterload and augment forward flow. Inotropic support with dopamine/dobutamine may be required in patients with cardiogenic shock who are manifesting hypoperfusion. Patients who do not respond to medical therapy and require intra-aortic balloon pumping require emergent valve surgery. Mitral valve repair is preferable to mitral valve replacement, because maintenance of subvalvular continuity improves postoperative LV function.

2.9.4 Mitral stenosis
Mitral stenosis (MS) is almost always rheumatic in origin. Other rare causes include left atrial myxoma, obstructing thrombus, malignant carcinoid, lupus, congenital defects, rheumatoid arthritis, and micropolysaccharidoses.

Isolated MS is associated with an impairment of left ventricular diastolic filling, with elevated left atrial pressure and volume, leading to pulmonary hypertension. The left ventricle is protected and contractility is normal.

Long-standing, severe pulmonary hypertension can lead to pulmonary vascular fibrosis, which may become irreversible.

Clinical features of MS include dyspnea and decreased exercise tolerance as a result of an increased left atrial pressure and the inability to achieve a significant increase in cardiac output with exertion. The development of atrial fibrillation with loss of the atrial kick and decreased filling time leads to a dramatic worsening of symptoms. Atrial embolic events as well as hemoptysis are common presentations of MS. Physical findings in MS include:

- elevated jugular venous pressure in the presence of pulmonary hypertension;
- right ventricular heave may be present; normal apical impulse;
- accentuated P_2 as a result of pulmonary hypertension;
- loud S_1;
- diastolic rumbling murmur sometimes with pre-systolic accentuation as a result of atrial contraction.

In severe MS, a decrease in cardiac output can make the murmur inaudible. In these cases, the signs of right ventricular failure are very prominent. The electrocardiogram (EKG) shows evidence of left atrial enlargement (P mitrale) and may have a rightward QRS complex with other signs of right ventricular hypertrophy. Left atrial enlargement and prominent pulmonary vasculature can be seen on chest X-ray.

Echocardiography allows for evaluation of mitral valve pathology and can evaluate left atrial size and the presence of a thrombus as well. Echocardiography can reveal a thick and unusually calcified mitral valve with decreased leaflet mobility in addition to left atrial enlargement. The severity of MS can be determined by planimetry of the valve orifice (*Table 2.6*).

Therapy includes controlling ventricular rate and maintenance on restoration of sinus rhythm. Digoxin and diuretics can provide substantial symptomatic relief along with negative chronotropic agents to control heart rate and anti-arrhythmic agents to maintain sinus rhythm. Chronic anticoagulation is usually required as a result of atrial fibrillation and mitral stenosis association with thromboembolism. Surgical therapy provides definitive therapy for patients who are moderately symptomatic with severe MS. Surgical options include valve replacement, commissurotomy and balloon valvulotomy. The choice of therapy depends on the degree of subvalvular complication and concomitant mitral regurgitation and other clinical characteristics.

Table 2.6 Severity of mitral stenosis in relation to mitral valve area

Normal mitral valve area	4–6 cm^2
Trivial MS	>2.0 cm^2
Mild MS	1.5–2.0 cm^2
Moderate MS	1.0–1.5 cm^2
Severe MS	<1.0 cm^2

MS, mitral stenosis.

2.9.5 Aortic stenosis

Aortic stenosis (AS) is the most common isolated valvular lesion and is most often caused by degeneration and calcification, or a congenital bicuspid valve in patients under the age of 70, or a tricuspid valve in persons over the age of 70. Degenerative AS caused by 'wear and tear' is characterized by calcification of the aortic side of the valve preventing the cusps from opening normally.

AS manifests as a fixed obstruction to left ventricular outflow leading to left ventricular pressure overload. This increase in wall stress and left ventricular hypertrophy occurs as a compensatory response. Hypertrophy decreases left ventricular compliance, and increases left ventricular diastolic pressure. Although cardiac output at rest is usually normal in these patients, because of the outflow track obstruction there is limitation of stroke volume augmentation during exertion. Increased left ventricular mass and wall stress increases myocardial oxygen consumption. A decrease in the aortic pressure distal to the obstruction and an increased left ventricular diastolic pressure causes a decrease in coronary perfusion pressure and myocardial oxygen supply. This can result in subendocardial ischemia, further decreasing left ventricular compliance and systolic performance. In the later stages of AS, systolic function deteriorates and left ventricular dilation occurs.

Classical presenting symptoms of AS include angina, syncope and heart failure, usually exercised-induced. Presentation of AS in the ICU include pulmonary edema, angina, severe hypotension and low cardiac output states. Physical findings include:

- delayed and diminished carotid upstroke;
- sustained apical impulse;
- an ejection click, soft A_2, loud S_4;
- a harsh systolic ejection murmur at the base, peaking later with increased severity of AS.

EKG shows left ventricular hypertrophy with strain and may show interventricular conduction delays or atrio-ventricular blocks. Echocardiography can determine the severity of stenosis by evaluating the degree of thickening, calcification, and excursion of aortic valve. Pulse Doppler can provide an accurate assessment of both mean and peak gradients across the stenotic valve (*Table 2.7*). Doppler examination permits estimation of the trans-valvular pressure gradient and calculation of the aortic valve area. Although catheterization remains the standard for determining valve area, echocardiographically determined aortic valve area correlates well with catheterization results. Aortic catheterization should be reserved for the symptomatic patient being

considered for valvular surgery. In addition, catheterization is performed as part of the workup to provide information about concomitant coronary artery stenosis.

Management of patients with AS involves maintaining an adequate preload to sustain cardiac output. Prompt fluid resuscitation should be instituted for hypovolemia. Preload and afterload reduction are contraindicated in the patient with known AS. Excess fluid administration, however, may result in pulmonary edema as a result of impaired left ventricular diastolic compliance. As atrial systole makes an important contribution to fill in the noncompliance left ventricle in AS, efforts should be used to maintain a normal sinus rhythm. When symptoms develop in a patient with moderate to severe AS, valve replacement is required.

2.9.6 Aortic regurgitation

The most common causes of acute aortic regurgitation are acute infective endocarditis, acute aortic dissection, spontaneous chordal rupture, or tears of myxomatous valve leaflets, and valve destruction from blunt or perforating chest trauma.

Hemodynamically significant acute aortic regurgitation (AR) presents with manifestations of left ventricular diastolic pressure overload as a result of a high-pressure regurgitant flow into a noncompliant, nondilated LV. This increased diastolic pressure is transmitted to the left atrium and the pulmonary venous system. Although left ventricular preload is increased, the ventricle is able to dilate enough to maintain a sufficient stroke volume to compensate for the regurgitate flow. Compensatory tachycardia commonly occurs to maintain cardiac output. Rapidly declining aortic diastolic pressure along with increasing left ventricular end-diastolic pressure reduces coronary perfusion pressure, which, when combined with decreased diastolic filling time owing to tachycardia, presents the potential for subendocardial ischemia.

Table 2.7 Severity of aortic stenosis in relation to aortic valve area

Normal aortic valve area	3–4 cm²
Trivial AS	>1.3 cm²
Mild AS	1.1–1.3 cm²
Moderate AS	0.7–1.0 cm²
Severe AS	≤0.7 cm²
Critical AS	≤0.5 cm²

AS, aortic stenosis.

Clinical features of AR include:

- wide pulse pressure with a 'water hammer' pulse;
- inferior and lateral displacement of the apical impulse;
- a soft A_2;
- a third heart sound;
- a high-pitched blowing decrescendo early diastolic murmur along with a systolic murmur caused by increased flow across the aortic valve;
- an apical diastolic murmur.

In patients with acute AR, many of the above signs may be greatly attenuated or absent. Doppler echocardiograph is essential for accurate and rapid evaluation of AR in the hemodynamically unstable patient. Valvular vegetations or prolapse caused by leaflet tears can be diagnosed, as can aortic annular dilation. Transesophageal echo is highly useful in cases of suspected ascending aortic dissection or aneurysms, and in evaluation of the aortic route in patients with endocarditis and suspected aortic ring abscesses.

Management of patients with acute AR and pulmonary edema includes reducing elevated left ventricular preload with diuretics and nitrate. Afterload reduction to improve flow and reduce regurgitant fraction with ACE-inhibitors, hydralazine or nitroprusside is also indicated[14]. Intra-aortic balloon pumping worsens AR and is contraindicated. Bradycardia increases regurgitant fraction and should be avoided. Atrial pacing may be useful to increase heart rate in normotensive patients, and inotropes may be useful if concurrent hypotension or a low output state are present. AR frequently responds to medical therapy and aortic valve surgery can be undertaken electively. However, patients with ascending aortic dissection with acute AR should be treated acutely with antihypertensives and beta-blockers to decrease aortic wall stress. Pulmonary edema as a result of infective endocarditis and severe AR is also an indication of surgical intervention particularly when the vegetation is large (>1 cm), when the infection involves a prosthetic valve or if the aortic root is involved.

References

1. **Ross, J., Jr** (1979) Afterload mismatch and preload reserve: a conceptual framework for the analysis of ventricular function. *Prog. Cardiovasc. Dis.* **14**: 255–264.
2. **Hands, M.E., Rutherford, J.D., Muller, J.E., et al.** (1989) The in-hospital development of cardiogenic shock after myocardial infarction: incidence, predictors of occurrence, outcome and prognostic factors. *J. Am. Coll. Cardiol.* **14**: 40–46.
3. **Schaffer, J., Tews, A., Langes, K., et al.** (1987) Relationship between myocardial norepinephrine content and left ventricular function. An endomyocardial biopsy study. *Eur. Heart J.* **8**: 748.
4. **Gregoratos, G., Cheitlan, M.D., Conill A., et al.** (1998) ACC/AHA guidelines for implantation of cardiac pacemakers and antiarrhythmia devices. *J. Am. Coll. Cardiol.* **31**: 1110–1114.
5. **Chen, L.K., Teerlink, J.R. and Goldschlager, N.** (1997) Pacemaker emergencies. In: *Cardiac Intensive Care* (ed. D.L. Brown). Philadelphia, PA: W.B. Saunders, pp. 405–426.
6. **Vasan, R.S., Benjamin, E.J. and Levy, D.** (1995) Prevalence, clinical features, and prognosis of diastolic heart failure: An epidemiologic perspective. *J. Am. Coll. Cardiol.* **26**: 1565–1574.
7. **Wilson, J.R., Rayos, G., Yeoh, T.K., et al.** (1995) Dissociation between exertional symptoms and circulatory function in patients with heart failure. *Circulation* **92**: 47–53.
8. **Francis, G.S., Goldsmith, S.R., Levine, T.B., et al.** (1984) The neurohumoral axis in congestive heart failure. *Ann. Intern. Med.* **101**: 370–377.
9. **Seward, J.B., Khandheria, B.K., Oh, J.K., et al.** (1988) Transesophageal echocardiology: Technique, anatomic correlations, implementation and clinical applications. *Mayo Clin. Proc.* **63**: 649.
10. **Kimmelstiel, C., Udelson, J., Smith, J., et al.** (1998) Current concepts in the treatment of patients with heart failure. *ACC Curr. J. Rev.* **7**: 39–43.
11. **The Digitalis Investigation Group** (1997) The effect of digoxin on mortality and morbidity in patients with heart failure. *N. Engl. J. Med.* **336**: 525–533.

12. **Dittrich, H.C., Chow, L.C. and Nicol, P.H.** (1989) Early improvement in left ventricular diastolic function after relief of chronic right ventricular pressure overload. *Circulation* **80:** 823–830.

13. **DePace, N.L., Nestico, P.F. and Morganroth, J.** (1985) Acute severe mitral regurgitation: Patho-physiology, clinical recognition, and management. *Am. J. Med.* **78:** 293.

14. **Miller, R.R., Vismara, L.A., DeMara, A.N., *et al.*** (1976) Afterload reduction therapy with nitroprusside in severe aortic regurgitation: Improved cardiac performance and reduced regurgitant volume. *Am. J. Cardiol.* **38:** 564.

Chapter 3

Oxygen transport and tissue oxygenation

William T. McGee, MD, MHA
and Paul Jodka, MD

Contents

3.1 Introduction

Physicians frequently evaluate indices of organ function as an endpoint of therapy. In the angina patient, relief of pain and resolution of ischemic electrocardiographic changes are viewed as success of antianginal therapy. Similarly, in renal disease, maintenance of adequate urine output, a normal creatinine and blood urea nitrogen (BUN) are useful global physiologic measures of renal health. Normal organ function implies at a minimum adequate blood flow and oxygen (O_2) delivery. When disease intervenes, however, organ function may deteriorate. As illness progresses and subsequent organ function deteriorates to a critical stage, a variety of technologies are instituted in the critical care unit to prevent immediate death. Nonetheless, many patients continue to deteriorate and can die as a result of the gradual decline of all organ function. Multisystem organ failure in the critically ill results from failure of adequate oxygen and other nutrients to be delivered to tissues. Methods of determining adequate tissue oxygenation are crucial to the practice of medicine within the intensive care environment. It is critical to differentiate between organ dysfunction as a result of primary disease and organ dysfunction as a result of failure of the oxygen transport system.

Since the mid-1970s, it has been common to utilize invasive hemodynamic monitoring to delineate pulmonary artery pressures, pulmonary capillary wedge pressure, and cardiac output. However, these measurements merely define the determinants and indices of cardiac function, but do not provide information on the distribution of blood flow or the adequacy of peripheral tissue oxygenation and utilization. Critical illness ultimately results in the breakdown of the normal peripheral mechanisms of blood flow distribution, oxygen delivery, and oxygen utilization.

Data obtained during pulmonary artery catheterization allow evaluation of the oxygen delivery system and the global utilization of oxygen by the body. Evaluation of mixed venous oxygen and its general relationship to tissue oxygenation can at least assure us that bulk O_2 delivery, which we have significant ability to manipulate in the ICU, is not the cause of organ dysfunction and ultimately death.

3.2 Calculating oxygen transport

3.2.1 Oxygen delivery

The adequacy of tissue oxygenation depends upon the balance between the oxygen transported to cells and the oxygen requirement determined by their metabolic activity. Bulk oxygen transport also known as oxygen delivery and frequently abbreviated as DO_2 is simply the amount of oxygen carried within the blood multiplied by the blood flow or cardiac output[1]:

$$O_2 \text{ transport } (DO_2) = \text{cardiac output (CO)} \times \text{arterial oxygen content } (CaO_2)$$

Arterial oxygen content (CaO_2) is the amount of oxygen carried in 100 ml of blood, which includes oxygen chemically bound to hemoglobin as well as a small portion of oxygen dissolved in the plasma.

Quantitatively,

$$CaO_2 = (1.36 \times \text{g of hemoglobin} \times O_2 \text{ saturation } [SaO_2]) + (PaO_2 \times 0.003).$$

$PaO_2 \times 0.003$ represents the dissolved fraction of oxygen in plasma and is usually of insignificant quantity.

In a normal patient (with a hemoglobin content of 15 g and an arterial oxygen saturation of 99%)

$$CaO_2 = (1.36 \times 15 \times 0.99) + (100 \times 0.003)$$
$$= 20.1 \text{ ml } O_2 \text{ per 100 ml of blood}$$
$$\text{or } 20.1 \text{ ml dl}^{-1}.$$

Then

$$DO_2 = 5 \text{ l min}^{-1} \text{ (normal cardiac output)} \times 20.1 \text{ ml } O_2$$

per 100 ml $\times$ 10 dl l^{-1} (correction factor for the difference in units between CO and CaO_2).

Thus, a normal DO_2 is 1000 ml O_2 min^{-1}[1]. DO_2 may be indexed by body surface area and reported as DO_2I. Normal DO_2I in a 1.73 m^2 individual would be 575–600 ml O_2 min^{-1} m^{-2}.

DO_2 is the amount of oxygen that normally leaves the heart each minute and is delivered to the tissues. The distribution of this oxygen is determined in a complex manner by autoregulation of the arterioles and capillary beds in the periphery. Tissues that require large amounts of oxygen will open capillary beds, thus increasing the amount of oxygen delivered to the tissues. Similarly, tissues that have low metabolic activity close capillary beds, thus preventing wasted blood flow.

When supply is deficient, oxygen utilization is limited by decreased availability. Metabolism becomes anaerobic, lactic acid is produced, and a metabolic acidosis will result. Prolonged declines in O_2 delivery are associated with lactic acidosis, organ dysfunction and ultimately death.

3.2.2 Oxygen consumption (VO_2)

Oxygen is utilized by the mitochondria to produce energy for the cells. The quantity of oxygen extracted from the capillaries as blood passes to the venous side is defined as oxygen consumption. Oxygen consumption varies as the metabolic needs of the tissues change. Oxygen consumption can be measured directly by determining the difference between the quantity of inspired and expired oxygen. This may be done rather easily under laboratory conditions when the patient is breathing room air, or in the operating room with a closed-circuit anesthetic delivery system. Under clinical conditions in the ICU, direct oxygen consumption measurements are difficult, require specialized equipment, and are fraught with multiple sources of error[2,3]; indirect measurements are more practical.

Oxygen consumption (VO_2) may be calculated indirectly by the Fick equation, which states that oxygen consumption equals the difference between arterial oxygen delivery and venous oxygen return. The quantity of oxygen returned in venous blood to the right side of the heart can be calculated in a manner similar to the calculation for DO_2. Venous oxygen

return equals venous return (VR) × venous oxygen content (CvO_2). The calculation for CvO_2 utilizes the same general formula as for calculating CaO_2, i.e.

$$CvO_2 = (\text{hemoglobin} \times 1.36 \times \text{mixed venous oxygen saturation } [SvO_2]) + (PvO_2 \times 0.003).$$

The values for SvO_2 and PvO_2 are measured from mixed venous blood drawn from the pulmonary artery using the pulmonary artery catheter. The PvO_2 and SvO_2 in a normal healthy human are approximately 40 mmHg and 75%, respectively:

$$CvO_2 = (15 \times 1.36 \times 0.75) + (40 \times 0.003)$$

which equals 15 ml of oxygen per 100 ml of blood. Venous return in steady-state conditions is equal to the cardiac output, a normal venous return is 5 l min^{-1}, and therefore

$$\text{normal venous oxygen return} = 5 \text{ l min}^{-1} \times$$
$$15 \text{ ml dl}^{-1} \times 10 \text{ dl l}^{-1} \text{ (correction factor)}$$
$$= 750 \text{ ml } O_2 \text{ min}^{-1}.$$

As the normal oxygen delivery is 1000 ml min^{-1} and a normal venous oxygen return is 750 ml min^{-1}, the difference between these two, 250 ml min^{-1}, is the amount of oxygen extracted, i.e. the oxygen consumption (*Figure 3.1*). The process of consuming oxygen is assumed to occur completely at the capillary bed. Oxygen consumption equals oxygen delivery minus oxygen return or

$$(CO \times CaO_2) - (VR \times CvO_2).$$

As $CO = VR$ in the steady state,

$$O_2 \text{ consumption } (VO_2) = CO \times (CaO_2 - CvO_2).$$

This is just a restatement of the Fick equation. Determining oxygen consumption in this way requires accurate measurement of cardiac output, hemoglobin, PaO_2, SaO_2, PvO_2, and SvO_2, all of which are clinically available with a pulmonary artery catheter and a laboratory or bedside blood gas machine. Utilization of the Fick equation and $C(a\text{-}vO_2)$ can provide important information about the balance

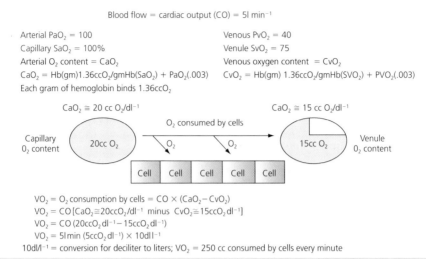

Blood flow = cardiac output (CO) = 5l min^{-1}

Arterial PaO$_2$ = 100
Capillary SaO$_2$ = 100%
Arterial O$_2$ content = CaO$_2$
CaO$_2$ = Hb(gm)1.36ccO$_2$/gmHb(SaO$_2$) + PaO$_2$(.003)
Each gram of hemoglobin binds 1.36ccO$_2$

Venous PvO$_2$ = 40
Venule SvO$_2$ = 75
Venous oxygen content = CvO$_2$
CvO$_2$ = Hb(gm) 1.36ccO$_2$/gmHb(SVO$_2$) + PVO$_2$(.003)

CaO$_2$ ≅ 20 cc O$_2$/dl^{-1}

O$_2$ consumed by cells

CaO$_2$ ≅ 15 cc O$_2$/dl^{-1}

Capillary O$_2$ content
20cc O$_2$
O$_2$ O$_2$
15cc O$_2$
Venule O$_2$ content

Cell Cell Cell Cell Cell

VO$_2$ = O$_2$ consumption by cells = CO × (CaO$_2$ − CvO$_2$)
VO$_2$ = CO [CaO$_2$ ≅ 20ccO$_2$/dl^{-1} minus CvO$_2$ ≅ 15ccO$_2$ dl^{-1}]
VO$_2$ = CO (20ccO$_2$ dl^{-1} − 15ccO$_2$ dl^{-1})
VO$_2$ = 5l min (5ccO$_2$ dl^{-1}) × 10dl l^{-1}
10dl/l^{-1} = conversion for deciliter to liters; VO$_2$ = 250 cc consumed by cells every minute

Figure 3.1 Normal oxygen transport, giving normal values for oxygen consumption and venous oxygen content.

between oxygen delivery and oxygen consumption[3]. Like DO$_2$, VO$_2$ may be indexed by body surface area and reported as VO$_2$I.

3.2.3 Oxygen extraction

As a tissue increases its metabolic activity, oxygen delivery is increased by an increase in flow. This may occur globally (i.e. by cardiac output) or locally (i.e. by an increase in flow (recruitment of capillary beds through autoregulation)). The increase in blood flow and therefore oxygen delivery is sometimes unable to meet the increased need secondary to higher metabolic activity. In these instances, oxygen extraction at the capillary level can increase. This results in a decrease in the oxygen saturation of the venous blood (SvO$_2$) leaving the capillaries. If this decrease occurs globally, or if it occurs regionally in a large volume of capillary beds, venous saturation of blood in the pulmonary artery (SvO$_2$) will decrease. An increasing C(a-vO$_2$) or a decreasing SvO$_2$ or PvO$_2$ implies that peripheral oxygen utilization has exceeded the body's capacity to supply oxygen by increasing flow[4]. However, this ability to extract oxygen at the capillary bed is limited. The oxygen extraction ratio (O$_2$ ER) is a convenient measure of global oxygen extraction. It is calculated by dividing the VO$_2$ by the DO$_2$. Normal values are 24–28%.

3.3 Balancing oxygen supply and demand

An oxygen supply/demand imbalance may occur for four basic reasons:

(i) a critical deficiency in one or more of the components of oxygen delivery (i.e. acute pump failure, hypoxemia or acute anemia);

(ii) an increase in metabolic demand that exceeds oxygen transport reserves;

(iii) blockage of normal cellular oxygen metabolism;

(iv) adequacy of total oxygen supply, but inadequate distribution to regional vascular beds.

In these circumstances, cells develop anaerobic metabolism in an attempt to manufacture energy in the absence of oxygen. This is a situation that cannot be maintained. If the metabolic need of the tissues does not decrease or if the oxygen delivery cannot increase, the cells supplied by these capillary beds will undergo ischemic death. A common example of this phenomenon occurs within muscle vascular beds during exercise. Although blood flow to exercising muscle increases tremendously, the metabolic activity of muscle cells demands more oxygen than can be supplied through increased blood flow alone. Oxygen extraction in exercising muscle therefore increases tremendously. Nonetheless, oxygen demand is still greater than the additional amount supplied by increased oxygen extraction. Therefore, exercising muscle enters an anaerobic phase and lactic acid is produced. This is a physiologic condition that can be maintained only for short periods of time, after which the muscle loses function. In this case, the organ dysfunction generally is beneficial, in that less exercise can be performed, the metabolic demands fall accordingly, and the supply/demand balance is restored.

In critically ill patients with diseases such as sepsis, adult respiratory distress syndrome (ARDS) or major trauma, oxygen supply/demand may not be autoregulated efficiently, and may result in the gradual onset of multisystem organ failure and death. The mechanisms by which this occur are not simple and remain poorly understood[1,4].

3.4 Clinical factors influencing oxygen supply

Adequate oxygen delivery implies a normal or compensated cardiopulmonary system. *Table 3.1* depicts the effects of separately altering the

components of oxygen transport. These calculations are oversimplistic, inasmuch as normal compensatory mechanisms adjust for individual deficiencies. Increases in heart rate and contractility or decreases in afterload will increase cardiac output when changes in hemoglobin or oxygen saturation decrease oxygen transport. Normally, cardiac output will begin to rise if hemoglobin drops below 10 g dl⁻¹, and is doubled when hemoglobin drops to 5 g dl⁻¹. The mechanism of increased flow is in part due to an increase in contractility, but is primarily caused by increases in heart rate and a drop in afterload. This is the result of alterations in blood viscosity, which occur in acute anemia. In chronic anemia, cardiac output returns toward baseline, and tissue oxygenation is maintained by an increase in red blood cell 2,3-diphosphoglycerate (2,3-DPG). This change in 2,3-DPG facilitates the release of oxygen from hemoglobin at the capillary level[5] (*Figure 3.2*).

3.4.1 Oxygen saturation

Increasing arterial oxygen saturation increases oxygen transport in a linear fashion. Oxygenation is usually thought to be sufficient if PaO_2

Table 3.1 Normal oxygen supply and demand and effects of low cardiac output, anemia and arterial desaturation on mixed venous (PvO_2) and (SvO_2)

DO_2 variable	Normal	Low cardiac output = 2.5 l min⁻¹	Anemia Hb = 7.5 g dl⁻¹	Arterial desaturation SaO_2 = .75 (PaO_2 = 40)
Arterial O_2 content (CaO_2) (ml dl⁻¹)	20	20	10	15
O_2 transport (CaO_2) (ml O_2 min⁻¹)	1000	500	500	750
minus O_2 consumption (VO_2 min⁻¹)	−250	−250	−250	−250
equals venous return (ml O_2 min⁻¹)	750	250	250	500
divided by CO (dl min⁻¹)	÷50	÷25	÷50	÷50
equals venous O_2 content				
(CvO_2) (ml dl⁻¹)	15	10	5	10
(a-v)O_2 content ($C(a-v)O_2$) (ml dl⁻¹)	5	10	5	5
Mixed venous O_2 saturation (SvO_2)	0.75	0.50	0.50	0.50
Mixed venous PO_2 (PvO_2) (torr)	40	27	27	27

Hb = 15 g dl⁻¹; SaO_2 = 1.0; cardiac output = 5 l min⁻¹; VO_2 = 250 ml min⁻¹. Other components of O_2 delivery are assumed to remain constant for this illustration.

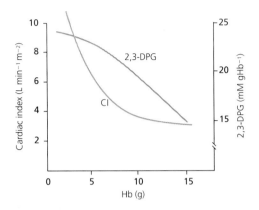

Figure 3.2 Effect of anemia on cardiac index and 2,3-DPG. Reproduced with permission from *The New Journal of Medicine* (1972) **286**: 412.

equals 60 torr because the oxyhemoglobin dissociation curve is horizontal beyond that point. However, a PaO$_2$ of 60 mmHg is still 7% less than complete hemoglobin saturation, and in patients with marginal oxygen transport, an increase of 7% may represent a crucial increase in oxygen supply. A PaO$_2$ above 100 mmHg increases the amount of dissolved oxygen in plasma but results in a quantitatively negligible increase in transported oxygen in most circumstances. However, the availability of dissolved oxygen becomes increasingly important in severe anemia, as might occur acutely with massive bleeding or in a Jehovah's Witness who refuses to accept transfusion. If the hemoglobin is 3 g dl^{-1}, then raising the PaO$_2$ from 100 mmHg to 500 mmHg will increase oxygen delivery by 33%. If blood transfusions are delayed, this therapeutic maneuver may be life saving.

3.4.2 Hemoglobin concentration

An obvious clinical maneuver to increase oxygen transport is to raise serum hemoglobin levels. Practically, this is limited by rheologic considerations of blood viscosity and cell deformability. Raising hemoglobin levels above 10–11% generally offers no clearcut increase in total cellular oxygen delivery and may compromise oxygen delivery when hemoglobin rises to polycythemic levels (>18 g %) owing to increased viscosity and sludging. If serum hemoglobin levels are less than 10%,

significant increases in oxygen transport can be obtained by transfusion; whether this improves outcome remains controversial.

3.5 Determinants of oxygen consumption

Oxygen consumption is stable in patients at rest but often is increased markedly in the ICU population as a result of fever, stress, cytokine release or other alterations of basal metabolic rate. Oxygen consumption varies in proportion to body temperature, with a 10–13% increase per degree centigrade elevation above normal[6]. Likewise, VO$_2$ decreases approximately 7% per degree centigrade below normal[7]. Shivering may increase VO$_2$ by over 100%[8].

The typical metabolic response to illness and injury results in significant elevations of VO$_2$ above normal. Moderate surgical trauma produces a 10–30% increase in VO$_2$, a 50% increase may accompany severe infections, and as much as a 100% increase is seen with large full-thickness burns[9]. Typical ICU procedures such as chest physiotherapy have been shown to increase VO$_2$ by 35%[10].

A commonly overlooked source of increased oxygen consumption involves the work of breathing. Normally, spontaneous ventilation at rest accounts for 1–3% of resting oxygen consumption. Critically ill patients with decreased pulmonary compliance or tachypnea may utilize as much as 25–40% of oxygen transport to maintain the energy required for spontaneous ventilation[11] (*Figure 3.3*). Intubation and mechanical ventilation can be important tools in balancing oxygen supply and demand in the critical patient.

3.6 Critical factors influencing cellular oxygen utilization

The most commonly recognized deficiency of cellular oxygen utilization accompanies cyanide poisoning, which uncouples oxidative phosphorylation. Impairment of oxygen utilization is also seen in shock, trauma, ARDS, sepsis, and multiple organ failure.

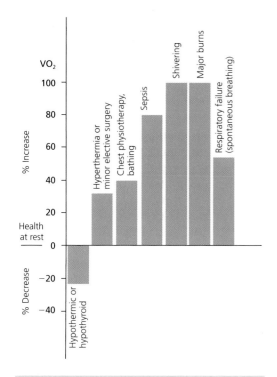

Figure 3.3 Changes in oxygen consumption (VO$_2$) in varying clinical disease states; percentages are averages, as wide ranges may be seen for each pathologic state.

Oxygen diffuses from the capillaries into the interstitium along a pressure gradient that decreases in direct proportion to the distance traveled. The farther oxygen has to travel, the less available it is to cells[5]. When the number of open capillary beds is inappropriately low for the metabolic need, areas distant from the capillary membrane may become hypoxic. As blood flows along the capillary, a progressive drop in capillary PO$_2$ results.

The administration of large volumes of crystalloid solutions to adequately resuscitate critically ill patients can result in tissue edema. This edema may cause decreased tissue PO$_2$, which probably is the result of increased inter-capillary distance. Interstitial edema, when accompanied by increased tissue pressure, may also impede capillary blood flow. Capillary occlusion may alter capillary pattern and density, increase intercapillary distances, and

influence microcirculatory shunting of blood. Mediators of the inflammatory cascade could also initiate or aggravate this pathophysiology. Metabolic uncoupling may occur at the cellular level if endogenously produced mediators disrupt oxidative phosphorylation.

3.7 **Evaluation of tissue oxygenation**

In healthy humans at rest, the quantity of oxygen delivered to all tissues is in excess of that required by metabolic demand. With stress and disease, however, oxygen consumption may increase markedly whereas supply is limited. An essential aspect of care of the critically ill is to define the point at which tissue oxygenation fails, so that therapy may be instituted to optimize oxygen transport.

Hemodynamic monitoring focuses on the central circulation as a means of deriving information on the adequacy of the oxygen transport system. The component parts of this system (lung, heart, hemoglobin, vascular conduits, and cellular oxygen consumption) must be individually evaluated.

3.7.1 Mixed venous oxygen tension (PvO$_2$)

There is currently no 'gold standard' for evaluation of global or regional tissue oxygenation. Mixed venous oxygen tension (PvO$_2$) is the most reliable, single physiologic indicator of the overall balance between oxygen supply and demand[3]. The driving force that transports oxygen out of the capillaries is the partial pressure gradient between capillary PO$_2$ and cellular PO$_2$. End-capillary oxygen tension reflects tissue oxygen tension and the balance between blood flow, capillary density, oxygen content, and oxygen consumption.

PvO$_2$ is the flow-weighted average oxygen tension of the capillary effluent from the entire body, and therefore reflects whole-body supply/demand balance. Some investigators prefer utilizing mixed venous oxygen saturation (SvO$_2$), which when measured directly incorporates alterations in oxyhemoglobin dissociation and more accurately reflects the quantity of oxygen released from hemoglobin. The PvO_2 and the SvO_2 from a specific organ bed may be significantly lower or higher than the global PvO_2 or SvO_2 measured in the pulmonary artery. For instance, the SvO_2 from the heart normally is 30% whereas that from the skin is 90%. These differences are indicative of the different resting metabolic rates, proportional non-nutrient blood flow, and basal oxygen extraction between the heart and the skin. Oxygen saturation in the superior vena cava is slightly lower than that in the inferior vena cava, which drains organs such as the spleen, kidney, and resting mesentery with lower oxygen extraction. In shock states, inferior vena caval saturation decreases and superior vena caval saturation becomes higher than the SvO_2, emphasizing the effect of vascular redistribution[12].

It is crucially important to recognize that the PvO_2 is a mixture of venous effluent from all perfused beds. It may be normal in spite of small (in relation to the entire vascular system) areas of severe ischemia. Also, PvO_2 will not be affected by areas of complete non-perfusion. When flow is distributed according to metabolic need, PvO_2 and SvO_2 correlate well with oxygen reserve and tissue oxygenation. If flow is maldistributed or if the microcirculation malfunctions, interpretation of PvO_2 and SvO_2 as indicators of tissue oxygenation becomes problematic.

In flow-deficient states an increased oxygen extraction maintains tissue oxygenation until the oxygen reserve is exhausted. Which level of PvO_2 is indicative of an exhausted oxygen reserve and consequent tissue ischemia? All oxygen-bound hemoglobin is not extractable. Available evidence indicates that 30–35% of such oxygen is unavailable for tissue consumption[13]. In a group of patients with cardiopulmonary disease, Kasnitz found a threshold PvO_2 of 28 mmHg below which lactic acidosis occurred and survival decreased. In this study, PvO_2 predicted lacticacidemia and death more accurately than did PaO_2 or cardiac output[14].

3.7.2 Lactic acid and PvO_2

The presence of lactic acidosis in critically ill patients is considered a marker of poor prognosis[15]. In particular, the failure of serially measured lactate levels to decline portends a bad outcome in a variety of clinical settings and evaluation of such trends in lactate clearance has been found to have greater prognostic utility than oxygen-derived variables[16–18]. Although lactic acidosis is typically a marker of anaerobic metabolism, not all instances of lactate elevation are necessarily associated with tissue hypoperfusion and cellular hypoxia[19]. Lactate levels represent the balance of lactate production and utilization and may be altered in a variety of critical illnesses. In sepsis, for example, increased glycolytic flux combined with impaired pyruvate utilization[20] is probably one of several mechanisms giving rise to elevated lactate levels in the absence of frank oxygen deprivation (*Figure 3.4*). For practical purposes, one must still first determine adequacy of resuscitation of patients with lactic acidosis before ascribing this finding to complex metabolic alterations induced by a given disease process.

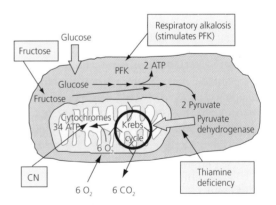

Figure 3.4 Lactic acidosis is most commonly the result of conversion of excess pyruvate to lactate in the face of anaerobic conditions that foreclose metabolism via the Krebs cycle. Other causes of lactic acidosis include use of fructose rather than glucose as a substrate, stimulation of phosphofructokinase (PFK)$_9$, thiamine deficiency and cyanide toxicity.

Simmons found the best predictor of anaerobiosis and hyperlacticacidemia to be a critical PvO_2 of 27 mmHg[21]. Others have argued that a PvO_2 of approximately 20 mmHg is the crucial level below which cellular function deteriorates, because in healthy maximally exercising humans, PvO_2 reaches a plateau at 20 mmHg[22]. However, the relevancy of these data to the stress of disease states is questionable. Maximal exercise is a physiologic state of progressive oxygen debt, anaerobiosis, and increasing acidosis, which cannot be maintained for more than short periods of time. In states of depressed myocardial function, the correlation of PvO_2 with lactic acidosis has been better than the correlation of any other index, including cardiac output[23].

The PvO_2 and SvO_2 are normally about 40 mmHg and 75%, respectively. These values indicate that under normal circumstances, 25% of the oxygen bound to hemoglobin is consumed by normal metabolic activity. When the PvO_2 drops to 28 mmHg, the saturation is 50%. Because of the steep slope of the oxyhemoglobin dissociation curve at partial pressures of oxygen in this range, a mere 12 mmHg drop in PvO_2 reflects a doubling of oxygen extraction. This additional oxygen extraction, for practical purposes, reflects the remaining oxygen reserves below which metabolic derangement begins. Therefore, as the PvO_2 decreases from 40 mmHg to 28 mmHg, progressive exhaustion of oxygen reserve occurs. PvO_2 below 28 mmHg and SvO_2 values below 50% imply oxygen deficits that must be corrected if survival is expected.

A low or decreasing SvO_2 is associated with a poor prognosis in respiratory failure, myocardial infarction, and traumatic shock[10,14]. Some evidence suggests that in chronic hypoxemia or chronic low-flow states, unusually low PvO_2 may be tolerated without gross metabolic dysfunction[24], possibly as a result of enzymatic adaptation, or enhanced microcirculatory regulation[25].

3.8 Influence of loss of vasoregulation

Although the PvO_2 always indicates oxygen supply/demand balance for perfused tissues, the use of PvO_2 to mark a critical threshold below which anaerobic metabolism is or is not found depends on intact vasoregulation, the absence of significant interstitial edema, normal capillarity, and the absence of microcirculatory obstruction. Normal or high PvO_2 may be misleading in disease states such as sepsis, cirrhosis of the liver, and ARDS, as well as other capillary leak syndromes that may be associated with functional systemic shunts[26]. The mechanism of systemic shunting may be related to differential capillary bed flow rates, inappropriate capillary density, capillary–venule back diffusion of oxygen, or cellular inability to consume oxygen. The shunting of capillary blood can have a profound effect on mixed venous oxygen tension (*Figure 3.5*). Therefore, a normal, high or rising PvO_2 may coexist with tissue oxygen deprivation and anaerobiosis in these pathologic states. Diagnostically, an elevated or increasing PvO_2 may be an early indication of disease characterized by functional systemic shunts.

Therapeutic maneuvers that increase DO_2 may be judged according to their effect on VO_2. A two-phase relationship has been proposed, with an initial direct relationship giving way to a plateau at the point of critical O_2 delivery (*Figure 3.6*). The VO_2 plateau despite increasing DO_2 implies satisfaction of cellular oxygen requirements. This will be discussed more fully in Section 3.10.

3.9 Continuous mixed venous oxygen saturation in clinical medicine

The capability for continuous monitoring of SvO_2 has been incorporated into pulmonary artery catheters as an early indicator of significant clinical deterioration. In patients being

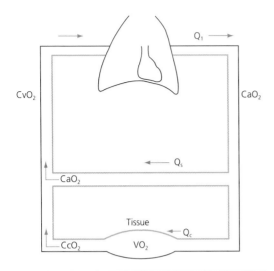

Figure 3.5 Two-compartment model of systemic circulation. Q_t, cardiac ouput; Q_s, blood flow shunted from arterial to venous circuit; Q_c, tissue capillary blood flow; CaO_2, arterial oxygen content; CvO_2, mixed venous oxygen content; CcO_2, oxygen content of blood leaving the tissue compartment. As all oxygen consumption (VO_2) occurs in the tissue compartment, the blood leaving the shunt compartment has the composition of arterial blood and will have a profound effect on CvO_2. From: Mill, M.J. (1982) Tissue oxygenation in clinical medicine: an Historical Review, The International Anesthesia Research Society. Reproduced with permission from *Anesthesia and Analgesia*, Lippincott, Williams & Wilkins.

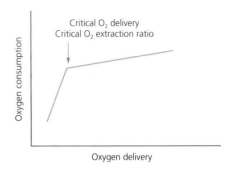

Figure 3.6 Beyond the inflection point A, oxygen consumption is independent of delivery. Increasing oxygen delivery beyond this would not be expected to have clinical utility. Before reaching this plateau (during active resuscitation of shock patients) restoring oxygen delivery is a primary goal during resuscitation of critically ill patients.

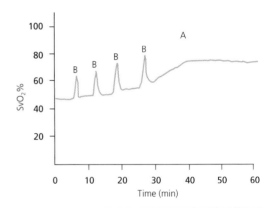

Figure 3.7 Trauma victim with hypovolemic shock, showing the effect of successive fluid boluses (B) and ultimate maintenance of normal SvO_2 once volume resuscitation is complete (A). The increase in SvO_2 from 50% to 75% implies that oxygen transport doubled during this successful resuscitation.

weaned from intraaortic balloon pumps, changes in mixed venous oxygen saturation occur almost instantaneously with changes in the balloon inflation interval[27]. In patients maintained on AV sequential pacemakers, changes to ventricular pacing that are accompanied by a significant decrease in cardiac output may be ascertained immediately by a drop in the mixed venous oxygen saturation[28]. The SvO_2 in hypovolemic shock will increase dramatically after a fluid bolus and thereafter will be sustained when higher filling pressures are maintained[29] (*Figure 3.7*). Therapeutic manipulations (e.g. ventilator changes) often not associated with hemodynamic perturbations may be recognized within minutes when utilizing continuous SvO_2 monitoring[30]. Cost savings

may result from decreased utilization of arterial blood gas studies.

3.10 Goal-directed therapy with DO_2 and VO_2

Defining what constitutes adequate (or optimal) global DO_2, the relationship of oxygen consumption (VO_2) to delivery (DO_2) in critical illness, and how to detect inadequate DO_2 (either globally or regionally), has been the subject of debate for a number of years. In most circumstances, physicians utilize trends in hemodynamic parameters (e.g. Blood Pressure (BP), Cardiac output/cardiac index (CO/CI), PCWP), oxygen transport variables (DO$_2$, arterial/mixed venous O$_2$ contents), oxygen consumption variables (VO$_2$, O$_2$ ER), end-organ function, and serial laboratory assessments (e.g. arterial lactate level) to arrive at a composite impression as to the adequacy of tissue oxygenation. Monitors of regional (e.g. gastric tonometry) and cellular perfusion and oxygen utilization are being developed but have not yet found widespread application for reasons of technical feasibility and need for further validation.

3.10.1. DO$_2$/VO$_2$ in critical illness

Available experimental data suggest that VO$_2$ is normally maintained at a relatively stable and unchanging level over a wide range of normal or elevated DO$_2$ values (supply-independent VO$_2$). However, as DO$_2$ is progressively reduced, a DO$_2$ value is reached below which compensatory mechanisms fail and VO$_2$ becomes dependent on DO$_2$ (supply-dependent VO$_2$) (*Figure 3.6*)[31]. This DO$_2$ value is referred to as the critical (or threshold) O$_2$-delivery value. At this point, any further reduction in DO$_2$ results in an oxygen supply–demand mismatch with resultant widespread tissue hypoxia, conversion to anaerobic metabolism, and generation of lactic acidosis. The point at which this occurs is difficult to predict in humans, as maintenance of 'adequate' global DO$_2$ values may not preclude regional oxygen supply–demand imbalances.[32] Few human studies have actually identified the critical DO$_2$[31,33], and cellular dysoxia as well as lactate generation in critical illness probably involve mechanisms beyond simple disturbances in bulk O$_2$ flow[19,20].

Certain disease states, such as ARDS and sepsis, may raise the critical value of DO$_2$ and alter the DO$_2$–VO$_2$ relationship and cellular oxygen utilization, resulting in a state of 'pathological' delivery-dependent VO$_2$ with the risk of concomitant 'occult' tissue hypoxia

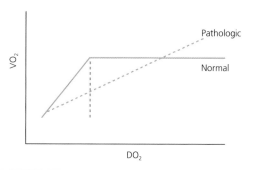

Figure 3.8 The oxygen delivery (DO$_2$) and oxygen consumption (VO$_2$) relationship in normal (continuous line) and pathologic (dashed line) conditions. Under normal conditions, as DO$_2$ decreases, VO$_2$ remains relatively constant until the critical VO$_2$ (dashed vertical line), at which point VO$_2$ decreases as DO$_2$. In contrast, in pathologic conditions, pathologic dependence of VO$_2$ and DO$_2$ is characterized by higher critical DO$_2$ and a much wider range of dependence of VO$_2$ on DO$_2$.

in the face of normal global DO$_2$ values (*Figure 3.8*)[34,35]. Furthermore, observational data[36] suggest that survivors of surgical critical illness manifest significantly elevated levels of DO$_2$ and VO$_2$. Several investigators have explored the effect of interventions aimed at achieving such 'supranormal' (or 'survivor') hemodynamic patterns and DO$_2$ values on outcome in a variety of clinical settings[37–42] based on assumptions that critical illness induces pathologic supply-dependent oxygen consumption and that raising DO$_2$ to supranormal values prevents or reverses occult tissue hypoxia. In high-risk surgical patients the results of such an approach instituted preoperatively are associated with a survival advantage[43,44]. Interventions to raise DO$_2$ included (depending on study design) the use of fluids, blood products, and catecholamines to achieve predetermined hemodynamic and/or DO$_2$ end-points (most commonly CI > 4.5 l m^{-2} Body surface area (BSA), DO$_2$ > 600 ml min^{-1} m^{-2}).

The results of the trials of supranormal DO$_2$ in mixed populations of critically ill patients have suggested either no benefit[37,42] or even a higher mortality in the treatment group as compared with the control group[40].

Meta-analysis of available trials involving supranormal DO_2 confirms lack of efficacy of this intervention if there is a delay between the insult and institution of therapy, but also concedes that there may be some benefit to a select group of patients in whom it is begun preoperatively[45]. It is of interest that these trials have suffered from significant 'crossover' of patients between study groups where 'control' patients spontaneously achieved the study patients' supranormal hemodynamic values, and 'study' patients were unable to reach the hemodynamic goals expected of them by study design. Such crossovers tend to obscure any real treatment effect (should it exist) but may simply reflect a difference in cardiopulmonary reserve between survivors and non-survivors, as a better outcome is associated with the ability to sustain an elevated CI/DO_2 (regardless of assignment to study or control group). Further methodologic problems found in studies evaluating supranormal DO_2 include inconsistencies in study design involving the timing of interventions, lack of standardization of cointerventions, use of retrospective subgroup analysis as well as lack of double-blinded design[39,46].

3.11 Summary

A primary goal of critical care medicine is to optimize oxygen delivery to cells and tissues. Based on available data from trials involving supranormal DO_2 strategies, there is insufficient evidence to support using predetermined supraphysiologic hemodynamic or oxygen transfer values as empiric endpoints of therapy. Mixed venous oxygen remains a valuable indicator of the balance between global oxygen delivery and utilization in most clinical situations. In general, a low or decreasing SvO_2 indicates an imbalance between oxygen consumption and oxygen delivery and warrants investigation. A stable SvO_2 suggests that global oxygen transport is balanced to oxygen consumption. However, no single laboratory or clinical data point can be taken in isolation as an indication that the oxygen supply–demand relationship is ideal or adequate. Rather, a thorough assessment of the adequacy of perfusion and oxygen delivery requires integration of serial physical examination findings with trends in hemodynamic parameters, oxygen consumption variables, end-organ function, and laboratory data such as lactate level.

Essential equations

$$O_2 \text{ transport } (DO_2) = \text{cardiac output (CO)} \times \text{arterial oxygen content } (CaO_2)$$

$$CaO_2 = (1.36 \times g \text{ of Hb} \times O_2 \text{ saturation} (SaO_2)) + (PaO_2 \times 0.003)$$

$$\text{normal: Hb} = 15; SaO_2 = 99\%; PaO_2 = 100\%; CO = 5 \text{ l min}^{-1}$$

$$CaO_2 = (1.36 \times 15 \times 0.99) + (100 \times 0.003) = 20.1 \text{ ml } O_2 \text{ dl}^{-1}$$

$$DO_2 = 5 \text{ l min}^{-1} \times 20.1 \text{ ml } O_2 \text{ dl}^{-1} \times 10 \text{ dl l}^{-1} \text{ (correction factor)}$$

$$DO_2 = 1000 \text{ ml } O_2 \text{ min}^{-1} \text{ (leaving the heart)}$$

$$\text{venous oxygen return} = \text{venous return (VR)} \times \text{venous oxygen content } (CvO_2)$$

$$CvO_2 = (1.36 \times Hb \times SvO_2) + (PvO_2 \times 0.003)$$

$$\text{normal Hb} = 15 \ SvO_2 = 75\% \ PvO_2 = 40 \text{ VR} = 5 \text{ l min}^{-1}: SvO_2 + PvO_2$$

sampled from pulmonary artery

$$CvO_2 = (1.36 \times 15 \times 0.75) + 40 \times 0.003) = 15 \text{ ml } O_2 \text{ dl}^{-1}$$

$$\text{venous oxygen return} = 5 \text{ l min}^{-1} \times 15 \text{ ml } O_2 \text{ dl}^{-1} \times 10 \text{ dl (correction factor)}$$

$$\text{venous oxygen return} = 750 \text{ ml } O_2 \text{ min}^{-1} \text{ (returning to right heart)}$$

$$\text{oxygen consumption } (VO_2) = (\text{oxygen delivery } [DO_2] - \text{venous oxygen return})$$

$$VO_2 = (CO \times CaO_2) - (VR \times CvO_2), \text{ as CO} = VR$$

$$VO_2 = CO \times (CaO_2 - CvO_2) \times 10 \text{ THE FICK EQUATION}$$

$$VO_2 = CO \times C(a\text{-}vO_2) \times 10.$$

References

1. Finch, C.A. and Lenfant, C. (1972) Oxygen transport in man. *N. Engl. J. Med.* **286**: 407.

2. Ultman, J.S. and Bursztein, A. (1981) Analysis of error in the determination of respiratory gas exchange at varying FiO$_2$. *J. Appl. Physiol.* **50**: 210–216.

3. Browning, J.A., Linbert, S.E., Turney, S.Z. and Chodoff, P. (1982) The effects of a fluctuating FiO$_2$ on metabolic measurements in mechanically ventilated patients. *Crit. Care Med.* **10**: 82–85.

4. Kandel, G. and Aberman, A. (1983) Mixed venous oxygen saturation: its role in the assessment of the critically ill patient. *Arch. Intern. Med.* **143**: 1400–1402.

5. Woodson, R.D. (1979) Physiological significance of oxygen dissociation curve shifts. *Crit. Care Med.* **7**: 368.

6. Beisel, W., Wannemacher, R.W. and Neufield, H.A. (1980) Relation of fever to energy expenditure. In: *Assessment of Energy Metabolism in Health and Disease.* Ross Laboratories, Columbus, OH, p. 144.

7. Harris, E.A., Scalye, E.R. and Squire, A.W. (1971) Oxygen consumption during cardiopulmonary bypass with moderate hypothermia in man. *Br. J. Anaesth.* **43**: 1113.

8. Rodriquez, J.L., Weissman, L., Damask, M.C., *et al.* (1983) Physiologic requirements during rewarming: suppression of the shivering response. *Crit. Care Med.* **11**: 490.

9. Kinney, J.M., Duke, J.H., Long, C.L., *et al.* (1970) Tissue fuel and weight loss after injury. *J. Clin. Pathol.* **23**(Suppl. 4): 65–72.

10. Weissman, C., Kemper, M., Damask, M.C., *et al.* (1984) Effect of routine intensive care interactions on metabolic rate. *Chest* **86**: 815–818.

11. Aubier, M., Viires, N., Syllie, G., *et al.* (1982) Respiratory muscle contribution to lactic acidosis in low cardiac output. *Am. Rev. Respir. Dis.* **126**: 648.

12. Lee, J., Wright, F., Barber, R., *et al.* (1972) Central venous oxygen saturation in shock. *Anesthesiology* **36**: 472.

13. Bryan-Brown, C., Back, S., Makabali, G., *et al.* (1973) Consumable oxygen availability of oxygen in relation to oxyhemoglobin dissociation. *Crit. Care Med.* **1**: 17.

14. Kasnitz, P., Druger, G.L., Torra, F. and Simmons, D.H. (1976) Mixed venous oxygen tension and hyperlactatemia. Survival in severe cardiopulmonary disease. *JAMA* **236**: 570.

15. Cady, L.D., Jr, Weil, M.H., Afifi, A.A., *et al.* (1973) Quantitation of severity of critical illness with special reference to blood lactate. *Crit. Care Med.* **1**: 75.

16. Singarajah, C. and Carlson, R.W. (1998) A review of the role of blood lactate measurements in the ICU. *J. Intensive Care Med.* **13**: 218–228.

17. Friedman, G., Berlot, G., Kahn, R.J. and Vincent, J.-L. (1995) Combined measurements of blood lactate concentrations and gastric intramucosal pH in patients with severe sepsis. *Crit. Care Med.* **23**: 1184–1193.

18. Bakker, J., Coffernils, M., Leon, M., Gris, P. and Vincent, J.-L. (1991) Blood lactate levels are superior to oxygen-derived variables in predicting outcome in human septic shock. *Chest* **99**: 956–962.

19. Simmons, D.H., Alpas, A.P., Tashkin, D.P. and Coulson, A. (1978) Hyperlactatemia due to arterial hypoxemia or reduced cardiac output, or both. *Am. Phys. Soc.* **45**(2): 195.

20. Bevegard, S., Holmgren, A. and Johnsson, B. (1960) The effect of body position on the circulation at rest and during exercise, with special reference to the influence on the stroke volume. *Acta Physiol. Scand.* **29**: 279.

21. De La Roche, A.G., Edmonds, J.F., Williams, W.G., *et al.* (1978) Importance of mixed venous oxygen saturation in the care of critically ill patients. *Can. J. Surg.* **21**: 227.

22. Hotchkiss, R.S. and Karl I.E. (1992) Reevaluation of the role of cellular hypoxia and bioenergetic failure in sepsis. *JAMA* **267**: 1503–1510.

23. Fink, M.P. (2001) Cytopathic hypoxia—mitochondrial dysfunction as mechanism contributing to organ dysfunction in sepsis. *Crit. Care Clinics* **17**(1): 219–237.

24. Schlichtig, R., Cowden, W.L. and Chaitman, B.R. (1986) Tolerance of unusually low mixed venous oxygen saturation: adaptations in the chronic low cardiac output syndrome. *Am. J. Med.* **80**: 813–818.

25. Robin, E.D. (1980) Of men and mitochondria: coping with hypoxic dysoxia. *Am. Rev. Respir. Dis.* **122**: 617.

26. Danek, S.J., Lynch, J.P., Weg, J.G., *et al.* (1980) The dependence of oxygen uptake on oxygen delivery in the adult respiratory distress syndrome. *Am. Rev. Respir. Dis.* **122**: 387.

27. Gore, J. (1984) Use of continuous monitoring of mixed venous saturation in the CCU. *Chest* **86**: 757.

28. Baele, P.L., McMichan, J.C., March, H.M., *et al.* (1982) Continuous monitoring of mixed venous oxygen saturation in critically ill patients. *Anesth. Analg.* **61**: 513.

29. McMichan, J.C. (1983) Continuous monitoring of mixed venous oxygen saturations. In:

Continuous Measurement of Blood Oxygen Saturation in the High Risk Patient, Vol. 1 (ed. J.F. Schweiss). Beach International Inc., San Diego, CA: 1–29.

30. **Nelson, L.D.** (1987) Continuous venous oximetry in surgical patients. *Ann. Surg.* **203**: 329–333.

31. **Ronco, J.J., Fenwick J.C., Tweeddale M.G.,** *et al.* (1993) Identification of the critical oxygen delivery for anaerobic metabolism in critically ill septic and nonseptic humans. *JAMA* **270**(14): 1724–1730.

32. **Marik, P.E.** (1993) Gastric intramucosal pH, a better predictor of multiorgan dysfunction syndrome and death than oxygen-derived variables in patients with sepsis. *Chest* **104**: 225–229.

33. **Shibutani, K., Komatsu T., Kubal K.,** *et al.* (1983) Critical level of oxygen delivery in anesthetized man. *Crit. Care Med.* **11**: 640–643.

34. **Astiz, M.E., Rackow E.C., Falk J.L.,** *et al.* (1987) Oxygen delivery and consumption in patients with hyperdynamic septic shock. *Crit. Care Med.* **15**(1): 26–28.

35. **Danek, S.J., Lynch J.P., Weg J.G., and Dantzker D.R.** (1980) The dependence of oxygen uptake on oxygen delivery in the adult respiratory distress syndrome. *Am. Rev. Resp. Dis.* **122**: 387–395.

36. **Shoemaker, W.C., Montgomery, E.S., Kaplan, E. and Elwyn, D.H.** (1973) Physiologic patterns in surviving and nonsurviving shock patients: use of sequential cardiorespiratory variables in defining criteria for therapeutic goals and early warning of death. *Arch. Surg.* **106**: 630–636.

37. **Alia, I., Esteban A., Gordo F.,** *et al.* (1999) A randomized and controlled trial of the effect of treatment aimed at maximizing oxygen delivery in patients with severe sepsis or septic shock. *Chest* **115**: 453–461.

38. **Hayes, M.A., Timmins, A.C., Yau, E.H.S., Palazzo, M., Watson, D. and Hinds, C.J.** (1997) Oxygen transport patterns in patients with sepsis syndrome or septic shock: Influence of treatment and relationship to outcome. *Crit. Care Med.* **25**: 926–936.

39. **Tuchschmidt, J., Fried, J., Astiz, M. and Rackow, E.** (1992) Elevation of cardiac output and oxygen delivery improves outcome in septic shock. *Chest* **102**: 216–220.

40. **Hayes, M.A., Timmins, A.C., Yau, E.H.S., Palazzo, M., Hinds, C.J. and Watson, D.** (1994) Elevation of systemic oxygen delivery in the treatment of critically ill patients. *N. Engl. J. Med.* **330**: 1717–1722.

41. **Yu, M., Burchell, S., Hasaniya, N.,** *et al.* (1998) Relationship of mortality to increasing oxygen delivery in patients (50 years of age: A prospective, randomized trial. *Crit. Care Med.* **26**: 1011–1019.

42. **Gattinoni, L., Brazzi L., Pelosi P.,** *et al.* (1995) A trial of goal-oriented hemodynamic therapy in critically ill patients. *N. Engl. J. Med.* **333**: 1025–1032.

43. **Boyd, O., Grounds, M.R. and Bennett, D.E.** (1993) A randomized clinical trial of the effect of deliberate perioperative increase of oxygen delivery on mortality in high-risk surgical patients. *JAMA* **270**: 2699–2707.

44. **Shoemaker, W.C., Appel, P.L., Kram, H.B., Waxman, K. and Lee, T.** (1988) Prospective trial of supranormal values of survivors as therapeutic goals in high-risk surgical patients. *Chest* **94**: 1176–1186.

45. **Heyland, D., Cook, D., King, D.,** *et al.* (1996) Maximizing oxygen delivery in critically ill patients: a methodologic appraisal of the evidence. *Crit. Care Med.* **24**: 517–524.

46. **Yu, M., Levy, M.M., Smith, P., Takiguchi, S.A., Miyasaki, A. and Myers, S.A.** (1993) Effect of maximizing oxygen delivery on morbidity and mortality rates in critically ill patients: a prospective, randomized, controlled study. *Crit. Care Med.* **21**: 830–838.

Chapter 4

Acid–base disorders

Ali Al-Khafaji, MD,
Marcus J. Hampers, MD and
Howard L. Corwin, MD

Contents

4.1 Introduction

Acid–base abnormalities are common in the intensive care unit. Most metabolic and physiologic processes in the body require the pH to be within a narrow range of 7.35–7.45. To achieve a normal acid–base balance, the interaction between the respiratory, renal and buffering systems should be intact. When there is an acid–base abnormality, the buffer system will be the first to respond by altering hydrogen ions. The lungs will remove the carbon dioxide and the kidneys will excrete acidic urine. This is a very well-orchestrated process, the net result of which will be a normal acid–base balance.

4.2 Basic concepts and definitions

Normal arterial blood gas values are pH 7.35–7.45, PCO_2 35–45 mmHg, and HCO_3 22–26 mequiv l^{-1}.

There are four primary acid–base disorders:

- metabolic acidosis: decreased pH and decreased HCO_3;

- respiratory acidosis: decreased pH and increased PCO_2;
- metabolic alkalosis: increased pH and increased HCO_3;
- respiratory alkalosis: increased pH and decreased PCO_2.

4.2.1 Compensatory response (*Figure 4.1*)
For each acid–base disorder, there is a compensatory response mediated by the kidneys or the lungs that tends to bring the pH back towards normal (*Table 4.1*). It is important to note that compensation does not fully correct the primary acid–base disorder.

4.2.2 Buffer system
A buffer is any substance that can reversibly bind to H^+ to neutralize the effect:

$$buffer + H^+ \Leftrightarrow H\ buffer.$$

A free H^+ combines with a buffer to form a weak acid that, depending on the concentration of H^+, can remain as an unassociated complex or dissociate back to H^+ and buffer. In plasma and interstitial fluid, bicarbonate

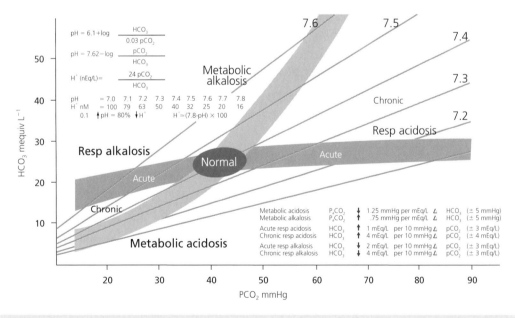

Figure 4.1 Acid–base nomogram can be used to predict pH changes with changes in bicarbonate or PCO_2. Reprinted with permission from Mark Graber, M.D., VA Medical Center, Northport, NY. In: *The Kidney Kard* 3rd Edition (1995).

Table 4.1 Causes of respiratory alkalosis

Primary disorder	pH	Compensatory response
Metabolic acidosis (⇓ HCO_3)	<7.35	⇓ PCO_2
Metabolic alkalosis (⇑ HCO_3)	>7.45	⇑ PCO_2
Respiratory acidosis (⇑ PCO_2)	<7.35	⇑ HCO_3
Respiratory alkalosis (⇓ PCO_2)	>7.45	⇓ HCO_3

(HCO_3), proteins and phosphate compounds are the major buffer system, whereas in the red blood cells, hemoglobin serves as the major buffer. An acid–base buffer system works to prevent changes in pH when either acid or base is added. The ratio of acid to base, along with an equilibrium constant (pK), defines the free H^+ concentration of the solution. This relationship is expressed by the Henderson–Hasselbalch equation: pH = pK + log (base/acid).

The pK of a buffer system identifies the pH at which the concentration of acids and bases in that system is equal. In acidosis, the base member of the buffer pair will accept an H^+, altering the ratio of acid–base leading to an increase in pH. In alkalosis, on the other hand, an acid member of the buffer pair donates H^+, altering the acid–base ratio leading to a decrease in pH.

4.2.3 Role of the respiratory system

Carbon dioxide (CO_2) is formed continually in the body by different intracellular metabolic processes. PCO_2 plays an important role in the acid–base regulation. Referring to the Henderson–Hasselbalch equation, an increase in PCO_2 decreases the pH whereas a decrease of PCO_2 increases the pH. By adjusting the PCO_2 up or down, the lungs can effectively regulate the pH.

4.2.4 Role of the renal system

The kidneys control acid–base balance by excreting either acidic or basic urine. There are three mechanisms by which the kidneys regulate acid–base balance: reabsorption of filtered bicarbonate (HCO_3^-) ions, generation of new bicarbonate ions and secretion of hydrogen (H^+) ions.

4.2.5. Anion gap

The anion gap (AG) represents the difference between the major plasma cations and anions, and reflects usually unmeasured anions such as sulfate. The normal value of AG is 8–16 mequiv l^{-1};

$$\text{anion gap} = [Na^+] - ([Cl^-] + [HCO_3]).$$

The calculation of the AG is essential in the work-up of acid–base disorders. Anion gap is decreased in hypoalbuminemia, multiple myeloma, and bromide intoxication. The anion gap is increased in some types of metabolic acidosis (see below).

4.2.6 Urinary anion gap

The urinary anion gap (UAG) is expected to be negative in patients with metabolic acidosis. A positive UAG in a patient with acidosis reflects a problem with urinary acidification ability of the kidneys. The UAG is calculated as follows:

$$UAG = (Na^+ + K^+) - Cl^-.$$

4.2.7 Osmolal gap

The normal plasma osmolality ranges from 280 to 295 mOsm kg^{-1}. The calculated plasma osmolality accounts for the most prevalent solutes contributing to the osmolality:

$$\text{osmolality (mOsm } kg^{-1}) = 2(Na^+ \text{ mequiv } l^{-1}) + \text{glucose}/18 + \text{BUN}/2.8$$

where glucose and BUN are measured in mg dl^{-1}. If the measured plasma osmolality exceeds the calculated plasma osmolality by more than 10 mOsm kg^{-1} then unmeasured solutes are present. A high osmolal gap is seen in methanol and ethylene glycol intoxication.

4.3 Approach to acid–base abnormalities

In analyzing acid–base abnormalities, the following approach is helpful:

- Determine the pH: acidosis when pH is less than 7.35 versus alkalosis when pH is greater than 7.45.
- Calculate the anion gap. If the anion gap is high, then this suggests certain types of metabolic acidosis (see *Table 4.2*).
- Determine the PCO_2. PCO_2 is high with respiratory acidosis or as compensation to metabolic alkalosis. PCO_2 is low with respiratory alkalosis or as compensation to metabolic acidosis.
- Determine the HCO_3. HCO_3 is high with metabolic alkalosis or as compensation to respiratory acidosis. HCO_3 is low with metabolic acidosis or as compensation to respiratory alkalosis.
- Assess compensatory response to every acid–base abnormality. If the appropriate compensatory response is not present, a mixed acid–base disorder is present.
- Remember that the compensatory response should not fully correct the primary acid–base disorder. Overcompensation suggests a mixed acid–base disorder.

4.4 Metabolic acidosis

Metabolic acidosis is characterized by low pH (<7.35) and low HCO_3 (<22 mequiv l^{-1}). Metabolic acidosis develops by the addition of acid, loss of a base, or the failure of the kidneys to excrete sufficient net acid to replenish the HCO_3 used to buffer acids. Metabolic acidosis can be either anion gap or non-anion gap. Causes of metabolic acidosis are listed in *Table 4.2*.

4.4.1 Compensatory mechanism
The compensatory response to metabolic acidosis is hyperventilation, which results in a decrease in PCO_2. For each 1 mequiv decrease in HCO_3^- the PCO_2 will fall by 1–1.5 mmHg.

Table 4.2 Causes of metabolic acidosis

Increased anion gap metabolic acidosis
Ketoacidosis including diabetic, alcoholic and starvation
Lactic acidosis
Uremia
Salicylate intoxication
Methanol intoxication
Ethylene glycol intoxication
Paraldehyde intoxication

Normal anion gap metabolic acidosis
Diarrhea
Urinary diversion
Ileostomy
Pancreatic fistula
Surgical drainage
Cholestyramine
Renal tubular acidosis
Normal saline infusion
Carbonic anhydrase inhibitors
Following respiratory alkalosis
Parenteral nutrition

4.5 Anion gap metabolic acidosis

4.5.1 Diabetic ketoacidosis (*Figure 4.2*)
Diabetic ketoacidosis is characterized by the presence of hyperglycemia, low insulin levels, hyperglucagonemia, high catecholamine levels and, subsequently, the overproduction of ketoacids (acetoacetic acid and β-hydroxybutaric acid) and metabolic acidosis. Patients may present with hyperventilation, vomiting, abdominal pain and sometimes shock and coma. Hyponatremia, hyperkalemia, hyperosmolarity, ketonurea and elevated BUN and creatinine are often present. The treatment of diabetic ketoacidosis consists of replacing insulin by i.v. infusion, hydration with normal saline, and correcting electrolyte abnormalities. Replacing insulin stops excessive gluconeogenesis and also stops mobilization of fatty acids, which are the precursors of ketones. The need for bicarbonate in the treatment of metabolic acidosis in diabetic ketoacidosis has been debated and, if used at all, should be reserved for patients with severe metabolic acidosis despite adequate hyperventilation.

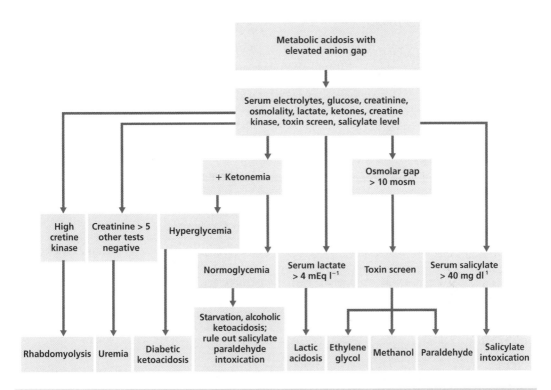

Figure 4.2 Diagnostic algorithm for metabolic acidosis with elevated anion gap. Adapted from Breyer, M.D. and Jacobson, H.R. (1989) Approach to the patient with metabolic acidosis or metabolic alkalosis. In: *Textbook of Internal Medicine* (ed. W. Kelley), p. 926. With permission from Lippincott, Williams & Wilkins.

4.5.2 Alcoholic ketoacidosis

Alcoholic ketoacidosis occurs in alcoholics who usually have poor nutrition. This is probably due to insulin deficiency caused by hypoglycemia induced by fasting. Patients may have had several episodes of vomiting and might also present with metabolic alkalosis. The diagnosis of alcoholic ketoacidosis is made when the patient presents with anion gap metabolic acidosis, history of chronic alcohol use, ketonemia, high osmolar gap and variable plasma glucose levels[1]. The treatment for alcoholic ketoacidosis consists of dextrose infusion and fluid deficit correction[2]. Treatment with bicarbonate is not required for this condition.

4.5.3 Starvation ketoacidosis

Starvation ketoacidosis occurs because of a switch to lipolysis and gluconeogenesis as the sole source of calories. In starvation, as in patients with alcoholic ketoacidosis, patients have low insulin levels induced by hypoglycemia and the associated increase in glucagon, epinephrine, cortisol and growth hormone stimulate lipolysis with release of fatty acids. Treatment will include proper nutrition and a dextrose infusion. Treatment with bicarbonate is not required for this condition.

4.5.4 Lactic acidosis

Lactic acid is produced by most tissues and carried to the liver to be oxidized and converted back to glucose via gluconeogenesis. Lactic acidosis can be divided into type A and type B. The causes of each are listed in *Table 4.3*.

Type A lactic acidosis is generally due to tissue hypoperfusion from any cause such as seen in cardiogenic, hypovolemic, and septic shock. On the other hand, type B is not associated with tissue hypoperfusion and is usually due to

Table 4.3 Causes of lactic acidosis

Type A	Type B
Shock	**Drugs and toxins**
Severe hypoxia	Epinephrine, norepinephrine
Convulsions	Salicylates
Severe heart failure	Ethanol, methanol and ethylene glycol
Severe anemia	Biguanides
Vigorous exercise	
Cyanide poisoning	**Diseases**
Hypothermic shivering	Diabetes
	Renal failure, hepatic failure
	Malignancies
	Iron deficiency
	Severe infection

impaired lactate clearance as a result of hepatic failure. Patients with type A lactic acidosis have a worse prognosis as compared with patients with type B. A distinctive type of lactic acidosis called D-lactic acidosis occurs as a result of bacterial overgrowth in patients with small bowel resection or patients with jejunoileal bypass[3]. Serum lactate can be used as a prognosticator in patients with shock: with serum lactate above 9 mmol l^{-1}, the mortality is more than 75%[4].

Treatment of lactic acidosis consists of treating the underlying problem. Patients with shock should receive adequate fluid resuscitation, antibiotics and vasopressor support.

The use of bicarbonate therapy in lactic acidosis is controversial[5,6]. There is no evidence that the use of bicarbonate in the treatment of lactic acidosis improves outcome. In fact, its use may have several side effects, which include hyperosmolality[7], hypernatremia[7], volume overload[7], hypocalcemia[8], worsening intracellular acidosis[9,10] and transient increase in intracranial pressure[11].

Some argue against the use of bicarbonate regardless of the pH value[12]. Other buffer solutions that potentially can be used in the treatment of metabolic acidosis include the following.

Carbicarb

This is a mixture of sodium bicarbonate and disodium carbonate in a 1:1 ratio. Carbicarb does not produce the significant increase in PCO_2 seen with the use of sodium bicarbonate and thus might not cause worsening intracellular acidosis. The risks of hypervolemia, hyperosmolality and hypernatremia are the same as when sodium bicarbonate is used. Carbicarb has not been extensively evaluated for human use.

Tromethamine

Tromethamine (THAM) is an amino alcohol that buffers acids and CO_2 by its amine (NH_2). THAM has a buffering capacity without the generation of CO_2 and thus does not worsen intracellular acidosis. THAM toxicity causes hypoglycemia, respiratory depression and hyperkalemia. THAM has been used to treat severe acidosis caused by sepsis, diabetic ketoacidosis and renal tubular acidosis[13]. THAM use remains unproven in the treatment of metabolic acidosis.

Dichloroacetate

Dichloroacetate (DCA) is a buffer compound that increases the activity of pyruvate dehydrogenase and thus promotes the clearance of lactate. A large, multicenter, placebo-controlled trial in patients with lactic acidosis failed to show improving hemodynamics or outcome with the use of DCA[14].

4.5.5 Renal failure

Renal failure is usually associated with metabolic acidosis as a result of the inability of the kidney to produce ammonia. There is retention of sulfate and phosphate, leading to an increased anion gap. The aim should be to keep the pH and the HCO_3 level near normal to limit progressive bone disease. The acidosis is usually nonprogressive and relatively asymptomatic. Oral sodium bicarbonate can be used as a treatment for the acidosis.

4.5.6 Salicylate intoxication

Acute salicylate intoxication causes two acid–base abnormalities, respiratory alkalosis and an anion gap metabolic acidosis. Respiratory alkalosis occurs as a result of hyperventilation caused by direct effect of salicylate on the respiratory center. Toxicity is considered mild after acute ingestion of less than 150 mg kg^{-1}, moderate after ingestion of 150–300 mg kg^{-1}, and severe after ingestion of 300 mg kg^{-1} or more. The diagnosis of salicylate intoxication is based upon obtaining a history, performing a physical examination, and obtaining laboratory testing. Patients may present with hyperventilation, fever, nausea, vomiting, dehydration, tinnitus, vertigo, stupor and coma. The laboratory tests might show hyperglycemia or hypoglycemia, hypokalemia, hypouricemia, coagulation abnormalities and ketosis. Salicylate levels above 100 mg dl^{-1} indicate severe intoxication. Treatment for salicylate intoxication consists of the following:

- supportive measures: these include cooling blankets for the fever, hydration, close monitoring of the pH, coagulation indices and replacement of potassium;
- elimination of salicylate:

(i) induction of emesis and administration of charcoal;
(ii) alkaline diuresis: indicated for salicylate levels above 40 mg dl^{-1} and achieved by the use of 100 mequiv of sodium bicarbonate in 1 l of dextrose water infused at a rate of 10–15 ml kg^{-1} h^{-1}; the goal of therapy is a urine pH of 7–8;
(iii) hemodialysis: indicated when the serum salicylate level is above 100 mg dl^{-1} 6 h after ingestion, refractory acidosis, seizure, renal failure and pulmonary edema.

4.5.7 Methanol intoxication

Methanol is metabolized to formic acid via alcohol dehydrogenase. Formic acid is usually responsible for the anion gap metabolic acidosis. Methanol metabolism is represented as follows:

$$\text{methanol} \xrightarrow{\text{alcohol dehydrogenase}} \text{formic acid} \xrightarrow{\text{folate}}$$

$$CO_2 + H_2O.$$

Patients with methanol intoxication may present with blurred vision, lethargy, tachypnea, confusion, nausea, vomiting, depressed mental status, and, in severe intoxication, convulsions and coma. The diagnosis is made by the history of ingestion, an anion gap metabolic acidosis, high osmolal gap, and the finding of a high blood methanol level.

The treatment of methanol toxicity consists of:

- Gastric lavage and charcoal if the patient presents soon after ingestion.
- Increasing the metabolism of formic acid by using folinic acid 50 mg i.v. followed by folic acid 1 mg kg^{-1} i.v. every 4 h for six doses.
- Decreasing the metabolism of methanol to formic acid by the administration of ethanol. Ethanol will compete with methanol for alcohol dehydrogenase. A 10% ethanol solution is administered at a rate of 8–10 ml kg^{-1} and should be titrated to achieve a blood alcohol level of 100–150 mg dl^{-1}. Ethanol infusion should be continued until the methanol level is below 10 mg dl^{-1} and there is resolution of the anion gap and the metabolic acidosis.
- Fomepizole (4-methylpyrizole), an alcohol dehydrogenase antagonist, can be used instead of ethanol. Fomepizole 15 mg kg^{-1} i.v. is followed by 10 mg kg^{-1} i.v. every 12 h for four doses. This is followed by 15 mg kg^{-1} i.v. every 12 h until the methanol level is less than 20 mg dl^{-1}.
- Correction of metabolic acidosis using sodium bicarbonate 1–3 mequiv kg^{-1} infused i.v. to achieve normal pH.

- Hemodialysis is indicated when the methanol level is more than 50 mg dl^{-1} or in the presence of renal failure and persistent visual symptoms.

4.5.8 Ethylene glycol intoxication

Ethylene glycol is metabolized to glycoldehyde via alcohol dehydrogenase. Glycoldehyde is further metabolized to toxic compounds such as formic acid, oxalic acid, glycine, and ketoaldehyde. Patients present with lethargy, coma, convulsions, tachypnea, tachycardia, and renal failure. Hyperkalemia, hypocalcemia, anion gap metabolic acidosis, and a high osmolal gap are usually found. Diagnosis is made by a history of ingestion of ethylene glycol and the presence of oxalate crystals in urine. Treatment consists of the following:

- Gastric lavage if the patient presents soon after ingestion.
- Fomepizole can be used, using the same dose as in methanol intoxication. It should be continued until the ethylene glycol level is less than 20 mg dl^{-1}.
- Ethanol infusion to compete for alcohol dehydrogenase as used for methanol.
- Correcting the metabolic acidosis with sodium bicarbonate as with methanol toxicity.
- Pyridoxine 100 mg IV qd and thiamine 100 mg i.v. qd.
- Hemodialysis is indicated when the ethylene glycol level is more than 50 mg dl^{-1}, and there is persistent acidosis and renal failure.

4.6 Normal anion gap metabolic acidosis (*Figure 4.3*)

It is best to classify normal anion gap metabolic acidosis into three groups.

4.6.1 Acidosis owing to bicarbonate loss

Examples include diarrhea, fistula drainage, and villous adenoma. These are characterized by a negative urinary anion gap. Treatment with fluid, bicarbonate, and potassium is recommended as needed.

4.6.2 Addition of acid

In this group, the addition of acid (hydrochloric) precursors such as ammonium chloride and arginine hydrochloride produces acidosis. Administration of arginine, histidine, or lysine in parenteral nutrition may result in non-anion gap acidosis.

4.6.3 Renal tubular acidosis (RTA)

Renal tubular acidosis is divided into the following.

Type 1 or distal RTA

This is characterized by the inability to maximally acidify the urine regardless of the level of serum HCO$_3$. Distal RTA is a primary idiopathic disorder although it may have causes as shown in *Table 4.4*.

The diagnosis is made when there is a non-anion gap metabolic acidosis with inability to acidify the urine and the presence of hypokalemia.

Treatment consists of sodium bicarbonate (1–3 mequiv kg^{-1} day^{-1}).

Type II or proximal RTA

This is characterized by reduction of the renal capacity to reabsorb HCO$_3$. It can be an isolated defect or part of Fanconi syndrome (glycosurea, aminoacidurea, hypouricemia and hypophosphatemia). Secondary causes of proximal RTA are listed in *Table 4.5*.

Patients with proximal RTA rarely develop severe acidosis and plasma bicarbonate is usually maintained at levels higher than 15 mequiv l^{-1}. Diagnosis is made as follows. After administration of i.v. sodium bicarbonate to

Table 4.4 Causes of distal RTA

Amphotericin B
Lithium
Toluene
Analgesics use
Nephrocalcinosis
Chronic infection

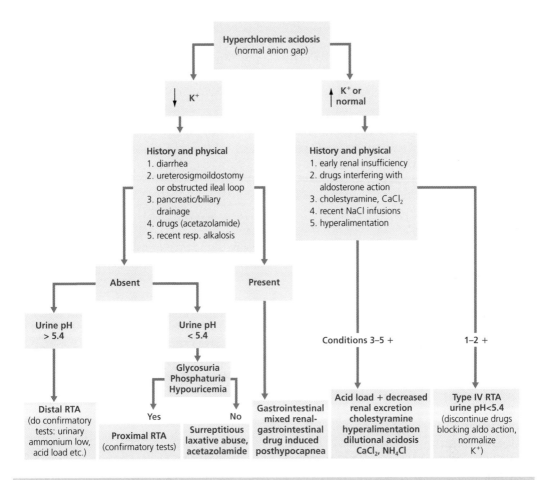

Figure 4.3 Diagnostic algorithm for hyperchloremic metabolic acidosis. Adapted from Breyer, M.D. and Jacobson, H.R. (1989) Approach to the patient with metabolic acidosis or metabolic alkalosis. In: *Textbook of Internal Medicine* (ed. W. Kelley). With permission from Lippincott, Williams & Wilkins.

reach a normal plasma bicarbonate level, urine pH and fractional excretion of bicarbonate is measured. In proximal RTA, urine pH is greater than 7.0 and fractional excretion of bicarbonate is greater than 15%. Treatment consists of bicarbonate therapy (10–15 mequiv kg^{-1} day^{-1}), and potassium supplementation and thiazide diuretics may be used.

Type IV RTA (hyporeninemic hypoaldosteronism)

Aldosterone promotes potassium and hydrogen secretion and sodium reabsorption in distal tubules. This disorder is of unknown etiology and is characterized by the presence of hyperkalemia, low plasma aldosterone, low renin level and a normal gap metabolic

Table 4.5 Causes of proximal RTA

Carbonic anhydrase inhibitors

Lead

Outdated tetracycline

Multiple myeloma

Amyloidosis

SLE, Sjögren's syndrome

Chronic active hepatitis

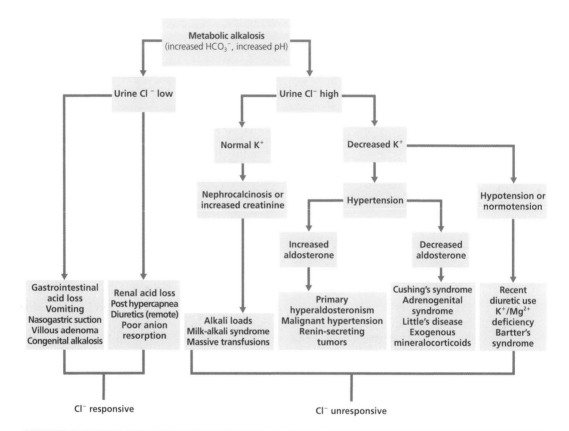

Figure 4.4 Diagnostic algorithm for metabolic alkalosis. Adapted from Breyer, M.D. and Jacobson, H.R. (1989) Approach to the patient with metabolic acidosis or metabolic alkalosis. In: *Textbook of Internal Medicine* (ed. W. Kelley). With permission from Lippincott, Williams & Wilkins.

acidosis. Acidosis develops as a result of impaired acid excretion from decreased ammonia formation secondary to hyperkalemia and aldosterone deficiency. In many patients, the hyperkalemia is mild and well tolerated. The liberal use of salt intake combined with diuretic, potassium restriction, sodium bicarbonate 1–3 mequiv kg^{-1} day^{-1} and fludrocortisone 0.1–0.5 mg p.o. day^{-1} is considered the treatment of choice.

4.7 Respiratory acidosis

Primary respiratory acidosis is a condition characterized by low pH (<7.35) and high PCO_2. Respiratory acidosis can occur with any condition that causes decreased alveolar venti-

lation. Respiratory acidosis can be acute or chronic and the causes are listed in *Table 4.6*.

Patients with acute respiratory acidosis present with decreased mentation, restlessness, agitation, headache, tachycardia, tremors, and, in severe cases, coma.

4.7.1 Compensatory mechanism
The compensatory response to respiratory acidosis is achieved through increased bicarbonate reabsorption and increased ammonia excretion by the kidney. The compensation for respiratory acidosis is predictable as follows:

- acute respiratory acidosis: HCO_3 will increase by 1 mequiv l^{-1} for each 10 mmHg increase of PCO_2 above 40 mmHg;

Table 4.6 Causes of respiratory acidosis
Airway obstruction, acute or chronic
Respiratory center depression
Neuromuscular diseases
Mechanical underventilation
Circulatory collapse
Restrictive defects

Table 4.7 Causes of metabolic alkalosis
Gastrointestinal losses of hydrogen ions Vomiting Gastric suctioning
Renal hydrogen ion losses Loop or thiazide diuretics Mineral corticoid excess Renal compensation for chronic respiratory acidosis Hypercalcemia
Hypokalemia
Alkali loading HCO_3 administration Excessive antacid use

- chronic respiratory acidosis: HCO_3 will increase by 3.5 mequiv l^{-1} for each 10 mmHg increase of PCO_2 above 40 mmHg.

The renal compensation for respiratory acidosis usually occurs over several days and in general, the compensated serum bicarbonate does not exceed 35 mequiv l^{-1}.

Treatment for respiratory acidosis is directed towards correcting the primary cause and improving alveolar ventilation. The use of bicarbonate is rarely indicated.

4.8 Metabolic alkalosis (*Figure 4.4*)

Metabolic alkalosis is a condition characterized by high pH (>7.45) and a high HCO_3 (>26). Because there are few symptoms associated with mild to moderate metabolic alkalosis, treatment is generally not required urgently. However, when the plasma pH rises above 7.55, treatment should be initiated. Metabolic alkalosis results from three general processes: (i) loss of hydrogen ions from either the stomach or kidney; (ii) exogenous bicarbonate administration; (iii) loss of extracellular bicarbonate free fluid, so-called 'contraction alkalosis'. Common causes are listed in *Table 4.7*.

Metabolic alkalosis is a relatively common problem in the ICU. Before initiating treatment, it is helpful to classify the metabolic alkalosis as either chloride resistant or chloride sensitive. Chloride responsive alkaloses are those that result from the concomitant loss of chloride with hydrogen. This is observed most commonly with gastrointestinal or renal losses of hydrogen ions (listed above).

Although the history is usually sufficient to suggest the cause of a metabolic alkalosis, and whether or not it will be chloride responsive, the diagnosis can be established by measuring urinary chloride concentration. Generally, if the urine chloride is less than 20 mequiv l^{-1}, the alkalosis is chloride responsive. Conversely, if the urine chloride is greater than 20 mequiv l^{-1}, the alkalosis is generally chloride resistant. Common causes are listed in *Table 4.8*.

Whenever possible, the underlying cause for the metabolic alkalosis should be addressed (e.g. continuous nasogastric suctioning, diuresis). The majority of chloride responsive alkaloses may be treated with normal saline and potassium chloride. Such therapy corrects volume contraction (if present), and repletes chloride and potassium stores. The rate of administration of normal saline should be based upon the clinical evaluation of the patient's volume status. The administration of potassium chloride should not exceed 20 mequiv h^{-1}.

4.8.1 Correction of metabolic alkalosis

Therapy with acetazolamide (250 mg IV) should be considered in those patients who are volume replete and/or those patients in whom large sodium and potassium loads are not tolerated. Acetazolamide is a carbonic anhydrase inhibitor, which acts to block renal bicarbonate resorption. In severe cases of metabolic alkalosis, which are unresponsive

Table 4.8 Causes of metabolic alkalosis	
Urine chloride <20 mEq l⁻¹	**Urine chloride >20 mEq l⁻¹**
Gastric suctioning	Mineralocorticoid excess
Vomiting	Hypokalemia
Diuretic use (recent)	Diuretic use (ongoing)
Post-hypercapnea	Bartter syndrome
Exogenous alkali loading	Exogenous alkali loading

to saline and potassium chloride administration, hydrochloric acid may be administered. The rate of acid administered depends on the calculated bicarbonate excess, calculated as 0.5 (body weight)(observed HCO_3 – desired HCO_3). In patients with renal failure and severe metabolic alkalosis, treatment may require either hemodialysis or continuous veno-venous hemofiltration with dialysis (CVVHD). Chloride-rich dialysis solutions are typically used.

Chloride resistant alkaloses are less common in the ICU, and treatment is directed at correcting the underlying cause (e.g. treating primary hyperaldosteronism). Potassium chloride treatment is helpful in those patients who are hypokalemic.

4.8.2 Compensatory mechanism
The compensatory response to metabolic alkalosis is variable and often not significant.

4.9 Respiratory alkalosis

The diagnosis of a pure respiratory alkalosis is made when the $PaCO_2$ decreases and a concomitant decrease in the serum bicarbonate is observed. Respiratory alkalosis is common in the ICU and is often due to iatrogenic overventilation. Acute respiratory alkalosis in which serum pH rises above 7.55 may result in life-threatening cardiovascular dysfunction, cardiac arrythymias, decreased cerebral blood flow, bronchospasm and posthyperventilation hypoxia. Common causes of respiratory alkalosis are listed in *Table 4.9*.

The treatment of a respiratory alkalosis should be aimed at the underlying cause. In the patient who is being iatrogenically overventilated, minute ventilation should be adjusted.

4.9.1 Compensatory mechanism
The compensatory response to respiratory alkalosis is achieved through increased HCO_3 excretion by the kidney.

- Acute respiratory alkalosis: HCO_3 will decrease by 2 mequiv l⁻¹ for each 10 mmHg decrease of PCO_2 below 40 mmHg.
- Chronic respiratory alkalosis: HCO_3 will decrease by 5–7 mequiv l⁻¹ for each 10 mmHg decrease of PCO_2 below 40 mmHg.

Table 4.9 Causes of respiratory alkalosis
Mechanical overventilation
Hypermetabolic states
Fever
Sepsis
Thyrotoxicosis
Anxiety and fear
CNS lesions
Hepatic failure
Hormones
Epinephrine
Progesterone
Drugs
Salicylate intoxication
Shock
Interstitial lung disease

4.9.2 Mixed acid–base disorders

Mixed acid–base disturbances are common in the critically ill patient. Although the diagnosis is formally made by analyzing the patient's arterial blood gas and serum electrolytes, the history remains an important diagnostic tool. There are few absolute rules in determining a mixed acid–base disturbance. It should be noted that compensation, whether metabolic or respiratory, never overcorrects, and rarely restores a normal pH.

References

1. **Wrenn, K.D., Slovis, C.M., Minion, G.E. and Rutkowski, R.** (1991) The syndrome of alcoholic ketoacidosis. *Am. J. Med.* **91**: 119.
2. **Miller, P.D., Heinig, R.E. and Waterhouse, C.** (1987) Treatment of alcoholic acidosis. The role of dextrose and phosphorus. *Arch. Intern. Med.* **139**: 67.
3. **Bustos, D., Ponse, S., Pernas, J.C.,** *et al.* (1994) Fecal lactate and the short bowel syndrome. *Dig. Dis. Sci.* **39**: 2315–2319.
4. **Peretz, D.L., Scott, H.M. and Duff, J.** (1965) The significance of lactic acidemia in the shock syndrome. *Ann. N. Y. Acad. Sci.* **119**: 1133–1141.
5. **Stacpoole, P.W.** (1986) Lactic acidosis: The case against bicarbonate therapy. *Ann. Intern. Med.* **105**: 276–279.
6. **Narins, R.G. and Cohen, J.J.** (1987) Bicarbonate therapy for organic acidosis: The case for its continued use. *Ann. Intern. Med.* **106**: 615–618.
7. **Mattar, J.A., Well, M.H., Shubin, H.,** *et al.* (1974) Cardiac arrest in critically ill: II. 8. Hyperosmolal states following cardiac arrest. *Am. J. Med.* **56**: 162–168.
8. **Cooper, D.J., Walley, K.R., Wiggs, B.R. and Russell, J.A.** (1990) Bicarbonate does not improve hemodynamics in critically ill patients who have lactic acidosis: A prospective, controlled study. *Ann. Intern. Med.* **112**: 492–498.
9. **Bersin, R.M. and Arieff, A.I.** (1988) Improved hemodynamic function during hypoxia with carbicarb: A new agent for the management of acidosis. *Circulation* **77**: 227–233.
10. **Shapiro, J.I.** (1990) Functional and metabolic responses of isolated hearts to acidosis: Effect of sodium bicarbonate and carbicarb. *Am. J. Physiol.* **258**: H1835.
11. **Huseby, J.S. and Gumprecht, D.G.** (1981) Hemodynamic effects of rapid bolus hypertonic sodium bicarbonate. *Chest* **79**: 552–554.
12. **Forsythe, S.M. and Schmidt, G.A.** (2000) Sodium bicarbonate for the treatment of lactic acidosis. *Chest* **117**: 260–267.
13. **Nahas, G.G., Sutin, K.M. and Fermon, C.** (1998) Guidelines for the treatment of acidemia with THAM. *Drugs* **55**: 191.
14. **Stacpoole, P.W., Wright, E.C., Baumgartner, T.G.,** *et al.* (1992) A controlled clinical trial of dichloroacetate for the treatment of lactic acidosis in adults. *N. Engl. J. Med.* **327**: 1564–1569.

Chapter 5

Bedside hemodynamic monitoring

Jay S. Steingrub, MD

Contents

5.1 Introduction

Bedside hemodynamic monitoring can provide beneficial clinical information when patients are carefully selected, if the resulting data are interpreted accurately, and if the procedure is properly performed. When the above criteria are met, hemodynamic monitoring provides precise and quantitative information that can help confirm what was clinically suspected, help select appropriate therapeutic interventions and assist in following-up patients' response to treatment. With hemodynamic monitoring, variables such as preload, afterload, contractility, and heart rate can be altered by various therapeutic interventions. The clinical value of invasive hemodynamic monitoring has been generally accepted for numerous clinical conditions including shock associated with myocardial infarction, sepsis, major trauma, acute respiratory failure, cardiogenic or noncardiogenic pulmonary edema, and management of perioperative patients (*Table 5.1*). The purpose of this chapter is to review and illustrate the detailed physiologic information that can be obtained from both pulmonary artery catheterization (PAC) and central venous pressure (CVP) monitoring. We will also consider limitations inherent in pulmonary artery monitoring, and address risk versus benefit.

5.2 Central venous monitoring

Monitoring central venous pressure or right arterial pressure measurements along with urine output, blood pressure and physical examination provided information for the management of acutely ill patients before the introduction of pulmonary artery catheterization in the early 1970s. Normal right atrial pressure is approximately 0–6 mmHg. The pressure is low because pressure produced during ventricular systole is blocked by the closed tricuspid valve. It should be noted that the atria do not have systolic or diastolic pressure. A right atrial pressure tracing has 'a', 'c' and 'v' waves during each cardiac cycle (*Figure 5.1*).

The 'a' wave is produced by atrial contraction, the 'c' wave reflects initiation of isovolemic ventricular contraction, and the 'v' wave representing right ventricular contraction. The 'a' wave follows a simultaneously recorded electrocardiographic P wave by about 80 ms and usually precedes the wave. The 'v' waves coincide with the T wave of the EKG.

The CVP measurement is an accurate measure of right ventricular end-diastolic pressure, but when used to predict left ventricular end-diastolic pressure (LVEDP) assumes that the right and left ventricular end-diastolic pressures are normally close and directional changes are similar. An increase in CVP is assumed to be followed by an increase in left ventricular end-diastolic pressure. Widespread availability of the pulmonary artery catheter has prompted a re-evaluation of CVP measurements. Previously accepted as an adequate guideline for managing shock and hypovolemia, poor or absent correlation was observed when comparing pulmonary artery wedge pressure (PAWP) with CVP in critically

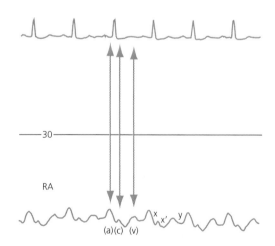

Figure 5.1 Normal right atrial pressure waveform. The rhythm is sinus. The mean right atrial pressure is 6 mmHg. The 'a' wave (a) is the dominant positive pressure wave. The right atrial 'c' wave (c) occurs immediately following the QRS complex. The right atrial 'v' wave occurs on the downslope of the electrocardiographic T wave.

Table 5.1 Pulmonary artery catheter indications and findings

Disorder	Hemodynamic profile	Comments
Ischemic RV dysfunction	Increased RA, decreased SV, decreased CO, decreased AP, RA ≥ PCWP	Steep y descent RV diastolic dip and plateau (square root sign) Volume loading may unmask hemodynamic changes
Acute mitral regurgitation	Increased PCWP, prominent 'v' waves, sometimes reflecting onto the PA tracing as well	'v' waves may not always differentiate mitral regurgitation from ventricular septal rupture
Acute ventricular septal rupture	Oxygen step-up from PA to RV	RV forward output exceeds LV forward output Early recirculation on the thermodilution curve
Shock		
Cardiac	Increased PCWP, decreased SV	decreased CO, decreased AP, increased SVR
Hypovolemic	Decreased or low-normal PCWP, decreased SV, decreased CO, decreased AP, increased SVR	Orthostatic tachycardia
Early septic	Increased PA, increased PVR, increased CO, decreased AP, decreased SVR	In later stages, SVR is elevated and cardiac output is lowered
Noncardiac pulmonary edema	Decreased or normal PCWP normal or increased CO	Normal heart size
Massive pulmonary embolism	Decreased SV, decreased CO, decreased AP, increased PA, increased PVR, normal PCWP	PCWP is normal despite elevated pulmonary artery systolic and diastolic pressures
Chronic precapillary pulmonary hypertension	Increased RA, increased RV, systolic pressure, increased PA, increased PVR, normal PCWP	Left-sided pressures are often normal Pulmonary arterial and RV systolic pressures may reach systemic levels
Acute cardiac tamponade	Increased RA, increased PCWP, RA = PCWP, decreased SV, decreased CO, decreased PA	Paradoxical pulse Blunted y descent Prominent x descent on RA tracing
Constrictive pericarditis	Increased RA, increased PCWP, dip and plateau in RV pressure, 'M'- or 'W'-shaped jugular venous pressure with preserved x and steep y descent	Paradoxical pulse is rare Positive Kussmal's sign is common May simulate ischemic RV dysfunction or restrictive cardiomyopathy
Restrictive cardiomyopathy	Findings are similar to those described for constrictive pericarditis, but PAWP may be higher than RA; difference between PCWP and RA may be exaggerated by exercise	Simulates constrictive pericarditis; however, PA systolic pressure is usually >50 mmHg and diastolic plateau is less than one-third peak RV systolic pressure; other tests are often needed for differentiation from constrictive pericarditis
Tricuspid regurgitation	Increased RA, increased RV end-diastolic pressure	Blunted x descent, prominent 'v' wave, steep y descent Ventricularization of RA pressure

ill patients[1]. The CVP will not reflect LVEDP when the pumping function of either ventricle is selectively depressed.

5.2.1 Conditions where CVP may not reflect LVEDP

Clinical entities that may contribute to a discrepancy between CVP and LVEDP readings include diseases that may cause or contribute to the development of acute right ventricular decompensation such as pulmonary embolism, hypoxic pulmonary vasoconstriction, primary pulmonary hypertension, acute respiratory distress syndrome, positive pressure ventilation, valvular stenosis, tricuspid insufficiency, septal defects, and septic shock. Any given value of PAWP can be associated with a wide range of CVP values. Ischemia, heart disease, and cardiomyopathies may result in a higher left ventricular end-diastolic pressure (PAWP) for a given blood volume on the left side of the heart, when compared with the right ventricular system. CVP measurements may also be unreliable in predicting the amount of fluid treatment in liver disease, sepsis or burns. However, CVP measurements may be helpful in predicting transfusion requirements in healthy adults with hemorrhage shock[2]. Generally speaking, if the CVP is known to correlate with the PAWP in an individual patient, than CVP determinations are useful. Furthermore, in the absence of cardiopulmonary dysfunction, CVP still remains a reliable assessment of right and left heart volume status. However, in critical illness when right and left ventricular function is so disparate that absolute CVP readings and changes are unreliable and mislead estimates of left heart filling, pulmonary artery catheters may be used to provide further monitoring.

5.3 Pulmonary artery catheterization

The pulmonary artery catheter measures pulmonary artery pressure (systolic, diastolic), right atrial and ventricular filling pressures, and PAWP, and allows sampling of true mixed venous blood and measurement of cardiac output. The objective of hemodynamic monitoring and its derived physiological parameters is assessment of left and right ventricular function by quantitatively expressing both the output and the filling pressures of both ventricles.

5.3.1 Apparatus

The pulmonary artery catheter is a balloon tipped flow directed catheter that allows rapid access to the central venous circulation and the right heart to secondary and tertiary divisions of the right or left pulmonary artery. Standard catheters are constructed from polyvinyl chloride and coated with heparin to reduce catheter thrombogenicity. The length of the catheter is approximately 110 cm, with an external diameter of 7 or 7.5 French (1 French = 0.0335 mm) in standard catheters. The balloon at the tip when inflated guides the catheter from the greater intrathoracic veins through the right atrial and ventricular chambers into the pulmonary artery. Balloon capacity varies according to catheter size, from 0.5 to 1.5 ml. Conventionally, the balloon is inflated with air, but filtered carbon dioxide can be used in situations such as right to left intracardiac shunt where balloon rupture might cause a systemic embolus into the arterial system. For best results, the catheter should be positioned in the large pulmonary artery from which it can consistently flow into wedge position. The goal is to obstruct the distal vessel passively, but not to distend it. The most commonly used catheters are multilumen, incorporating one lumen to allow balloon inflation, a distal lumen that opens at the catheter tip for measurement of pulmonary artery and PAWP and for sampling of pulmonary artery mixed venous blood, and a proximal lumen 30 cm from the catheter tip for CVP measurements used for injection of a thermal indicator for thermal dilution cardiac output measurements, fluid and drug administration. A fourth lumen (VIP or vasoactive infusion port) allows for additional fluid and drug administration. A wire terminates in a thermistor bead, 3.5–4.0 cm proximal to the tip of the catheter, and provides an electrical connection to the cardiac output computer. The thermistor measures pulmonary artery blood temperature and allows thermodilution cardiac output measurements.

5.3.2 Insertion site

The right internal jugular vein is considered a preferred site because of its direct access to the right atrium and right ventricle. The left sub-clavian vein is preferred to the left internal jugular vein route because of potential damage of the thoracic duct. The broad anatomic curve of the left subclavian vein allows easier catheter passage into the right atrium. If the right subclavian vein anatomy has a sharp curve into the thoracic cavity before entering the superior vena cava, this may predispose to technical difficulties and catheter kinking. The internal jugular approach is associated with both a more rapid placement and an appreciable lower incidence of pneumothorax compared with the subclavian approach. Major disadvantages with the subclavian approach include the significant higher rate of iatrogenic pneumothorax and difficulty in applying pressure for hemostasis in those patients encountering coagulopathy problems. The femoral vein approach may have some enhanced risks of deep vein thrombosis and resultant embolism[3].

5.3.3 Techniques of insertion

The Seldinger technique allows for venous puncture with a small needle, followed by a wire to secure the position and provide a path for a vein dilator and side arm introducer. As a general guide, after achieving venous access, the right atrium should be reached about 15–20 cm from the jugular vein and 10 cm from the subclavian vein (*Table 5.2*). The balloon when inflated to its recommended volume (usually 1.5 ml of air) protrudes over the catheter tip and decreases the risk of endomyocardial stimulation and induction of arrhythmias during passage of the catheter tip through the right ventricle. Initially, the balloon remains deflated until the catheter tip is in the intrathoracic location, with the correct location indicated by increased respiration-related pressure variation. Once in the right atrium, the balloon is inflated to its recommended volume. The catheter is then smoothly advanced under continuous electrocardiographic and pressure monitoring across the tricuspid value through the right ventricle and pulmonary artery and into the pulmonary wedge position. This occurs when the balloon occludes the distal pulmonary artery segment. Characteristic pressure changes accompany its passage across each chamber. Generally, a catheter should reach the pulmonary artery within 50–55 cm if advanced from the internal jugular vein, and within 65–70 cm if inserted via the femoral vein. If substantially greater lengths are required to reach the pulmonary artery, catheter coiling in the right atrium or ventricle should be suspected. Occasionally, the catheter tip reverses direction after crossing the pulmonary valve and comes to lie in the papillary muscles of the right ventricle. This positioning results in a damped pressure that often simulates a pulmonary capillary wedge tracing. In the absence of flow, pressure rapidly equilibrates and the pressure tracings from the distal orifice of the catheter will reflect left atrial pressure if certain conditions are fulfilled. Wedge position may be assumed if: (i) balloon inflation and deflation are consistently accompanied by disappearance and reappearance of pulmonary artery pressure; (ii) catheter obstruction and damping artifact are excluded; (iii) wedge tracings show an appropriate wave form; (iv) withdrawn blood has an oxygen saturation equal to or greater than that of systemic arterial blood with the balloon inflated. The normal pressure ranges and waveforms recorded within each chamber and vessels have certain specific characteristics (*Figure 5.2*).

5.3.4 Proper positioning

Proper positioning within a pulmonary artery should be confirmed by waveform analysis at least once daily, and if possible before each balloon inflation. When proper positioning can

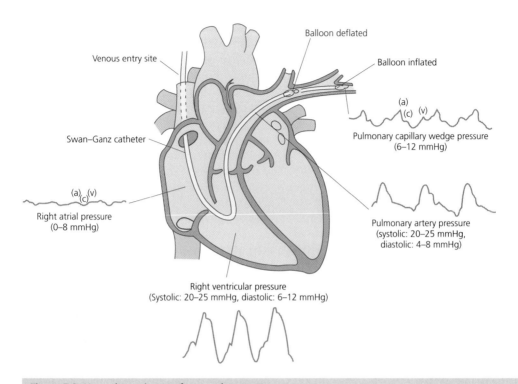

Figure 5.2 Hemodynamic waveform and pressures.

be confirmed, repeat wedge measurements may be obtained by full balloon inflation. In other settings, the balloon should be slowly inflated (in increments of 0.2–0.5 ml of air) while the pulmonary artery pressure is continuously monitored.

Wedge tracings obtained at substantially less than full inflation volumes suggest distal migration of the catheter tip. Such migration may result from a combination of forward thrusting

of the catheter with each heart beat and loop shortening caused by catheter softening.

Poor wedging may also result from patient movement with resultant catheter displacement, or from the administration of PEEP or other forms of mechanical ventilation. The term overwedge refers to a pressure tracing that continues to rise, eventually exceeding the limits of the scale. Balloon inflation causes the distal lumen to impact the pulmonary artery intima and occlude the distal lumen. The distal lumen pressure rises because the catheter is flushed at a continuous rate of 3 ml h^{-1} with the pressure generated to reach 300 mmHg to flush the catheter. In *Figure 5.3*, the tracing suggests that the catheter is positioned too distal into the pulmonary artery, which increases the risk of perforation.

5.3.5 Pulmonary artery wedge pressure measurements

Under normal conditions, the PAWP reflects left atrial and left ventricular end-diastolic

Table 5.2 Catheter insertion sites

Location	Distance from skin to vena cava/RA junction (cm)
Internal jugular	15–20
Superior vena cava	10–15
Femoral vein	30
Right antecubital fossa	40
Left antecubital fossa	50

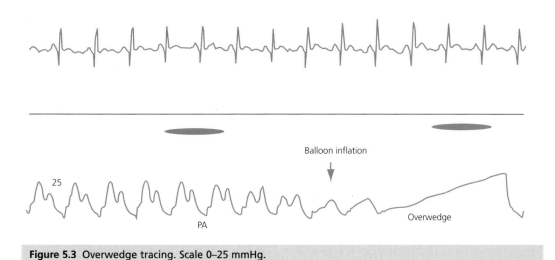

Figure 5.3 Overwedge tracing. Scale 0–25 mmHg.

pressure. Continuous PAWP monitoring is impractical because prolonged obstruction of the artery is likely to cause endothelial damage and hence the possibility of pulmonary artery rupture, and/or infarction. We recommend keeping wedge time to a minimum of 8–15 s and suggest that pressures be recorded over no more than 2–4 respiratory cycles.

The positive and negative swings in intrathoracic pressures associated with all forms of respiration directionally influence intraluminal pulmonary vascular pressures. During spontaneous breathing, intraluminal pressure is lower in inspiration than in expiration. However, during mechanical ventilation, pressures on inspiration exceed those of expiration. Intrathoracic pressures are closest to zero during end-expiration regardless of whether the patient is breathing spontaneously or being mechanically ventilated. Thus, all pressures should be measured at end-expiration to minimize the influence of intrathoracic pressure swings. Carefully measured end-expiratory pulmonary diastolic pressures can be substituted for mean PAWPs whenever wedge tracings are unobtainable, as end-expiratory pressures are often most accurate. In the absence of elevated pulmonary vascular resistance, pulmonary artery diastolic pressure usually approximates the wedge pressure (less than

2–4 mmHg difference). This relationship is essentially fixed through the physiologic range of pressure. For example, if the initial PAWP is 12 mmHg and the pulmonary artery diastolic pressure is 15 mmHg, when left ventricular failure causes the PAWP to increase to 20 mmHg, the pulmonary artery diastolic pressure would then be approximately 23 mmHg. This gradient will remain fixed unless lung disease becomes more severe or an acute process occurs during the pressure monitoring. The wedge pressure should not be greater than the pulmonary artery diastolic pressure. In the presence of pulmonary hypertension as with pulmonary embolic disease, pulmonary fibrosis, ARDS, or reactive pulmonary hypertension, pulmonary artery diastolic pressure (PADP) may markedly exceed mean PAWP and is an unreliable index of left ventricular function.

5.3.6 PAWP and left atrial pressure

PAWP tracing is very similar to the right atrial pressure wave form but reflects mechanical events of the left atrium. In the wedge position, blood flow is stopped and central pulmonary pressure occluded so that the catheter tip senses pressure transmitted backward through the static column of blood from the pulmonary veins. The major clinical value of the PAWP is that it usually approximates left atrial pressure (LAP), intracavitary LVEDP (filling pressure) and by extension, left ventricular end-diastolic volume (preload). However, this assumption is correct only if the pulmonary vascular system distal to the catheter tip (the pulmonary capillaries and veins) remains freely patent, and provides a direct blood-filled vascular connection between the catheter tip and the left atrium, serving essentially as a direct extension of the catheter (*Figure 5.4*). In essence, vascular pressure equilibrates along the continuous column of blood that has no flow. The PAWP is a useful approximation of LVEDP because during the diastole, the PAWP, pulmonary venous pressure, left atrial and left ventricular pressure equalize in patients with a normal mitral valve and normal left ventricular function. This relationship is found in most clinical settings, but there are important exceptions.

5.4 Validity of measurements

Because LVEDV is difficult to measure routinely at the bedside, PAWP measurements are considered a reasonably accurate estimate of LVEDP and thus ventricular preload. LVEDP is a major determinant of LVEDV, with the preload directly determining the force of cardiac contraction for any given level of muscle contractility. The above relationship implies the following assumptions: (i) LVEDP is directly

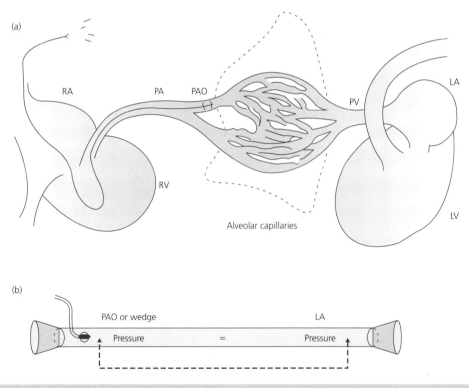

Figure 5.4 (a) Simplified representation of the pulmonary artery catheter in the 'wedge' or pulmonary artery occlusion (PAO) position. With the balloon inflated, no flow exists. (b) By analogy to a 'closed pipe' system, equal pressure readings are found for the wedge pressure, pulmonary venous (PV) pressure, and left atrial (LA) pressure. Adapted from Sprung, C.L., Rackow, E.C. and Civetta, J.M. (1983) Direct measurements and derived calculations using the pulmonary artery catheter. In: *The Pulmonary Artery Catheter: Methodology and Clinical Applications* (ed. Sprung, C.L.). Baltimore: University Park Press, Baltimore, MD, pp. 105-1-40.

related to LVEDV; (ii) LVEDP and LAP equalize at end-diastole; (iii) intrathoracic pressures do not influence the measurement of pressures within the pulmonary vasculature; (iv) PAWP is accurately measured. Although these assumptions are valid in a healthy population, they may not be so in critically ill patients. The correlation between pressure and volume can be altered by the PA catheter tip location, increased airway pressure (PEEP), hypovolemia, and alterations in ventricular compliance[4].

Two principal factors, pulmonary artery catheter position and alterations in pressure during the respiratory cycle, may affect pulmonary artery pressure values and in particular PAWP, as indices of left ventricular filling pressure. As discussed, the validity of PAWP as a measure of pulmonary venous pressure and LAP assumes an uninterrupted column of blood between the balloon and the pulmonary veins. West *et al.* showed that there exists a marked variation in blood flow within the lung as a result of the interrelationship between alveolar and vascular pressures and the effect of gravity[5]. As shown in *Figure 5.5*, the conceptually upright lung is divided into zones based on relationship among alveolar (PA), pulmonary artery (Pa), and pulmonary venous pressures (Pv). In the upper zone (zone 1) near the lung apex, where alveolar pressure commonly exceeds pulmonary, arterial, and venous pressures, pulmonary capillaries are usually closed and no blood flow occurs. This effectively precludes PAWP reflection of left atrial pressure. In the central lung areas (zone 2), alveolar flow is primarily determined by the balance between arterial and alveolar pressures only, because in these zones, alveolar pressure commonly exceeds pulmonary venous pressure. Balloon inflation and catheter wedging will convert a zone 2 situation into a zone 1 situation by preventing blood flow. Thus, if the catheter is lodged in either zone 1 or zone 2, PAWP will not reflect mean LAP, but rather alveolar pressure. In the lower zone (zone 3), the gravity-dependent area of the lung, capillaries remain open, because both pulmonary artery and venous pressures exceed alveolar

pressures. As a result, there is free communication between the left atrium and pulmonary arteries. Only in zone 3 will a patent vascular channel act as an open conduit between the catheter lumen and the left atrium, and blood flow here remains constant. Fortunately, most of the lung is in zone 3 when a patient is supine; flow directed catheters will usually enter zone 3 because most blood is flowing to this area. Non-zone 3 catheter placement is most likely to occur in hypovolemic patients and in those with elevated intra-alveolar pressure. One should keep in mind, however, that these zones are not defined anatomically, but rather the division is physiologic and the zone sizes may change. For example, during spontaneous breathing in the supine position, the majority of the alveolar capillary units normally will fall in zone 3 throughout the respiratory cycle. The extent of zone 1 or 2 will increase when alveolar pressure rises relative to pulmonary venous pressures as during hypovolemia or mechanical ventilation with PEEP. Because PEEP both augments alveolar pressure and reduces venous return, its application tends to diminish the zone 3 region. When vascular pressures decrease as in hemorrhagic shock, or PEEP elevation raises alveolar pressure, zone 3 may be converted into zone 1 or zone 2. In zone 1 and 2, the PA catheter measures predominantly alveolar pressure with the balloon inflated instead of left atrial pressure. It may be necessary to refloat the catheter under new physiologic conditions or to increase zone 3 via volume expansion to re-obtain a true wedge position. Therefore, only if the catheter tip is located in zone 3 will PAWP truly reflect left atrial pressure. A lateral chest radiograph may confirm the catheter tip location at or below the left atrium. What is important to remember is that as long as the catheter tip remains below the left atrium, zone 3 conditions will exist, despite even high levels of PEEP. A sudden increase or decrease in PEEP level should not influence the PAWP. The pulmonary catheter tip position may be less important in the patient with pulmonary parenchymal injury, as many of these patients have non-compliant lungs, thereby reducing transmission of alveolar pressure to the pulmonary vasculature. For further confirmation of the correct tip position, pressure and wave form data should be examined. In a non-zone 3 position, wedge pressure can exceed PADP, with marked respiratory variations being seen in the wave form in the absence of cardiac influences, such as the 'a' or 'v' waves.

5.5 Intrathoracic pressure changes during spontaneous respiration

Although LVEDP (PAWP) is an intravascular pressure, the LVEDP is not the only determinant of LVEDV. Transmural pressure is defined as the net distending pressure of the left ventricle and is a true estimation of LVEDP without the effects of pressures extrinsic to the heart (juxtacardiac pressure)[6]. When we refer to the PAWP as an index of the left ventricular preload, in actuality, transmural pressure results from subtracting the juxtacardiac pressure from intracavitary pressure (LVEDP).

Juxtacardiac pressure, the pressure surrounding the heart, is approximated by measuring the intrathoracic pressure (intrapleural). During normal spontaneous breathing, the cyclic changes in intrathoracic pressure are transmitted to the intravascular pressure tracing, manifesting a fluctuating baseline reflecting both inspiratory troughs and expiratory peaks relating to the respiratory cycle. Large fluctuations in intrapleural pressure are attributed to alterations in ventilatory patterns. These intrapleural swings are due to positive pressure ventilation, labored respiratory efforts, coughing and valsalva maneuvers. These fluctuations can cause either over- or underestimations of LVEDP (PAWP). During periods of respiratory distress such as in non-cardiac or cardiac pulmonary edema, pressure swings between inspiration and expiration can also result in corresponding alterations in wedge pressure measurements during different parts of the respiratory cycle. Pressure readings obtained at end expiration provide a standard reference point for following hemodynamic changes

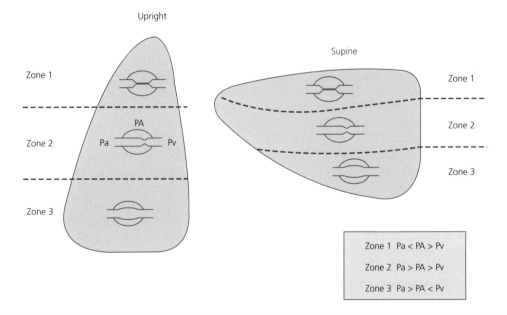

Figure 5.5 Lung zones characterize the relationship among pulmonary alveolar pressure (PA), pulmonary artery pressure (Pa) and pulmonary venous pressure (Pv). Wedge pressure reflects Pv only when Pv exceeds PA (zone 3).

and for subsequent therapeutic interventions. Digital read-out displays average measurements over time, making it difficult to measure end-expiratory pressures accurately. PAWP measurements should therefore be taken at end expiration with graphic tracings preferred over digital readouts. In patients on ventilators, a course of short-acting paralysis should be considered if end-expiratory pressure readings are thought to be artificially high because of marked respiratory variations[7].

5.6 Positive end-expiratory pressure (PEEP)

As the major pressure surrounding the heart and intrathoracic vessels is a juxtacardiac pressure (approximated by intrathoracic/intrapleural pressure (Ppl)), the effects of PEEP on transmural pressure can affect the relationship of PAWP to LVEDV. PEEP can alter ventricular distensibility by increasing intrapleural pressure and decreasing venous return. With an increase in Ppl, the increment may be transmitted to pulmonary vessels and heart, resulting in an elevated measured PAWP in the presence of a normal intravascular volume (LVEDV). Transmural pressure, and not PAWP, reflects the patient's intravascular volume status in such situations. PEEP application during mechanical ventilation, resulting in a positive Ppl, may cause a decrease or no alteration in transmural pressure and a disproportionate elevation in LVEDP (PAWP) relative to LVEDV. Transmural pressure can be obtained by insertion of a small esophageal balloon to measure mid-esophageal pressure. Esophageal pressure is subtracted from the PAWP and the transmural pressure is determined. A more practical approach is to estimate Ppl and subtract it from the measured PAWP, although estimates of Ppl are prone to error.

In clinical studies in which Ppl was measured in patients with acute respiratory distress syndrome, intrapleural pressure does not usually become positive with levels of PEEP below 10 cm of water[8]. At PEEP levels of 10 cm of water or less, transmural pressure accurately reflects PAWP. At PEEP levels above 10 cm of water, there tends to be an increase in disparity between PAWP, LAP, and LVEDP. The more compliant the patient's lungs, the greater the effect of Ppl will be reflected on the cardiovascular structures, and the higher will be the recorded mean PAWP as a result of perivascular and pericardial compression. The degree to which PEEP is transmitted to the pleural space and heart varies with the individual. Therefore, simply substracting the PEEP level from the PAWP measurement may not help. Even knowledge of the intrathoracic pressure itself may not help, as PEEP transmission varies within the thorax[9].

It is more important to assess alterations and trends in PAWP relative to medical therapy rather than attaching excessive significance to isolated measurements of PAWP. Temporary disconnection of PEEP from the ventilator is no longer recommended and is in fact discouraged, as hemodynamics may become destabilized. It may also leave the patient at increased risk for severe hypoxemia, alveolar collapse and increased intrapulmonary shunt[10].

5.7 Ventricular compliance

LVEDV is determined by both the transmural pressure and ventricular compliance. Compliance is defined as volume change per unit pressure change. In the steady state, under conditions of an unaltering compliance, the left ventricular volume–pressure relationship is curvilinear (*Figure 5.6*). With increasing compliance, LVEDV can increase with minimal change in LVEDP (PAWP). With compliance decreasing, LVEDP (PAWP) increases with minimal changes in LVEDV. Different compliance curves for various disease states with acute therapeutic interventions may alter left ventricular compliance. Factors that decrease ventricular compliance include myocardial ischemia, left ventricular hypertrophy, hypertension, cardiac tamponade, aortic stenosis, right to left interventricular septal shifts, constrictive cardiomyopathies, and inotropes. Ventricular compliance

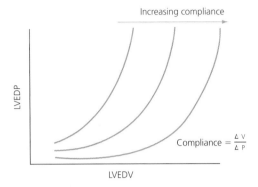

Increasing compliance

LVEDP

Compliance = $\frac{\Delta V}{\Delta P}$

LVEDV

Figure 5.6 Ventricular compliance curve. The relationship between LVEDV and LVEDP is dependent on compliance. A measure of LVEDP can represent different pathologic states of LVEDV, reflecting left ventricular preload.

increases are associated with vasodilators, congestive cardiomyopathy, left to right interventricular septal shifts, and mitral and aortic regurgitation.

Left ventricular compliance is affected not only by left ventricular filling, intrinsic stiffness properties and extrinsic therapeutic interventions, but also by right ventricular diastolic volume (see Chapter 2). As a result of the two ventricles being physically coupled by the interventricular septum and pericardium, the end-diastolic volume curve of either ventricle is dependent upon the diastolic volume of the other. Therefore, any increase in right ventricular volume will impose limitations on LVEDV, which in turn will be reflected in an increase in LAP, LVEDP, or PAWP.

The clinical implications of changes in left ventricular compliance contribute to possible alterations in PAWP without parallel changes in LVEDV. Variations of PAWP may reflect only a shift in the left ventricular pressure–volume relationship rather than a change in the left ventricular end-diastolic volume (preload). This is important when interpreting a given PAWP at the bedside in relation to LVEDV. For example, in a known hypertensive patient with a decreased left ventricular compliance, optimal preload will require a higher LVEDV than would be necessary in a normal state.

A decrease in ventricular compliance always results in an increase in LVEDP. This explains the development of hydrostatic pulmonary edema in patients with diastolic dysfunction and hypertension with normal LVEDV. Therefore, it is essential to assess whether a change in PAWP indicates a change in left ventricular compliance or reflects an actual change in LVEDV. By serial measurements of cardiac output and PAWP, a Frank–Starling curve can be plotted that depicts a relationship between volume (cardiac output) and pressure (PAWP) in a given patient (see *Chapter 2, Figure 2.1*). Based on the curve, cardiac output can be optimized by the infusions of fluids to increase preload, diuretics to decrease preload, inotropes to alter cardiac output, or vasodilators to reduce pulmonary and systemic vascular resistance. Echocardiography is capable of estimating LVEDV and may serve as a non-invasive technique of preload estimation if PAWP measurements are unreliable or lack correlation with clinical status.

5.8 Limitations of pulmonary artery wedge pressure

A pressure gradient normally should not develop between pulmonary veins and the left atrium. Occlusion of the pulmonary veins (tumor, vasculitis, fibrosis, atrial myxoma) can cause pulmonary venous pressure to exceed LAP. PAWP closely correlates with LAP and LVEDP only over a range of approximately 5–25 mmHg. Above 25 mmHg, the LAP tends to be higher than PAWP. The left atrial pressure in turn is essentially identical to LVEDP when the left ventricle has not been chronically diseased. With chronic lung disease, left ventricular end-diastolic pressure is usually higher than the left atrial pressure. In this instance, use of the peak 'a' wave of the wedge pressure rather than the mean PAWP may reduce the disparity between wedge and LVEDP. *Table 5.3* describes conditions in which PAWP is greater or less than LVEDP.

Valvular heart disease can alter the LAP–LVEDP relationship. With mitral insufficiency, retrograde transmission of ventricular

Table 5.3 Conditions in which PAWP is greater or less than LVEDP

PAWP > LVEDP
- Mitral stenosis
- Left atrial myxoma
- Pulmonary venous obstruction
- High intra-alveolar pressure (continuous positive pressure ventilation)

PAWP < LVEDP
- Stiff left ventricle
- High (>25 mmHg) LVEDP

systole can cause LAP to exceed LVEDP. With mitral stenosis, LAP exceeds LVEDP. Aortic insufficiency causes a reverse pressure gradient with LVEDP greater than LAP as a result of continued retrograde ventricular filling from the aorta. As discussed previously, an alteration in left ventricular compliance can cause a disparity between LAP and LVEDP. Physiologically, LVEDP is rate dependent, with bradycardia increasing LVEDP and tachycardia decreasing LVEDP.

5.9 Thermodilution cardiac output

Thermodilution cardiac output (TCO) is widely used as a method for determining cardiac output in the ICU. Clinical studies verify that there is good correlation between TCO determination and the Fick method performed randomly in the respiratory cycle. Determination of cardiac output via thermodilution requires measuring the patient's blood temperature and the temperature of a known volume of fluid (indicator) injected into the right atrium through the proximal port of a pulmonary artery catheter with temperature change detected distally by a thermistor located 4 cm from the catheter tip. This technique needs a constant blood flow during the period of indicator flows from the right atrium to the thermistor. A cardiac output microprocessor solves the indicator dilution equation (Stewart Hamilton equation). When the injectate is injected rapidly as an indicator

bolus into the circulation, the solution becomes thoroughly mixed with blood in the pulmonary artery and the temperature change is sensed by the thermistor. The computer will then process the change in temperature and produce a record of the temperature change over time, resembling a skewed bell-shaped curve (*Figure 5.7*). The area under the curve (indicator dilution curve) represents the denominator of the Stewart Hamilton equation and thus determines cardiac output. When cardiac output is low, more time is required for the temperature to return to baseline, producing a larger area under the curve. With high cardiac output, the cooler injectate travels faster through the heart and the temperature returns to baseline faster. This produces a small area under the curve. Certain conditions may prevent appropriate mixing or directional flow of the indicator solution. Intracardiac shunts, tricuspid insufficiency, cardiac arrhythmias, and mechanical ventilation with PEEP can alter the accuracy of TCO by affecting beat-to-beat cardiac ejection. TCO appears to have an inaccuracy of approximately 12% for single measurements and 8% for values averaged over three measurements. Because many of the derived hemodynamic indices and planned therapies are dependent on accuracy of TCO measurements, one needs to recognize the limitations in TCO calculations. Room temperature injectate is probably as accurate as iced injectate except during hypothermia. The average of three consecutive TCO measurements performed randomly during respirations will reflect a valid cardiac output measurement. When multiple measurements are performed for each cardiac output determination, a change of at least 15% between determinations should occur before clinical significance is attached[11].

5.10 Derived hemodynamic parameters

Several important hemodynamic parameters may be derived using data obtained by

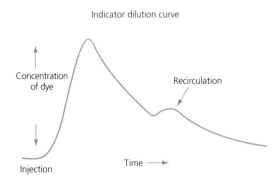

Indicator dilution curve

Concentration of dye

Recirculation

Injection

Time

Figure 5.7 Thermodilution cardiac output curve. Adapted with modification from Tobin, M.J. (ed.) (1998) *Principles and Practice of Intensive Care Monitoring*. Reproduced with permission from McGraw–Hill, New York.

pulmonary artery catheterization. Calculations of these parameters and their normal values are included in *Table 5.4*. Understanding these physiologic measurements may assist in defining specific hemodynamic patterns for a variety of clinical situations. Disorders for which hemodynamic profiles have been established include the following.

5.10.1 Acute mitral regurgitation
This presents as elevations in left atrial pressure and PAWP, large 'v' waves in PAWP tracings and, at times, inflated 'v' waves in pulmonary artery pressure tracings. In this situation, the left ventricle will eject blood into a normal-sized and relatively non-compliant left atrium causing a giant 'v' wave in the wedge pressure tracing. This large 'v' wave elevates the mean pulmonary venous pressure, resulting in heart failure. Acute mitral insufficiency is one example in which the pulmonary end-diastolic pressure is actually lower than the mean PAWP. The transient reversal of pulmonary blood flow that accompanies the left atrial 'v' wave can cause highly oxygenated blood to enter the pulmonary artery and the mistaken diagnosis of a left to right intraventricular shunt. When severe, this syndrome often leads to profound hemodynamic disturbance and shock.

5.10.2 Acute right ventricular infarctions
These are seen in patients with ischemic right ventricular dysfunction, and in as many as 40% of patients with inferior infarctions, although the clinical recognition is often sketchy and inadequate. In patients with right ventricular dysfunction related to ischemia or to an increased right ventricular afterload, low cardiac output and shock may develop. The treatment and prognosis of shock secondary to a right ventricular infarct is different from that of shock caused by severe left ventricular dysfunction. The characteristic hemodynamic profile of acute right ventricular infarction or dysfunction includes an elevated right atrial pressure that equals or exceeds the PAWP, a steep y descent, and a right ventricular pressure tracing that may show a diastolic dip and plateau (square root sign). These findings can be detected in approximately 50% of patients with acute ischemic right ventricular dysfunction. In other patients with this disorder, volume loading may be necessary to unmask hemodynamic abnormalities.

5.10.3 Acute ventricular septal rupture
The diagnosis for acute ventricular septal rupture can be confirmed by the detection of oxygen saturation step-up between the right atrium and the right ventricle of 10%. With small defects, intracardiac pressures are usually normal, but with large defects and associated left to right shunt, the left atrial pressure and LVEDP are usually elevated. Larger defects are associated more frequently with congestive heart failure, arrhythmias or pulmonary hypertension development.

5.10.4 Septic shock
The characteristic profile of septic shock is manifested by an elevated cardiac output and a low system vascular resistance. In early shock, the profile can reveal a low PAWP, occasional increases in pulmonary vascular resistance, and a low, normal or hyperdynamic CO state, depending on the underlying volume status. In the later stages of septic shock, it is not uncommon to observe an increase in

Table 5.4 Cardiovascular and respiratory parameters (measured and calculated)

	Abbreviation	Formula	Unit	Normal
Volume-related variables				
Mean arterial pressure	MAP	DP + 1/3pp	mmHg	93
Central venous pressure	CVP	(measured)	cm H_2O	10
Stroke volume	SV	(CO/HR) × 1000	ml min^{-1}	50–70
Stroke index	SI	(CI/HR) × 1000	ml min^{-1} m^{-2}	35–50
Hemoglobin	Hgb	(measured)	g %	12
Mean pulmonary arterial pressure	MPAP	(measured)	mmHg	15
Pulmonary artery wedge pressure	PCWP	(measured)	mmHg	6–12
Flow-related variables				
Cardiac output	CO	(measured)	l min^{-1}	4–7
Cardiac index	CI	CO/BSA	l min^{-1} m^{-2}	2.5–4
Left ventricular stroke work index	LVSWI	(MAP–PCWP) × SVI × 0.0136	g-m m^{-2} per beat	40–70
Right ventricular stroke work index	RVSWI	(PAP–CVP) × SVI × 0.0136	g-m m^{-2} per beat	4–8
Resistance				
Systemic vascular resistance index	SVRI	(MAP – CVP)/CI × 79.92	dyne-s cm^{-5}	1500–2600
Pulmonary vascular resistance index	PVRI	(MPAP – PCWP)/CI × 79.92	dyne-s cm^{-5}	45–225
Oxygen transport				
Arterial pH	pH	(measured)	—	7.4
Arterial CO_2 tension	$PaCO_2$	(measured)	mmHg	40
Mixed venous O_2 tension	$P\bar{v}O_2$	(measured)	mmHg	40
Arterial O_2 saturation	SaO_2	(measured)	%	99
Arterial O_2 content	CaO_2	1.36 (Hg)(SqO_2) + 0.003 (PaO_2)	ml O_2 dl^{-1}	20
Mixed venous O_2 content	$C\bar{v}O_2$	1.36 (Hg)($S\bar{v}O_2$) + 0.003 (PqO_2)	ml O_2 dl^{-1}	15
O_2 availability	O_2 avail.	CaO_2 × CI × 10	ml min^{-1}	500–700
O_2 consumption	VO_2	CaO_2 × CI × 10	ml min^{-1}	200–250
O_2 extraction	O_2 ext.	(CaO_2 – $C\bar{v}O_2$)/CaO_2	%	25–32%
Rate pressure product	RPP	HR × SBP	–	12000

systemic vascular resistance and a decrease in cardiac output.

5.10.5 Non-cardiac pulmonary edema

Distinguishing non-cardiac pulmonary edema from edema secondary to cardiac disorders is often difficult because in both instances patients are critically ill, have severe arterial blood gas abnormalities and have chest X-ray findings of generally interstitial and alveolar infiltrates. Hydrostatic pulmonary edema from congestive heart failure usually is characterized by a high CVP and PAWP recording and a decreased CO along with an associated increase in systemic vascular resistance. Non-cardiac permeability pulmonary edema is frequently associated with a high CO and a PAWP typically low to normal, but the latter may be elevated because of fluid overload or associated acute pulmonary hypertension. Distinguishing between the two types of edema is crucial because therapeutic strategies and overall prognosis differ markedly.

5.10.6 Acute massive pulmonary embolism

This can produce a clinical picture simulating that of cardiogenic shock. Although pulmonary vascular resistance is markedly increased, the PAWP is usually low or normal in these patients. The CVP, the right ventricular systolic and diastolic pressures, and PA systolic pressures are also elevated. The mean pulmonary artery pressure is in the range of 20–40 mmHg with right ventricular and pulmonary artery systolic pressure exceeding 50 mmHg.

5.10.7 Acute cardiac tamponade

This produces diastolic compression, which impairs ventricular filling. The hemodynamic profile reveals a low stroke volume, a falling cardiac output with normal systolic function, equalization of right and left side filling pressures, and a prominent systolic x descent and blunted y descent on right atrial pressure monitoring. However, in postoperative cardiac surgical patients where the pericardium has been

left open, classic equalization of pressures may not be present.

5.10.8 Tricuspid regurgitation

This is associated with an elevated CVP and right ventricular end-diastolic pressure. Characteristically, the mean CVP demonstrates a rise or no fall with inspiration, an absent or diminished x descent and a prominent early 'v' wave. As the tricuspid regurgitation becomes more severe, the CVP pressure tracing will increasingly resemble the right ventricular pressure tracing.

5.10.9 Constrictive pericarditis

This, like tamponade, produces diastolic equalization and elevation of right- and left-sided filling pressures. A characteristic 'm'- or 'w'-shaped CVP tracing can be detected with a preserved systolic x descent and a prominent early diastolic y descent.

5.11 **Risk versus benefit**

The information provided by hemodynamic monitoring can help identify patients most responsive to treatment and monitor closely the patient's response to therapy in the critical care setting. Although the information obtained with pulmonary artery catheterization is not readily available by other means, it has never been clearly demonstrated that PAC improves survival in critically ill patients. Well-designed, randomized controlled trials are still needed to resolve this point. Dysrhythmias, such as premature ventricular depolarization or conduction abnormalities, are the most common complications, occurring in 13–78% of patients[12].

Although several organizations have published guidelines for the use of PAC, the recommendations are based on the experience and beliefs of the expert panels rather than on a critical appraisal of the available evidence. Furthermore, the guidelines have never been prospectively evaluated. If we employ PAC without having effective therapy for the underlying disease, other than with supportive care, the catheter should not be expected to affect outcome. Therefore, the need arises for more investigations into the mechanisms of critical illnesses and the clinical applications of new therapies.

References

1. **Swan, H.J.C.** (1974) Central venous pressure monitoring is an outmoded procedure of limited practical value. In: *Controversies in Internal Medicine* (eds F.J. Ingelfinger, R.V. Ebert, M. Finland, *et al.*). W.B. Saunders, Philadelphia, PA, pp. 185–193.
2. **Northfield, T.C. and Smith, T.** (1970) Central venous pressure in clinical management of acute gastrointestinal bleeding. *Lancet* **2:** 584–586.
3. **Merrer, J., De Jonghe, B., Golliott, F.,** *et al.* (2001) Complications of femoral and subclavian venous catheterization in critically ill patients. A randomized controlled trial. *JAMA* **286:** 700–706.
4. **Biondi, J.W., Schulman, D.S. and Matthay, R.A.** (1988) Effects of mechanical ventilation on right and left ventricular function. *Clin. Chest Med.* **9:** 55.
5. **West, J.B., Dollery, C.T. and Naimark, A.** (1964) Distribution of pulmonary blood flow in isolated lung: Relation to vascular and alveolar pressures. *J. Appl. Physiol.* **19:** 713–724.
6. **Quinn, R. and Marini, J.J.** (1983) Pulmonary artery occlusion pressure; clinical physiology, measurement, and interpretation. *Am. Rev. Respir. Dis.* **128:** 319–326.
7. **Schuster, D.P.** (1984) Accuracy of pulmonary artery and wedge pressures. *Crit. Care Med.* **12:** 695–696.
8. **Marini, J., O'Quinn, R., Culver, B.W. and Butler, J.** (1982) Estimation of transmural cardiac pressures during ventilation with PEEP. *J. Appl. Physiol.* **53:** 384–391.
9. **Jardin, F., Genevray, B., Brun-Ney, D. and Bourdarias, J.P.** (1985) Influence of lung and chest wall compliances on transmission of airway pressure to the pleural space in critically ill patients. *Chest* **86:** 653–658.
10. **Kumar, A., Falke, K.J., Geffin, B.,** *et al.* (1970) Continuous positive-pressure ventilation in acute respiratory failure. Effects on hemodynamics and lung function. *N. Engl. J. Med.* **283:** 1430.
11. **Ellis, R., Gold, J., Rees, R.,** *et al.* (1972) Computerized monitoring of cardiac output by thermal dilution. *JAMA* **220:** 507–511.
12. **Shah, K.B., Rao, T.L.K., Laughlin, S. and El-Etz, A.A.** (1984) A review of pulmonary artery catheterization in 6,245 patients. *Anesthesiology* **61:** 271–275

Chapter 6

Shock in the intensive care unit

Jay S. Steingrub, MD

Contents

6.1 Introduction

Shock is common among critically ill patients; as many as 20–25% of all ICU admissions are shock related. Although the diagnosis of shock should be suspected in any patients with signs of altered tissue perfusion, commonly the clinical diagnosis is often established when hypotension develops. Variables determining outcome for a patient in shock include age, pre-existing medical conditions, severity and type of injury, and the length of time that elapses before initiation of resuscitation that can limit the effectiveness of compensatory responses. Traditionally, shock has been estimated by the oxygen retention of pulmonary artery blood (mixed venous O_2) and the degree of lactic acidosis. Because the partial pressure of mixed venous O_2 may not reflect oxygen delivery in patients with sepsis or acute respiratory distress syndrome (ARDS), oxygen delivery is better assessed by measuring cardiac output, hemoglobin concentration, and arterial and mixed venous blood gases.

Ineffective tissue perfusion causes cellular and tissue ischemia as a result of an imbalance in the supply and demand of oxygen and nutrients. This is clinically recognized as the syndrome of shock. The progression of shock can be categorized into three stages. During the early stage, several compensatory responses directed towards maintaining specific organ perfusion (heart and brain) are initiated; the effectiveness of these compensatory responses depends on the rate and degree of intravascular volume depletion. During the second stage, both microvascular and cellular injuries are observed. In the final stage, decompensated shock develops, manifested by irreversible organ damage.

6.2 Pathophysiology

Compensatory mechanisms preserve cerebral and coronary circulation at the expense of skin, skeletal muscle, renal, and splanchnic circulation. A decrease in arterial pressure secondary to cardiac output depression stimulates a compensatory autonomic response. Baroreceptor reflexes are stimulated by high-pressure stretch receptors located in the carotid sinus, aortic arch, and splanchnic circulation[1]. Volume receptors located in the right atrium trigger reflex pathways in the setting of hypovolemia. Sympathetic nervous system activation causes arteriole vasoconstriction and redistribution of blood flow away from skeletal muscles and splanchnic beds. Sympathetic outflow will also augment heart rate and myocardial contractility and cause venoconstriction, thus increasing venous return. Increases in sympathetic nervous system discharge cause adrenomedullary hormone release, catecholamine release, and activation of the renin–angiotensin axis[2]. Both the renin–angiotensin system and vasopressin increase vasomotor tone, predominantly in the mesenteric bed. Angiotensin II increases aldosterone release and sympathetic outflow; vasopressin stimulates both catecholamine release and myocardial contractility. Ongoing ischemia at the cellular level can facilitate both humeral and proinflammatory reactions (cytokines, nitric oxide), which can further compromise circulatory abnormalities, leading to end-organ damage and death.

6.3 Specific shock syndromes

Unless the underlying cause is determined, shock can be viewed as a dynamic state with several major etiologies potentially leading to progressive end-organ damage. To identify the underlying cause, one must first determine whether shock is central or peripheral in origin. Shock can be further categorized into four categories. Central causes of shock resulting in impairment in cardiac emptying include cardiogenic shock (pump failure) and obstructive shock (impaired blood flow). Peripheral causes of shock are attributed to alterations at the vascular blood level, and include hypovolemic shock (inadequate blood volume) and distributive shock (abnormal distribution of available blood volume) (*Table 6.1*).

Table 6.1 Mechanisms of shock

Central	Peripheral
Cardiogenic shock	**Hypovolemic shock**
Pump failure	Inadequate blood volume
• Myocardial infarction	• Hemorrhage/bleeding
• Cardiomyopathy	• Capillary leak
• Arrhythmias	• Burns
• Post-cardiopulmonary bypass	
• Myocarditis	
• Intrinsic depression SIRS related	
• Valvular dysfunction	
Obstructive shock	**Distributive shock**
Blood flow impairment	Blood volume maldistribution
• Pulmonary hypertension	• Sepsis/inflammatory
• Pulmonary/air embolism	• Anaphylaxis
• Tension pneumothorax	• Spinal cord injury
• Positive pressure ventilation	• High spinal anesthetic
• Dissecting aneurysm	• Adrenal insufficiency
• Tamponade	
• Ball valve thrombosis	
• Mediastinal tumors	

6.4 Hypovolemic shock

6.4.1 Clinical signs and symptoms

This category of shock is caused by visible or occult hemorrhage and non-traumatic diseases including non-hemorrhagic hypovolemic shock. Inadequate circulatory blood volume can be secondary to massive sequestration of 'third-space' fluid in burns, soft tissue injuries, bowel obstruction, and acute inflammatory disorders such as pancreatitis. An increase in capillary permeability resulting in hypovolemia is observed in both sepsis and anaphylactic shock; however, these clinical syndromes have other additional mechanisms that explain shock. This shock state can occur abruptly or gradually through several stages, depending on the severity of hypovolemia and the rate of its development. The diagnosis of hypovolemic shock relies on the identification of symptoms and signs of inadequacy of tissue perfusion in the appropriate clinical setting (*Table 6.2*). Poor skin turgor, dry mucous membrane, hyperthermia, elevated hematocrit, low central venous pressures, or pulmonary artery

Table 6.2 Monitoring tissue perfusion

Clinical assessment

Invasive blood pressure monitoring

Cardiac output

Continuous pulse oximetry

Cardiac filling pressure

Lactate levels

Gastric tonometry

Oxygen delivery and extraction (from mixed venous blood gases)

Clinical
  Pulse rate
  Skin color
  Temperature
  Capillary refill
  Urinary output
  Anion gap
  Mental status

wedge pressure (PAWP), hypernatremia, and glucosuria are common findings. With an increase in blood or fluid loss, heightened sympathetic tone becomes apparent, manifested by increasing heart rate and respiratory rates, decreased capillary refill and narrowing of pulse pressure. An altered mental status is usually a late clinical manifestation (*Table 6.3*).

Blood volume is approximately 7% of the body weight in an adult (5 l in a 70 kg patient) and 8–9% in a child. Patients are usually asymptomatic with blood volume deficits of less than 10% (approximately 500 ml). Sympathetic vasoconstriction and tachycardia will maintain both blood pressure and cardiac output while secretion of renin–angiotensin, vasopressin and aldosterone contributes toward compensation. Orthostatic blood pressure changes are usually observed when blood loss approximates 15–20% of the vascular volume (750–1000 ml), resulting in a decrease in left ventricular preload with a subsequent decrease in stroke volume (SV) and cardiac output (CO). During this stage, compensatory arteriolar and venous vasoconstriction results in an increase in diastolic pressure and a narrowing of pulse pressure. Blood volume deficits of greater than 25% (approximately 1250 ml) or at least 1.5 l in a 70 kg patient will cause a decrease in systolic and diastolic pressure, cardiac output and tissue perfusion. When significant hypovolemia is suspected because of traumatic or non-traumatic mechanisms, fluid therapy should be initiated regardless of the systolic blood pressure.

6.4.2 Therapy

Therapy for hypovolemic shock includes rapid restoration of circulating volume with blood, crystalloid or colloid fluids as indicated (see Chapter 7). The initial resuscitation fluids used in hypovolemic or hemorrhagic shock should be IV isotonic crystalloid solutions, either lactated Ringer's solution or isotonic 0.9% saline. These fluids provide transient expansion of the intravascular space as well as correction of electrolyte abnormalities.

Controversy persists regarding the use of

Table 6.3 Signs of hypoperfusion

Organ	Clinical signs
Neurologic	Altered mental status (agitation, coma)
Metabolic	Hyperthermia/hypothermia, respiratory alkalosis, metabolic acidosis
Pulmonary	Hypoxemia, tachypnea
Cardiac	Tachycardia, arrhythmias, ischemia, hypotension
Renal	Oliguria (output ≤ 0.5 cc kg^{-1} h^{-1})

colloid solutions (hetastarch, albumin) as an acute resuscitative fluid in hypovolemic shock. Although both colloid and crystalloid solutions are equally effective in resuscitation, the volume of crystalloid infused is usually twice to four times the total volume of colloid required to achieve the target end point.

Blood loss of 15–30% of blood volume (70 ml kg^{-1}) in a healthy, uncomplicated patient can be corrected with crystalloids alone. Usually, a loss of greater than 30% (2000 ml) of blood volume in the presence of hypovolemic shock will require both crystalloid and blood products to restore both intravascular volume and oxygen carrying capacity. Generally, healthy well-resuscitated hemodynamically stable patients tolerate hematocrits of approximately 21–25%. Older patients with underlying heart disease and patients with shock may require higher hematocrits. Practice guidelines suggest that replacement of red cells is usually indicated at hemoglobin levels below 7 g dl^{-1} and unnecessary at hemoglobin levels above 10 g dl^{-1}. At intermediate values, the need for transfusions should be evaluated on a case-by-case basis. A large study in a mixed group of ICU patients showed no benefit of transfusion to a hemoglobin level of 10 g dL^{-1} versus 7 g dl^{-1} [13]. In this trial, the use of the lower hemoglobin level trigger for transfusion resulted in improved survival. When considering blood transfusions to improve oxygenation in critically ill patients, stored blood may be less effective than fresh blood.

6.4.3 Blood components in hemorrhagic shock

Rapid blood infusion can be accompanied by coagulopathy and usually attributed to the consumption of platelets. Platelet infusions are helpful if the platelet count is less than 100,000. One pooled pack of platelets (eight units) increases platelet count by 80,000 cells mm^{-3}. Factor depletion usually occurs later than platelet loss. In general, one unit of fresh frozen plasma (FFP) is generally required for every 6 units of packed red blood cells (PRBC), but replacement can be guided by coagulation monitoring. Cell saver devices should be considered when feasible. FFP infusion might be helpful if the prothrombin time (PT) and/or activated partial thromboplastin time (APTT) are prolonged (>11/2 times control). Administration of component therapy prophylactically during resuscitation has no benefit, but exposes the patient to the risks of hepatitis and other blood-borne pathogens.

6.4.4 Evaluation of response

The clinical response to fluid or blood administration should be evaluated by following systolic blood pressure, pulse rate, and signs of organ perfusion (capillary refill, mental status, urine output >0.5 cc kg^{-1} h^{-1} in adults).

Additional bolus infusions should be employed based on the assessment. Monitoring of therapy may be enhanced by central venous catheterization, which assesses right ventricular filling pressures. Trends in the central venous pressure (CVP) measurements are more valid than absolute numbers. Placement of a pulmonary artery catheter (PAC) should be considered if the CVP is persistently elevated in the presence of shock or pulmonary edema, or if increasing vasopressor dosing is required. The PAC allows for assessment of left ventricular filling pressures, mixed venous blood samples, and cardiac output (*Table 6.4*). Arterial monitoring allows for the accurate monitoring of arterial pressure and access for blood sampling.

Patients may require vasopressors to maintain blood pressure while fluid and blood resuscitation are in progress. Ongoing vasopressor requirements after fluid resuscitation is complete may indicate ongoing concurrent losses, distributive shock, or complications such as pump failure, myocardial infarction or tamponade. The presence of lactic acidosis suggests inadequate fluid resuscitation.

6.4.5 Oxygen and mechanical ventilation

Most patients in hypovolemic shock should receive supplemental oxygen and may require

Table 6.4 Pulmonary artery catheterization and shock diagnosis

Diagnosis	PAWP	CO
Cardiogenic shock	↑↑	↓↓
Acute ventricular septal defect	↑ or N	↓↓
Acute mitral regurgitation	↑↑	↓↓
Right ventricular infarction	↓ or N	↓↓
Extracardiac obstructive shock		
Pericardial tamponade	↑↑	↓ or ↓↓
Massive pulmonary emboli	↓ or N	↓↓
Hypovolemia	↓↓	↓↓
Distributive shock		
Septic	↓ or N	↑↑ or N
Anaphylaxis	↓ or N	↑ or N

↑↑ or ↓↓ indicates moderate to severe increase or decrease; ↑ or ↓ indicates mild to moderate increase or decrease; N, normal; PAWP, pulmonary artery wedge pressure; CO, cardiac output.

mechanical ventilation. In hypovolemic shock, positive pressure ventilation will frequently decrease preload, causing a decrease in cardiac output and systemic oxygen delivery (DO_2) (See Section 2.2.4 and *Figure 2.1*).

6.5 Distributive shock

In distributive shock, patients characteristically have both hypotension and maldistribution of blood flow. Causes of distributive shock includes anaphylaxis, sepsis, spinal cord injury, drug actions, and endocrine emergencies such as thyroid storm. Patients with distributive shock frequently develop extravasation of intravascular volume secondary to intracapillary leak. A decreased resistance to flow, a maldistribution of flow, and relative hypovolemia characterize the underlying pathophysiology. Intravascular monitoring of these patients will show a decrease in mean arterial pressure, a decreased or normal PAWP, an increase in cardiac output (post fluid resuscitation) and a reduction in systemic vascular resistance. Sepsis and anaphylaxis are the two most common causes of distributive shock. The incidence of shock in patients with Gram-negative bacteremia is approximately 40%, with mortality rates ranging from 30 to 40%[4]. In 1991, experts in the discipline of critical care medicine proposed new definitions for sepsis and the adverse sequelae of sepsis. Sepsis was defined as a continuum of injury response, ranging from sepsis to septic shock, to multi-organ dysfunction syndrome[5]. The proposed definitions for the systemic inflammatory response syndrome (SIRS) and sepsis were evaluated in a prospective trial. The mortality rate increased with increasing number of SIRS criteria or the patients developed more severe adverse sequelae. The mortality rate increased progressively as the patients manifested two SIRS criteria (7%), three SIRS criteria (10%), four SIRS criteria (17%), sepsis (16%), severe sepsis (20%) and septic shock (46%)[6]. The diagnosis of septic shock is defined as sepsis plus organ dysfunction and evidence of persistent hypotension requiring vasopressor support to maintain blood pressure

(*Table 6.5*). Both Gram-negative and Gram-positive bacteria, viruses, and fungi can trigger the clinical syndrome, which typically occurs over a period of hours or days.

Anaphylactic shock, another etiology of distributive shock, occurs more acutely than septic shock, has a shorter duration, and is produced when patients are exposed to foreign substances or when substances enter the blood stream causing various endogenous mediators to be released. The cardiovascular abnormality of distributive shock is treated by restoring intravascular volume, increasing systemic vascular resistance with vasopressors and treating the underlying etiology.

6.5.1 Diagnosis of distributive shock
Identification and eradicating the source of sepsis is the mainstay of therapy in septic shock. Most patients presenting with severe sepsis usually have a pulmonary, genitourinary, primary blood stream, intra-abdominal or intravenous catheter as a source of infection. In approximately 75% of patients with presumed sepsis, an infectious etiology can be isolated, usually divided between Gram-positive and Gram-negative organisms[7].

Specimens for Gram staining and cultures should be obtained from multiple sites, ideally before antibiotics are administered. However, the need for aggressive therapy may render it impossible to collect specimens immediately, and early antibiotic administration offers an outcome advantage. Blood cultures should be obtained from two different sites. In those patients with an indwelling venous or arterial catheter, specimens should be collected through each port of the catheter. At least one blood specimen should be collected through the catheter port to rule out catheter-related bacteremia. A minimum of two and a maximum of three sets of blood cultures should be obtained for each episode of suspected bacteremia. No interval is required between taking sets of blood cultures.

Sputum specimens can be obtained following instillation of 3% saline, or can be obtained through nasotracheal or endotracheal sampling. The specimens should contain

Table 6.5 ACCP/SCCM consensus conference definitions of sepsis, severe sepsis, and septic shock*

Systemic inflammatory response syndrome (SIRS). The systemic inflammatory response to a wide variety of severe clinical insults, manifested by two or more of the following conditions:
- temperature >38°C or <36°C
- heart rate >90 beats min⁻¹
- respiratory rate >20 breaths min⁻¹ or $PaCO_2$ <32 mmHg
- white blood cell count >12,000 mm⁻³, <4000 mm⁻³, or >10% immature (band) forms

Sepsis. The systemic inflammatory response to a documented infection. In association with infection, manifestations of sepsis are the same as those previously defined for SIRS. It should be determined whether they are a direct systemic response to the presence of an infectious process and represent an acute alteration from baseline in the absence of other known causes for such abnormalities. The clinical manifestations would include two or more of the following conditions as a result of a documented infection:
- temperature >38°C or <36°C
- heart rate >90 beats min⁻¹
- respiratory rate >20 breaths min⁻¹ or $PaCO_2$ <32 mmHg
- white blood cell count >12,000 mm⁻³, <4000 mm⁻³, or >10% immature (band) forms

Severe sepsis/SIRS. Sepsis (SIRS) associated with organ dysfunction, hypoperfusion, or hypotension. Hypoperfusion and perfusion abnormalities may include, but are not limited to, lactic acidosis, oliguria, or an acute alteration in mental status

Sepsis (SIRS)-induced hypotension. A systolic blood pressure <90 mmHg or a reduction of ≥40 mmHg from baseline in the absence of other causes for hypotension

Septic shock/SIRS shock. A subset of severe sepsis (AIRS) and defined as sepsis (SIRS)-induced hypotension despite adequate fluid resuscitation along with the presence of perfusion abnormalities that may include, but are not limited to, lactic acidosis, oliguria, or an acute alteration in mental status. Patients receiving inotropic or vasopressor agents may no longer be hypotensive by the time they manifest hypoperfusion abnormalities or organ dysfunction, yet they would still be considered to have septic (SIRS) shock

Multiple organ dysfunction syndrome (MODS). Presence of altered organ function in an acutely ill patient such that homeostasis cannot be maintained without intervention

*From Bone, R.C., Balk, R.A., Cerra, F.B., *et al.* (1992) American College of Chest Physicians/Society of Critical Care Medicine Consensus Conference: Definitions for sepsis and organ failure and guidelines for the use of innovative therapies in sepsis. Reproduced with permission from: *Chest* **101**: 1644–1655.

fewer than 10 squamous epithelial cells per high-power field and have more than 25 leukocytes per high-power field to differentiate contamination or colonization from true infection (see Chapter 16).

Urine samples should not be obtained from a closed collection container. A syringe and small gauge needle can be used to obtain urine sample directly from the catheter tubing. Although the presence of large numbers of bacteria in the urine indicates infection, it does not necessarily indicate that the infection arose in the urinary tract.

The clinical situation will determine which other specimens to collect. A stool specimen for *Clostridium difficile* cytotoxic assay should be sent if diarrhea develops in patients receiving antibiotics. If meningitis is suspected, lumbar puncture specimens should be sent for cell count, culture, glucose testing, and testing for bacterial antigen levels. Fluid collections found on radiologic exams should be aspirated and sent for Gram staining and culture. Differentiation of infected material from hematoma or inflammatory fluid is not possible on the basis of radiology alone. The pH of the fluid obtained may be a sensitive marker. Ultrasound is the modality of first choice in the diagnosis of intra-abdominal infection, but CT scan should be considered in the presence of diffuse post-operative ileus.

6.5.2 Antibiotic therapy

Antimicrobial therapy remains the primary treatment for patients with sepsis. Antibiotic choices are dictated by the initial source of infection, the patient's underlying immunologic status and/or whether the infection is nosocomial or community acquired. Retrospective data shows that early administration of appropriate antibiotics reduces the mortality in patients with bloodstream infections with Gram-negative sepsis[8]. In the majority of cases, empiric therapy should begin as soon as the diagnosis of sepsis is considered. Although initial empiric therapy may require more than one antibiotic to cover potential pathogens, once a pathogen is isolated, monotherapy is adequate for most infections. Monotherapy with carbapenem antibiotics is as effective as combination therapy with a β-lactam and an aminoglucoside for the empiric treatment of non-neutropenic patients with severe sepsis. Monotherapy with a third- or fourth-generation cephalosporin is as effective as combination therapy with a β-lactam plus an aminoglycoside in non-neutropenic severe sepsis[9]. Fluoroquinolones are highly effective for the treatment of documented Gram-negative bacteremia, but evidence for their use as a single-agent treatment of severe sepsis is lacking. Third- and fourth-generation cephalosporins and carbapenem antibiotics are equally effective as empiric therapy in patients with severe sepsis. The indiscriminate use of vancomycin is to be avoided to limit the risks. Antifungal therapy is recommended for patients with candidemia. It should not be used on a routine basis as empiric therapy in patients with severe sepsis. Double antibiotic therapy is commonly employed in those patients with suspected pseudomonas infections, enterococcal infections, febrile neutropenic patients, and severe intra-abdominal infections, but monotherapy may be equally appropriate (see Chapter 16). Empiric therapy is recommended for those patients with cul-ture negative sepsis. Changing antibiotic regimens is appropriate in patients with ongoing culture negative sepsis who do not respond to the initial empiric regimen. Antibiotics are usually continued for up to 2 weeks, except in cases of osteomyelitis and endocarditis.

6.5.3 Hemodynamic support

In distributive shock, secondary to sepsis, peripheral vasodilation is associated with hypotension and abnormal distribution of blood flow. Increased capillary permeability causes tissue edema and relative intravascular volume depletion. Fluid retention and signs of organ hypoperfusion are common in patients with sepsis, despite a characteristic high cardiac output. Myocardial contractility is depressed with global left and right ventricular dilatation. Studies suggest that lactic acidosis and low oxygenation are strong predictors of multi-organ system dysfunction and death in septic patients[10].

Aggressive fluid resuscitation is the mainstay of therapy for septic shock. Intravascular volume depletion and hypotension can often be reversed with fluid administration alone. Ventricular performance improves with fluid resuscitation, with the ventricle accommodating an increase in volume without any increase in pressure as a result of an increased ventricular compliance in severe sepsis. Fluid requirements during the initial resuscitation phase are large, with up to 10 l of crystalloid being required during the first 24 h. Adequate fluid resuscitation is essential before initiating vasoactive therapy. Despite aggressive fluid resuscitation, a subset of patients with septic shock remain hypotensive and progress to end-organ dysfunction. These patients may benefit from the use of vasopressor therapy (see Chapter 8). Although the benefit of pulmonary artery catheterization (PAC) in the management of septic shock remains unproven, the clinical evaluation of intravascular volume of septic patients is extremely difficult. Pulmonary artery catheterization may allow more appropriate employment of fluids and vasoactive drug therapy[11].

6.5.4 Adrenal insufficiency and septic shock

Acute adrenal insufficiency should be suspected in patients who fail to respond to vasopressors in septic shock. The incidence of adrenal insufficiency may be 20–25%[12]. A low-dose ACTH (cortrosyn) stimulation test (1–2 μg) and a trial of stress doses of hydrocortisone (100 mg every 8 h) pending test results is suggested when adrenal insufficiency is suspected in septic shock[13]. A rapid and dramatic improvement in hemodynamics following the infusion of hydrocortisone within a few hours of administration can be observed. If the ACTH (cortrosyn) stimulation test cannot be performed immediately, dexamethasone (2 mg) should be given and the test performed within 12 h. Corticosteroids should not be used in severe sepsis or septic shock at high doses (30 mg kg^{-1}) and for a short course (1–2 days). However, steroids may be used during refractory septic shock, but not during severe sepsis without shock or mild shock. They should be used at low doses (<100 mg hydrocortisone three times a day) for 5–10 days and then with subsequent tapering of the dose according to the hemodynamic status. The results of a large trial suggest that low dose steroids can reduce 28-day mortality in septic shock[14]. Several factors may explain the recent positive effect of steroids during sepsis. These include the treatment of relative adrenal insufficiency and the potentiation of adrenergic receptivity in addition to the anti-inflammatory effect.

6.5.5 Complications of septic shock

Acute renal failure is a significant complication in patients with sepsis, with the mortality rate of patients who develop acute tubular necrosis greater than 50%[15]. Typical findings include oliguria and azotemia. Urinary sodium excretion may be below 20 mequiv l^{-1} and urinary osmolality may be increased (>450 mOsm kg^{-1}). It is important that all patients with sepsis be aggressively resuscitated to prevent this complication. Although renal dose dopamine is widely used in preventing or ameliorating acute renal failure in patients with sepsis, data show that low-dose dopamine does not improve the survival or prevent the need for dialysis in patients with ischemic or toxic acute tubular necrosis[16]. In non-oliguric patients with sepsis, dopamine may enhance diuresis without an alteration in creatinine clearance. Continuous renal replacement therapies (CRRT) have been successfully used in the management of patients who have sepsis and oliguria despite aggressive resuscitation. CRRT allows more precise volume control, causes less hemodynamic instability, provides for greater continuous clearance and compared with intermittent hemodialysis provides a more stable metabolic control[17]. There are no controlled studies comparing the morbidity or mortality of patients treated with CRRT versus conventional intermittent hemodialysis.

Acute respiratory failure frequently precipitates intubation and the need for mechanical ventilation in sepsis. Tachypnea, associated with alveolar hyperventilation, is frequently seen in early sepsis. Hypoxemia is commonly observed, but may be masked by hyperventilation. Ventilation–perfusion mismatch and shunt are the usual causes of hypoxemia. Other pulmonary manifestations include respiratory muscle dysfunction and bronchoconstriction. The most common cause of acute lung injury or ARDS is sepsis, with a mortality rate reported to be as high as 40–60%[18]. ARDS is extensively reviewed in Chapter 14.

Central nervous system changes in severe sepsis include disorientation, seizures, lethargy or obtundation. Symptoms and signs of encephalopathy including non-focal neurologic findings may be seen. Evidence of polyneuropathy, including muscle weakness, wasting, and impaired deep tendon reflexes are part of the syndrome of critical care polyneuropathy.

Hematologic failure is another hallmark of severe sepsis. Leukocytosis is the most common hematologic manifestation, but some patients may be leukopenic. Thrombocytopenia and coagulation abnormalities are often seen. Sepsis is the most common cause of disseminated intravascular coagulation (DIC), occurring in 10–20% of patients with Gram-negative bacteremia and 70% of patient with septic shock[19]. DIC is the most important independent predictor of ARDS, multi-organ system dysfunction and death. DIC and sepsis can present either as a hemorrhagic syndrome or, less commonly, as a microvascular thrombosis leading to tissue ischemia and end-organ damage. The treatment of DIC remains controversial. There is no conclusive evidence that heparin treatment reduces the morbidity or mortality associated with DIC.

Blood component therapies are potentially hazardous in the treatment of patients with DIC. Components such as fibrinogen may become a substrate for higher levels of fibrin degradation products, which will further impair homeostasis. The administration of FFP and platelets should be restricted to patients with acute hemorrhage plus a prolonged prothrombin time and/or a severe decrease in platelet count, respectively.

Transfusion of red blood cells in patients with sepsis may cause microcapillary occlusion and tissue ischemia. Transfusions of red blood cells have also been shown to be immuno-suppressive and to increase the risk of post-operative infections and organ failure in surgical patients. A recent study did not demonstrate any benefit of increasing the transfusion threshold from 7 to 10 g dl^{-1} in the treatment of sepsis[3].

Abnormal gastric emptying or adynamic ileus are the most common gastrointestinal problems. Stress ulceration was a common problem before employment of prophylactic H$_2$-blockers or sucralfate. Transient extreme elevations in serum transaminase levels may follow an episode of severe shock or hypotension. Recent data suggest that early enteral nutrition, particularly with immune enhancing diets, may improve the hormonal, metabolic and immunologic derangements that occur in critically ill patients with sepsis[20]. In those patients who do not tolerate gastric tube feedings, post-pyloric feedings should be considered.

A variety of cardiovascular manifestations are observed in severe sepsis, the most common being tachycardia. Frequently, ejection fractions are depressed, the right and left ventricles are dilated, and the diastolic pressure–volume relationships are altered. Initially, before shock onset, the skin is warm, the pulse volume is increased, and pulse pressure is increased. Cardiac output is usually normal or elevated, and systemic vascular resistance (SVR) is commonly decreased. Despite cardiac output elevations, serum lactate levels are often elevated with progressive shock.

6.5.6 Sepsis trials

The systemic inflammatory response syndrome may result from a variety of physiologic insults such as infections, trauma, and pancreatitis. Sepsis is characterized by a constellation of clinical signs including tachycardia, fever, hyperthermia and tachypnea. These clinical signs result from the release of inflammatory mediators including cytokines, proteases, and eicosanoids, which are a component of the body's normal physiologic response to the aforementioned insults. The excessive release of these inflammatory mediators results in the development of diffuse capillary injury, intravascular coagulation with microvascular thrombosis, and multi-organ failure, a condition frequently called severe SIRS or in the presence of infection, severe sepsis. Over the past few years a number of therapeutic interventions aimed at inhibiting or reducing the extent of the body's inflammatory response have undergone extensive phase III trials. These therapies have met with only limited success and none have resulted in a statistically significant improvement in 28 day mortality rates. Anti-endotoxin therapies have been investigated in large populations of adult patients with presumed sepsis[21,22]. Although initial results were encouraging, particularly in patients with Gram-negative sepsis, larger clinical trials have shown no benefit. Several clinical trials have been evaluated with monoclonal anti-TNF (tumor necrosis factor) antibodies in severe sepsis populations[23,24]. No benefit has been found with any anti-TNF alpha therapy in patients in septic shock.

Ibuprofen, a powerful anti-inflammatory agent, failed to demonstrate any effect on mortality, shock or acute respiratory failure, in a large multi-center trial[25]. Additional studies are needed to determine whether some patients, for example those with hypothermia, could benefit from the drug. More recently, investigations have looked at the complex interaction between the inflammation and coagulation systems. Pro-inflammatory cytokines activate coagulation cascades, in particular via an effect upon tissue factor, which is a key player in the coagulation cascade. They can also reduce fibrinolysis and profoundly reduce the levels of protein C and antithrombin III, which are important anti-coagulant agents[26]. Antithrombin III inhibits several coagulation factors of the extrinsic pathways such as factors IXa, XIa and XIIa, in addition to factors Xa, IIa and plasmin. Activated protein C inhibits factors Va, VIIIa, and plasminogen activator inhibitor I (PAI-1). The overall net effect during sepsis is a marked procoagulant balance. In human studies, both antithrombin III and protein C levels are sharply decreased and mortality of septic patients is inversely correlated with the levels of these two products. Recently, several trials have evaluated the compounds antithrombin III, protein C and tissue factor protein inhibitor in the treatment of severe sepsis and septic shock. A large multicenter prospective trial has recently been completed and showed no significant improvement in survival with the employment of antithrombin III in severe sepsis[27]. A recently completed phase III trial with recombinant Activated Protein C (rhAPC) showed a significant reduction in 28 day mortality in severe sepsis patients. The data also revealed a 20% relative risk reduction when employing rhAPC compared with placebo[28]. Tissue factor protein inhibitor (TFPI) is another endogenous anticoagulant that inhibits the extrinsic pathway of blood coagulation triggered by activation of tissue factor in sepsis. TFPI complexes with tissue factor, factor VIIa and factor Xa to inhibit thrombin generation and fibrin formation. A phase III multicenter trial is currently under way to evaluate the efficacy of this compound in severe sepsis[29].

The definition of sepsis and septic shock used in most clinical trials has not included consideration of the length of time that the process has been present nor its anatomic site. Even though recent clinical trials have targeted specific mediators including endotoxin, Il-1 or TNF-alpha, which are postulated to have a pivotal role in the inflammatory cascade leading to organ system failure and sepsis, the presence of excessive levels of these mediators was not required for entry into the study. Therefore, the lack of a requirement to recruit demonstrably infected patients with elevated plasma levels of endotoxin or of cytokines may have adversely affected outcome in trials examining immunomodulatory agents in sepsis. Although a meta-analysis combining most of the clinical trials using anti-inflammatory agents has suggested that benefit in survival could be achieved with such therapies, the magnitude of such effect was small[30].

6.6 Anaphylactic shock

Anaphylaxis is a systemic form of immediate hypersensitivity that may progress to shock. It is a true medical emergency that is associated with a mortality rate approaching 10%. Anaphylactic shock is classically triggered by antigenic stimuli that initiate a sequence of events mediated by IgE, which results in the release of potent mast cells and basophil-derived biochemical mediators. The parenteral route of drug administration is most commonly implicated in severe reactions, but oral, topical and inhalational exposure can all cause anaphylaxis (Table 6.6). Anaphylactoid reactions present similarly to anaphylactic reactions, but unlike the latter are not IgE mediated. Among the agents eliciting mediator release independent of IgE are iodinated contrast materials, dextran, and some local anesthetics.

Most cases of true anaphylaxis are related to the use of antibiotics, primarily penicillin and cephalosporins. An acute allergic reaction develops in as many as 40 out of every 100,000

Table 6.6 Etiologies of anaphylaxis

IgE mediated
Antibiotics
Foods
Insect venom
Foreign proteins (hormones, enzymes)
Industrial chemicals

Non IgE mediated (anaphylactoid)
Iodinated contrast materials
Dextran
Dialysis membranes
Blood products

patients treated with penicillin[31]. The administration of radiocontrast agents is the most common cause of serious anaphylactoid reactions, with a rate of 1 per 1000 to 1 per 14,000 procedures[32]. Classic antibody-mediated anaphylaxis can also occur as a result of stings from bees, wasps, and hornets. Activation of the complement system has been suggested as the cause of anaphylaxis associated with the use of dialysis membranes.

Mediators released with anaphylactic reactions increase microvascular permeability and bronchial reactivity, clinically manifested by airway obstruction (laryngeal edema), impaired pulmonary gas exchange and hypovolemic shock. Activation of the complement system coagulation cascade via IgG and IgM antibody exposure to antigens will produce additional adverse systemic effects.

6.6.1 Clinical presentation

The presentation of anaphylaxis is characteristically acute and will vary depending on the rate of absorption of the offending stimuli, portal of entry and the patient's degree of hypersensitivity. A reaction may occur within minutes and in most instances the signs and symptoms begin within 1 h of exposure. Occasionally, clinical findings may appear many hours after exposure, and may be recurrent. Generally, the more rapid the onset and progression of features, the more severe the reaction. Physical findings are highly variable and may include diffuse erythema and pruritis. If swelling involves the tongue or the lips, swallowing may be compromised and it may become difficult to keep a patent airway. Laryngeal, epiglottic or airway edema may result in acute obstruction that is often characterized by respiratory stridor. Involvement of the lower airway leading to shortness of breath, wheezing and chest tightness is also common. Patients with anaphylactic shock may be susceptible to pneumothoraces and acute pulmonary emphysema produced by forced expiration against a closed edematous glottis. Signs of circulatory shock may characterize severe cases of anaphylaxis and may include hypotension and tachycardia, respiratory arrest, oliguria, and altered mental status. If hypotension persists beyond the first few minutes, established anaphylactic shock is present. Persistent hypotension during anaphylaxis is attributed to an increased vascular permeability with leakage of plasma proteins, which results in hypovolemia and vasodilation. Increased microvascular permeability secondary to this type of distributive shock may cause hemoconcentration. Supraventricular or ventricular cardiac arrhythmias may occur secondary to either myocardial ischemia or elevation of circulatory catecholamine levels. Periorbital and perioral angioedema can be seen. Recent physical activity, ethanol ingestion and beta-adrenergic blocker therapy appear to exacerbate anaphylactic reactions. Crampy abdominal pain, nausea, vomiting, and diarrhea may also be present in patients who have anaphylaxis. Conditions that may mimic anaphylaxis include vasovagal episodes, acute cardiac and pulmonary events, carcinoid syndrome attacks, monosodium glutamate toxicity, and drug overdose.

6.6.2 Management of anaphylaxis

The treatment of anaphylaxis should be priority based, and physicians should be aware of the proper steps in its management. Most patients with anaphylaxis respond to initial therapy, although they may display prolonged persistent reactions despite appropriate therapy. A biphasic anaphylactic reaction may be observed with a reoccurrence of anaphylactic symptoms within 12–24 h after an initial favorable response to therapy. Continuous monitoring with electrocardiogram is important, as dysrhythmias are characteristic of these reactions, and may accompany therapy with bronchodilators, epinephrine, and other catecholamines.

The initial management of anaphylaxis should include the establishment of a patent airway, removal or reduction of systemic absorption of the toxin, pharmacological support with epinephrine and the establishment of an appropriate circulating blood volume with fluid resuscitation. Retained stingers from bees, wasps, or yellow jackets must be removed completely. A proximal constricting band can be applied to delay the absorption of venom if the site of evenomization is an extremity. It should be tightened sufficiently to impair venous flow from the involved area without impeding arterial flow to the distal extremity. Local epinephrine injection may produce localized vasoconstriction and retard system absorption. The employment of suctioning kits to remove the snake venom is controversial. These efforts are probably ineffective if more than 30 min have elapsed since the evenomization and may produce further tissue injury or enhance venom absorption.

A plan to provide sequential therapy for patients with acute anaphylaxis should be instituted rapidly and systematically and include stabilizing the patient's airway, administering parenteral epinephrine, and initiating treatment to correct hypotension. With increasing bronchospasm or laryngeal edema, endotracheal intubation should be recommended or if not possible, emergent cricothyroidotomy.

Parenteral epinephrine therapy is the standard treatment for anaphylactic crisis. Epinephrine inhibits further mediator release from basophils and mast cells, reducing bronchoconstriction, increasing vascular tone and improving cardiac output. Two concentrations are available: a 1:1000 solution (1.0 mg ml^{-1}) and a 1:10,000 solution (0.1 mg ml^{-1}). Epinephrine therapy should be monitored, as it may produce life-threatening dysrhythmias and enhance ventricular irritability. Epinephrine should be given parenterally for severe reactions in a dose of 3–5 ml of a 1:10,000 solution (0.3–0.5 mg). Although epinephrine can be instilled into the tracheobronchial tree via an endotracheal tube or directly through the cricothyroid membrane, the absorption of epinephrine is less predictable by this route. Subcutaneous or intramuscular epinephrine may be injected in a dose of 0.3–0.5 ml of a 1:1000 solution (0.3–0.5 mg). Repeated dose of epinephrine may be employed at 15 min intervals if symptoms persist and if adverse effects have not been observed. A continuous infusion of epinephrine at 0.05–2.0 µg kg^{-1} min^{-1} can be titrated to response.

Patients with a history of radiocontrast allergy should receive a prophylactic regimen before undergoing diagnostic radiographic testing[33]. The use of nonionic low-osmolality radiocontrast media may minimize the likelihood of an adverse reaction (*Table 6.7*).

Fluid therapy reverses the significant hypovolemia in anaphylaxis secondary to an increase in vascular permeability. In cases of mild anaphylaxis, intravenous fluids may not be required, as abnormalities in vascular permeability remain minor. Isotonic crystalloid fluids or colloidal fluids are preferred, as they produce the most rapid expansion in the intravascular space. When the patient remains hypotensive despite fluid replacement and epinephrine, pharmacologic support should be instituted (see Chapter 8). Pure alpha-adrenergic stimulation is to be avoided, as it may enhance

Table 6.7 Prophylactic therapy for radiocontrast sensitivity

Prednisone (50 mg) 13 h, 7 h, and 1 h before exposure
Diphenhydramine (50 mg) IM. or orally, 1 h before exposure

Emergent procedure
Hydrocortisone (200 mg) IV immediately and 4 h post procedure
Diphenhydramine (50 mg) before exposure

mediator release. However, if circulatory shock persists, alpha-adrenergic agents may need to be employed to maintain organ perfusion.

Beta agonists and oxygen therapy should be initiated if bronchospasm persists despite epinephrine therapy. Aminophylline is a bronchodilator that is useful in the management of patients who continue to exhibit bronchospasm after initial treatment with epinephrine. Most bronchodilators have associated significant toxic effects including life-threatening dysrhythmias and seizures. Nebulized epinephrine can be used in mild laryngeal edema, but has no role in the treatment of severe edema, stridor, and respiratory distress.

Corticosteroids are recommended for anaphylactic shock to delay recurrent episodes by inhibiting a secondary wave of mediator release. Methylprednisolone may be given intravenously at doses of 60–125 mg at 4–6 h intervals for 24 h and then tapered to prevent relapse. Therapies for anaphylaxis may be less effective in patients with asthma or those with a history of using beta-adrenergic blocking agents. These conditions decrease the responsiveness of bronchial smooth muscle to therapy and there is a potential for unopposed alpha adrenergic stimulation and severe hypertension in those patients given epinephrine while receiving beta-adrenergic block agents. In these situations, glucagon can be administered at a rate of 5–15 ml min^{-1}.

Antihistamines are not very helpful in the initial management of anaphylaxis, but may be administered while the patient is being stabilized. Non-selective antihistamines inhibit histamine (H_1 and H_2) receptors, thus blocking the systemic effects of H_1 receptor mediated increase in vascular permeability and bronchoconstriction. These agents may be tried in patients who fail to respond to the initial treatment of anaphylaxis. Diphenhydramine, an H_1 antagonist, may be given parenterally in doses of 25–50 mg at 4–6 h intervals. Theoretically, cimetidine, an H_2 antagonist, may also be given intravenously (300 mg) and repeated at 6–8 h intervals in patients with anaphylactic shock.

6.7 Cardiogenic shock

Cardiogenic shock includes conditions that cause failure of the heart as a pump and result in hypoperfusion of body organs. Impairment of diastolic function, systolic function or combination of these impairments can cause the heart to fail as a pump. However, the majority of patients in cardiogenic shock have sustained marked depression of ventricular systolic dysfunction, associated with a decrease in stroke volume and cardiac output. Cardiogenic shock is most commonly a consequence of myocardial ischemia and/or infarction. Complications of an infarction include pump failure, ruptured ventricular wall or septum and disrupted papillary muscle. Other potential causes include cardiomyopathy, arrhythmias, and valvular heart disease. Pulmonary artery catheterization in the setting of cardiogenic shock will classically show a low cardiac index (≤ 1.8 l min^{-1} m^{-2}) and an elevated pulmonary artery wedge pressure (18–25 cm H_2O). Approximately 10–15% of all patients with acute myocardial infarction will develop cardiogenic shock within 1 week of the initiating event[34]. In about 50% of this subset, this occurs within the first 48 h of an infarction. Clinically, patients commonly present with hypotension, tachypnea, a deceased pulse pressure, diaphoresis, cool extremities, and altered mental status. Cardiac examination may reveal tachycardia with an S_3 and/or S_4 gallop.

The recognition of cardiogenic shock is frequently delayed because of confusion regarding the shock syndrome in general. Although the diagnosis of cardiogenic shock is based on evidence of hypoperfusion of organs, some of the more established signs of shock such as hypotension and oliguria may not be present during its early phases or in shock of mild to moderate severity. The clinical manifestations of hypotension and oliguria usually indicate advanced disease and/or decompensation. Pharmacological interventions can be tailored by the evaluation of hemodynamic profiles via pulmonary artery catheterization.

6.7.1 Clinical presentations of cardiogenic shock

Approximately 20% of post-infarction shock patients manifest low ventricular filling pressures (low PAWP). The treatment goal is to improve systemic hypoperfusion and to normalize systemic blood pressure by augmenting stroke volume and cardiac output via fluid resuscitation with IV normal saline. Left ventricular filling pressures (PAWP) should generally be augmented from 12 mmHg or less to target pressures of 15–18 mmHg. A Frank Starling curve can be helpful to guide therapy in an individual patient. Fluid administration should be undertaken cautiously to avoid the development of acute volume overload or pulmonary edema. In those patients who do not display adequate perfusion after fluid infusion therapy, pharmacological support is usually required (see Chapter 8).

The majority of patients with post infarction cardiogenic shock will present with a normal to high PAWP, mild to moderate systemic hypotension, low to normal cardiac output and systemic hypoperfusion. Systemic hypoperfusion may occur in the presence of left ventricular filling pressures (PAWP) of 15 mmHg or more, systemic systolic pressures of between 70 and 100 mmHg and decreased stroke volume and cardiac output. Inotropic therapy aimed at improving ventricular contraction is the most direct and effective form of therapy in this subset of patients. Dobutamine is the preferred agent in these circumstances. In the presence of left ventricular dysfunction, high left ventricular filling pressures, mild to moderate hypotension and reduced peripheral perfusion, dobutamine (2–15 µg kg^{-1} min^{-1}) improves ventricular performance, stroke volume and cardiac output, decreases ventricular filling pressures, normalizes systemic blood pressure, and improves peripheral perfusion. Dobutamine can be titrated by increments of 2–3 µg kg^{-1} min^{-1} every 15–30 min until the clinical targets are met. Milrinone, an agent with both inotropic and vasodilatory actions, can also reduce both left- and right-sided filling pressures while improving cardiac output.

6.7.2 Severe cardiogenic shock

Severe cardiogenic shock presents with markedly elevated left ventricular filling pressure (high PAWP), decreased stroke volume and cardiac index (often <1.8 l min^{-1} m^{-2}), marked hypotension (systolic pressure <70 mmHg), and evidence of organ hypoperfusion. The mortality rate in this group of patients can be greater than 90%. Either dobutamine or milrinone may be inappropriate as first line pharmacologic therapy, as both drugs can cause marked hypotension owing to vasodilation. Initial therapy for severe shock should include an agent that acts as a vasopressor. Dopamine is both an inotrope and vasopressor at higher doses and will generally elevate blood pressure to levels acceptable for brain, kidney, and cardiac perfusion. Renal and cerebral perfusion require systolic blood pressures of greater than 75–80 mmHg, whereas coronary perfusion requires a systemic diastolic pressure of 60 mmHg or more. If escalating doses of dopamine do not increase blood pressure, or unacceptable tachycardia occurs, employment of a more selective alpha-adrenergic agonist such as norepinephrine is warranted despite the increased afterload effect and increasing myocardial oxygen demand.

6.7.3 Intraaortic balloon counterpulsation

With failed medical therapy, intraaortic balloon counterpulsation (IABC) should be considered. In patients with an identifiable, reversible cause of cardiogenic shock, IABC is a form of bridge therapy, providing hemodynamic support until more definitive intervention (angioplasty, bypass surgery) is pursued. IABC effectively improves tissue and coronary perfusion through its effects on decreasing afterload, with subsequent improvement in LV performance and decreasing myocardial oxygen consumption. IABC is specifically indicated in acute mitral regurgitation, or ventricular septal rupture. Hemodynamic stabilization should be followed by a diagnostic cardiac catheterization, angioplasty and/or a surgical procedure.

6.8 Obstructive shock

This category of shock involves impedance to the flow of blood resulting in a decrease in cardiac filling. The causes involve mechanisms other than primary myocardial or valvular dysfunction. Etiologies include impaired diastolic filling (cardiac tamponade, constrictive pericarditis, pneumothorax), and an increase in right or left ventricular afterload (massive pulmonary embolism, acute pulmonary hypertension, aortic dissection). The differential diagnosis is extremely important in this shock state, as a physical intervention (surgery, pericardiocentesis, or chest tube insertion) may reverse the condition and can be life saving. Disorders that impede blood flow are often overlooked and must always be considered in appropriate settings. Maintenance of intravascular volume is extremely important in patients with obstructive shock. Fluid resuscitation may temporarily enhance the cardiac output and hypotension. Diuretics should be avoided in this type of shock. Inotropes and/or vasopressors probably have a minimal, often temporary role in the management of a patient with obstructive shock.

6.8.1 Cardiac tamponade

Tamponade is caused by the accumulation of fluid in the pericardial space under abnormally increased pressure (*Table 6.8*). Although physicians tend to diagnose tamponade in the presence of hypotension, a decrease in blood pressure is usually a preterminal development that is often preceded by an increase in the central venous pressure and a decreasing cardiac output. Central venous pressures are always elevated, except in situations of 'low-pressure' tamponade, which is due to pericardial effusion in the presence of intravascular volume depletion. Equalization of right- and left-sided filling pressures is present in tamponade when the pericardial infusion is not loculated. Echocardiography is the most appropriate technique for diagnosing pericardial effusion in the ICU setting, but computer tomography and magnetic resonance imaging

(MRI) are appropriate diagnostic intervention when echocardiography is inconclusive. Tamponade is assumed to be present when there is a moderate or large pericardial effusion in the presence of a central venous pressure greater than approximately 15 mmHg. Fluid resuscitation will not usually precipitate pulmonary edema in these patients, as congestion is completely limited to the systemic venous compartment rather than in the lungs. Classically, chronic tamponade does not reduce coronary blood flow or induce ischemic myocardial dysfunction. The myocardial function appears to be normal in this shock state. Vasodilators and venodilators are not beneficial in the treatment of cardiac tamponade.

6.9 Shock states

The four categories of shock reviewed here are not mutually exclusive and in many cases, shock may have several causes as the clinical situation progresses. For example, hypovolemic shock may precipitate ischemia, or septic shock may induce volume depletion through third spacing of capillary fluid. One needs to evaluate each of the determinants of

Table 6.8 Etiology of pericardial tamponade

- Post-operative hemorrhage (cardiac surgery)
- Anticoagulation
- Esophageal perforation post-sclerotherapy
- Mechanical ventilation induced barotrauma
- Perforation of heart by indwelling catheter
- Internal jugular or subclavian vein puncture
- Balloon angioplasty perforation of coronary vessels
- Myocardial infarction
- Uremia
- Idiopathic pericarditis
- Neoplastic pericarditis
- Traumatic pericarditis

perfusion pressure when trying to identify precipitating or aggravating factors leading to shock.

References

1. Bond R.F. and Green, H.D. (1969) Cardiac output redistribution during bilateral common carotid occlusion. *Am. J. Physiol.* **216**: 393.
2. Davis, J.O. and Freeman, R.H. (1976) Mechanisms regulating rennin release. *Physiol. Rev.* **56**: 1.
3. Hebert, P.C., Wells, G., Blanchman, M.A., *et al.* (1999) A multicenter, randomized, controlled clinical trial of transfusion requirements in critical care. Transfusion Requirements in Critical Care Investigators, Canadian Critical Care Trials Group. *N. Engl. J. Med.* **340**: 409–417.
4. Abraham, F., Wunderink, R., Silverman, H., *et al.* (1995) Efficacy and safety of monoclonal antibody to human tumor necrosis factor alpha in patients with sepsis syndrome. *JAMA* **273**: 934–941.
5. Bone, R.C., Balk, R.A., Cerra, F.B., *et al.* (1992) American College of Chest Physicians/Society of Critical Care Medicine Consensus Conference: Definitions for sepsis and organ failure and guidelines for the use of innovative therapies in sepsis. *Chest* **101**: 1644–1655.
6. Rangel-Frausto, M., Pittet, D., Costigan, M., *et al.* (1995) The natural history of the systemic inflammatory response syndrome (SIRS). *JAMA* **273**: 117–123.
7. Fisher, C.J., Dhainaut, J.F., Opal, S.M., *et al.* (1994) Recombinant human interleukin I receptor antagonist in the treatment of patients with sepsis syndrome. Results from a randomized, double-blind, placebo-controlled trial. *JAMA* **271**: 1836–1843.
8. Taylor, F.B., Change, A.C., Peer, G.T., *et al.* (1991) DEGR-factor Xa blocks disseminated intravascular coagulation initiated by *Escherichia coli* without preventing shock or organ damage. *Blood* **78**: 364–8.
9. Extermann, M., Regamey, C., Humair, L., *et al.* (1995) Initial treatment of sepsis in non-neutropenic patients: ceftazidime alone versus 'best guess' combined antibiotic therapy. *Chemotherapy* **41**: 306–315.
10. Tuchschmidt, J., Fried, J., Swinney, R. and Sharma, O.M. (1989) Early hemodynamic correlates of survival in patients with septic shock. *Crit. Care Med.* **17**: 719–723.
11. Task Force of the American College of Critical Care Medicine, Society of Critical Care Medicine (1999) Practice parameters for hemo-dynamic support of sepsis in adult patients in sepsis. *Crit. Care Med.* **27**: 639–660.
12. Soni, A., Pepper, G.M., Wyrwinski, P.M., *et al.* (1995) Adrenal insufficiency occurring during septic shock: Incidence, outcome, and relationship to peripheral cytokine levels. *Am. J. Med.* **98**: 266–271.
13. Rasmuson, S., Olsson, T. and Hagg, E. (1996) A low dose ACTH test to assess the function of the hypothalamic–pituitary–adrenal axis. *Clin. Endocrinol.* **44**: 151–156.
14. Annane, D. (2000) Effects of the combination of hydrocortisone (HC)–fludro-cortisone (FC) on mortality in septic-shock. *Crit. Care Med.* **28**(12 Suppl.): A46.
15. Brivet, F.G., Kleinknecht, D.J., Loirat, P. and Landais, P.J.M. (1996) Acute renal failure in intensive care units—causes, outcome and prognostic factors of hospital mortality: a prospective, multicenter study. *Crit. Care Med.* **24**: 192–198.
16. Olson, D., Pohlman, A. and Hall, J.B. (1996) Administration of low-dose dopamine to non-oliguric patients with sepsis syndrome does not raise intramural gastric pH no improve creatinine clearance. *Am. J. Respir. Crit. Care Med.* **154**: 1664–1670.
17. Davenport, A., Will, E.J. and Davidson, A.M. (1993) Improved cardiovascular stability during continuous modes of renal replacement therapy in critically ill patients with acute hepatic and renal failure. *Crit. Care Med.* **21**: 328–338.
18. Kollef, M.H. and Schuster, D.P. (1995) The acute respiratory distress syndrome. *N. Engl. J. Med.* **332**: 27–34.
19. Kreger, B.E., Craven, D.E. and McCabe, W.R. (1980) Gram-negative bacteremia. IV. Re-evaluation of clinical features and treatment in 612 patients. *Am. J. Med.* **68**: 344–355.
20. Bower, R.H., Cerra, F.B., Bershadsky, B., *et al.* (1995) Early enteral administration of a formula (Impact) supplemented with arginine, nucleotides, and fish oil in intensive care unit patients: results of a multicenter, prospective, randomized, clinical trial. *Crit. Care Med.* **23**: 436–449.
21. Calandra, T., Glauser, M.P., Schellekens, J., *et al.* (1988) Treatment of Gram-negative septic shock with human IgG antibody to *Escherichia coli* J5: a prospective, double-blind, randomized trial. *J. Infect. Dis.* **158**: 312–319.
22. McCloskey, R.V., Straube, R.C., Sanders, C., *et al.* (1994) Treatment of septic shock with human monoclonal antibody HA-1A. A randomized, double-blind, placebo-controlled trial. CHESS Trial Study Group. *Ann. Intern. Med.* **121**: 1–5.

23. **Abraham, E., Wunderink, R., Silverman, H., et al.** (1995) Monoclonal antibody to human tumor necrosis factor alpha (TNF Mab): efficacy and safety in patients with the sepsis syndrome. *JAMA* **273**: 934–941.

24. **Abraham, E., Anzueto, A., Gutierrez, G., et al. for the NORASEPT II Study Group** (1998) Monoclonal antibody to human tumor necrosis factor alpha (TNF MAb) in the treatment of patients with septic shock: a multi-center, placebo controlled, randomized, double-blind clinical trial. *Lancet* **351**: 929–933.

25. **Bernard, G.R., Wheeler, A.P., Russell, J.A., et al.** (1997) The effects of Ibuprofen on the physiology and survival of patients with sepsis. *N. Engl. J. Med.* **336**: 912–918.

26. **Vervloet, M.G., Thijs, L.G. and Hack, C.E.** (1998) Derangements of coagulation and fibrinolysis in critically ill patients with sepsis and septic shock. *Semin. Thromb. Hemost.* **24**: 33–44.

27. **Riess, H.** (2000) Antithrombin in severe sepsis. 'New' indication of an 'old' drug. *Intensive Care Med.* **22**: S471–S481.

28. **Bernard, G.R., Vincent, J.L., Laterre, P.F., et al.** (2001) Recombinant human Protein C World-wide Evaluation in Severe Sepsis (PROWESS) study group: Efficacy and safety of recombinant human activated protein C for severe sepsis. *N. Engl. J. Med.* **344**: 699–709.

29. **Abraham, E.** (2000) Coagulation abnormalities in acute lung injury and sepsis. *Am. J. Respir. Cell Mol. Biol.* **22**: 401–404.

30. **Zeni, F., Freeman, B. and Natanson, C.** (1997) Anti-inflammatory therapies to treat sepsis and septic shock: a reassessment. *Crit. Care Med.* **25**: 1095–1100.

31. **Carlson, R.W., Bowles, A.L. and Haupt, M.T.** (1986) Anaphylactic, anaphylactoid and related forms of shock. *Crit. Care Med.* **2**: 347–372.

32. **Sim, T.C.** (1992) Anaphylaxis: How to manage and prevent this medical emergency. *Postgrad. Med.* **92**: 277–296.

33. **Lasser, E.C., Berry, C.C., Talner, L.B., et al.** (1987) Pretreatment with corticosteroids to alleviate reactions to intravenous contrast material. *N. Engl. J. Med.* **317**: 845.

34. **Bengston, J.R., Kaplan, A.J., Pieper, K.S., et al.** (1992) Prognosis in cardiogenic shock after acute myocardial infarction in the interventional era. *J. Am. Coll. Cardiol.* **20**: 1482.

Chapter 7

Fluid resuscitation in the ICU

Laurie A. Loiacono, MD

Contents

7.1 Introduction

Recognition and treatment of fluid imbalance is particularly important in the critically ill patient, especially as the normal homeostatic mechanisms (thirst, salt craving, renal elimination) may be bypassed or inoperative. Unrecognized fluid imbalance in this patient population can lead to severe metabolic derangements and shock states. Hypovolemia is a common cause of circulatory shock; patients can become relatively or absolutely volume depleted as the result of hemorrhage, fluid shifts ('third-spacing'), obligate osmotic diuresis, sweating, therapeutic maneuvers or acute vasodilatation (i.e. SIRS or sepsis). The differential diagnosis of clinical shock states is covered in Chapter 6; common clinical situations that often require aggressive fluid resuscitation are listed in *Table 7.1*. Timely recognition and treatment of fluid deficits can affect patient survival and minimize associated morbidity such as development of acute renal failure, acute lung injury and adult respiratory distress syndrome, myocardial infarction, mesenteric ischemia, stroke, and multisystem organ dysfunction. This chapter will highlight principles of resuscitation and the advantages and disadvantages of various replacement fluids.

7.2 Definitions

Acute resuscitation—fluid administration that restores intravascular volume.
Albumin—a relatively low molecular weight serum protein present in plasma, which accounts for approximately three-quarters of normal plasma colloid osmotic pressure. Albumin can be manufactured into a protein-based solution and administered as a colloid volume expander.

Chronic resuscitation—fluid administration directed toward maximizing and monitoring end-organ perfusion.
Colloid—a solution composed of osmotically active molecules that are relatively impermeable to capillary membranes and therefore create an osmotic gradient (or pressure) across a membrane.
Colloid osmotic pressure (COP)—the fluid diffusion pressure created across a capillary membrane by differences in protein concentration on either side of the membrane.
Crystalloid—an electrolyte-based solution of osmotically inactive particles that freely equilibrate across capillary membranes.
Donnan forces—electrostatic forces generated across a membrane by large, negatively charged osmotically active protein molecules that determine differential ion concentrations and total water flux across that membrane between two compartments.
Hetastarch—a synthetic colloid composed of hydroxyethyl-substituted branched chain amylopectin molecules supplied in normal saline solution (typically *c.* 310 mOsm l^{-1}) as Hespan™ or in balanced electrolyte solution as Hextend™.
Hydrostatic pressure—the pressure created across a membrane by fluid flow through a space.
Hypertonic—a solution that has an osmolarity higher than plasma (typically >300 mOsm l^{-1}).
Hypotonic—a solution that has an osmolarity lower than plasma (typically <270–280 mOsm l^{-1}). Hypotonic solutions include half-normal saline solution.
Isotonic—a solution that has an osmolarity similar to plasma (typically 280–300 mOsm l^{-1}). Isotonic solutions include lactated Ringer's and normal saline solutions.

Table 7.1 Common circulatory shock states requiring aggressive fluid resuscitation

Hypovolemic states	Distributive shock states with ongoing fluid loss
Hemorrhage	Pancreatitis
GI loss (diarrhea, vomiting)	SIRS
Ascitic leak	Sepsis
	Anaphylaxis

Osmolarity—a measure of the number of osmotically active particles in a solution.
Resuscitation—the restoration of adequate and oxygenated tissue perfusion in an effort to avoid tissue loss or injury.
Total osmotic pressure (TOP)—the fluid diffusion pressure created by the COP plus Donnan forces of the cation concentrations in solution.

7.3 Physiology of resuscitation

Although the pathophysiology of various shock states will vary significantly, the principles of physiologic support are remarkably consistent. Restoration of tissue oxygenation *and* perfusion are paramount for tissue preservation and recovery from shock. Acute tubular necrosis (ATN) and acute lung injury can occur following even transient periods of significant hypotension. In shock, circulating catecholamines constrict prearteriolar capillary sphincters, globally decreasing capillary perfusion and potentially producing significant tissue hypoperfusion and injury. Although the insult may be brief, end-organ effects can be prolonged or irreversible, and are probably related to these microcirculatory changes that occur to preserve macrovascular circulating blood flow.

7.3.1 Fluid compartments
Water comprises about 60% of body weight, but intravascular volume is only a small portion (about 10%) of total body fluid (*Figure 7.1*). Two-thirds of total body water (TBW) is intracellular and contains plasma and proteins responsible for intracellular metabolism. One-third of TBW is extracellular in a 3:1, interstitial (extravascular):intravascular distribution. Fluid moves between the intracellular and extracellular spaces across *cell membranes* and fluid moves between intravascular and extravascular spaces across *capillary membranes*.

7.3.2 Semipermeable membranes; fluid dynamics
Healthy *cell membranes* are semipermeable; therefore fluid shifts between the intracellular

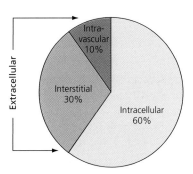

Figure 7.1 Major compartmental distribution of total body fluid.

and extracellular compartments occur only with free water, by osmosis, and in response to differences in transmembrane solute and ion concentration gradients. Electrolytes, most solutes and proteins do not freely cross the cell membrane unless the cell is injured or dying. Cations cross only through ATP-driven Na^+–K^+ pumps. Therefore, differences between intracellular and extracellular protein and total electrolyte concentrations (osmolarity) will determine fluid flux across cell membranes, facilitating cellular hydration, dehydration or swelling.

Healthy *capillary membranes* are freely permeable to water and electrolytes but not proteins. Fluid flux between the intravascular and extravascular (interstitial) space is therefore more dependent on transcapillary protein concentration gradients (i.e. COP) and transcapillary electrolyte concentrations are less significant, under normal physiologic conditions. In addition, because there is a 'driving' flow (or hydrostatic pressure) through capillaries (Pc), transcapillary fluid dynamics are more complex and other forces need to be considered.

The differences in permeability between cell and capillary membranes dictate in large part how different types of resuscitative fluids redistribute after administration (*Figure 7.2*). Infused isotonic fluids such as normal saline and Ringer's lactate are initially contained within the intravascular space but over time will equilibrate with the extracellular space

101

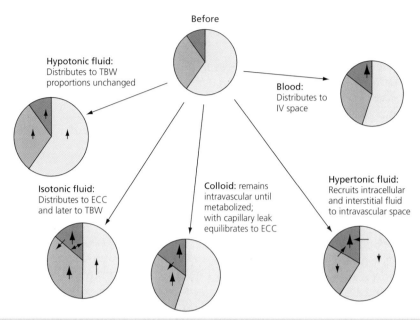

Figure 7.2 Redistribution of resuscitative fluids. Differences in permeability between cell and capillary membranes. ECC, extracellular compartment; TBW, total body water.

(intravascular and interstitial water) across the electrolyte-permeable capillary membranes. The intracellular space is less affected because cell membranes are *not* freely permeable to electrolytes. Hypotonic solutions, on the other hand, rapidly distribute to a volume approximating total body water because *both* cell and capillary membranes are permeable to free water. Dextrose-containing solutions such as D5W have sufficient osmolarity to avoid hemolysis of red blood cells when initially infused, but act as hypotonic solutions once the osmotic component (glucose) is metabolized. Replenishing lost intravascular fluid (plasma and/or whole blood) requires roughly four times the desired replacement volume as crystalloid, and larger amounts of hypotonic solutions. Compartmental redistribution of fluid begins within minutes.

7.3.3 Starling's principle
In 1896, Starling first described factors that influence the transfer of fluid across capillary membranes[1]. The Starling equation describes four forces that govern transcapillary flow:

$$Qf = Kf[(Pc - Pi) - \sigma(COPc - COPi)].$$

- Qf is total flow across the capillary membrane;
- Kf is the filtration coefficient (the rate of filtration min^{-1} mmHg^{-1} per 100 g tissue; varies from one tissue to another);
- Pc is capillary hydrostatic pressure (tends to force fluid out of the vascular space, varies from one end of the capillary to the other; mean Pc is *c.* 17 mmHg (see *Figure 7.4* (below));
- Pi is interstitial hydrostatic pressure (tends to draw fluid out of the vascular space, is usually negative; *c.* −6.3 mmHg);
- σ is the protein osmotic reflection coefficient (a measure of the ability of the capillary membrane to block protein movement; normal average is 0.9 for systemic capillaries and 0.7 for pulmonary capillaries but may decrease as low as 0.4 in leaky capillary states);

- COPc is the capillary, or plasma, osmotic pressure (tends to retain fluid in the capillary, the only Starling force that returns intravascular fluid, normally *c.* 28 mmHg with 19 mmHg from protein and 9 mmHg from cations in solution);
- COPi is the interstitial osmotic pressure (tends to retain fluid in the interstitial space, normally *c.* 5 mmHg).

Figure 7.3 is a diagrammatic representation of capillary anatomy with transmembrane pressures and flows indicated.

7.3.4 Acute versus chronic resuscitation
It is generally understood that an 'absolute' and/or 'relative' blood volume deficit is the primary defect in shock states. Because of the catecholamine, cytokine and complement release that occurs early in shock, it is helpful to separate *acute* from *chronic* resuscitative needs. We will exclude cardiogenic shock states from this discussion, as they are to be discussed in Chapters 6 and 8.

The primary need in early hypovolemic and distributive shock is for rapid intravascular volume expansion. Aggressive fluid therapy with the goal of restoring hemodynamic stability will minimize subsequent organ dysfunction. The composition of the fluid therapy is less important than the physical need to support right heart filling (preload) leading to support of cardiac output and restoration of tissue oxygenation or perfusion. Generally, blood loss (i.e. hemorrhage) is replaced with blood when possible, plasma loss (i.e. ascites) is replaced with plasma or colloid, and electrolyte loss (i.e. vomiting or diarrhea) is replaced with crystalloid.

Over the subsequent several hours to days, a post-shock reactive systemic inflammatory response ensues and capillary membranes become leaky to fluid and protein. Now the 'intravascular availability' of the fluid therapy becomes more important and more consideration should be given to the resuscitative fluid composition. It is in this later phase

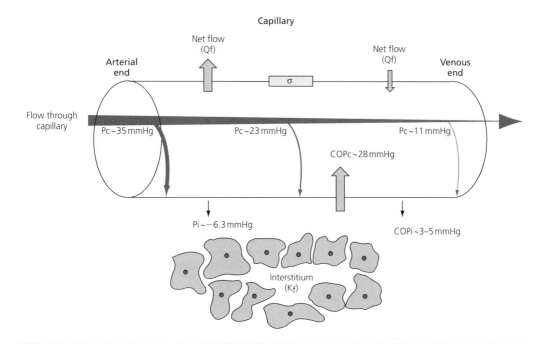

Figure 7.3 Diagrammatic representation of capillary anatomy with transmembrane pressures and flow represented.

of shock and/or shock recovery where 'chronic resuscitation' is necessary, not only to meet basic maintenance fluid needs but also to replace the insensible intravascular fluid losses that occur to the extravascular space as a result of fluid equilibration across leaky capillary membranes. In this chronic phase of resuscitation colloids tend to have a physiologic advantage over more rapidly equilibrating edemagenic crystalloids.

Defining 'the optimum resuscitative fluid' is difficult and controversial. When compared with crystalloid, are colloids or hypertonic fluids more effective in maintaining the integrity of intravascular volume, minimizing edema formation, better preserving interstitial osmolarity, and decreasing subsequent morbidity and mortality? Are there advantages if colloids are given earlier and more consistently throughout the resuscitative period from shock states? Are there advantages or disadvantages to colloids and hypertonic solutions other than osmotic support? As none of these questions have been conclusively answered, clinical practice tends to be variable.

7.4 Strategy

7.4.1 Initiation of circulatory support

Resuscitation begins with the 'ABCs': Airway, Breathing, and Circulation. Circulation implies the process of evaluating, establishing and maintaining adequate perfusion via cardiovascular support. Intravenous access needs to be established in anticipation of large fluid volume requirements. Patients with significant traumatic injuries or expected fluid shifts as the result of major thoracic and abdominal procedures should have at least two large-bore (18 gauge or larger) peripheral lines. Alternatively, central access can be established via the subclavian, internal jugular or femoral veins (see Chapter 5) with a wide variety of catheters ranging from single-, double- and triple-lumen CVP lines to large-bore (usually 8 or 9 French) Cordis transducers, combined introducer–triple lumen catheters, or

Quinton-type catheters normally used for dialysis.

7.4.2 Endpoints of fluid therapy

Clinical criteria used to define the goals of fluid therapy are broadly defined because of the difficulties in standardizing and controlling study populations. Most clinicians would consider a patient to be adequately resuscitated when the following criteria are met:

- PaO_2 of 60–65 mmHg or more;
- pH greater than 7.25;
- Hematocrit (Hct) greater than 24%, higher with myocardial ischemia or organ failure;
- mean arterial pressure (MAP) ≥ 60 mmHg;
- urine output of 0.5 cm^3 kg^{-1} or more in adults (in the absence of acute or chronic renal failure);
- well-perfused, warm extremities;
- oxygen delivery greater than 150 ml min^{-1} m^{-2}.

It is possible, however, to meet some or all of these goals without adequate fluid resuscitation. An alpha-adrenergic agent such as norepinephrine or phenylephrine (see Chapter 8) will vasocontrict peripheral vessels and raise blood pressure, even if filling pressures are inadequate. Although this therapy would accomplish the goal of a MAP greater than 60 mmHg, it does so at the expense of peripheral perfusion, and may ultimately result in lactic acidosis and organ failure.

Absolute central venous pressure or pulmonary artery occlusion pressure goals can be misleading because of variations in individual patient physiology. Although conclusions about end-diastolic volumes can be drawn from measured pressures, such conclusions may be erroneous if pressure–volume relationships (i.e. compliance) are altered. In general, low filling pressures (i.e. CVP < 5, PCWP < 8) suggest inadequate preload in patients with clinical symptoms of shock. Fluid challenges are helpful in assessing volume replacement needs. To detect changes, fluid boluses (preferably crystalloid) have to be of sufficient volume (>500 ml in adults), rapidly infused (within 10 min) and carefully monitored (with the clinician at bedside). Physical examination, central venous and/or PCWP, cardiac output, urine output, and arterial pressure give clues to the adequacy of fluid resuscitation. Following a fluid bolus, small (<3 mmHg), transient changes in filling pressures with improved cardiac output or blood pressure indicate ongoing fluid needs. Sustained or large (>7 mmHg) increases in filling pressures without improved output mark the point at which circulatory overload becomes a risk.

Fluid resuscitation can be tailored to the particular patient's physiology based on the generation of a Starling curve. Clinically, the relationship between filling pressures and cardiac output is plotted. (In the absence of a PA catheter, CVP can be plotted against arterial blood pressure.) *Figure 7.4* displays such a curve based on data from a patient before and after adequate fluid resuscitation. Pressor agents should be withheld until preload has been adequately addressed. The risks of over-resuscitation include hydrostatic pulmonary edema and diffuse tissue edema. In most cases, however, even gross fluid overload is a temporary problem, as much of the fluid will diffuse into the interstitial space within hours, or can be managed via diuresis or dialysis. The risks of inadequate fluid resuscitation (organ failure) tend to be more permanent and more devastating.

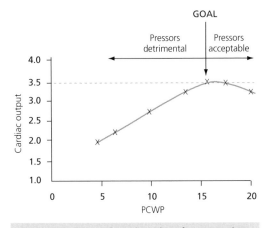

Figure 7.4 A curve based on data from a patient before and after adequate fluid resuscitation.

7.5 Red blood cells (RBCs)

Whole blood is the ideal fluid for replacement of intravascular volume deficits, but because of high demand for specific component therapy and technical difficulty in long-term storage of whole-blood preparations, RBCs are most commonly provided as citrate anticoagulated packed RBCs. RBCs should be used to (i) replace blood loss secondary to hemorrhage and (ii) individually maximize oxygen-carrying capacity in critically ill patients. Whereas a hemoglobin of 7–8 g dl^{-1} is generally adequate for stable preoperative patients[1], this level may be insufficient in the critically ill patient with circulatory compromise and high oxygen consumption.

When rapid, high-volume (>100 ml min^{-1}) citrated RBC infusions are required (i.e. massive gastrointestinal (GI) bleed or trauma-related hemorrhage), acute hypocalcemia can occur as the result of citrate intoxication[2]. Clinical symptoms include skeletal muscle hyperexcitability, ST-T segment changes, depressed cardiac output, hypotension, electromechanical dissociation, and ventricular fibrillation. Intravenous calcium replacement will correct these clinical symptoms, and should be guided by serum ionized calcium levels in these typically hypoproteinemic peri- or post-resuscitative patients.

Other transfusion-related risks are listed in *Table 7.2*.

7.6 Crystalloid products

Crystalloid solutions are electrolyte-based solutions of osmotically inactive particles that freely equilibrate across capillary, but not cell, membranes. They can be mixed and administered with or without dextrose solution. Addition of 5% dextrose to isotonic solutions will tend to increase the solution's osmolarity by approximately 250 mOsm l^{-1}. Dextrose-containing solutions are seldom used for volume resuscitation, because (i) dextrose freely equilibrates between the intracellular and extracellular spaces and is therefore of no value in terms of osmotic support, and (ii) patients in stressed

Table 7.2 Most common acute blood transfusion risks

Hemolytic transfusion reactions (immediate)
Delayed transfusion reactions (3–21 days post-transfusion)
Cytokine-mediated febrile reactions
Allergic reactions
Graft vs. host disease
Post-transfusion purpura
Metabolic disturbances (hypokalemia, hypothermia)
Immunosuppression
Infection (hepititis, HIV, EBV/CMV)

states will be glucose intolerant and can become hyperglycemic. Crystalloid solutions typically used for volume resuscitation are either isotonic or hypertonic (see definitions).

7.6.1 Isotonic solutions (NS and LR)

The two most commonly used isotonic solutions are 0.9% normal saline solution (NS) and lactated Ringer's solution (LR).

- 0.9% normal saline solution contains 9 g l^{-1} NaCl. It has an osmolarity of 308 mOsm l^{-1} (154 mequiv l^{-1} Na and 154 mequiv l^{-1} Cl). There is a risk of hyperchloremic acidosis with rapid and/or prolonged administration of isotonic saline[3–5].
- Ringer's lactate contains 6 g of sodium per liter. It has an osmolarity of 273 mOsm l^{-1} (130 mequiv l^{-1} Na$^+$, 109 mequiv l^{-1} Cl$^-$, 3 mequiv l^{-1} Ca^{2+}, 4 mequiv l^{-1} K$^+$, and 28 mequiv l^{-1} lactate). There is less risk of hyperchloremic acidosis than with normal saline, and the potential advantage of a buffer effect on any ongoing acidosis once the lactate in solution is converted to acetate in patients with preserved liver function.

Advantages of isotonic solutions

- Do not promote intracellular–extracellular shifts.
- Effective immediate volume expansion in acute resuscitation.
- Readily available in most situations.
- Low cost.

Disadvantages of isotonic solutions

- Freely equilibrate between the intravascular and interstitial spaces over time leading to diminished intravascular volume. This occurs particularly rapidly in hypoproteinemic patients. The intravascular 'availability' of these solutions as a result of rapid equilibration is, therefore, only a few hours.
- Larger volumes, compared with colloids, are required to achieve the same physiologic endpoints. Typically, crystalloid at 2–4 times the volume of colloid or Hetastarch is required for a comparable physiologic effect during resuscitation[6].
- Resuscitation with crystalloids has been shown to produce a rapid and sustained drop in plasma COP that is significantly more severe than the post-resuscitative drop in COP seen with colloid or HS[7].

7.6.2 Hypertonic solutions—risks and benefits

Hypertonic solutions (HS) facilitate the redistribution of fluid between the intracellular and extracellular compartments. HS infusions tend to rapidly 'recruit' intracellular water into the extracellular or intravascular space, maintaining relatively consistent serum sodium levels while simultaneously volume expanding the intravascular space. Smaller volumes of HS are therefore effective in meeting resuscitative goals when compared with isotonic fluid options. The most commonly used hypertonic solutions are hypertonic saline solution (HSS) and hypertonic albuminated fluid (HALF). Hypertonic solutions are well studied in burn resuscitation[8,9] and their use in trauma resuscitation and following neurotrauma or neurosurgery shows promise in terms of decreasing post-resuscitative morbidity[10].

- Hypertonic saline (HS) is a 3% sodium chloride solution that contains 513 mequiv l^{-1} Na, 513 mequiv l^{-1} Cl buffered to a pH of 5.0 using hydrochloric acid. It has an osmolarity of 1027 mOsm l^{-1}.
- Hypertonic albuminated fluid (HALF)[11] contains 240 mequiv l^{-1} Na, 120 mequiv

l^{-1} Cl, 120 mequiv l^{-1} lactate, plus 1.5 g l^{-1} albumin.

Advantages of hypertonic solutions

- Effective immediate volume expansion in acute resuscitation.
- Lower volumes of resuscitation required to reach physiologic endpoints than with isotonic fluids[11].
- Less cellular edema post-resuscitation, therefore less risk to injured nerve tissue in brain and spinal cord[10].

Disadvantages of hypertonic solutions

- Risk of severe hypernatremia, especially with HSS.
- Risk of hyperchloremic acidosis.
- Risk of cellular dehydration and secondary injury.
- More expensive than isotonic fluids.
- Requires central venous access for administration, because of intolerance of peripheral veins to the chemical stress of hypertonic solutions.

7.7 Cell-free colloids

Colloid solutions contain large molecules that are relatively impermeable to capillary membranes and therefore have a significant intravascular 'availability' post-administration.

7.7.1 Albumin

Albumin (5% or 25%) solutions

These solutions are prepared from heat-treated donor plasma and have less than 0.5% risk of adverse reaction (i.e. urticaria, fever, chills). In normal plasma, albumin provides about 80% of the plasma COP. Approximately 40% of the body's albumin pool is intravascular, and 60% is extravascular in tissue stores (about one-third of the extravascular tissue stores is in the skin)[12]. However, in situations of physiologic stress and critical illness, endogenous albumin levels drop precipitously, owing to capillary leak and/or increased breakdown in the catabolic state[13].

The 5% albumin solution contains 50 g l^{-1} albumin mixed in NSS and has a COP of about 20 mmHg. The 25% albumin solution contains 240 g l^{-1} albumin in buffered diluent containing 130–160 mequiv l^{-1} Na and has a COP of about 100 mmHg.

Advantages of albumin solutions

- Lower volumes of resuscitation than isotonic solution are needed to reach physiologic endpoints[14].
- Physiologic support of COP[14].
- Intravascular effects can last up to 24 h[14] depending on patient's pre-perfusion status[15].

Disadvantage of albumin solutions

- More expensive than crystalloids.

7.7.2 Hetastarch

Hetastarch is a synthetic colloid solution composed of hydroxyethyl-substituted branched-chain amylopectin molecules (each with an average molecular weight of 6.9×10^4, similar to that of an albumin molecule). The 6% solution of Hetastarch in NSS contains 60 g l^{-1} colloid, 154 mequiv l^{-1} Na, and 154 mequiv l^{-1} Cl. It has an osmolarity of approximately 310 mOsm l^{-1} and a COP of approximately 30 mmHg. Hetastarch molecules are either degraded in the liver or excreted in the stool and urine.

Advantages of Hetastarch

- Lower volumes of resuscitation than isotonic solution are needed to reach physiologic endpoints[15].
- Physiologic support of COP.
- Intravascular effects can last 24–36 h.
- Non-toxic and non-antigenic.
- Useful in Jehovah's Witnesses, who will not accept albumin.

Disadvantages of Hetastarch

- May impair coagulation when given in high volumes (i.e. >1.5 l per resuscitation episode or 20 ml kg^{-1} day^{-1}).

- More expensive than crystalloids.
- Risk of hyperchloremic acidosis when administered in large volumes, as a result of the solution containing normal saline[4].

7.7.3 Hetastarch with electrolytes (Hextend)

A 6% Hetastarch, formulated in a physiologically balanced crystalloid carrier similar to lactated Ringer's solution, is marketed under the brand name Hextend. The crystalloid carrier more closely resembles the ionic composition of normal plasma. It contains physiologic levels of sodium (143 mequiv l^{-1}), chloride (124 mequiv l^{-1}) and calcium (5 mequiv l^{-1}), and slightly lower than normal physiologic levels of potassium (3 mequiv l^{-1}) and magnesium (0.9 mequiv l^{-1}). Hextend also contains a subphysiologic level of dextrose (0.99 g l^{-1}) and 28 mequiv l^{-1} lactate, which provides a source of bicarbonate in patients with normal lactate metabolism. In contrast to 6% Hetastarch with saline, the Hetastarch in electrolyte solution is associated with less intraoperative calcium administration, and lower mean estimated blood loss[16]. The additional buffering capability may also reduce or eliminate the prolongation of thromboelastogram clot time seen with large volumes of Hetastarch–saline administration[16].

7.7.4 Dextrans

The dextrans are solutions of high molecular weight polysaccharides that are manufactured from products of bacteria-mediated, enzymatic digestion of sucrose-containing media. Two dextran products are available for use in the United States.

Dextran 70 is a 6% solution of dextran in sodium chloride. It has a weight-average molecular weight (MW) of 7×10^4, is hypertonic when compared with blood, and retains approximately 20–25 ml of water per gram infused. Because of its high MW, intravascular retention is excellent and generally lasts longer than 24 h before degradation in the viscera (to carbon dioxide and water) or excretion into the urine or gut.

Dextran 40 is a 10% solution of dextran in sodium chloride. It has a weight-average MW of 4×10^4, is hypertonic and has an equivalent COP *in vitro* to 17% albumin solution. However, because of its relatively low MW, dextran 40 molecules easily migrate across capillary membranes and are rapidly cleared via the kidneys. Sixty per cent of infused dextran 40 can be excreted in the urine within 6 h (in patients with normal renal function) and nearly 70% is excreted within 24 h following infusion[17]. Therefore, intravascular availability of dextran 40 is poor.

Advantages of dextrans

- Lower volumes of resuscitation than isotonic solution are needed to reach physiologic endpoints[15].
- Physiologic support of COP.

Disadvantages of dextrans

- Possibility of serious anaphylactoid reactions (incidence of about 5.3%).
- Rheologic effects can predispose to bleeding and coagulopathy (dextrans at large doses can coat platelets).
- Dextran 40 can contribute to acute renal failure in hypovolemic patients because the high rate of renal clearance in low flow states can result in increased tubular viscosity and obstruction[17].

7.8 Summary and conclusions

- Colloids and hypertonic solutions are more expensive, but also more efficient than crystalloids in correction of the absolute and relative volume deficit demonstrated early in shock states.
- Colloids and hypertonic solutions are less edemagenic than crystalloids when used early in resuscitation. This effect may minimize risks of post-resuscitative morbidity including wound healing and skin complications, non-cardiogenic pulmonary edema, and severely low plasma COP.

- Risks of colloids and hypertonic solutions are product specific—hemostasis is a concern with large volumes of Hetastarch, and the dextrans have a significant incidence of anaphylactoid reactions.
- Multivariate analyses have failed to show significant differences in efficacy of one colloid over another in the acute resuscitative setting.
- Isotonic crystalloids are the most cost-effective acute resuscitative fluid. However, in early shock, resuscitation with blood or colloids, although more expensive, helps preserve plasma COP and may be needed to maintain oxygen-carrying capacity.

7.9 Recommendations for fluid resuscitation in the ICU

- Evaluate the 'ABCs' and establish adequate IV access early.
- ALWAYS use only colloid, blood or isotonic fluids (NOT hypotonic fluids) for acute resuscitation from hypovolemic states.
- Resuscitate with colloids and/or blood whenever possible instead of isotonic crystalloids (particularly early in shock). This strategy acts to preserve plasma COP, maintain intravascular volume for longer periods, support oxygen-carrying capacity and minimize post-resuscitative edema.
- Remember to focus on resuscitative endpoints from the initiation of therapy, to minimize subsequent morbidity and mortality.
- Recognize that hypertonic solutions appear to be a good option for efficient short-term intravascular volume expansion but need to be administered via central venous lines.
- Monitor for infusion-related metabolic complications (i.e. hyperchloremic acidosis with saline-containing solutions, hypocalcemia with citrated blood products).
- Individualize therapy to individual patient physiology when possible (i.e. bedside Starling curve).

References

1. **Starling, E.H.** (1896) On the absorption of fluids from the connective tissue spaces. *J. Physiology* **9**: 312.
2. **Civetta, J.M.** (1979) A new look at the 'Starling' Equation. *Crit. Care Med.* **7**: 84.
3. **Lucas, C.E.** (1977) Resuscitation of the injured patient: the three phases of treatment. *Surg. Clin. N. Am.* **57**: 3.
4. **Tullis, J.L.** (1977) Albumin. *JAMA* **237**: 355.
5. **Rackow, E.C., Fein, I.A. and Leppo, J.** (1977) Colloid oncotic pressure as a prognostic indicator of pulmonary edema and mortality in the critically ill patient. *Chest* **72**: 709.
6. **Rackow, E.C., Falk, J.L. and Fein, I.A.** (1983) Fluid resuscitation in circulatory shock: a comparison of the cardiorespiratory effects of albumin, Hetastarch, and saline solutions in patients with hypovolemic and septic shock. *Crit. Care Med.* **11**: 839.
7. **Rackow, E.C., Fein, I.A. and Siegel, J.** (1982) The relationship of colloid osmotic pulmonary artery wedge pressure gradient to pulmonary edema and mortality in critically ill patients. *Chest* **82**: 433.
8. **Lowe, R.J., Moss, G.S., Jilek, J., et al.** (1977) Crystalloids vs. colloids in the etiology of pulmonary failure after trauma. A randomized trial in man. *Surgery* **81**: 676.
9. **Weaver, D.W., Ledgerwood, A.M., Lucas, C.E., et al.** (1978) Pulmonary effects of albumin resuscitation for severe hypovolemic shock. *Surgery* 1978; **113**: 387.
10. **Prough, D.S.** (2000) Acidosis associated with perioperative saline administration. Dilution or delusion? *Anesthesiology* **93**: 1167–1169.
11. **Waters, J.H. and Bernstein, C.A.** (2000) Dilutional acidosis following Hetastarch or albumin in healthy volunteers. *Anesthesiology* **93**: 1184–1187.
12. Dil. Acidosis. *Surg. Gynecol. Obstet.*
13. **Jarvela, K., Honkonen, S.E., Javela, T., Koobi, T. and Kaukinen, S.** (2000) The comparison of hypertonic saline (7.5%) and normal saline (0.9%) for initial fluid administration before spinal anesthesia. *Anesth. Analg.* **91**(6): 1461–1465.
14. **Jelenko, C., Wheeler, M.L., Callaway, B.D., Divilio, L.T., Bucklen, K.R. and Holdrege, T.D.** (1978) Shock and resuscitation II: Volume repletion with minimal edema using the 'HALFD' regimen. *JACEP* **7**(9): 326–333.
15. **Jelenko, C.** (1979) Fluid therapy and the HALFD method. *J. Trauma* **19**(Suppl.): 11.

16. **Gan, T.J.,** *et al.* (1999) Hextend, a physiologically balanced plasma expander for large volume use in major surgery: a randomized phase III clinical trial. *Anesth. Analg.* **88**(5): 992–998.

17. **Sumas, M.E., Legos, J.J., Nathan, D., Lamperti, A.A., Tuma, R.F. and Young, W.F.** (2001) Tonicity of resuscitative fluids influence outcome after spinal cord injury. *Neurosurgery* **48**(1): 167–172; discussion 172–173.

Chapter 8

Circulatory support

Thomas L. Higgins, MD

Contents

8.1 Introduction

Choosing the optimal pressor or inotrope in the hemodynamically unstable patient requires us to understand a number of issues, including which drugs affect specific adrenergic receptors and whether a drug is a full or partial agonist (*Table 8.1*). Catecholamines and sympathomimetics (drugs that mimic the effects of endogenous catecholamines) have traditionally been first line pharmacotherapy for shock states, but non-catecholamine agents such as milrinone may be particularly useful when catecholamine response is altered[1]. Catecholamines are not the only endogenous substances responsible for blood pressure homeostasis. Vasopressin may have a role in treating septic shock and vasodilation following cardiopulmonary bypass.

8.2 The sympathetic nervous system

Homeostatic control of blood pressure is mediated via the sympathetic nervous system. Sympathetic nerves originate in the spinal cord. Pre-ganglionic fibers generally exit to synapse with post-ganglionic neurons in the lateral or paravertebral ganglia. The pre-ganglionic fibers are cholenergic and secrete acetylcholine at their nerve endings. Post-ganglionic fibers, which terminate in vessels and visceral organs, primarily are adrenergic and secrete norepinephrine. Tyrosine is the basic building block for catecholamines (*Figure 8.1*). Through a series of reactions, tyrosine is hydrolyzed to dihydroxyphenylethylamine (DOPA) by the enzyme tyrosine hydroxylase and then decarboxylated to dopamine, which is transported and stored at nerve endings[2]. Dopamine is subsequently converted to norepinephrine and stored in vesicles in adrenergic nerves (see *Figure 9.4*). Sympathetic nerve stimulation causes norepinephrine vesicles to fuse to the membrane and be released into the synaptic cleft. Norepinephrine then crosses the synaptic cleft and binds at the alpha-1 receptor, activating a process that culminates in increased intracellular calcium and ultimately end-organ effects such as vasoconstriction. Simultaneously, some norepinephrine also binds at pre-synaptic alpha-2 receptors, inhibiting further norepinephrine release and ongoing sympathetic stimulation. Adrenergic receptor physiology provides insight into the employment of exogenous agonists in promoting vasoconstriction and use of alpha-2 agonists to lower blood pressure. Chapter 9 has additional details on alpha-adrenergic agonists and antagonists used for blood pressure control.

Table 8.1 Selectivity of catecholamines for adrenergic receptors at usual doses

Agent	Alpha$_1$	Alpha$_2$	Beta$_1$	Beta$_2$	Dopamine$_1$	Dopamine$_2$
Phenylephrine	++	0	0	0	0	0
Norepinephrine	+++	++	+++	+	0	0
Epinephrine	+++	+++	+++	++	0	0
Isoproterenol	0	0	+++	+++	0	0
Dopamine	0 to +++	0 to +	0 to +++	0 to ++	+++	++
Dobutamine	0 to +	0	+++	++	0	0
Fenaldopam	0	0	0	0	+++	0
Dopexamine	0	0	+	++	+++	++

+ to +++ indicate relative amounts of stimulation; these are not necessarily to scale between drugs. Some agents, particularly dopamine, have dose-dependent effects with alpha increasing at higher doses. 0, no effect.

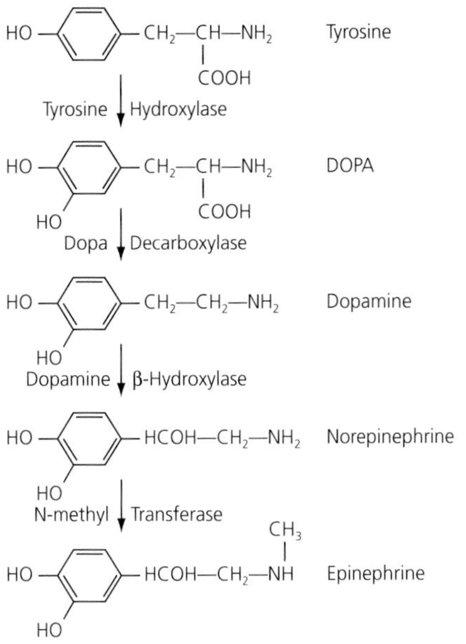

Figure 8.1 Synthetic pathway of catecholamines. Tyrosine from dietary sources is eventually synthesized into the endogenous catecholamines dopamine, norepinephrine and epinephrine. Substrate depletion impairs the body's ability to generate an appropriate catecholamine response. From: Chernow, B., Rainey, T.G. and Lake, C.R. (1982) Endogenous and exogenous catecholamines in critical care medicine. *Crit. Care Med.* **10**: 409–416. Reproduced with permission from Lippincott, Williams & Wilkins.

8.2.1 Adrenergic receptors

Properties of adrenergic receptors can be determined by radio-labeled binding, the effect of agonists and antagonists, and at a structural level. Although much more detail can be demonstrated experimentally, *Table 8.2* gives a clinically relevant summary for understanding adrenergic receptors. The alpha-1 adrenergic receptor controls blood pressure via vasoconstriction of arteries and arterioles. Alpha-adrenergic receptors also exist in the heart and are implicated in the genesis of cardiac arrhythmias; alpha-adrenergic receptor blockade has been shown to increase the threshold for epinephrine-induced arrhythmias[3]. The alpha-2 receptors on the pre-synaptic and post-synaptic membranes inhibit norepinephrine release and promote vasoconstriction, respectively. Beta-1 receptors mediate increases in heart rate, contractility, and conduction velocity. Beta-2 receptors mediate inotropy in the heart, and promote vasodilation in the lungs and peripheral vasculature. The dopamine 1 (DA-1) receptor produces both general and selective (renal and splanchnic) vasodilation, as well as specific effects on the renal proximal tubule and cortical collecting duct. DA-2 receptors, located on presynaptic

Table 8.2 Properties of adrenergic receptors

Receptor	Primary Location	Action
alpha$_1$	Postsynaptic	Vasoconstriction
alpha$_2$	Presynaptic Postsynaptic	Inhibits NE release Vaso- and veno-constriction
beta$_1$	Heart	Chronotropy and inotropy
beta$_2$	Lungs, vessels Myocardium	Broncho- and vasodilation Inotropy
DA$_1$	Postsynaptic smooth muscle Proximal tubule, cortical collecting duct	Peripheral vasodilation Increased RBF, natriuresis, diuresis
DA$_2$	Presynaptic nerve terminals Adrenal cortex Glomerulus	Vasodilation only if baseline norepinephrine levels elevated Decreased renal blood flow (RBF), glomerular filtration rate (GFR) and water excretion

nerve terminals, in the glomerulus and in the adrenal cortex, mediate peripheral vasodilation only if baseline norepinephrine levels are high at baseline. In contrast to DA-1 activation, DA-2 stimulation decreases renal blood flow, glomerular filtration rate and sodium and water excretion[4]. A patient's response to a given sympathomimetic agent depends on the dosage given as well as patient factors, so responses are not always predictable. In general, however, agonists produce relatively predictable results at relevant doses in most patients. Phenylephrine, for example, provides only alpha-adrenergic stimulation at usual doses, whereas isoproterenol provides only beta stimulation. Norepinephrine, epinephrine, dopamine and dobutamine have combined effects, which vary by infusion rate (*Table 8.1*). Fenoldopam, a relatively new agent, is highly selective for the DA-1 receptor.

8.3 Receptors and signal transduction

With the notable exceptions of steroids and thyroid stimulating hormone, most drugs and endogenous hormones are hydrophilic and can-

not easily cross cell membranes. A drug or a hormone must bind to a receptor on an extracellular surface. Signal transduction then generates a response from the cell by activating or inhibiting a secondary messenger.

Binding of a ligand to the extracellular surface of a receptor causes a change in membrane proteins resulting in an intracellular change (*Figure 8.2*). For example, binding of an alpha-1 agonist such as phenylephrine causes a change in the G_q protein activating phospholipase C to increase the intracellular concentrations of inositol 1,4,5-triphosphate (IP3) and diacetylglycerol (DAG). Alpha-2 agonists cause activation of an inhibitory G protein, inhibiting adenylyl cyclase and decreasing cyclic AMP concentrations within the cell. Conversely, beta-adrenergic agonists such as isoproterenol act through the G_s protein to stimulate adenylyl cyclase and increase cyclic AMP within the cell. Increased levels of cyclic AMP within the cell ultimately cause acceleration of heart rate or augmented cardiac contraction. *Figure 8.3* describes cyclic AMP metabolism by the enzyme phosphodiesterase F3. Two mechanisms thus exist for raising cyclic AMP levels within cells: stimulating the beta-adrenergic

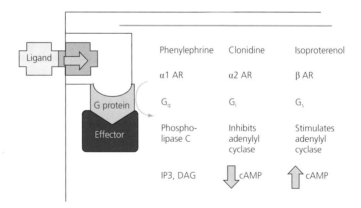

Figure 8.2 Signal transduction. Drugs or hormones (ligands) bind to extracellular adrenergic receptors (AR); an intermediary step of signal transduction, mediated by G proteins, is necessary to produce an action within the cell. IP3 (inositol 1,4,5-triphosphate) mobilizes calcium from intracellular stores. DAG (diacylglycerol) increases affinity of protein kinase C for intracellular calcium. cAMP (3',5'-cyclic adenosine monophosphate) is increased by the action of the G-stimulatory (Gs) protein, and decreased by the G-inhibitory (Gi) protein.

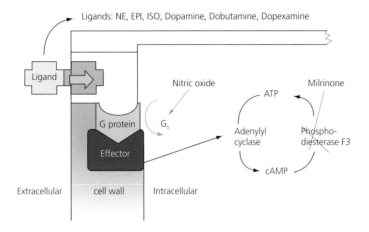

Ligands: NE, EPI, ISO, Dopamine, Dobutamine, Dopexamine

Ligand

Nitric oxide

ATP

Milrinone

G protein   G$_s$

Adenylyl cyclase

Phospho-diesterase F3

Effector

cAMP

Extracellular   cell wall   Intracellular

Figure 8.3 Generation of cyclic AMP. Intracellular increases in 3',5'-cyclic adenosine monophosphate (cAMP) result in increased inotropy and chronotropy. cAMP levels are increased through binding of adrenergic ligands and subsequent signal transduction. cAMP is broken down by phosphodiesterase F3, which is inhibited by the phosphodiesterase inhibitors amrinone and milrinone. This explains why phosphodiesterase inhibitors are effective in the presence of beta-adrenergic blockade, and also accounts for observed synergism in the clinical setting.

receptor and preventing the breakdown of cyclic AMP with a phosphodiesterase inhibitor such as milrinone. Inhibition of the phosphodiesterase pathway is particularly useful when receptor–effector coupling has been altered by sepsis[1] or other clinical conditions, or when access to the receptor is competitively blocked by agents (such as beta-adrenergic blockers) that prevent normal ligand–receptor binding.

8.4 Monitoring

Treatment with vasopressors or inotropes is justified when there is concern about the need to improve organ perfusion. Because our ability to monitor tissue perfusion is limited, we rely on non-specific findings such as oliguria, diminished arterial blood pressure and lactate generation. Depending on clinical circumstances, bedside examination, central venous pressure or PAC monitoring may help to establish the patient's volume status; echocardiography can demonstrate ventricular contractility and degree of ventricular filling. It is generally inappropriate to raise mean arterial pressure using pressor agents in a hypovolemic patient, unless such therapy is temporary while fluid resuscitation is under way. In a patient with hypoperfusion, the first question should be 'Is the volume status adequate?' (*Figure 8.4*). Hypovolemia should prompt fluid resuscitation, normally with crystalloid, but with blood if the hemoglobin level is already low (<7 g %) or is expected to drop further with aggressive volume repletion. Colloid solutions are rarely indicated for acute hypovolemia. Chapter 7 contains a more complete discussion of fluid choices in resuscitation.

Once volume status has been repleted, cardiac output should be reassessed. Inadequate cardiac output commonly reflects depressed ventricular function, resulting from ischemia, infarction, or sepsis-related myocardial depression. Other causes of acute decreases in cardiac output, such as cardiac tamponade, hypertrophic cardiomyopathy or pulmonary embolism, should be considered in the differential diagnosis. Inotropic support is contraindicated in the presence of hypertrophic cardiomyopathy, as increasing contractility with inotropes may worsen the obstruction. New presentation hypertrophic cardiomyopathy, which can be difficult to

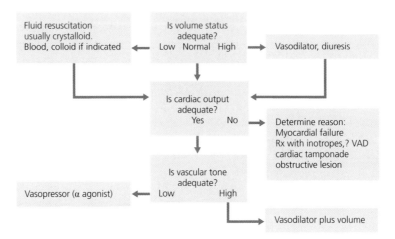

Figure 8.4 Algorithm for resuscitation. The patient's volume status must always be considered first, and then decisions made on the addition of inotropic or vasoconstrictive agents.

diagnose, requires a different therapeutic approach, including slowing the heart rate with a beta-adrenergic blocker, raising afterload, and providing adequate volume repletion. Myocardial failure secondary to most other causes will generally require inotropic support.

The final question to ask from a monitoring standpoint is whether or not vascular tone is adequate. A pulmonary artery catheter will allow calculation of systemic vascular resistance (SVR), which can guide titration of vasopressor support. SVR, however, is a calculated variable dependent on the vascular pressure gradient (MAP minus CVP) and the cardiac output. Under conditions of low cardiac output and low perfusion pressure, systemic vascular resistance might well be normal or low, prompting efforts to increase afterload, when in fact the underlying problem is inadequate cardiac output. Vasodilation may be apparent by clinical examination, although the classic picture of 'warm shock' can be modified when vascular disease is also present. Vasodilation responds to pressors, both alpha-adrenergic agonists such as norepinephrine and phenylephrine, and non-adrenergic agents such as vasopressin, discussed in section 8.8.

Inotropes and pressors are preferably administered through central lines because of the risk of IV infiltration, tissue necrosis and skin sloughing. If it is necessary to give an agent peripherally, the site should be carefully monitored. Phentolamine (5 mg in 10 cm³ normal saline) can be injected into areas of extravasation to limit tissue damage should infiltration occur with vasopressors.

8.5 Catecholamines and sympathomimetics

8.5.1 Phenylephrine (neo-synephrine)

This is an alpha-1 adrenergic agonist at conventional clinical doses, but activates the alpha-2- and beta-adrenergic receptors at 10-fold higher dose. Bolus doses of 50–100 µg IV increase systemic vascular resistance and typically improve perfusion pressure transiently. Infusions can be initiated at 0.5–1 µg kg^{-1} min^{-1} and titrated to clinical effect. Phenylephrine is usually mixed as 10–20 mg in 250 ml of D5W, but more concentrated mixtures may be used. Increased systemic vascular resistance from phenylephrine may cause reflex bradycardia, and this action of phenylephrine was once used to terminate supraventricular arrhythmias before the availability of more specific antiarrhythmics. Phenylephrine vasoconstricts renal, cutaneous and splanchnic vessels, but usually increases coronary perfusion as the result of improved diastolic perfusion pressure. However, phenylephrine is capable of constricting coronary vessels. Because phenylephrine has mostly alpha-1 effects, it is a useful agent in patients who develop tachyarrhythmias with norepinephrine or dopamine. Phenylephrine is compatible with a wide range of solutions and drugs, but incompatible with amphotericin B, azathiapine, gancyclovir, human insulin, pentamidine, and propofol. The bottom line is that phenylephrine is not as potent as norepinephrine or epinephrine, but can be extremely useful in the management of septic shock because it can selectively reverse vasodilating hypertension without causing undue cardiac stimulation.

8.5.2 Norepinephrine

Norepinephrine (Levophed) is primarily an alpha agonist, but stimulates beta receptors at doses as low as 2 µg min^{-1}. Norepinephrine is indicated for septic shock or severe vasodilation, once volume status is repleted. The standard mix for norepinephrine is 8 mg in 250 ml of D5W, but it is not uncommon to concentrate it further in patients requiring very high doses (see *Table 8.3*). The typical starting dose of norepinephrine is 0.1 µg kg^{-1} min^{-1}, increasing by 0.1 µg kg^{-1} min^{-1} every 5–10 min based on hemodynamic response. There is no upper limit to the dose of norepinephrine that can be used for short periods of time, but patients requiring very high doses (>2 µg kg^{-1} min^{-1}) for prolonged periods often have a refractory condition with poor likelihood of survival. Norepinephrine administration is associated with a poor outcome in patients with high degrees of organ failure or a delay of more than 1 day from ICU admission to norepinephrine therapy[5]. Norepinephrine infusion must be weaned slowly over 6–24 h to avoid abrupt hypotension. Norepinephrine is compatible with most anti-arrhythmics, other pressors and inotropes, heparin, and sedative agents such as midazolam and morphine sulfate. It is incompatible with aminophylline, amphotericin B, azathiaprine, furosemide, gancyclovir, insulin, lidocaine, barbiturates and sodium bicarbonate.

Norepinephrine's renal vasoconstricting properties have raised concern about its use in oliguric patients, yet the balance of evidence suggests that improvement in renal and cardiac perfusion with norepinephrine may outweigh the renal vasoconstrictive effects. Desjars *et al.*[6] evaluated norepinephrine at doses of 0.5–1 µg kg^{-1} min^{-1} in hyperdynamic septic patients who remained hypotensive despite volume expansion and dopamine therapy. Infusion of norepinephrine increased mean arterial pressure and systemic vascular resistance, decreased heart rate, and resulted in either unchanged or increased cardiac output in most patients. Urine flow increased to more than 0.5 ml min^{-1} when a critical renal perfusion pressure was reached as long as there was no pre-existing renal damage. In a subsequent study[7] the same authors showed that norepinephrine in doses up to 1.5 µg kg^{-1} min^{-1} does not produce deleterious effects on the kidneys as measured by serial analysis of creatinine, osmolar and free water clearance.

8.5.3 Dopamine

Dopamine is the immediate precursor in the metabolic pathway leading to the production of norepinephrine. Dopamine produces selective vasodilation in the renal and splanchnic circulations, but does not cross the blood–brain barrier. Its hemodynamic effects are variable, depending on dose utilized. Dopaminergic receptors are considered to be activated at doses less than 5 µg kg^{-1} min^{-1} but perhaps more accurately the 'dopaminergic' range should be considered to encompass 0.3–5 µg kg^{-1} min^{-1}, overlapping into the beta-adrenergic range. The beta-adrenergic range is classically described as 5–10 µg kg^{-1} min^{-1}, but tachycardia and arrhythmias may occur with lower doses, and an inotropic effect can be seen with as little as 2 µg kg^{-1}

Table 8.3 Typical starting and high-end doses

Agent and preparation			Typical starting doses (80 kg patient)			High-end doses (80 kg patient)*		
Drug	Typical mixture	Concentration	μg kg⁻¹ min⁻¹	μg min⁻¹	cm³ h⁻¹	μg kg⁻¹ min⁻¹	μg min⁻¹	cm³ h⁻¹
Norepinephrine	8 mg/250 ml D5W	32 μg cm⁻³	0.1	8	15	1.6	128	240
Epinephrine	4 mg/250 ml D5W	10 μg cm⁻³	0.05	4	15	1	80	300
Phenylephrine	20 mg/250 ml D5W	80 μg cm⁻³	0.5	40	30	5	400	300
Dopamine (renal)	400 mg/250 ml D5W	1600 μg cm⁻³	0.5	40	1.5	5	400	15
Dopamine (beta)	800 mg/250 ml D5W	3200 μg cm⁻³	3	240	4.5	10	800	15
Dopamine (alpha)	800 mg/250 ml D5W	3200 μg cm⁻³	10	800	15	40	3200	60
Dobutamine	500 mg/250 ml D5W	2000 μg cm⁻³	5	400	12	40	3200	96
Isoproterenol	2 mg/500 ml D5W	4 μg cm⁻³	0.025	2	30	0.25	20	300
Fenoldopam	10 mg/250 ml NS or D5W	40 μg ml⁻¹	0.025	2	3	0.3	24	40
Milrinone	50 mg/250 ml NS or D5W	200 μg ml⁻¹	0.375	30	9	0.750	60	18

*Drugs should generally be concentrated when used at these doses to reduce fluid load.

min⁻¹. Vasoconstrictive effects as a result of alpha receptor activation generally occur at doses greater than 10 μg kg⁻¹ min⁻¹, but in septic patients much higher doses may in fact be necessary to achieve vasoconstriction. Clinically, some patients may demonstrate blood pressure changes even at very low doses of dopamine.

Dopamine increases renal sodium excretion independently of its effects on renal blood flow, probably through inhibition of tubular solute reabsorption. Schaer et al.[8] randomized animals to receive dopamine 4 μg kg⁻¹ min⁻¹ or placebo while at the same time receiving escalating doses of norepinephrine. Renal blood flow increased gradually with escalating doses of norepinephrine alone, reaching a 10% increase over baseline at the highest dose. However, when dopamine was combined with norepinephrine, renal blood flow increased approximately 40%. Renal vascular resistance increased with norepinephrine alone, but decreased with the addition of dopamine. Dopamine has been associated with a functional improvement in acute oliguria post cardiopulmonary bypass[9], decreased renal impairment with orthotopic liver transplantation[10] and a dose-dependent increase in urine output in oliguric uvolemic surgical intensive care patients[11]. Despite these observations, well-conducted outcome studies showing dopamine's advantage as a renal protective agent are still lacking, and no survival advantage has been documented[12]. Besides producing alpha- and beta-1-adrenergic activity, dopamine stimulates dopaminergic receptors on renal and splanchnic vessels. At high doses, it can precipitate myocardial ischemia and arrhythmias. Dopamine can be used independently to manage septic shock when the goal is to attain significant cardiac stimulation and moderate vasoconstriction. There are no data to confirm that low-dose dopamine clinically improves renal or splanchnic blood flow independent of other hemodynamic effects. The use of low-dose dopamine does not appear to improve survival or obviate the need for dialysis.[12]

8.5.4 Fenoldopam

Fenoldopam is a selective dopamine-1 (DA-1) agonist with no alpha- or beta-adrenergic effects. An increase in heart rate may be seen as a reflex response to dopaminergic mediated vasodilation and decreased blood pressure. Administration may cause dilation of the renal afferent and efferent arterioles and an increase in glomerular filtration rate, and an increased excretion of water and electrolytes. The drug is currently marketed as an alternative to IV. nitroprusside for acute blood pressure control. A starting dose of 0.1 μg kg⁻¹ min⁻¹ can be increased in 0.1 μg kg⁻¹ min⁻¹ increments every 20 min to a maximum dose of 1.7 μg kg⁻¹ min⁻¹. Fenoldopam increases sodium excretion in both normal and hypertensive individuals by increasing renal blood flow, inhibiting tubular reaborption of sodium, and possibly increasing glomerular filtration rate. Activation of the DA-1 receptor by either dopamine or fenoldopam can increase intraoccular pressure[13]; a relative contraindication in patients with glaucoma. Outcome studies regarding renal protective effects are under way. In normotensive volunteers given doses ranging from 0.03 to 0.3 μg kg⁻¹ min⁻¹, fenoldopam increased renal plasma flow (RPF) in a dose-dependent manner. At the lowest dose, this increase in RPF occurred in the absence of changes in mean arterial pressure or heart rate[14,15]. Fenoldopam has also been shown to reverse some of the adverse renal effects of PEEP[16].

Stimulation of the DA-1 (but not DA-2) receptor reduces gastric acid secretion and may reduce gastric ulcer formation. In an animal study, administration of fenoldopam decreased the incidence of gastric lesions, ulcer area, and mortality rate[17].

Fenoldopam is conjugated by liver enzymes before renal excretion, but is not dependent on the cytochrome P450 system. There are no toxic metabolites or known metabolic drug interactions, and no dosage adjustments are needed for renal or liver disease. Although not officially sanctioned for renal protective use, data suggest that doses of fenoldopam as low as 0.03–0.05 µg kg^{-1} min^{-1} (lower than the dose recommended for blood pressure reduction) may be effective.

8.5.5 Epinephrine

Epinephrine is an extremely potent alpha and beta-1 agonist with considerable beta-2 activity useful for treatment of bronchospasm, anaphylactic shock, septic or cardiogenic shock, asystole, or refractory hypotension. Reflex vagal effects are less intensive than with predominantly alpha agents. Epinephrine is a potent inotrope and increases stroke volume, coronary blood flow and heart rate, but may also be arrhythmogenic. Treatment of asystole requires the largest dose (1 mg or 10 cm^3 of a 1/10,000 solution) given by rapid IV infusion and repeated as necessary. High-dose bolus epinephrine (0.2 mg kg^{-1}) has been promoted as treatment for refractory asystole, but is not currently recommended by Advanced Cardiac Life Support (ACLS) guidelines. An advantage of epinephrine in patients lacking vascular access is that the drug can be given via the endotracheal route using approximately twice the i.v. dose diluted in normal saline or distilled water.

More conventionally, continuous infusions of epinephrine are used for treatment of refractory hypotension and septic or cardiogenic shock. Initial IV infusion rates for septic or cardiogenic shock begin at 1 µg min^{-1} (0.01 µg kg^{-1} min^{-1}), but refractory hypotension can require a starting dose of 0.05 µg kg^{-1} min^{-1} (4 µg min^{-1}) and may go 10–20–fold higher (see *Table 8.3*). Selective activation of the beta receptor occurs at lower doses, but receptor selectively is lost and then reversed in favor of alpha receptors at high doses. The danger of excessive infusion rates or rapid infusion is a precipitous rise in blood pressure, which could theoretically result in cerebral hemorrhage. Epinephrine is incompatible with alkaline solutions and becomes unstable if the pH is higher than 5.5. Like norepinephrine, epinephrine is compatible with most anti-arrhythmics (except lidocaine), and most sedatives and neuromuscular blocking agents (exceptions being barbiturates and propofol).

Epinephrine is incompatible with aminophyline, amphotericin B, some antibiotics and sodium bicarbonate. Like other catecholamines, epinephrine has a short half-life, with metabolism by catecholamine-*o*-methyl transferase (COMT) and monoamine oxidase (MAO). Caution should be exercised when administering catecholamines to patients who have previously received MAO inhibitors.

8.5.6 Dobutamine

Dobutamine (Dobutrex) possesses only small amounts of alpha-receptor activity, and produces mostly beta-receptor stimulation of the heart. Compared with dopamine, dobutamine increases cardiac output with less tachycardia and smaller increases in arterial and pulmonary pressures. It may be better tolerated than dopamine in the setting of heart failure, because of its pulmonary vasodilating effects. The expected hemodynamic responses of dobutamine can be altered by preoperative beta-adrenergic blockade[18]. Sepsis may also alter the expected response, if alpha-adrenergic (vasoconstrictive) responses do not balance the beta-2 vasodilatory response. Usual hemodynamic actions of dobutamine at infusion rates of 2–10 µg kg^{-1} min^{-1} include an increase in cardiac output and stroke volume, little or no change in heart rate, and a decrease in pulmonary capillary wedge pressure and systemic vascular resistance. Dobutamine may produce substantial systemic and pulmonary vasodilation in the clinical setting, an effect that can be used to advantage in patients with pulmonary hypertension or right ventricular failure. Dobutamine is the preferred agent in the setting of hypoxemic respiratory failure and normotensive left ventricular failure, especially post-myocardial infarction, because additional vasoconstriction is not necessary in these situations and may actually worsen right ventricular function. Synergistic effects have been noted when combining dobutamine and phosphodiesterase inhibitors[19]. Dobutamine may also be given concurrently with norepinephrine if the expected decrease in SVR results in unacceptable hypotension.

Combination therapy with an α-agonist significantly improves mean pressure, cardiac index and left ventricular stroke-work index in dobutamine-resistant septic shock[20].

8.5.7 Isoproterenol

Isoproterenol (Isuprel) acts almost exclusively on the beta-adrenergic system. By increasing cutaneous and muscular vasodilation, the drug may redistribute blood to nonessential areas, resulting in significant hypotension. Isoproterenol was once utilized in therapy of cardiac failure because of its effects on inotropic activity and its potential for increasing cardiac output by augmenting preload and reducing afterload. With the availability of phosphodiesterase inhibitors, isoproterenol is now rarely used other than for management of bradyarrhythmias. Isoproterenol is generally mixed 1–4 mg in 250 ml of D5W or normal saline and titrated in the range of 0.05–0.5 $\mu g\ kg^{-1}\ min^{-1}$.

8.5.8 Dopexamine

Dopexamine is principally a dopaminergic and beta-2 agonist[21]; it is not yet available in the United States. Hemodynamic effects at doses of 1–6 $\mu g\ kg^{-1}\ min^{-1}$ include decreased mean arterial pressure and systemic vascular resistance; increased heart rate by reflex action; improved organ blood flow to cardiac, hepatic, splanchnic, and renal beds; and increased inotropy via beta-2 cardiac stimulation[22]. Dopexamine at lower doses (0.5–2.0 $\mu g\ kg^{-1}\ min^{-1}$) may have utility in promoting gut mucosal blood flow in high-risk patients[23], via direct splanchnic vasodilation.

8.6 Alterations in adrenergic response

A variety of factors influence the expected response of adrenergic receptors to endogenous and exogenous catecholamines (*Table 8.4*). Mild acidosis increases catecholamine synthesis and secretion, but severe acidosis (pH < 7.10) is associated with decreased cardiac contractility, diminished cardiac output, and a

Table 8.4 Alterations in catecholamine function

Acid–base status	Downregulation (stimulation)
Age	Electrolyte disorder
Alpha-blockers	Hemodilution
Anesthetics or opioids	Hypothermia
Beta-blockers	Individual variation
Calcium channel blockers	Sepsis
Congestive heart failure	Substrate depletion
Denervation	Surgical stress
Diabetes mellitus	Upregulation (blockade)

systemic vasoconstrictive response. Acidosis also may produce difficulty with defibrillation[24]. Alkalosis decreases catecholamine secretion, inhibits sympathetic nervous system activity, and results in decreased vasoconstrictive ability, accentuated vasodilation, and a propensity to ventricular dysrhythmias[24]. In untreated shock states, acidosis is more common, but alkalosis can result from overaggressive buffer therapy. Many clinicians choose to treat metabolic acidosis when arterial pH values are substantially below 7.25 but tolerate mild degrees of acidosis rather than risk overcorrection and alkalosis.

8.6.1. Receptor upregulation and downregulation

Tachyphylaxis, or a reduction in the expected response to an agonist with repeated use, is familiar to anyone who has overused over-the-counter nasal decongestants. Tachyphylaxis appears to be mediated either by uncoupling of receptors from G proteins, or a net internalization of hormone-receptor complexes within the cell[25], a process called 'downregulation' (*Figure 8.5*). Upregulation, an increase in the number of receptors per cell, occurs following chronic receptor blockade (*Figure 8.6*). This phenomenon becomes especially important if the chronic blockade is suddenly terminated,

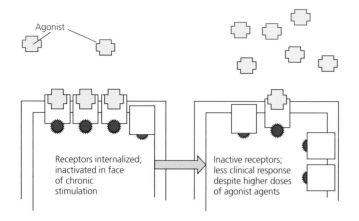

Figure 8.5 Downregulation (internalization and inactivation of adrenergic receptors) occurs after chronic stimulation. Higher doses of agonist agents are required to obtain the desired effect.

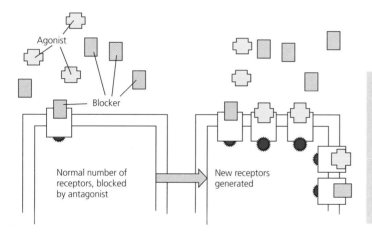

Figure 8.6 Upregulation occurs following chronic blockade. New receptors are generated; if the blocking agent is suddenly withdrawn (as might happen with cessation of chronic antihypertensive beta-adrenergic blocking agents), an exaggerated clinical response will be seen with subsequent stimulation.

as the more numerous and now unoccupied receptors can generate an exaggerated clinical response. For example, when propranolol therapy is withdrawn perioperatively, an increased response to isoproterenol can be seen during the next 12–48 h; clinical withdrawal of beta blockade can precipitate undesirable tachycardia.

8.6.2 Electrolyte disorders and adrenergic response

Adrenergic receptor action is a calcium-dependent process, and the level of serum electrolytes modulates the activity of the endogenous sympathetic system and exogenous pharmacologic agents. Within a relevant range, left ventricular contractility varies directly with blood-ionized calcium levels[26].

Normal circulating calcium concentrations are needed for adequate myocardial performance and maintenance of vascular tone. Patients with Gram-negative infection, however, may develop hypocalcemia as a result of parathyroid gland dysfunction and/or vitamin D insufficiency[27]. Concerns have been raised, however, over calcium administration in sepsis, because increased mortality has been noted in calcium-treated animals with endotoxic shock[28].

Hypophosphatemia is also common in critically ill patients and contributes to respiratory insufficiency, erythrocyte and leukocyte dysfunction, metabolic acidosis, and central nervous system dysfunction. Maintenance of normal levels of 2,3–diphosphoglycerate requires normal phosphate metabolism.

Correction of hypophosphatemia improves myocardial function possibly via improving intracellular availability of ATP[29].

Hypomagnesemia is another common finding in the critically ill. Magnesium has a permissive action on parathyroid hormone (PTH) release, and thus, hypomagnesemia may contribute to hypocalcemia.

8.7 Bypassing the adrenergic receptor

8.7.1 Phosphodiesterase inhibitors
Phosphodiesterase inhibitors (PDIs) prevent the breakdown of cAMP and increase intracellular cAMP levels (see *Figure 8.3*). Selective phosphodiesterase inhibitors include amrinone, milrinone, enoximone and a number of experimental agents; all raise intracellular cAMP levels by inhibiting phosphodiesterase F_3. Because the PDIs act intracellularly and bypass both the adrenergic receptor and the calcium channel, they can reverse the cardiopressant effects of drugs such as verapamil and propranolol[30]. Administration of the PDI amrinone significantly improves cardiac index, pulmonary capillary wedge pressure and right atrial pressure, and decreases systemic vascular resistance and pulmonary vascular resistance in low output states[31]. Amrinone may also have advantages over the alpha-adrenergic agents in restoring intracellular calcium levels toward normal[32]. Dobutamine and amrinone at equipotent doses produce similar effects on cardiac index, pulmonary capillary wedge pressure, mean right atrial pressure, heart rate, systemic vascular resistance, and mean arterial pressure[33]. The addition of amrinone to 15 µg kg^{-1} min^{-1} of dobutamine has an additional synergistic effect, resulting in continued increase in ejection fraction[34]. Combination therapy with dopamine and amrinone has also been described in the setting of refractory low-output syndrome after open heart surgery[35].

8.7.2 Milrinone
Milrinone is a chemical relative of amrinone with higher potency and fewer side effects.

Milrinone is more cost effective and is largely supplanting amrinone, although both drugs remain available in the United States. Milrinone is given as a 50–75 µg kg^{-1} i.v. bolus, followed by a 0.3–0.75 µg kg^{-1} min^{-1} infusion. Hypotension, tachycardia, atrial fibrillation, and atrial bigeminy can occur, as with amrinone, but milrinone is associated with a lower incidence of fever and thrombocytopenia. In patients with congestive heart failure, both milrinone and dobutamine improve cardiac index, but dobutamine increases myocardial oxygen consumption, whereas milrinone does not[36].

8.8 Vasopressin

The body's response to stress includes release of epinephrine, cortisol, corticotropin, renin and vasopressin. Vasopressin is released in response to decreased blood volume, increased plasma osmolality, and pain. Endogenous release of vasopressin corresponds with the return of spontaneous circulation after cardiopulmonary resuscitation[37], leading to speculation that exogenous vasopressin might be useful in shock. Experimentally, vasopressin increases vital organ flow more than epinephrine[38]. Synergistic effects of vasopressin plus epinephrine have been noted in a porcine cardiopulmonary resuscitation model[39]. Vasopressin has also been shown to reverse intractable hypotension in the late phase of hemorrhagic shock in dogs[40].

Clinical studies in humans are limited[41]. Increases in mean arterial pressure and systemic vascular resistance are observed when vasopressin is infused in septic, but not cardiogenic shock, patients[42]. In septic trauma patients, infusion of vasopressin at 0.04 U min^{-1} increased blood pressure and systemic vascular resistance and increased ability to wean from pressors[43]. Vasopressin has also been used in a bolus dose of 40 U (*c.* 0.5 U kg^{-1}) to restore spontaneous cardiovascular function in patients failing IV epinephrine and defibrillation[44].

As discussed earlier, responsiveness to beta stimulation is reduced in sepsis and severe heart failure. Although milrinone may improve inotropy and reduce afterload in this situation, it is often associated with unacceptable hypotension. One recent approach has been to combine vasopressin with milrinone, as the afterload increasing effects of vasopressin are offset by milrinone and the hypotensive effects of the milrinone may be specifically inhibited by vasopressin[45].

Large-scale trials are necessary before the routine use of vasopressin can be recommended, and it is not currently FDA-approved for this indication. However, synthetic vasopressin (DDAVP, desmopressin) is readily available for other indications and the literature supports initial doses in the range of 0.01–0.07 U min^{-1}, with upward titration as needed. Appropriate monitoring should be carried out to ensure that the increase in afterload does not adversely decrease cardiac output. In addition to the expected effect of increased afterload, there is the possibility of coronary and mesenteric vasoconstriction, which argues for continuous EKG monitoring.

8.9 Weaning pharmacologic support

The rapidity with which pharmacologic support can be weaned from the patient in shock must be individualized, and depends on the length of inotropic therapy, patient characteristics and the half-lives of the agents used. For catecholamines, which have short half-lives (minutes), titration can be rapid, with decreases of 10–25% on a half-hour or hourly basis, relying on clinical monitoring to determine the end point of weaning. The PDIs have longer half-lives (50 min for milrinone, >200 min for amrinone) and can be decreased by 50–100% acutely, but require a longer period of observation (6–8 h) before further weaning is attempted.

8.9.1 Removal of monitoring and ICU discharge

Despite the extremely high mortality rate with circulatory shock, some patients demon-strate hemodynamic improvement, which may either be dramatic or gradual over a period of a week or more. Surviving patients often have multi-organ system dysfunction or continued respiratory support needs. The pulmonary artery catheter should be removed when the cardiac index has been stable and the information gained from the catheter no longer outweighs the risk of leaving it in place. Most patients can be weaned from inotropic support without a pulmonary artery catheter in place, although continued central venous monitoring and arterial monitoring are usually helpful. Removal of central venous lines often depends more on vascular access requirements for medication and total parenteral nutrition rather than the need for CVP readings.

The patient is ready for ICU discharge when hemodynamics have been stable for an extended period of time (12–24 h) and when the likelihood of emergent return to the ICU from the 'floor' is small. Beware that the phosphodiesterase inhibitors have a longer 'tail-end' effect; 36–48 h of post-infusion monitoring may be more appropriate in these patients. Discharge criteria also depend on the hospital's facilities and nursing staffing ratios, including availability of monitoring on a ward or intermediate level unit.

8.10 Summary

Pharmacologic support is most effective when intravascular volume is repleted and the patient's acid–base status is normal. Catecholamines are chosen on the basis of inotropic and peripheral vasoconstrictive effects; combination therapy may be needed to address both inotropic and pressor needs. Catecholamine response may be altered by the patient's premorbid condition, acidosis, prolonged drug therapy (downregulation), and hypothermia. Although the catecholamines and phosphodiesterase inhibitors are at present the approved therapeutic options, vasopressin is emerging as a valuable adjunct, particularly in sepsis.

References

1. Matsuda, N., Hattori, Y., Akaishi, Y. *et al.* (2000) Impairment of cardiac β-adrenoceptor cellular signaling by decreased expression of G_{sa} in septic rabbits. *Anesthesiology* **93**: 1465–1473.

2. Karamian, A. (1984) Physiology of the nervous system: The autonomic nervous system. In: *Physiology for the Anesthesiologist*, 2nd Edn (eds N. Goudsozin and A. Karamian). Appleton Century Crofts, Norwalk, CT, p. 328.

3. Maze, M., Haywood, E. and Gaba, D.M. (1985) Alpha-1 adrenergic blockade raises epinephrine arrhythmic threshold in halothane anesthetized dogs in a dose dependent fashion. *Anesthesiology* **63**: 611.

4. Carey, R.M., Siragy, H.M., Ragsdale, N.V., *et al.* (1990) Dopamine-1 and dopamine-2 mechanisms in the control of renal function. *Am. J. Hypertension* **3**: 595–635.

5. Abid, O., Akca, S., Haji-Michael, P., *et al.* (2000) Strong vasopressor support may be futile in the intensive care unit patient with multiple organ failure. *Crit. Care Med.* **28**: 947–949.

6. Desjars, P., Pinaud, M., Potel, G., *et al.* (1987) A reappraisal of norepinephrine therapy in human septic shock. *Crit. Care Med.* **15**: 134–137.

7. Desjars, P., Pinaud, M., Bugnon, D. and Tasseau, F. (1989) Norepinephrine therapy has no deleterious renal effects in human septic shock. *Crit. Care Med.* **17**: 426–429.

8. Schaer, G.L., Fink, M.P. and Parrillo, J.E. (1985) Norepinephrine alone versus norepinephrine plus low-dose dopamine enhanced renal blood flow with combination pressor therapy. *Crit. Care Med.* **13**: 492–496.

9. Davis, R.F., Lappas, D.G., Kirklin, J.K., *et al.* (1982) Acute oliguria after cardiopulmonary bypass renal functional improvement with low-dose dopamine infusion. *Crit. Care Med.* **10**: 852–856.

10. Polson, R.J., Park, G.R., Lindop, M.J., *et al.* (1987) The prevention of renal impairment in patients undergoing orthotopic liver grafting by infusion of low dose dopamine. *Anaesthesia* **42**: 15–19.

11. Flancbaum, L., Choban, P.S. and Dasta, J.F. (1994) Quantitative effects of low-dose dopamine on urine output in oliguric surgical intensive care unit patients. *Crit. Care Med.* **22**: 61–66.

12. Chertow, G.M., Sayegh, M.H., Allgren, R.L., *et al.* (1996) Is the administration of dopamine associated with adverse or favorable outcomes in acute renal failure? *Am. J. Med.* **101**: 49–53.

13. Brath, P.C., MacGregor, D.A., Ford, J.G. and Prielipp, R.C. (2000) Dopamine and intraocular pressure in critically ill patients. *Anesthesiology* **93**: 1398–1400.

14. Mathur, V.S., Swan, S.K., Lambrecht, L.J., *et al.* (1999) The effects of fenoldopam, a selective dopamine receptor agonist, on systemic and renal hemodynamics in normotensive subjects. *Crit. Care Med.* **27**: 1832–1837.

15. Murphy, M.B., McCoy, C.E., Weber, R.R., *et al.* (1987) Augmentation of renal blood flow and sodium excretion in hypertensive patients during blood pressure reduction by intravenous administration of the dopamine$_1$ agonist fenoldopam. *Circulation* **78**: 1312–1318.

16. Poinsot, O., Romand, J.-A., Favre, H. and Suter, P.M. (1993) Fenoldopam improves renal hemodynamics impaired by positive end-expiratory pressure. *Anesthesiology* **79**: 680–684.

17. Desai, J.K., Goyal, R.K. and Parmar, N.S. (1999) Characterization of dopamine receptor subtypes involved in experimentally induced gastric and duodenal ulcers in rates. *J. Pharmacol.* **51**: 187–192.

18. Tarnow, J. and Komar, K. (1988) Altered hemodynamic response to dobutamine in relation to the degree of preoperative β-adrenoreceptor blockade. *Anesthesiology* **68**: 912.

19. Uretsky, B.F., Lawless, C.E., Verbalis, J.G., *et al.* (1987) Combined therapy with dobutamine and amrinone in severe heart failure. *Chest* **92**: 657–662.

20. Martin, C., Vivland, X., Arnaud, S., *et al.* (1999) Effects of norepinephrine plus dobutamine or norepinephrine alone on left ventricular performance of septic shock patients. *Crit. Care Med.* **27**: 1708–1713.

21. Vincent, J.-L., Reuse, C. and Kahn, R.J. (1989) Administration of dopexamine, a new adrenergic agent, in cardiorespiratory failure. *Chest* **96**: 1233.

22. Poelaert, J.I.T., Mungroop, H.E., Koolen, J.J. and Van den Berg, P.C.M. (1989) Hemodynamic effects of dopexamine in patients following coronary artery bypass surgery. *J. Cardiothorac. Anesth.* **3**: 441–443.

23. Byers, R.J., Eddleston, J.M., Pearson, R.C., *et al.* (1999) Dopexamine reduces the incidence of acute inflammation in the gut mucosa after abdominal surgery in high-risk patients. *Crit. Care Med.* **27**: 1787–1793.

24. Barton, M., Lake, C.R., Rainey, T.G. and Chernow, B. (1982) Is catecholamine release pH mediated? *Crit. Care Med.* **10**: 751–753.

25. Lefkowitz, R.J., Caron, M.G. and Stiles, G.L. (1984) Mechanisms of membrane-receptor regulation. *N. Engl. J. Med.* **310**: 1570–1576.

26. **Lang, R.M., Fellner, S.K., Neumann, A., et al.** (1988) Left ventricular contractility varies directly with blood ionized calcium. *Ann. Intern. Med.* **108:** 524–529.

27. **Zaloga, G.P. and Chernow, B.** (1987) The multifactorial basis for hypocalcemia during sepsis. *Ann. Intern. Med.* **107:** 36.

28 **Malcolm, D.S., Zaloga, G.P. and Holaday, J.W.** (1989) Calcium administration increases the mortality of endotoxic shock in rats. *Crit. Care Med.* **17:** 900.

29. **O'Connor, L.R., Wheeler, W.S. and Bethune, J.E.** (1977) Effect of hypophosphatemia on myocardial performance in man. *N. Engl. J. Med.* **297:** 901.

30. **Makela, V.H.M. and Kapur, P.A.** (1987) Amrinone and verapamil–propranolol induced cardiac depression during isoflurane anesthesia in dogs. *Anesthesiology* **66:** 792.

31. **Goenen, M., Pedemonte, O., Baele, P. and Col, J.** (1985) Amrinone in the management of low cardiac output after open heart surgery. *Am. J. Cardiol.* **56:** 33B.

32. **Auffermann, W., Stefenelli, T., Wu, S.T., et al.** (1991) Influence of positive inotropic agents on intracellular calcium transients. Part I. Normal rat heart. *Am. Heart J.* **118:** 1219–1227.

33. **Benotti, J.R., McCue, J.E. and Alpert, J.S.** (1985) Comparative vasoactive therapy for heart failure. *Am. J. Cardiol.* **56:** 1B.

34. **Sundram, P., Reddy, H.K., McElroy, P.A., et al.** (1990) Myocardial energetics and efficiency in patients with idiopathic cardiomyopathy: response to dobutamine and amrinone. *Am. Heart J.* **119:** 891.

35. **Olsen, K.H., Kluger, J. and Fieldman, A.** (1988) Combination high dose amrinone and dopamine in the management of moribund cardiogenic shock after open heart surgery. *Chest* **94:** 503.

36. **Grose, R., Strain, J., Greenberg, M. and Lejemtel, T.H.** (1986) Systemic and coronary effects of intravenous milrinone and dobutamine in congestive heart failure. *J. Am. Coll. Cardiol. 7:* 1107.

37. **Lindner, K.H., Strohmenger, H.U., Ensinger, H., et al.** (1992) Stress hormone response during and after cardiopulmonary resuscitation. *Anesthesiology* **77:** 662–668.

38. **Eichinger, M.R. and Walker, B.R.** (1994) Enhanced pulmonary arterial dilatation to arginine vasopressin in the chronically hypoxic rat. *Am. J. Physiol.* **267:** H2413–H2429.

39. **Mulligan, K.A., McKnite, S.H., Lindner, K.H., et al.** (1997) Synergistic effects of vasopressin plus epinephrine during cardiopulmonary resuscitation. *Resuscitation* **35:** 265–271.

40. **Morales, D., Madigan, J., Cullinane, S., et al.** (1999) Reversal by vasopressin of intractable hypotension in the late phase of hemorrhage shock. *Circulation* **100:** 226–229.

41. **Mets, B., Michler, R.E., Delphin, E.D., et al.** (1998) Refractory vasodilation after cardiopulmonary bypass for heart transplantation in recipients on combined amiodarone and angiotensin-converting enzyme inhibitor therapy: A role for vasopressin administration. *J. Cardiothorac. Vasc. Anes.* **12:** 326–329.

42. **Landry, D.W., Levin, H.R., Gallant, E.M., et al.** (1997) Vasopressin deficiency contributes to the vasodilation of septic shock. *Circulation* **95:** 1122–1125.

43. **Malay, M.B., Ashton, R.C., Landry, D.W., et al.** (1999) Low-dose vasopressin in the treatment of vasodilatory septic shock. *J. Trauma Infect. Crit. Care* **47:** 699–705.

44 **Lindner, K.H., Prengel, A.W., Brinkman, A., et al.** (1996) Vasopressin administration in refractory cardiac arrest. *Ann. Intern. Med.* **124:** 1061–1064.

45. **Gold, J., Cullinane, S., Chen, J., et al.** (2000) Vasopressin in the treatment of milrinone-induced hypotension in severe heart failure. *Am. J. Cardiol.* **85:** 506–509.

Chapter 9

Hypertensive urgencies and emergencies

Thomas L. Higgins, MD

Contents

9.1 Introduction

Hypertensive urgencies and emergencies can account for ICU admission or prolonged critical care length-of-stay. Interventions to control blood pressure elevations in the ICU range from simple sedation and analgesia to multi-drug IV regimens. Most blood pressure elevation can be controlled over the course of several hours with oral agents, given if necessary via orogastric or feeding tube. Hypertensive emergencies require immediate aggressive intervention while avoiding overtreatment and consequent hypotension. For malignant hypertension, it is recommended to lower the MAP by about 25% over the first 2–4 h, while keeping the diastolic blood pressure above 100 mmHg. Initial therapy should be instituted while searching for an underlying cause (*Tables 9.1–9.3*). Although there are no studies showing an outcome benefit with a particular treatment regimen, an understanding of the pathophysiology causing the hypertension can help rationalize the choice of antihypertensives.

9.2 Definitions

Hypertension is frequently defined as systolic blood pressure in excess of 160 mmHg, and/or diastolic pressure above 90 mmHg. Perioperative hypertension is defined as an increase of more than 20% over preoperative levels[1]. The importance of any given blood pressure reading, however, will vary by age, gender, and clinical circumstances.

Hypertensive crisis is a severe elevation of blood pressure and may be urgent or emergent. Accelerated hypertension, also called hypertensive urgency, is defined by diastolic blood pressures greater than 120 mmHg without evidence of end-organ injury. Malignant hypertension or hypertensive emergency is accelerated hypertension with evidence of end-organ damage, typically a necrotizing vasculitis that results in small-vessel occlusion. The presence of retinopathy helps distinguish malignant from accelerated hypertension. Patients with either accelerated or malignant

Table 9.1 Medical causes of hypertension

Essential hypertension
Renal disease
- Acute or chronic renal failure
- Renovascular hypertension

Endocrine-related disorders
- Hypoglycemia
- Hyperthyroidism
- Pheochromocytoma (diagnosed or latent)
- Catecholamine-secreting tumors
- Hyperparathyroidism
- Acromegaly
- Myxedema
- Cushing's syndrome
- Carcinoid syndrome
- Renin-secreting tumors

Myocardial ischemia or infarction

Medication related
- Rebound: clonidine, beta blockers
- Monoamine oxidase inhibitors
- Tricyclic antidepressant

Other
- Obesity
- Advanced age
- Pregnancy (preeclampsia or eclampsia)
- Oral contraceptives
- Alcohol or opioid withdrawal
- Polyarteritis nodosa
- Hypercalcemia
- Increased intracranial pressure

hypertension may have nonspecific symptoms such as headache and blurred vision, and cardiac symptoms are common. Nausea, vomiting and focal neurologic deficits are uncommon. Hypertensive encephalopathy is a central nervous system vasculopathy usually seen in patients with chronic hypertension. Headache, nausea, vomiting, blurred vision and confusion are common findings with hypertensive encephalopathy; focal neurologic deficits may also occur.

Medical emergencies commonly associated with hypertension include acute renal failure, pulmonary edema, eclampsia, cerebral ischemia, cerebral hemorrhage, angina, pheochromocytoma, monoamine oxidase (MAO) inhibitor crisis, cocaine overdose, and antihypertensive withdrawal syndrome. Postoperative hypertension occurs in 3–6% of

Table 9.2 Surgical and anesthetic events associated with hypertension

Surgical causes

Cardiac surgery
- Myocardial revascularization
- Valve repair or replacement
- Heart transplantation

Vascular surgery
- Aortic aneurysm resection
- Aortic coarctation
- Carotid endarterectomy

Neurosurgical procedures
- Neurovascular procedures
- Increased intracranial pressure
- Autonomic hyperreflexia

Abdominal surgery
- Endocrine tumors
- Liver transplantation
- Renal surgery and transplantation
- Urologic surgery

Obstetric surgery
- Eclampsia
- Preeclampsia
- Hypertension of pregnancy

Radical neck dissection

Anesthetic causes

Intravenous agents
- Opioids (meperidine or pethidine)
- Ketamine
- Neuroleptic agents
- Opioid antagonists

Anesthetic emergence
- Metabolism of intravenous agents
- Rebound from induced hypotension

Regional anesthesia
- Systemic absorption of epinephrine
- Tourniquet pain

Endotracheal intubation

Residual intraoperative medications
- Vasopressor effect
- Anticholinergics

Preoperative medications
- Monoamine oxidase inhibitors
- Tricyclic antidepressants
- Illicit drugs
- Nonprescription drugs

Discontinuation of preoperative medication
- Beta blocker therapy
- Clonidine

Table 9.3 Quick differential checklist for hypertension in the ICU

- Hypoxemia
- Hypercarbia
- Acidosis
- Pain
- Anxiety
- Shivering
- Hypervolemia
- Hypovolemia
- Ventilator dyssynchrony or stimulation from endotracheal tube
- Distended bladder, stomach, or intestine

patients following non-cardiac surgery[1,2], and up to 50% following myocardial revascularization[3]. Postoperative hypertension is a significant risk factor for myocardial ischemia, heart failure and cerebrovascular events. Pain, bladder distention, hypothermia with shivering, and intolerance of endotracheal intubation can trigger hypertension as patients emerge from anesthesia. Patients may also experience respiratory difficulties related to airway obstruction or prior sedation and neuromuscular blockade, resulting in hypercapnia, hypoxemia, or acidosis, which further increases sympathetic tone. The increased sympathetic nervous system activity results in both alpha-1-mediated vasoconstriction increasing vascular resistance and venous return, and beta-1-receptor-mediated increases in the heart rate.

Hypotension is subnormal arterial blood pressure, but the precise level at which a patient might be considered hypotensive is situation-specific. Mean arterial pressures of 60 mmHg or lower can be seen normally in healthy, young individuals who are asleep or sedated, but pressures this low raise concern in most critically ill patients. In individuals with chronic hypertension, hypertrophy of the arterial musculature limits the ability of vascular beds to vasodilate when MAP drops. Hypertensive individuals have a rightward shift in their cerebral autoregulatory curve (*Figure 9.1*), and may develop symptoms of ischemia even at pressures more than adequate for normotensive patients. Tissue perfusion depends on the resistance of the vascular bed, so a MAP of 60 mmHg may produce sufficient flow in the presence of vasodilation, whereas a MAP of 100 mmHg could be inadequate in the presence of severe vasoconstriction. End-organ assessment (cerebral function, myocardial function, urine output, peripheral skin temperature) tempers the clinical interpretation of hypotension. Common causes of low blood pressure are hypovolemia, decreased venous and/or arterial tone, and decreased cardiac output. Chapter 8 more fully describes shock states and the interactions between blood pressure, myocardial function, and systemic vascular resistance.

9.3 Physiology of blood pressure control: MAP = SVR × CO

Systemic vascular resistance is determined primarily by the state of vascular smooth muscle tone, which in turn depends on input from the adrenergic and renin–angiotensin systems as well as local control from vascular endothelium (*Figure 9.2*). Cardiac output is determined by heart rate and stroke volume. Stroke volume in turn is determined by cardiac preload, afterload and myocardial contractility. The circulatory system has highly sophisticated mechanisms for maintaining mean arterial

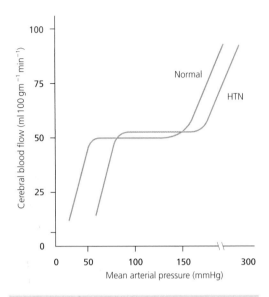

Figure 9.1 Cerebral autoregulation. HTN, hypertension.

pressure in the normal range. These control mechanisms (*Table 9.4*) may be categorized as short-term, intermediate, or long-term. Rapidly acting control mechanisms (seconds to minutes) rely on baroreceptor and chemoreceptor feedback to regulate central nervous system responses. Baroreceptors are located in the walls of large arteries in the thoracic and cervical regions, most notably in the aorta and the internal carotid artery. As blood pressure increases, stretch of nerve endings signals for inhibition of the medullary vasoconstrictive center, enhancement of vagal tone, and ultimately peripheral vasodilation, diminished heart rate, and diminished force of myocardial contraction. The baroreceptor response adapts to persistent pressure changes over a 24–48 h period, limiting its utility in chronic hypertension[4]. Baroreflex failure rarely occurs, but may present as severe labile hypertension and/or hypotension with elevated plasma catecholamine levels[5].

Chemoreceptors respond to decreased oxygen supply and accumulation of excess hydrogen ion[6]. Unlike the baroreceptors, which are active in the normal blood pressure range, chemoreceptors do not respond until

Table 9.4 Blood pressure adaptation and control mechanisms

Adaptation	Onset	Peak effect	Duration	Feedback
Short term				
Baroreceptor	<15 s	30 s	2–4 days	Pressure
Chemoreceptor	<15 s	60 s	Prolonged	PO_2, PCO_2, pH
Central nervous system	<15 s	Minutes	Prolonged	Ischemia
Intermediate				
Stress relaxation	30 s	Days	Prolonged	Pressure
Capillary fluid shift	8 min	Days	Prolonged	Pressure
Renin-angiotension	2 min	45 min	Prolonged	Pressure
Long Term				
Blood volume	5–120 min	Days	Prolonged	Renal

PCO_2, partial pressure of carbon dioxide, PO_2, partial pressure of oxygen

the mean arterial pressure falls well below 80 mmHg, arterial PO_2 falls below normal, or arterial CO_2 or hydrogen ion concentration rises significantly. Under these conditions, nerve transmission to the medullary center results in sympathetic excitation and vagal inhibition[7]. In addition, stretch receptors located in the systemic and pulmonary arteries recognize increased venous return, and will cause reflex vasodilation[8].

Intermediate mechanisms of blood pressure control involve hormonal mechanisms active over minutes to hours. Acute hypotension stimulates adrenal release of the endogenous vasoconstrictor norepinephrine, and triggers renin release leading to afferent renal arteriolar

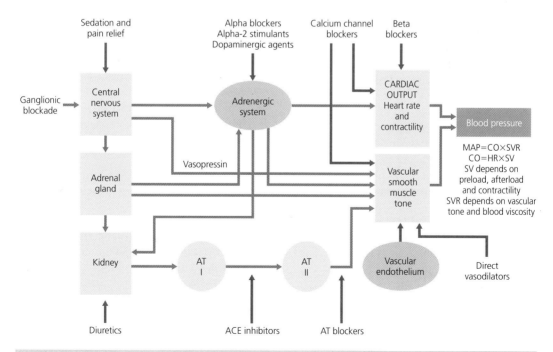

Figure 9.2 Blood pressure control. SV = stroke volume, SVR = systemic vascular resistance, AT = angiotensin, ACE = angiotensin converting enzyme.

vasodilation and efferent vasoconstriction. Persistent low mean arterial pressure, however, results in increased levels of angiotensin, which ultimately constricts afferent arterioles and decreases glomerular blood flow. Angiotensin I is inactive, but is converted in the lungs to active angiotensin II. Inhibitors of angiotensin-converting enzyme (ACE) are therefore useful antihypertensives. Hypotension also stimulates hypothalamic secretion of vasopressin, which has direct vasoconstrictive effects, and also plays a role in renal tubular fluid reabsorption. Further intermediate regulation occurs as a result of relaxation of capacitance vessels[9].

Long-term regulation (hours to days) of blood pressure involves the renin–angiotensin system, and adrenal cortical release of aldosterone[10]. Structural changes associated with chronic hypertension include cardiac hypertrophy, diminished left ventricular distensibility, diastolic dysfunction, and arterial muscular hypertrophy.

9.4 Monitoring considerations

Mean arterial pressure (MAP) is typically the same in all large arterial vessels in a supine patient, with only a small gradient between the aorta and a radial arterial line. Gradients may increase following hypothermia and rewarming, as in cardiac surgery[11]. Systolic and diastolic pressures, however, vary by location, and systolic pressure tends to rise in the periphery owing to the influence of reflected waves (*Figure 9.3*). Automated sphygmomanometry (e.g. Dynamap) and manual cuff pressures are inaccurate when cuff width is less than two-thirds of arm circumference. Use of a narrow cuff, and presence of atherosclerotic vessels both tend to overestimate true blood pressure.

Arterial cannulation is indicated with hemodynamic instability or shock, malignant hypertension, concurrent oxygenation problems, or when frequent blood sampling is required. Complications of arterial line placement include local hemorrhage, infection, and thrombosis. Large catheter size relative to vessel size[12], low cardiac output, pre-existing

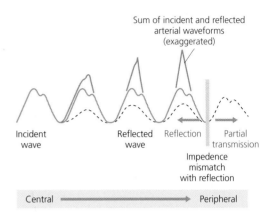

Figure 9.3 Influences of reflected waves.

vascular disease and vasopressors all increase the risk of arterial thrombosis.

9.5 Agents to decrease blood pressure

Figure 9.2 demonstrates the points at which pharmacologic agents act to influence blood pressure. Antihypertensive agents can be categorized by their mechanisms of action:

- direct vasodilation (e.g. sodium nitroprusside, hydralazine);
- autonomic ganglia blockade (e.g. trimethaphan);
- alpha-adrenergic blockade (e.g. phentolamine);
- alpha-2-adrenergic stimulation (e.g. clonidine);
- beta blockade (e.g. esmolol, propranolol, metoprolol);
- combined alpha and beta blockade (e.g. labetalol);
- calcium channel blockade (e.g. nicardipine, isradipine, nifedipine);
- ACE inhibition (e.g. captopril, enalaprilat);
- angiotersin III receptor antagonists (e.g. Iosartan);
- diuresis (e.g. furosemide, bumetanide, thiazide diuretics);
- sedation and/or analgesia.

The wide variety of effective agents makes it possible to individualize therapy based on urgency, routes of access, and presence of contraindications to specific drugs (*Table 9.5*). Direct vasodilators, particularly sodium nitroprusside, tend to be the most rapidly acting and effective agents, but require close titration and have undesirable side effects, including tachyphylaxis. The more indirect the mechanism of blood pressure reduction, the longer it may take to achieve a satisfactory result in a hypertensive emergency. A typical approach is to use sodium nitroprusside, hydralazine or fenoldopam for immediate control of acute hypertension, while also starting a longer-acting agent, one that can be given orally and outside a closely monitored setting. Patients may not respond to a single agent, so combinations of agents with differing mechanisms of action are frequently necessary. Beta-adrenergic antagonists or combined alpha and beta blockers prevent and treat the reflex tachycardia that can occur following peripheral vasodilation. Labetalol and beta blockers, however, are relatively contraindicated in patients with bronchospastic disease or high-degree atrioventricular conduction block. Nitroglycerine is useful in the presence of coronary insufficiency, and loop diuretics and nitroglycerine together are indicated when pulmonary edema is also present. Afterload reduction with an ACE inhibitor may be appropriate with heart failure or when the renin system is activated, but ACE inhibitors should be avoided in patients with bilateral renal artery stenoses or renal artery stenosis with a solitary kidney. Centrally acting agents, particularly clonidine, are helpful in the presence of excess sympathetic discharge, as may be seen with head injury or substance withdrawal. However, these agents also tend to cloud mental status and amplify the effects of opioids. *Table 9.6* outlines considerations for therapy in specific disease states.

9.5.1 Direct vasodilators

Nitroprusside (Nipride) acts directly on arterioles and venules by decreasing the tone of vascular smooth muscle, resulting in reduced afterload and less increase in preload compared with other vasodilators. Nitroprusside has an immediate onset of action and effects dissipate in 2–3 min. The solution, typically mixed as 50 mg of nitroprusside in 250 cm³ of D5W, must be protected from light; deeply discolored solutions lack potency and should be discarded. Nitroprusside should be given by infusion pump. The usual starting dose is 0.1–0.3 µg kg^{-1} min^{-1}, but doses may be rapidly titrated based on patient response to a maximum acute dose of 10 µg kg^{-1} min^{-1} for 10 min or less. Sustained infusions should not exceed 3 µg kg^{-1} min^{-1}, particularly with hepatic or renal dysfunction. Extracardiac effects of sodium nitroprusside include increased renal blood flow (as a result of increased cardiac output) and reduced pulmonary artery pressure and pulmonary vascular resistance, which may alter regional blood flow in the lung, worsening the ventilation–perfusion ($\dot{V}/\dot{Q}$) ratio, and increasing dead space ventilation. Nitroprusside combines with hemoglobin to produce cyanomethemoglobin and cyanide ions. Cyanide combines with thiosulfate to produce thiocyanate, a reaction catalyzed by the liver enzyme rhodanase. Thiocyanate is then eliminated by the kidneys. Excess cyanide inhibits oxidative metabolism, which will present clinically as metabolic acidosis, increased mixed venous oxygen, and a reduced arterio-venous oxygen difference. Thiocyanate toxicity can also occur, especially with renal failure, but also if nitroprusside infusions are maintained for more than 72 h. Thiocyanate toxicity can present as delirium, headache, nausea, abdominal pain, muscle spasms or restlessness. Although thiocyanate levels can be measured, results are typically not available in a clinically relevant time frame. Increasing nitroprusside dose requirement, mental confusion and lactic acidosis should raise suspicion of toxicity. Administration of thiosulfate (150 mg kg^{-1}) provides sulfate donors facilitating the conversion of cyanide to thiocyanate[13]. Amyl nitrate (inhaled) or sodium nitrate (5 mg kg^{-1} intravenously) provides nitrate ions to convert hemoglobin to methemoglobin, which binds the cyanide molecule. Hydroxycobalamin

Table 9.5 Agents for control of hypertension in the ICU

Mechanism of action	Drug	Dosage	Onset	Duration of action	Indications	Contraindications	Side effects	Comments
Vascular smooth muscle relaxation	Sodium nitroprusside	IV: 0.3–10 µg kg^{-1} min^{-1} Usually ≤3 µg kg^{-1} min^{-1} Mix 50 mg per 100 ml	Immediate	2–3 min	Postoperative hypertension Hypertensive crisis General purpose	Pregnancy	Hypotension, nausea, and cyanide toxicity (increased with renal and hepatic insufficiency)	Invasive pressure monitoring recommended Shield from light
	Hydralazine	IV: 2.5–20 mg bolus i.m.: 20–40 mg q 4–6 h Oral: 10–50 mg q 6 h	15–30 min	IV.: 3–20 min Oral: 2–4 h	Postoperative hypertension	Severe coronary disease, lupus, aortic stenosis	Fluid retention, lupus-like rash, headache, positive Coombs' test	Tolerance may develop Ideal for eclampsia
	Nitroglycerin	IV: 5–100 µg min^{-1} Sublingual 0.15–0.5 mg	1–2 min	3–5 min	Myocardial ischemia or infarction	Septal hypertrophy, hemoglobinopathies	Bradycardia, tachycardia, methemoglobinemia, flushing, vomiting, headache	Rapid tachyphylaxis Venodilation at low doses
	Diazoxide	IV: 50–100 mg q 5–10 min, up to 600 mg Infusion: 30 mg min^{-1}	1–5 min	6–12 h	Postoperative hypertension	Diabetes, hyperuricemia, CHF	Hypotension, tachycardia, fluid retention, myocardial ischemia, hyperglycemia, nausea, vomiting, heart failure	Potentiated by beta blockers and diuretics
	Nitric oxide	Inhaled 15–30 ppm	Immediate	Seconds	Experimental			
Autonomic ganglia blockers	Trimethaphan	IV: 1–5 mg min^{-1}, titrate to effect. Mix 50 mg per 500cm^3 of normal saline (NS)	2–5 min	4–12 h	Postoperative hypertension	CAD, prostatism, cerebrovascular insufficiency, diabetes mellitus, glaucoma	Ileus, urinary retention, hypotension, blurred vision, dry mouth, angina, pupillary dilation	Invasive pressure monitoring recommended
Alpha blockers	Phentolamine	IV: 5–20 mg q 10 min	Immediate	2–10 min	Pheochromocytoma	CAD	Tachycardia, vomiting, angina, hypotension, miosis, dry mouth	
Combined alpha and beta blockers	Labetalol	IV: 10–80 mg q 10 min to 300 mg max. Infusion: 0.5–2 mg min^{-1}	5–10 min	3–6 h	General purpose	Heart block, asthma, bradycardia, heart failure, hypertension secondary to decreased cardiac output	Hypotension, heart failure, heart block, dizziness, nausea, phlebitis, bronchospasm, cardiac arrest if given with verapamil	Increases digoxin level, prolongs neuromuscular blockade of succinylcholine
Beta blocker	Esmolol	IV: load with 500 µg kg^{-1} over 1–2 min and infusion 50–200 µg kg^{-1} min^{-1}	<5 min	10–20 min	CAD w/o left ventricle dysfunction, aortic dissection w/o heart failure, post-operative hypertension related to increased sympathetic tone, hyperthyroidism	Asthma, heart block, sinus bradycardia, heart failure, cardiogenic shock, pregnancy	Heart failure, bronchospasm, heart block, hypotension, phlebitis, dizziness, urinary retention	Elevates digoxin level, prolongs neuromuscular blockade with succinylcholine, risk of fatal cardiac arrest if combined with verapamil

Table 9.5 Continued

Mechanism of action	Drug	Dosage	Onset	Duration of action	Indications	Contraindications	Side effects	Comments
Calcium antagonist	Isradipine	Oral: 2.5–20 mg b.i.d.	2–3 h	12+ h	Afterload reduction	Tight aortic stenosis	Headache, dizziness, edema	Diuretic effects
	Nifedipine	Sl: 10–20 mg q 15 min* Oral:10–20 mg t.i.d.	1–5 min 5–10 min	20–30 min 30–60 min	Has been used for acute BP control	Heart block, IV beta blockers w/o pacer backup	Headache, tachycardia, flushing, dizziness, hypotension, phlebitis or infarction	Watch for overshoot Rapid uncontrolled BP reduction can precipitate strokes
	Nicardipine	IV: 5–15 mg h−1	1–5 min	3–6 h	Myocardial ischemia or infarction	Severe aortic stenosis, hypersensitivity	Hypotension, tachycardia, nausea, minimal myocardial depression	
	Nimodipine	PO: 60 mg q 4 h	1–2 h	4–6 h	Subarachnoid hemorrhage	Pregnancy, hepatic impairment	Edema, hypotension, headache, ileus, nausea, abnormal liver function	Can administer through NG tube
Centrally acting	Clonidine	IV: 0.1–0.2 mg, PO 0.2 mg q 6 h, transdermal patch max. 2.4 mg day−1	30 min–1 h	6–8 h	Rebound hypertension following discontinuation of clonidine	Heart block, bradycardia, sick sinus syndrome	Drowsiness, sedation, dry mouth, augments opioids, nightmares, restlessness	Reduce dose in elderly, cerebrovascular or cardiovascular disease; rebound phenomena
	Methyldopa	IV: 250–200 mg q 6 h	up to 4 h	12–24 h	Postoperative hypertension	Pheochromocytoma, hepatic disease, MAO inhibitors	Drowsiness, hypotension, fever, positive Coombs' test, chronic hepatitis, lupus-like syndrome	
Converting enzyme inhibitors	Enalaprilat	IV: titrated 0.625–1.25 mg q 6–8 h	10–15 min	6–24 h	Hypertension related to renal artery stenosis	Pregnancy, renal failure, bilateral renal stenosis	Cough and angioedema, fever urticaria hypotension, pancytopenia	
Dopaminergic stimulation	Fenoldopam	IV: 0.1 μg kg−1 min−1 titrated up at 0.1 μg kg−1 increments q 20 min Maximum dose 1.7 μg kg−1 min−1	4 min	20 min	Postoperative hypertension, hypertensive crisis	Glaucoma	Increased intraocular pressure, headache, flushing, nausea, asymptomatic EKG ST-changes	

*Not FDA approved. CAD, coronary artery disease; CHF, congestive heart failure; MAO, monoamine oxidase; NG, nasogastric.

Table 9.6 Considerations for specific hypertensive situations

Clinical situations	Treatment goals	Preferred agents
Acute aortic dissection	Reduce pressure gradient across lesion; reduce inotropy	Nitroprusside plus beta blocker; or labetalol
Acute left ventricular dysfunction or CHF	Afterload reduction while preserving inotropy. Consider milrinone or dobutamine to provide both simultaneously	ACE inhibitor, nitroprusside or nitroglycerin Beta blockers may paradoxically improve output by slowing rate
Catecholamine-induced crisis (MAO inhibition, cocaine overdose, clonidine or opiate withdrawal)	Block alpha and beta simultaneously (see separate entry for pheochromocytoma)	Labetalol, nitroprusside + beta blocker, phentolamine
Eclampsia and severe pre-eclampsia	Avoid nitroprusside, trimethaphan (fetal CNS toxicity); enalaprilat and nimodipine relatively contraindicated	Magnesium sulfate if seizures, hydralazine, labetalol, calcium channel blockers
Hypertensive encephalopathy	Avoid cerebral vasodilation with intracranial bleeding	Nicardipine
Intracranial hemorrhage, subarachnoid hemorrhage, increased ICP	Goal: MAP 80% of initial value, keep DBP <140 Avoid sedative effects (methyldopa, clonidine) Treat underlying causes of increased intracranial pressure	Labetalol; calcium channel blockers, esp. nimodipine
Ischemic stroke	Not clear if benefit to intervention Treat only if BP >180/105	Sodium nitroprusside Nicardipine Nimodipine
Myocardial ischemia	Reduce preload and heart rate; control pulmonary hypertension	Nitroglycerin, beta blockers and morphine
Perioperative hypertension	Avoid stress on fresh suture lines Avoid hypotension (risk of thrombosis) Consider possible physical causes and treat pain appropriately	Labetalol, nitroprusside Sedatives or analgesics
Pheochromocytoma	Unopposed beta blockade can precipitate crisis; block alpha first or simultaneously; add beta blockade to prevent tachycardia	Preoperative alpha blockade: phenoxybenzamine; acute treatment: phentolamine or labetalol
Postoperative cardiac surgery	Avoid vasodilators with subaortic stenosis or tight aortic stenosis	Labetalol, esmolol, nitroprusside, nicardipine, nitroglycerine
Thyroid storm	Control tachycardia while dealing with underlying hormone excess	Propylthiouracil (PTU) beta blockers

combines with cyanide to produce non-toxic cyanocobalamin. Hemodialysis can also eliminate thiocyanate.

Because of concerns about tachyphylaxis and toxicity, other antihypertensive agents should be added while acute hypertension is controlled with nitroprusside. Diuretics potentiate nitroprusside's effects by helping to eliminate pooled venous blood. Beta blockers counteract reflex tachycardia. When using nitroprusside for medical management of acute aortic dissection, beta blockade will also decrease shear forces across the dissection by reducing the pressure gradient between the heart and dilated peripheral vasculature.

Nitroglycerin relaxes smooth muscle in venules and arterioles. It is not a particularly potent antihypertensive in normal circumstances, but is often effective with acute volume overload. Reduction of venous return is a major cause of decreased blood pressure with nitroglycerin. Side effects associated with nitroglycerin include headache owing to meningeal vessel dilation, and methemoglobinemia, because nitroglycerin oxidizes hemoglobin. Nitroglycerin can be given sublingually (0.15–0.6 mg per dose), transdermally (2% ointment) or as a sustained-action patch, but the preferred method of administration in the ICU is IV infusion, typically a mix of 50 mg in 250 cm^3 of D5W initiated at 10 μg min^{-1} and titrated to patient response.

Hydralazine (Apresoline) is a direct-acting vasodilator with an onset of action of 3–20 min following IV administration, and a duration of action of 2–6 h. It is the drug of choice in eclampsia as it preserves myometrial blood flow. Hydralazine is relatively contraindicated as the sole antihypertensive agent in patients with severe coronary disease, because of the potential for precipitating reflex tachycardia. In addition, hydralazine has been reported to cause a lupus-like rash, fluid retention and headache. Typical IV doses of hydralazine are 5–10 mg q 4–6 h individualized to the patient's response. Oral doses are 10–50 mg p.o. q 6 h.

Fenoldopam is a vasodilator that acts by selective stimulation of dopamine DA-1 receptors. The drug has no effect at beta-adrenergic or dopaminergic DA-2 receptors. Fenoldopam can be safely given via a peripheral (as opposed to central) IV line. Its onset of action is rapid (within 4 min) and duration of action short. In contrast to nitroprusside, it induces diuresis and natriuresis[14]. Other advantages include lack of light-induced loss of potency, and absence of toxic metabolites[15]. Fenoldopam and nitroprusside both cause rapid and significant reduction in systolic blood pressure and systemic vascular resistance. In postoperative cardiac surgery patients, fenoldopam also results in increased cardiac index and stroke volume[16].

Other direct vasodilators include minoxidil and diazoxide. Minoxidil therapy can be initiated with 2.5–5 mg orally, and dose doubled every 6 h until blood pressure control is obtained. The effective dose can then be continued daily or b.i.d. Because of minoxidil's potent vasodilating effects, sympathetic nervous activation is likely and the drug's vasodilating effect may be antagonized by endogenous release of norepinephrine and angiotensin II. Fluid retention is a complication of minoxidil therapy requiring addition of a thiazide and/or loop diuretic.

Diazoxide is a direct arteriolar dilator with little effect on venous capacitance. Diazoxide has a long serum half-life (c. 30 h), which is further increased in patients with impaired renal function. Because the drug is bound to albumin, it must be given as a rapid IV bolus, typically 50–150 mg of diazoxide over 30 s. Diazoxide also causes sympathetic stimulation and fluid retention so its effects will be potentiated by sympatholytic agents and diuretics. Undesirable side effects of diazoxide include reduction in cerebral blood flow[17], increased blood glucose levels as a result of an inhibition of insulin release, and hyperuricemia. In hypertensive emergencies, the maximum effect of diazoxide is reached in 5 min and dissipates over the next 12 h.

9.5.2 Calcium channel blockers

Calcium channel antagonists reduce muscle contractility and thus inotropy and systemic vascular resistance by limiting calcium influx though slow channels in myocardium and smooth muscle cells. Nicardipine (Cardene) is a short-acting calcium channel antagonist. The initial rate of infusion is 5 mg h^{-1} up to a maximum dose of 15 mg h^{-1}. Nicardipine's onset of action is 1–5 min and its duration of action is 3–6 h. Because of its coronary vasodilatory effect, nicardipine is particularly useful for blood pressure control with concurrent myocardial ischemia or infarction. It has the potential side effects of tachycardia, nausea, and myocardial depression, and is contraindicated in patients with tight aortic stenosis and with hypersensitivity reactions. Nicardipine is effective as sodium nitroprusside following coronary bypass surgery, achieves a therapeutic response sooner, and requires less frequent dosage adjustment during maintenance therapy, with fewer episodes of severe hypotension compared with sodium nitroprusside[18].

Nifedipine (Adalat, Procardia) is a potent vasodilator and afterload reducing agent with mild inotrophic and chronotropic effects. A sublingual dose of 10–20 mg is effective in the management of acute hypertension[19], but more recent reports[20] recommend against this practice, because of the potential for overshoot and hypotension. Nicardipine is preferable to nifedipine because of a slower and more prolonged decrease in blood pressure. Relative contraindications to nifedipine include hypersensitivity, severe congestive heart failure, tight aortic stenosis, and renal insufficiency. Side effects include hypotension, tachycardia, syncope, platelet dysfunction, hepatotoxicity, and headache. In patients receiving digoxin, nifedipine increases serum digoxin levels.

Isradipine (Dynacirc) is a calcium channel antagonist similar to nifedipine that has been evaluated for sublingual use. At low doses, it produces vasodilation without affecting myocardial contractility. With normal ventricular function, isradipine's overload-reducing properties frequently lead to an increase in cardiac output. Blood pressure reduction occurs some 2–3 h following an oral dose of 2.5–20 mg, and the duration of action is 12 h or more, allowing twice-daily administration. Sublingual doses of 1.25–5 mg have an onset in 30 min and a duration of 2 h[21]. Intravenous isradipine via infusion (mean dose 18.6 µg min^{-1}) is effective and well tolerated in patients developing hypertension post coronary artery bypass grafting (CABG)[22].

Diltiazem (Cardizem) and Verapamil (Calan) relax smooth muscle and thus have antihypertensive effects, but have relatively greater effects on cardiac conduction, particularly in the setting of combined therapy with beta-blocking agents or digitalis. Nimodipine has been shown to improve outcome in patients with aneurysmal subarachnoid hemorrhage[23].

9.5.3 Adrenergic blocking agents

Esmolol (Brevibloc) is a short-acting cardioselective beta blocker indicated for control of supraventricular tachycardia. Esmolol has no reported antihypertensive effects in the absence of tachycardia or high catecholamine activity and is not recommended for first line treatment of hypertensive crisis. Numerous reports, however, attest to its utility when hypertension is associated with a hyperdynamic state. It has an onset of action of 3–5 min with a duration of action of 10–20 min. Esmolol is metabolized by red blood cell esterase and has an extremely short beta half-life (around 9 min). Dose-related hypotension occurs in 20–50% of patients when esmolol is given for heart rate control. The initial infusion dose of esmolol is 500 µg kg^{-1} over 1 min, followed by 50 µg kg^{-1} min^{-1}, and then titrated in the range of 50–200 µg kg^{-1} min^{-1} to the desired endpoint. Additional loading doses of 100 µg kg^{-1} over 1 min may be necessary. Although cardioselective, esmolol is still relatively contraindicated in patients with asthma, severe diabetes, high-degree heart block, sinus bradycardia, heart failure, and pregnancy. Like other beta-blocking agents, esmolol reduces systolic blood pressure by decreasing cardiac output. In severe hypertensive episodes where the elevated blood pressure results from high systemic vascular resistance, a decrease in cardiac output may significantly compromise organ perfusion, so the drug should be avoided when cardiac output is borderline or inadequate. This danger is somewhat offset by the very short half-life of esmolol. Beta-adrenergic blockers with longer half-lives include metoprolol, atenolol, and propranolol.

Labetalol (Normodyne, Trandate) is a combined alpha- and beta-adrenergic blocker, with more beta than alpha activity (a 7:1 relative activity ratio is commonly quoted). It is particularly useful in the management of acute hypertension, particularly that caused by catecholamine excess. Full effects occur within 5–10 min of IV injection. Because of the beta-adrenergic blocking effect, labetalol is unlikely to precipitate tachycardia when given for severe hypertension. Labetalol's metabolism is primarily hepatic, with less than 5% excreted unchanged via the kidneys. Bolus doses of 5–10 mg IV may be repeated or doubled at 10 min intervals until a maximum dose of 80 mg is reached. However, much higher doses (>500 mg) have been necessary in some patients[24]. It may also be administered as an infusion of 0.5–2 mg min^{-1}. Because of its beta-blocking properties, labetalol is relatively contraindicated in patients with congestive heart failure or bronchospastic disease. In patients with pheochromocytomas, paradoxic responses have occurred because of the relatively greater beta-blocking potential. Labetalol may also block the tachycardia associated with hypoglycemia and therefore, as with all beta-adrenergic blocking agents, should be used cautiously in patients receiving IV insulin or oral hypoglycemic agents. Side effects of labetalol include bradycardia, heart block, anaphylaxis, hypotension, and dizziness.

9.5.4 Alpha-adrenergic agents (*Table 9.7*)

An understanding of the subtypes of the alpha receptor clarifies the role of selective and non-selective agents in blood pressure control (*Figure 9.4*). Alpha-1 receptors, located on the post-synaptic membrane, mediate vasoconstriction. Blockade of these alpha-1 receptors

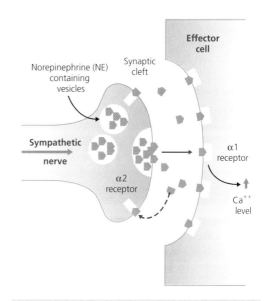

Figure 9.4 Sympathetic nerve terminal. NE, norepinephrine.

Table 9.7 Alpha-adrenergic agents

	Agonists	Antagonists
alpha-2	Guanfacine Guanabenz Clonidine α-Methylnorepinephrine	Yohimbine
alpha-1 and -2	Epinephrine Norepinephrine	Tolazoline Phentolamine Phenoxybenzamine (irreversible binding)
alpha-1	Phenylephrine Methoxamine	Labetalol [alpha and beta] Prazosin Doxazosin Terazosin

is an effective treatment for hypertension. Alpha-2 receptors, located on the pre-synaptic membrane, modulate the release of norepinephrine across the synaptic cleft. Stimulation of alpha-2 receptors thus reduces sympathetic stimulation and consequently blood pressure. Pressor agents such as epinephrine and norepinephrine stimulate both forms of receptors (see Chapter 8) whereas non-selective alpha-adrenergic blockers such as phentolamine and phenoxybenzamine block both types of receptors. More selective agents can be categorized by their relative binding infinity at the alpha-1 and alpha-2 receptor (*Table 9.5*). Simulation of central alpha-2 receptors diminishes sympathetic activity and drugs with alpha-2 selectivity tend to be sedating.

Clonidine (Catapres) is a centrally acting alpha-2-receptor agonist that modulates tonic and reflex blood pressure control, and lessens sympathetic outflow[25,26], resulting in lowered heart rate and blood pressure. Clonidine is administered in a dose of 0.1–0.2 mg intravenously and may be also administered orally via a nasogastric tube (0.1–0.3 mg twice daily) or by transdermal patch (3.5 cm^2 or 0.1 mg day^{-1}). The IV form has an onset of action of 30–60 min with a duration of action of 6–8 h. Doses higher than 0.4 mg have little additional benefit. Clonidine is contraindicated in patients with bradycardia, sick sinus syndrome, or heart block. The dose should be reduced in elderly patients and in patients with pre-existing cerebral or cardiovascular disease, because of exaggerated bradycardiac responses and potential for drowsiness and sedation. Clonidine is particularly useful in hypertension associated with substance withdrawal and with uncontrolled sympathetic discharges in neurosurgical patients. Clonidine can significantly decrease cerebral blood flow and one death from progressive cerebral infarction has been reported[27].

Dexmedetomidine (Precedex) is primarily marketed as a sedative agent. Like clonidine, dexmedetomidine acts at the alpha-2 adrenergic receptor, and enhanced sedation is noted when dexmedetomidine is co-administered with inhalation anesthetics, propofol, opioids, and benzodiazepines. Although hypotension is commonly seen during sedative treatment with dexmedetomidine, hypertension may also be seen, particularly with rapid bolus administration.

Alpha-methyldopa is a converted to an active metabolite that, like clonidine, acts as a potent alpha-2 receptor agonist. Because of the requirement for a metabolite to be formed, the onset of action may be delayed (4 h) and the action prolonged (up to 24 h). Alpha-methyldopa tends to cause sedation, impair mental judgment, and depress overall behavior. Roughly 25% of patients maintained on long-term methyldopa develop a positive direct Coombs test. In high doses, all of the alpha-2 agonists can stimulate peripheral vasoconstriction and cause hypertension. Thus, methyldopa should not be combined with clonidine, guanabenz, and guanfacine because of additive effects.

Phentolamine is an alpha-adrenergic blocker historically used in situations involving excess catecholamine levels such as pheochromocytoma and antihypertensive withdrawal syndrome. Its use has largely been supplanted by labetalol or the combination of nitroprusside plus a beta blocker. Phentolamine may cause tachycardia, angina, vomiting, and headache.

9.5.5 Angiotensin-converting enzyme (ACE) inhibitors

Enalaprilat is the IV form of enalapril with an onset of action in 10–15 min and a duration of action of 6–24 h. It is administered as a titrated dose of 0.625–1.25 mg every 6 h. Enalaprilat is indicated in the management of hypertension when oral ACE therapy is impractical, and in particular when the hypertension is related to unilateral renal artery stenosis. It is contraindicated in pregnancy, with a history of angioedema related to ACE inhibitors, and in renal failure as a result of bilateral renal artery stenosis or unilateral stenosis of a solitary kidney. Enalaprilat has been reported to provide a more favorable profile than nitroprusside even in patients with no demonstrable evidence of elevated plasma renin activity, suggesting that the mechanism for blood pressure control involves something more than the renin–angiotensin system[28].

A number of oral ACE inhibitors are available for clinical use, including captopril, enalopril, lisinopril, fosinopril, benazapril, and ramipril, the last three being prodrugs that must be converted to their active form by a functioning liver. Pressure reduction with the ACE inhibitors may initially be dramatic in patients with high renin levels, although subsequent doses tend to cause less hypotension. Volume-depleted patients typically manifest an exaggerated response. In patients with congestive heart failure, cardiac output should increase with afterload reduction[29]. Side effects of the ACE inhibitors include excessive hypotension, angioedema, impaired renal function, hypercalemia, and cough. In addition to ACE inhibitors, angiotensin receptor antagonists such as losartan are becoming available[30] but clinical experience in the ICU setting is sparse.

9.5.6 Adjunctive agents

In the critically ill patient, diuretics are generally avoided for the acute treatment of hypertension unless blood volume is elevated. Rapidly acting IV diuretics such as furosemide (Lasix) or bumetanide (Bumex) are useful when there is overt congestive heart failure or pulmonary edema. Diuretics are generally needed with long-term therapy to counteract renal sodium retention.

Sedative agents such as opioids, benzodiazepines, and propofol reduce blood pressure by controlling central stimulation, and may be useful adjuncts in blood pressure control, particularly in mechanically ventilated or agitated patients.

9.5.7 Ganglionic blockers

Trimethapham is a ganglionic blocking agent historically used for the treatment of hypertension in the setting of acute aortic dissection. Trimethapham reduces left ventricular ejection fraction and heart rate, but with the advent of beta-blocking drugs and combined alpha–beta-blocking agents such as labetalol, trimethopram is now rarely used. Side effects include urinary retention, paralytic ileus, midriasis, dry mouth, and development of tachyphylaxis.

9.6 Specific clinical considerations

An understanding of the pathophysiology in specific clinical conditions can guide the choice of agents (Table 9.6).

9.6.1 Acute aortic dissection

Medical management of acute aortic dissection involves rapid reduction of blood pressure to normal levels using IV sodium introprusside. The force and velocity of ventricular contractions and pulsatile flow affect the shear stress on the aortic wall. Unless contraindicated, a beta-blocking agent should be added to decrease myocardial contractility and the pressure on the aortic wall. If beta blockers are contraindicated, trimethaphan camsilate or urapidil can be substituted.

9.6.2 Excess circulatory catecholamines

Pheochromocytomas are the most common of the catecholamine-secreting tumors. Hypertension associated with these tumors may be silent or paradoxic in nature in up to 40% of patients[31]. Postoperative hypertension may be the initial clinical presentation of these tumors[32].

A hallmark feature of patients with these tumors is relative volume contraction. Hypotension is common following pheochromocytomas resection because of the removal of the continuous source of catecholamines in the presence of the adrenergic blockade given for preoperative preparation. Such hypotension may necessitate the administration of fluids to expand the intravascular volume as well as cautious administration of vasopressor agents. Excess circulatory catecholamines can also be seen in rebound hypertension following clonidine withdrawal, following ingestion of street drugs (cocaine, amphetamines, phencyclidine, LSD and weight loss drugs) and as a result of the interaction of MAO inhibitors with dietary tyramine (cheese, wine, certain beers). Beta-blocking agents should always be preceded by alpha blockade to avoid unopposed peripheral vasoconstriction[33].

9.6.3 Autonomic hyperreflexia

Quadraplegic or paraplegic patients with spinal cord injuries above the inhibitory splanchnic outflow level (T4 to T7) have a potential for acute sympathetic hyperactivity in response to stimuli below the level of the transsection. This generalized sympathetic activity results from reflex stimulation of the sympathetic neurons in the anterolateral column of the spinal cord below the transection level without the inhibitory modulation that comes from the higher centers in the central nervous system. This disorder occurs in 65–85% of quadraplegic and high-level paraplegic patients, often in response to bladder catheterization[34].

Hypertension in these patients is related to profound increases in systemic vascular resistance resulting from the sympathetically mediated vasoconstriction. Autonomic hyperreflexia is commonly associated with a reflex bradycardia mediated by the baroreceptor reflex. In addition, there may be a second reflex arc involving skeletal muscles that produce intense muscle spasm. Treatment of the hypertensive response in autonomic hyperreflexia is directed at reversing elevated systemic vascular resistance with sodium nitroprusside or ganglionic blocking agents such as trimethaphan[34,35].

9.6.4 Increased intracranial pressure

Marked elevation of intracranial pressure results in a reflex sympathetic response with peripheral vasoconstriction and hypertension. Through the baroreceptor-mediated response, this profound hypertension results in an accompanying reflex bradycardia. This combination of physiologic events is commonly referred to as the Cushing reflex. In addition to space-occupying lesions, other causes of

increased intracranial pressure include intracranial bleeding, cerebral edema, hypercapnia, and hypoxemia. Management is directed at the underlying mechanism responsible for the intracranial hypertension and may warrant immediate surgical intervention. Intracerebral pressure may be acutely lowered by reducing cerebral blood flow with deliberate hypocapnia via hyperventilation, and administering pharmacologic agents that reduce blood pressure without causing an associated vasodilation. Initially, mannitol which induces an osmotic diuresis, may increase intracranial pressure as a result of its effect on volume expansion. Pretreatment with furosemide helps prevent this effect. Pharmacologic blockade of alpha-1- or beta-1-adrenergic receptors reduces blood pressure with little effect on intracranial pressure, within the autoregulatory range[36]. Urapidil also blocks postsynaptic alpha-1 receptors without increasing cerebral blood flow. In the neurosurgical patient, early extubation should be considered, when possible, to avoid the stimulant effects of awakening while intubated[37].

Intracerebral hemorrhage causes a rise in intracranial pressure and thus higher mean arterial pressure for adequate perfusion. The resulting hypertension typically resolves spontaneously within 48 h, and although rapid reduction in blood pressure may prevent further bleeding, there is a risk of cerebral hypoperfusion. Patients with MAP lower than 145 mmHg and those whose MAP is controlled below 125 mmHg have a better outcome by retrospective analysis[38]. In these circumstances, blood pressure should be reduced only to 80% of the pre-treatment blood pressure level[39].

9.6.5 Acute ischemic stroke

Autoregulation of cerebral blood flow is impaired following cerebral infarction, resulting in excess perfusion through damaged tissue, edema, and compression of normal brain. On the other hand, local vasoconstriction may warrant a higher arterial pressure to perfuse jeopardized brain tissue in the peri-infarction zone. There are no controlled outcome studies suggesting that short-term lowering of blood pressure improves outcome in patients with acute ischemic stroke. In patients with diffuse stenosis of cerebral arteries, neurologic improvement may be seen with blood pressure elevation[40]. The benefits of acute blood pressure control in patients with acute stroke are questionable[41].

9.6.6 Thyrotoxicosis or thyroid storm

The stress of critical illness may contribute to the release of high levels of T_4 hormone from the thyroid gland into the circulation in patients with undiscovered hyperthyroidism. Thyroid storm is often associated with elevated levels of the T_4 hormone in comparison to the more frequent elevations of T_3 seen in thyrotoxicosis[42]. Patients with thyroid storm present in the perioperative setting with the signs of increased sympathetic tone and are commonly febrile, hypertensive, tachycardic, agitated, and confused. Increased oxygen demands placed on the heart may precipitate high output failure or uncover underlying ischemic heart disease, resulting in the acute onset of congestive heart failure. Treatment includes the management of the patient's hyperthermia, the administration of beta-adrenergic blockers and inhibitors of the synthesis and release of thyroid hormones (propylthiouracil, methimazole, and sodium iodide). In severe circumstances, active removal of the thyroid hormone from the circulation is indicated via plasmaphoresis or peritoneal dialysis[43,44].

9.6.7 Eclampsia and preeclampsia

Eclampsia and preeclampsia occur in approximately 10% of all late pregnancies and cause up to 20% of all maternal deaths[45]. These disorders are related to an immunologic reaction to the fetal tissue, resulting in placental vasculitis and subsequent ischemia, with release of uterine renin. Hydralazine is favored for control of blood pressure owing to minimal effects on uterine perfusion. Labetalol and nifedipine are acceptable alternatives[46] but diuretics, trimethaphan, nitroprusside and ACE inhibitors should be avoided. The hypertensive response usually abates postpartum, but persistent postpartum hypertension can occur as a result of increased sensitivity to endogenous or exogenous oxytocin and catecholamines. Oxytocin should be used sparingly, if at all, in the postpartum period to avoid prolonging the hypertension.

9.6.8 Acute renal ischemia

Acute renal ischemia can occur from the occlusion of renal arteries during major vascular surgery or following renal transplantation. The lack of blood flow and resulting ischemia of the juxtaglomerular apparatus increases renin secretion and subsequent conversion of angiotensin I to angiotensin II. If there is significant myocardial dysfunction and/or coronary artery disease, the increase in systemic afterload may be life-threatening. Hypertension following renal transplantation has been associated with stenosis of the renal artery anastomosis, rejection reactions, immunosuppressive therapy, and excessive renin release by the diseased kidneys[47]. Immunosuppressive therapy with steroids increases the arteriolar–systemic vascular resistance to endogenous catecholamines along with excess renin released from the diseased kidneys. Cyclosporine has been associated with an increase of sympathetic discharge[47]. Deterioration of renal function in the presence of elevated blood pressure requires immediate intervention to reduce systemic vascular resistance without compromising renal blood flow. Labetalol, calcium channel blockers, fenoldopam and nitroprusside with dosage adjustment are reasonable choices.

9.6.9 Volume overload

Between dialysis treatments, patients with chronic renal failure become hypervolemic as a result of inability to handle normal sodium and water excretion. These patients frequently have an exaggerated response to vasopressor therapy or volume replacement, owing to the chronically elevated renin levels and enhanced vascular responsiveness. Hypertension can be managed with vasodilators or ACE inhibitors temporarily until dialysis or ultrafiltration can be provided. Severe hypertension can precipitate acute left ventricular failure. Decreasing afterload will decrease the workload of the failing myocardium and improve cardiac function.

9.7 Medication-related hypertension

Ketamine causes stimulation of the sympathetic autonomic nervous system and inhibits the uptake of catecholamines by postganglionic neurons. Neuroleptics, such as droperidol and haloperidol, block dopamine-mediated peripheral vasodilation in the setting of sympathetic stimulation, vasopressor administration, or a catecholamine-secreting tumor. Acute clonidine withdrawal manifests with hypertension, starting within 18 h and lasting up to 3 days unless appropriate therapy, such as transcutaneous clonidine, is reinstituted. Narcotic withdrawal may be a result of either a patient's declining opioid blood level or the administration of narcotic antagonist such as naloxone. Use of opioid agonist-antagonists, such as pentazocine or nalbuphine, may also precipitate narcotic withdrawal and associated hypertension. Alcohol or sedative withdrawal may occur as a result of either decreased chronic level of use or abrupt withdrawal as may occur in the critical care setting. Symptoms of withdrawal from these agents include central nervous system excitation, diaphoresis, autonomic hyperactivity with associated hypertension, and tachycardia. Treatment with beta blockers or clonidine can reduce the profound sympathetic stimulation associated with withdrawal syndromes.

Abrupt preoperative discontinuation of beta blockers has been associated with pronounced rebound tachycardia and hypertension[48]. Such rebound episodes may be associated with the development of myocardial ischemia.

Monamine oxidase inhibitors are used as antidepressant agents because of their ability to block the oxidative deamination of catecholamine to vanillylmandelic acid. Inhibition of monamine oxidase causes an accumulation of norepinephrine, dopamine, epinephrine, and 5-hydroxytryptamine (5-HT) in sympathetic tissues. Use of indirect-acting sympathomimetic agents, such as ephedrine, or the narcotic meperidine has been associated with exaggerated hypertensive responses secondary to the triggered release of the catecholamines that have accumulated in the nerve terminals[49].

9.8 Conclusions

Although hypertensive emergencies are rare, they require immediate treatment to limit the threat to the cardiovascular system and to prevent end-organ injury. Aggressive IV therapy in an intensive care setting is indicated. At the same time, longer-acting oral agents can be started to limit the amount of time the patient must be on titratable IV drugs in a monitored setting. Postoperative hypertension, although not generally associated with end-organ damage, does increase stress on fresh suture lines and is frequently treated with IV agents. Hypertensive urgencies, manifested by elevated blood pressure without end-organ damage, may be treated with oral or IV agents, although outcome data showing the benefits of acute blood pressure reduction are not available. An accepted approach in these patients is to lower the blood pressure more gradually over a 24–48 h period and to avoid precipitous declines in blood pressure.

References

1. **Seltzer, J.L., Gerson, J.I. and Grogano, A.W.** (1980) Hypertension in the perioperative period. *N.Y. State J. Med.* **80**: 29.

2. **Gal, T.J. and Cooperman, L.H.** (1975) Hypertension in the immediate postoperative period. *Br. J. Anaesth.* **47**: 70.

3. **Estafanous, F.G., Tarazi, R.C., Viljoen, J.F. and Tawil, M.Y.** (1973) Systemic hypertension following myocardial revascularization. *Am. Heart J.* **85**: 732.

4. **Kreiger, E.M.** (1970) Time course of barorecep-tor resetting in acute hypertension. *Am. J. Physiol.* **8**: 486.

5. **Robertson, D., Hollister, A.S., Biaggioni, I., Netterville, J.L., Mosqueda-Garcia, R. and Robertson, R.M.** (1993) The diagnosis and treatment of baroreflex failure. *N. Engl. J. Med.* **329**: 1449–1455.

6. **Mancia, G., Lorenz, R.R. and Shepherd, J.T.** (1976) Reflex control of circulation by heart and lungs. *Int. Rev. Physiol.* **9**: 111.

7. **Malliani, A.** (1982) Cardiovascular sympathetic afferent fibers. *Rev. Physiol. Biochem. Pharmacol.* **194**: 10.

8. **Mark, A.L. and Mancia, G.** (1983) Cardiopul-monary baroreflexes in humans. In: *Handbook of Physiology, Volume 3* (eds J.T. Shepherd and F.M. Abboud). American Physiology Society, Bethesda, MD, p. 397.

9. **Brenner, B.M. and Laragh, J.H.** (1988) *Advances in Atrial Peptide Research.* Raven Press, New York.

10. **Guyton, A.C., Hall, J.E.** (1996) Dominant role of the kidneys in long term regulation of arte-rial pressure and in hypertension: The inte-grated system for pressure control. In: *Textbook of Medical Physiology,* 9th Edn. W.B. Saunders, Philadelphia, p. 221–237.

11. **Bazaral, M.G., Welch, M., Golding, L.A.R. and Badhwar, K.** (1990) Comparison of brachial and radial arterial pressure monitoring in patients undergoing coronary artery bypass surgery. *Anesthesiology* **73**: 38–45.

12. **Bedford, R.F.** (1977) Radial arterial function fol-lowing percutaneous cannulation with 18- and 20-gauge catheters. *Anesthesiology* **47**: 37–39.

13. **Cole, P.** (1978) The safe use of sodium nitro-prusside. *Anesthesia* **33**: 473.

14. **Post, J.B. and Frishman, W.H.** (1998) Fenoldopam: A new dopamine agonist for the treatment of hypertensive urgencies and emergencies. *J. Clin. Pharmacol.* **38**: 2–13.

15. **Brogden, R.N. and Markham, A.** (1997) Fenoldopam: A review of its pharmacodynamic and pharmacokinetic properties and intra-venous clinical potential in the management of hypertensive urgencies and emergencies. *Drugs* **54**(4): 634–650.

16. **Hill, A.J., Feneck, R.O. and Walesby, R.K.** (1993) A comparison of fenoldopam and nitro-prusside in the control of hypertension follow-ing coronary artery surgery. *J. Cardiothorac. Vasc. Anes.* **7**: 279–284.

17. **Pearson, R.M., Griffith, D.N.W., Wallard, M. and James, I.M.** (1979) Comparison of effects of cerebral blood flow of rapid reduction in systemic arterial pressure by diazoxide and lobetilol in hypertensive patients. *Br. J. Clin. Pharm.* **8**: 155S–198S.

18. **Halpern, N.A., Goldberg, M., Neely, C., et al.** (1992) Postoperative hypertension: A multi-center, prospective, randomized comparison between intravenous nicardipine and sodium nitroprusside. *Crit. Care Med.* **20**(12): 1637–1643.

19. **McAllister, R.G.** (1986) Kinetics and dynamics of nifedipine after oral and subliminal doses. *Am. J. Med.* **81**(Suppl.6A): 2–5.

20. **Grossman, E., Messerli, F.H., Grodzicki, T., et al.** (1996) Should a moratorium be placed on sublingual nifedipine capsules given for hyper-tensive emergencies and pseudoemergencies? *JAMA* **276**: 1328–1331.

21. **Saragoca, M.A., Portela, J.E., Plavnik, F., et al.** (1992) Isradipine in the treatment of hyperten-sive crisis in ambulatory patients. *J. Cardiovasc. Pharmacol.* **19**(Suppl. 3): S76–S78.

22. **Leslie, J., Brister, N., Levy, J.H., et al.** (1994) Treatment of postoperative hypertension after coronary artery bypass surgery: Double-blind comparison of intravenous israpidine and sodium nitroprusside. *Circulation* **90**(part 2): II-256–II-261.

23. **Wong, M.C.W. and Haley, E.C., Jr** (1990) Calcium antagonists: stroke therapy coming of age. *Stroke* **21**: 494–501.

24. **Atkin, S.H., Jaher, M.A., Beaty, P., et al.** (1992) Oral labetalol versus oral clonidine in the emerging treatment of severe hypertension. *Am. J. Med. Sci.* **303**: 9–15.

25. **Ghigrione, M., Calvillo, O. and Quintin, L.** (1987) Anesthesia and hypertension: the effect of clonidine on perioperative hemodynamics and isoflurane requirements. *Anesthesiology* **67**: 3.

26. **Flacke, J.W., Bloor, B.C., Flacke, W.E., et al.** (1987) Reduced narcotic requirement by cloni-dine with improved hemodynamic and adren-ergic stability in patients undergoing coronary artery bypass surgery. *Anesthesiology* **67**: 11.

27. **Spitalewitz, S., Porush, J.G. and Oguayha, C.** (1983) Use of oral clonidine for rapid titration of blood pressure in severe hypertension. *Chest* **83**(Suppl.): 404–407.

28. **Mirenda, J., Edwards, C.** (1991) Use of intra-venous enalaprilat for hypertension following myocardial revascularization. *Anesth. Analg.* **72**: 667.

29. **Turini, G.A., Bribic, M., Drunner, H.R., Waeber, B. and Gavras, H.** (1979) Improve-ment of chronic congestive heart failure by oral captopril. *Lancet* **1**: 1213–1215.

30. **Goodfriend, T.L., Elliott, M.E. and Catt, K.J.** (1996) Angiotensin receptors and their antago-nists. *N. Engl. J. Med.* **334**: 1649–1654.

31. **Cryer, P.E.** (1987) Diseases of the sympatho-chromaffin system. In: *Endocrinology and Metabolism*, 2nd Edn (eds Felig, P., Baxter, J.D., Broadus, A.E. and Frohman, L.A.). McGraw–Hill, New York, p. 651–692.

32. **Roizen, M.F., Horrigan, R.W., Koike, M.,** *et al.* (1981) A prospective randomized trial of four anesthetic techniques for resection of pheochromocytomas. *Anesthesiology* **57**: A43.

33. **Calhoun, D.A. and Opanl, S.** (1990) Treatment of hypertensive crisis. *N. Engl. J. Med.* **323**: 1177–1183.

34. **Abin, M.S.** (1990) Anesthesia for spinal cord injury. *Probl. Anesth.* **4**: 138–143.

35. **Schonwald, G., Fish, K.J. and Perkaash, I.** (1981) Cardiovascular complications during anesthesia in chronic spinal cord injured patients. *Anesthesiology* **55**: 550.

36. **Tietjen, C.S., Hurn, P.D., Ulatowski, J.A. and Kirsch, J.R.** (1996) Treatment modalities for hypertensive patients with intracranial pathology: Options and risks. *Crit. Care Med.* **24**: 311–322.

37. **Bruder, N. and Ravussin, R.** (1999) Recovery from anesthesia and postoperative extubation of neurosurgical patients: A review. *J. Neurosurg. Anesth.* **11**: 282–293.

38. **Dandapani, B.K., Suzuki, S., Kelly, R.E.,** *et al.* (1995) Relation between blood pressure and outcome in intracerebral hemorrhage. *Stroke* **26**: 21–24.

39. **Lavin, P.** (1986) Management of hypertension in patients with acute stroke. *Arch. Intern. Med.* **146**:66–68.

40. **Rordorf, G., Cramer, S.C., Efird, J.T.,** *et al.* (1997) Pharmacologic elevation of blood pressure in acute stroke: Clinical effects and safety. *Stroke* **28**: 2133–2138.

41. **Powers, W.J.** (1993) Acute hypertension after stroke. The scientific basis for treatment decisions. *Neurology* **43**: 461–467.

42. **Stehling, L.C.** (1974) Anesthetic management of the patient with hyperthroidism. *Anesthesiology* **41**: 585.

43. **Bennett, M.H. and Wainwright, A.P.** (1989) Acute thyroid crisis on induction of anesthesia. *Anaesthesia* **44**: 28.

44. **Lombardi, A., Chiovato, L. and Braverman, L.E.** (1991) Thyroid storm. In: *Intensive Care Medicine* (eds J.M. Rippe, R.S. Irwin, J.S. Alpert and M.P. Fink). Little, Brown, Boston, MA, p. 976.

45. **Assche, F., Spitz, B. and Vansteelant, L.** (1989) Severe systemic hypertension during pregnancy. *Am. J. Cardiol.* **63**: 22C.

46. **Rey, E., LeLorier, J., Burgess, E.,** *et al.* (1997) Report of the Canadian Hypertension Society Consensus Conference: 3. Pharmacologic treatment of hypertensive disorders in pregnancy. *Can. Med. Assoc. J.* **157**: 1245–1254.

47. **Stanek, B., Kovarik, J., Rasoul-Rockenschaub, S. and Silberbauer, K.** (1987) Renin–angiotensin–aldosterone system and vasopressor in cyclosporine treated renal allograft recipients. *Clin. Nephrol.* **8**: 186–189.

48. **Miller, R.R.** (1975) Propranalol withdrawal rebound phenomenon: exacerbation of coronary events after abrupt cessation of antianginal therapy. *N. Engl. J. Med.* **293**: 416.

49. **Stack, C.G., Rogers, P. and Linter, S.P.** (1988) Monamine oxidase inhibitors and anaesthesia. *Br. J. Anaesth.* **60**: 222.

Chapter 10

Acute myocardial infarction

Marc Schweiger, MD

Contents

10.1 Overview

Each year, in the United States approximately one million people sustain an acute myocardial infarction (AMI) with about one-quarter being fatal[1]. Almost all of these patients have underlying atherosclerosis with superimposed thrombus. The exception are patients with conditions in which myocardial oxygen demand exceeds the available supply (i.e. severe anemia, thyrotoxicosis). Although the incidence of AMI and its mortality have been decreasing, AMI remains the most common cause of death in Western society. The reason for the decreased incidence of acute myocardial infarction is presumably multifactorial. Awareness of risk factors for atherosclerosis, which include hypertension, cigarette smoking, diabetes mellitus, hyperlipidemia and a family history of premature coronary disease, has led to more aggressive treatment and prevention. Newer medical treatments and use of more aggressive forms of interventional therapy (percutaneous coronary intervention, coronary bypass surgery) may be partially responsible.

Previously, myocardial infarctions were categorized as either Q wave or non-Q wave. However, with our present understanding of the pathophysiology, the more appropriate terminology is ST elevation MI (STEMI—Q wave or transmural MI) and non-ST elevation MI (NSTEMI—non-Q wave or non-transmural MI). Although many of the treatment modalities are appropriate for both types of MI, certain treatments are appropriate for STEMI but inappropriate for NSTEMI and vice versa.

The acute coronary syndromes are a continuum from unstable angina to NSTEMI to STEMI. Fissure or rupture of the atherosclerotic plaque exposes the subendothelial matrix to substances that activate platelets and generate thrombin[2]. If the thrombus occludes the lumen (with platelets, thrombin and red blood cells), an STEMI occurs unless the distal territory of the blood vessel has adequate collateral blood flow. Patients with a non-occlusive thrombus typically have more platelet-rich thrombi and are more likely to present with either ST segment depression or T wave inversion. Elevation of cardiac enzymes defines patients with ST depression or T wave inversion who have an NSTEMI (*Figure 10.1*).

10.2 Diagnosis, definitions and triage

The history, physical examination, electrocardiogram and laboratory tests are the tools used to make the diagnosis and appropriately triage patients. The definition of a myocardial infarction requires the presence of symptoms suggestive of ischemia and either EKG evidence or enzyme evidence. EKG evidence requires the development of Q waves in two or more leads to retrospectively establish a diagnosis of STEMI[3].

10.2.1 Classic history

The classic history of MI discomfort involves a discomfort usually in the chest, often associated with diaphoresis, which may radiate into the arms or back (see *Table 10.1*). The discomfort may be localized to only the arms, back or jaw or may radiate to these areas. The description of the discomfort is usually a pressure,

Table 10.1 Differential diagnosis of chest discomfort

Cardiac	Non-cardiac
• Angina	• Esophageal disorders
• Acute MI	
• Aortic dissection	• Peptic ulcer
• Pericarditis	• Costochondritis
• Myocarditis	• Cervical disk
• Mitral valve prolapse	• Hyperventilation
	• Anxiety
	• Pulmonary embolism
	• Pulmonary hypertension
	• Pneumonia

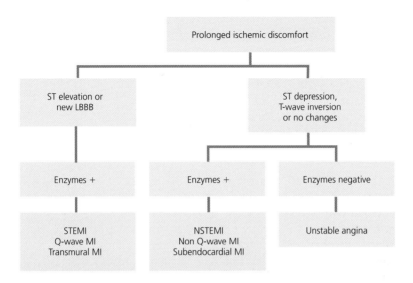

Figure 10.1 This shows the classification of patients who present with prolonged ischemic discomfort. Patients with ST segment elevation or a new left bundle branch block on their electrocardiogram will have, in the presence of + enzymes, an ST elevation myocardial infarction (also known as a Q Wave Myocardial Infarction or Transmural Myocardial Infarction). Patients without EKG changes or those with ST depression or T wave inversion will have a non ST-elevation myocardial infarction (also known as a Non-Q Wave Myocardial Infarction or Subendocardial Myocardial Infarction) if their cardiac enzymes are +, and unstable angina if their cardiac enzymes are negative.

burning or constricting sensation. It may be described as indigestion. Often patients will answer 'no' to the question of whether there is any pain but will answer in the affirmative to the question of whether there is discomfort. There is often associated nausea and vomiting. There are, however, many variations of presenting symptoms and some patients may not have any discomfort at all. In the intensive care unit setting patients may develop myocardial ischemia while intubated, sedated and paralyzed. Residual anesthesia or analgesics may lessen or eliminate the discomfort. Questions regarding any similar symptoms recently, previous cardiac history and presence of risk factors help in assessing the likelihood of ischemic pain when the presentation is not classic. Discomforts that last seconds are rarely ischemic. The differential diagnosis of chest discomfort is shown in *Table 10.1*.

10.2.2 Electrocardiogram

The electrocardiogram of patients with acute ST segment elevation MI will show new ST segment elevation (>1 mm in at least two contiguous leads) (*Figure 10.2*) or a new left bundle branch block. Patients presenting with a posterior wall myocardial infarction may present with a normal EKG. The electrocardiogram of patients with unstable angina or non-ST elevation MI will usually show ST segment depression or T wave inversion (*Figure 10.3*). The majority of patients presenting with ST segment elevation will evolve a Q wave myocardial infarction but some will develop a non-Q wave myocardial infarction. Patients presenting with ischemic discomfort at rest without ST segment elevation are likely to ultimately be diagnosed as unstable angina or non-Q wave myocardial infarction; a minority will develop a Q wave myocardial infarction.

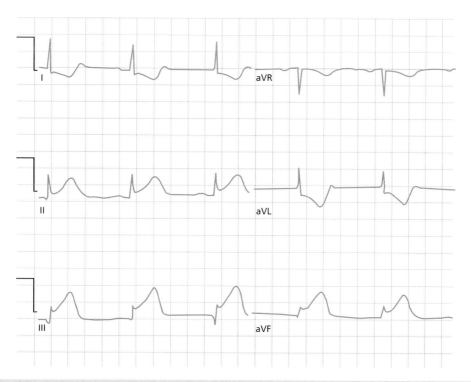

Figure 10.2 EKG showing changes of an inferior wall ST elevation myocardial infarction. Significant (>3 mm) ST elevation is noted in leads II, III and aVF.

10.2.3 Laboratory evidence

Laboratory evidence, particularly cardiac enzymes, is useful for diagnosis and prognosis. For patients presenting with rest chest pain without ST segment elevation, positive cardiac enzymes confirm the diagnosis of myocardial infarction. Troponin I and T are sensitive and specific markers for myocardial necrosis but do not elevate until 4–6 h following necrosis. Thus a negative early troponin requires an additional troponin 8–12 h after symptom onset. Troponins may remain elevated for up to 2 weeks and thus are useful in diagnosing recent MI. A significant number of patients presenting with ischemic pain without ST segment elevation are diagnosed as an NSTEMI because their troponin is positive whereas their Creatine Phosphokinase-Myocardial Band (CK-MB) is negative. In patients who present with unstable angina/non-ST segment elevation MI, troponins are also useful for risk stratification[4], as a positive troponin predicts recurrent myocardial infarction and mortality.[5] CK-MB, an isoenzyme of CK, although widely used, is not specific for myocardial necrosis, as some CK-MB is present in skeletal muscle. The diaphragm and esophagus are also sources of CK-MB, which may elevate following thoracic surgical procedures (see Chapter 24). CK-MB often does not elevate until more than 6 h after myocardial necrosis. The timing of the peak CK is useful in assessing reperfusion in ST elevation MI (earlier peak with successful reperfusion). Myoglobin is a specific but not sensitive marker of myocardial necrosis. It rises rapidly (>2 h) and returns to normal less than 24 h after myocardial necrosis. A negative myoglobin, 4–8 h following symptoms, in a patient with a non-diagnostic EKG effectively rules out myocardial necrosis. Previously utilized laboratory tests, such as serum glutamic oxaloacetic acid transferase (SGOT) and lactic dehydrogenase (LDH), have limited utility in the era of newer cardiac markers.

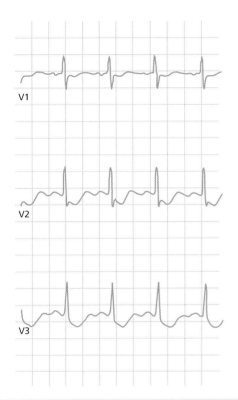

Figure 10.3 EKG showing significant ST segment depression in leads V2 and V3.

10.2.4 Triage decision

When evaluating patients with symptoms of acute coronary syndrome, the initial triage decision is determined by an EKG, which should be performed within 10 min of arrival. An EKG showing ST segment elevation or a new or presumably new left bundle branch block leads to an evaluation for reperfusion therapy. An electrocardiogram suspicious for ischemia, or ongoing ischemic pain without electrocardiographic changes, should prompt admission to a monitored bed. Should the pain appear classic and unrelenting, in the absence of EKG changes, the diagnosis of a posterior wall MI should be entertained and an echocardiogram may be useful in this situation (posterior wall akinesis in the absence of a previous MI history). The diagnosis of a myocardial infarction requires the presence of elevated cardiac enzymes. The electrocardiogram will distinguish a non-ST elevation MI from an ST elevation MI and the enzymes will distinguish a non-ST elevation MI from unstable angina.

10.3 Initial treatment of acute ischemic syndrome

10.3.1 Routine requirements

All patients with acute ischemic syndromes should undergo continuous EKG monitoring for arrhythmia detection[1,6]. Intravenous access must be established. Oxygen supplementation should be routine airway for O_2 saturation of 95% or more.

10.3.2 Nitroglycerine

All patients with acute ischemic chest pain should receive one sublingual nitroglycerine (generally 1/150 grain) unless the systolic blood pressure is less than 90 mmHg. Nitroglycerine should not be used in patients with right ventricular MI because these patients are extremely volume dependent and may become hypotensive with vasodilation. Only one sublingual nitroglycerine should routinely be given to patients with ST segment elevation MI. Intravenous nitroglycerine is recommended for patients with acute STEMI with persistent hypertension or congestive heart failure. In patients with STEMI, IV nitroglycerine should not be used in lieu of adequate analgesia. In patients with NSTEMI, sublingual NTG can be given 5 min apart $\times$ 3 followed by an IV nitroglycerine infusion for continued ischemic discomfort.

10.3.3 Morphine sulfate

This should be used to treat ischemic pain that does not respond promptly to sublingual nitroglycerine in patients with ST segment elevation MI. Morphine serves as an anxiolytic and analgesic. It also decreases arterial pressure and venous return. Morphine should be given in 2–4 mg increments every 5 min until the pain is controlled and the patient less anxious. The use of analgesia may make it difficult to assess pain relief in patients given thrombolytic therapy, but its use should not be

151

withheld. Side effects of morphine include hypotension, nausea and respiratory depression. Although these must be considered, adequate analgesia is a cornerstone of initial MI treatment. Patients experiencing an NSTEMI (or unstable angina—enzymes not yet back) should also receive IV morphine for pain not responding to nitrates, pulmonary congestion, or significant agitation. In the ICU setting where respiration is monitored and often controlled, fentanyl 50–100 µg IV is less likely to cause hypotension, as fentanyl does not cause histamine release.

10.3.4 Oral anti-platelet therapy

Aspirin has been shown to reduce mortality in patients with STEMI[7] when used alone or in combination with streptokinase. It also has been shown to decrease reocclusion and recurrent ischemic events following thrombolytic therapy. Aspirin works by inhibition of platelet activation via its inhibition of thromboxane A_2. Aspirin has also been shown to decrease risk in patients with unstable angina/non-ST segment elevation MI[8]. It is recommended that patients presenting with acute ischemic syndrome who have not been taking aspirin promptly receive a chewable aspirin, dose of 160 mg or 325 mg[1,6]. Patients can then be maintained on 75, 160 or 325 mg of aspirin daily. Patients who have an allergy to aspirin may be given either ticlopidine (Ticlid) or clopidogrel (Plavix), which inhibits ADP-mediated platelet activation. Clopidogrel has fewer reported side effects than ticlopidine. Clopidogrel is usually given in a dose of 75 mg day[-1]; however, this dosage has delayed efficacy and a loading dose of 300 mg is preferred in acute ischemic syndrome for aspirin intolerant patients.

10.3.5 Beta adrenergic-blocker therapy

For patients with STEMI, intravenous followed by oral beta blocker therapy reduces mortality in patients not receiving thrombolytic therapy[9], and reduces reinfarction and recurrent ischemia in patients receiving thrombolytic therapy[10]. Intravenous beta blockers are indi-

cated in patients with STEMI treated within 12 h, followed by oral therapy, unless there are contraindications such as bradycardia (heart rate <60), systolic pressure <100 mmHg, bronchospastic lung disease, second- or third-degree heart block, active congestive heart failure, or prolonged PR interval (>0.24 s). Patients are generally given 5 mg of metoprolol (lopressor) intravenously every 5 min for three doses provided their blood pressure and heart rate are within parameters. They are then generally started on 25 mg of metoprolol orally, which is increased as necessary to achieve an appropriate heart rate (and blood pressure) response. Beta-adrenergic blockers with intrinsic sympathomimetic activity (i.e. Pindolol) should be avoided. For patients admitted with acute ischemic syndrome without ST segment elevation, intravenous beta blockers should be given, in the absence of contraindications, if ongoing chest pain is present, followed by oral administration. *Table 10.2* shows properties of commonly used beta-adrenergic blockers.

10.3.6 Calcium channel blocker therapy

The role of calcium channel antagonism in acute myocardial infarction has been somewhat controversial. It is not first line therapy in patients with STEMI or NSTEMI. In patients with myocardial infarction, the use of non-hydropyridine calcium antagonists, verapamil or diltiazem, may be appropriate for patients, with ongoing ischemia or rapid ventricular response to atrial fibrillation, who are intolerant of beta blockers secondary to bronchospastic lung disease. These agents should not be used with ongoing congestive heart failure or significant heart block (second- or third-degree heart block or first-degree heart block with PR interval >0.24 s). Diltiazem (cardizem) may be added as standard therapy to patients with NSTEMI after 24 h and continued for 1 year in the absence of LV dysfunction or congestive heart failure[11]. Immediate-release dihydropyridine calcium channel blockers should never be given in the absence of a beta-adrenergic blocker but can in certain instances be given to

Table 10.2 Beta-adrenergic receptor antagonists

Agent	Selectivity	Agonist activity	Dose (usual)
Acebutolol (Sectral)	B$_1$	Partial	200–600 mg twice daily
Atenolol (Tenormin)	B$_1$	No	50–200 mg daily
Metoprolol (Lopressor)	B$_1$	No	25–100 mg twice daily
Bisoprolol (Zebeta)	B$_1$	No	10 mg daily
Betaxolol (Kerlone)	B$_1$	No	10–20 mg daily
Esmolol (Breviblock)	B$_1$	No	IV 50–300 mg kg^{-1} min^{-1}
Propranalol (Inderal)	None	No	10–40 mg 4 times daily
Nadalol (Corgard)	None	No	40–240 mg daily
Timolol (Blocadren)	None	No	10 mg twice daily
Labetalol (Normodyne)	Combined alpha and non-selective B	No	200–600 mg daily
Pindolol (Visken)	None	Yes	10–30 mg 3 times daily

patients with ongoing ischemia post-infarction who are receiving a beta blocker.

10.3.7 Angiotensin-converting enzyme inhibitors (ACEI)

These have been shown to reduce mortality in patients with a recent myocardial infarction. The benefit is most pronounced in patients with left ventricular systolic dysfunction[12]. Recent evidence suggests a benefit for patients with vascular disease and/or diabetes greater than 55 years of age[13]. Therefore in the absence of contraindications, ACEI therapy may be initiated in patients with acute myocardial infarction (STEMI or NSTEMI) early in their hospital course, particularly when there is known or suspected left ventricular dysfunction or continued hypertension.

10.3.8 Parenteral anticoagulants

These include unfractionated heparin, low molecular weight heparin, hirudin, and bivalirudin. Hirudin and bivalirudin are direct thrombin inhibitors. Bivalirudin has been approved for use in percutaneous coronary intervention. Hirudin is utilized in patients with heparin-induced thrombocytopenia. Unfractionated heparin or low molecular weight heparin, when added to aspirin, reduces the risk of recurrent MI or mortality in patients with unstable angina/NSTEMI by approximately 50%[14]. Unfractionated heparin inactivates thrombin through its action on antithrombin III and has a lesser effect on factor X$_a$ and IX$_a$. Unfractionated heparin does have limitations related to its non-specific binding to proteins, which leads to variable anticoagulation requiring frequent activated partial thromboplastin time (APTT) measurements and dose adjustments. Low molecular weight heparin has a more predictable anticoagulant response and a longer plasma half-life than unfractionated heparin, and is therefore easier to use than unfractionated heparin. Low molecular weight heparin has less of an effect on thrombin than unfractionated heparin, as the cross bridging between antithrombin and thrombin requires pentasaccharide containing chains of at least 18 saccharide units. Heparin-induced thrombocytopenia appears to be somewhat less common with low molecular weight heparin than unfractionated heparin.

Multiple clinical trials suggest that low molecular weight heparin is at least as effective as unfractionated heparin in the treatment of unstable angina/NSTEMI. Although some trials have suggested a clinical benefit of low molecular weight heparin over unfractionated heparin, other trials have revealed no benefit[14]. Trials comparing the various low molecular weight heparins have not been performed. The safety and efficacy of low molecular weight heparins in the catheterization laboratory and in concert with glycoprotein IIb/IIIa inhibition has not been adequately studied.

Patients with unstable angina/NSTEMI should receive either IV unfractionated heparin or subcutaneous low molecular weight heparin (*Table 10.3*). Unfractionated heparin is usually given as a weight-adjusted regimen with an initial bolus of 60–70 U kg^{-1} (maximum 5000 U) with an initial infusion of 12–15 U kg^{-1} h^{-1} (maximum 1000 U). Each institution should establish its own nomogram to achieve target aPTT (1.5–2.5 times control). Measurements should be made 6 h after a dosage change and used to adjust heparin dosing until the aPTT is therapeutic. When two consecutive aPTT results are therapeutic the next measurement can be made in 24 h unless a change in clinical condition ensues. Daily hemoglobin, hematocrit and platelet count measurements are suggested with patients on heparin. Most trials of unfractionated heparin in unstable angina/non-ST segment elevation myocardial infarction continued therapy for 2–5 days (it is the current practice to discontinue heparin after a percutaneous coronary intervention is performed). Mild thrombocytopenia occurs in 10–20% of patients receiving unfractionated heparin; severe thrombocytopenia (platelet count <100 000) occurs in 1–2% and usually occurs late (4–14 days after starting therapy). Fewer than 0.2% of patients experience heparin-induced thrombocytopenia with thrombosis[6]. Patients who develop heparin-induced thrombocytopenia should be given hirudin, a direct acting thrombin inhibitor, given as a bolus of 0.4 mg kg^{-1} IV over 15–20 s followed by an IV infusion of 0.15 mg kg^{-1} h^{-1} with a target aPTT of 1.5–2.5 times control.

Patients presenting with STEMI who are undergoing reperfusion therapy with alteplase or tenecteplase should receive a 60 U kg^{-1} bolus of heparin followed by a maintenance infusion of 12 U kg^{-1} h^{-1} (maximum 4000 U bolus and 1000 U h^{-1} infusion for patients weighing >70 kg), adjusting the aPTT to 1.5–2.0 times control for 24–48 h. Most physicians stop heparin after a successful percutaneous coronary intervention. Heparin can be continued for patients at high risk for systemic or venous thromboembolism.

Oral anticoagulation with warfarin is at present recommended only for patients with established indications such as atrial fibrillation, mechanical heart valves or left ventricular thrombus. Recently presented studies suggest a benefit for long-term high-dose coumadin in preventing late vessel occlusion but this needs confirmation in larger trials.

10.3.9 Glycoprotein IIb/IIIa antagonists

The glycoprotein IIb/IIIa receptor is the final common pathway for platelet aggregation. Platelet agonists activate the platelet and induce a conformational change in the IIb/IIIa receptor that increases its affinity to bind fibrinogen and von Willebrands factor. There are at present three intravenous glycoprotein IIb/IIIa receptor antagonists available for clinical use. The monoclonal antibody abciximab (ReoPro) has been extensively studied and has been clearly shown to reduce clinical events following percutaneous coronary intervention. Its efficacy, however, in unstable angina/NSTEMI has not been established. The small molecule glycoprotein IIb/IIIa antagonists, eptifibatide (integrelin) and tirofiban (aggrastat), have been shown in clinical trials to reduce recurrent events (predominantly recurrent myocardial infarction) in patients presenting with unstable angina/non-Q wave myocardial infarction[15,16]. It is recommended that these agents be administered, in addition to aspirin and unfractionated heparin, in patients with ongoing ischemia, high-risk features, or in whom a percutaneous coronary intervention is planned. High-risk features include positive serum markers, transient ST elevation or depression with chest pain, more than 20 min of rest pain, accelerating pain over the previous 24–48 h, age over 75 years, ischemia-induced congestive heart failure or mitral regurgitation, hypotension or sustained ventricular tachycardia[6] (*Table 10.3*).

10.4 Thrombolytic therapy

Reperfusion therapy with a thrombolytic agent is utilized for the treatment of acute STEMI (or new or presumably new left bundle branch block) in the presence of chest pain less than 12 h after onset of the most severe symptoms. Thrombolytic therapy is contraindicated in patients with NSTEMI. Thrombolytic therapy restores patency in the infarct artery and therefore reduces mortality and improves left ventricular function. It has the greatest benefit when given early after symptom onset. It is estimated that for every 1 h delay in administering thrombolytic therapy there is a loss of approximately 20 lives for every 1000 patients treated. Therefore it is important to educate patients to come to hospital promptly with symptoms of acute myocardial infarction, and it is incumbent on hospital emergency rooms to have a short 'door-to-needle' time.

Thrombolytic therapy has the advantage of universal hospital availability and thus, unlike primary angioplasty, can be offered expeditiously at all hospitals. There are, however, both absolute and relative contraindications to patient treatment with thrombolytic therapy. Absolute contraindications for thrombolytic therapy include: active internal bleeding, known intracranial neoplasm, and previous intracranial bleed. Relative contraindications include: elevated systolic blood pressure over 180 mmHg, diastolic blood pressure over 110 mmHg (note: blood pressure is the first reliable blood pressure taken after arrival to the emergency room), previous cerebrovascular event at any time, active peptic ulcer, pregnancy, non-compressible vascular puncture, prolonged (>10 min) CPR, recent (<3 weeks) major surgery, recent trauma (<4 weeks), recent internal bleeding (<4 weeks). Relative contraindications will vary depending on the availability and speed to alternative therapy (i.e. primary angioplasty) as well as the perceived risk to the patient of their myocardial infarction (i.e. speedy access to primary angioplasty would increase the threshold to utilize thrombolytic therapy in a patient with a relative contraindication; apparent large myocardial infarction early after symptom onset in a situation where transport for primary angioplasty is not

Table 10.3 Non-parental antithrombotic therapy	
Intravenous antiplatelet therapy	**Dose**
Eptifibatide (Integrilin)	180 µg kg^{-1} bolus followed by 2 µg kg^{-1} min^{-1} infusion
Tirofiban (Aggrastat)	0.4 µg kg^{-1} min^{-1} bolus over 30 min followed by 0.1 µg kg^{-1} min^{-1} infusion
Unfractionated heparin	UA/NSTEMI: 60–70 U kg^{-1} (max. 5000 U) bolus followed by 12–15 U kg^{-1} h^{-1} infusion (titrated to aPTT 1.5–2.5 times control)
	STEMI—with thrombolytic tenectepase (TNK): 60 U kg^{-1} bolus, infusion of 12 U kg^{-1} h^{-1} (max. 4000 U bolus, 1000 U h^{-1} infusion if weight >70 kg), adjusted to aPTT between 1.5 and 2 times control
Lovenox (Enoxaparin)	1 mg kg^{-1} subcutaneously every 12 h
Dalteparin (Fragmin)	120 IU kg^{-1} subcutaneously every 12 h (maximum 10 000 IU twice daily)

feasible would decrease the threshold to utilize thrombolytic therapy).

Table 10.4 shows characteristics of currently available thrombolytic agents. Retaplase and tenectaplase are derived from tissue plasminogen activator. Retaplase is a deletion mutant, tenectaplase a substitution mutant of the tPA molecule. With currently available agents, optimal flow (TIMI (thrombolysis in myocardial infarction) 3 flow) is established at 90 min in 35–60% of patients. Intracranial hemorrhage occurs in 0.5–1% of patients depending on the agent and patient population. Trials comparing the mortality for the various thrombolytic agents have been performed; alteplase was shown to decrease mortality compared with streptokinase[17], retaplase and streptokinase were shown to be equivalent[18], retaplase was not shown to be superior to alteplase[19], and tenectaplase and alteplase were shown to be equivalent with slightly less bleeding in the tenectaplase-treated patients[20].

Recently, preliminary trials of half-dose thrombolytic and glycoprotein IIb/IIIa inhibition therapy have been shown to achieve reperfusion more rapidly and improve TIMI 3 flow rates without an increase in bleeding[21]. At present, there are numerous ongoing trials involving combinations of thrombolytic therapy with all of the currently available glycoprotein IIb/IIIa inhibitors.

10.5 Primary angioplasty

Primary angioplasty has been compared with thrombolytic therapy in many small randomized clinical trials. A meta-analysis suggests a mortality benefit for patients treated with primary angioplasty[22]. The benefit of primary angioplasty appeared to attenuate over 6 months in the GUSTO III trial[23]. This may be related to restenosis or reocclusion of the dilated infarct artery causing lesion and may be obviated with the use of coronary stents and perhaps glycoprotein IIb/IIIa inhibitors. Primary angioplasty is not routinely available at many hospitals. The benefit of primary angioplasty is probably obtained when patients can be taken to the catheterization laboratory quickly (door-to-balloon time <90 min); however, the average door-to-balloon time in registry studies appears to be approximately 120 min[24]. This is of concern, as during this 'delay' there is unlikely to be improvement in flow. Future studies are likely to compare primary angioplasty with combined low-dose thrombolytic and glycoprotein IIb/IIIa inhibition therapy (with or without early coronary angiography and percutaneous intervention). Primary angioplasty does appear to be superior in patients less than 75 years old presenting with cardiogenic shock[25]. Primary angioplasty is also indicated in patients with

Table 10.4 Comparison of thrombolytic agents				
Characteristics	**Streptokinase**	**Alteplase (t-PA)**	**Retaplase (r-PA)**	**Tenectaplase (TNK-tPA)**
Immunogenicity	Yes	No	No	No
Fibrin specificity	+	++	+	+ + +
Plasma half-life	?	4–6 min	18 min	20 min
90 min TIMI 3 flow	30–35%	45–60%	50–60%	50–60%
Cost	+	+ + +	+ + +	+ + +
Dose	1.5 × 10⁶ over 60 min	15 mg infusion, up to 50 mg over next 30 min, up to 35 mg over next 60 min	10 + 10 MU; double bolus 30 min apart	0.5 mg kg⁻¹ IV bolus (not to exceed 50 mg)

contraindications to thrombolytic therapy. Patients with prior coronary artery bypass surgery may also benefit from primary angioplasty, as the benefit of thrombolytic therapy in this subset of patients is not well established. However, there may also be a great deal of difficulty in performing angioplasty on acutely occluded saphenous vein grafts. The use of stents in primary angioplasty has been shown to decrease the need for repeat procedure secondary to restenosis[26].

10.6 Lipid-lowering therapy

Guidelines have been established for the treatment of hypercholesterolemia in patients with known coronary artery disease. It is at present recommended that patients be treated to obtain an LDL cholesterol less than 100 mg dL^{-1} [27]. The mortality benefit seen in previous clinical trials begins to appear shortly after the initiation of therapy, suggesting a role for acutely treating patients with acute coronary syndromes to enhance plaque stabilization. The recently presented MIRACL trial[28] suggested a benefit at 4 months for patients with acute coronary syndrome treated immediately with aggressive lipid-lowering therapy.

10.7 Complications of myocardial infarction

10.7.1 Right ventricular infarction
This frequently accompanies inferior myocardial infarction. There is a characteristic hemodynamic pattern of elevated right sided filling pressures. Left ventricular filling pressures are normal or only minimally elevated. Cardiac output may be depressed. An increase in right atrial pressure with inspiration (Kussmal's sign) may be present. Patients presenting with an inferior wall myocardial infarction with signs of decreased cardiac output (hypotension) who have elevated right atrial pressure should be suspected of having a right ventricular infarction. The EKG will usually show an

inferior wall MI and right precordial leads will show ST segment elevation. Coronary angiography will generally show involvement of the proximal right coronary artery, although rarely there will be circumflex involvement. First-line therapy consists of aggressive fluid resuscitation guided by central hemodynamic monitoring. Intravenous fluid is administered until an increase in left ventricular filling pressure occurs, as indicated by an increase in pulmonary capillary wedge pressure. When fluid resuscitation fails to improve forward flow, inotropic stimulation is required (see Chapter 8). Dobutamine (usually 4–10 µg kg^{-1} min^{-1}) is administered to augment cardiac output. Besides providing inotropic support, dobutamine decreases pulmonary vascular resistance and reduces right ventricular afterload, thereby facilitating flow from the right heart to the left ventricle.

Right ventricular MI may be associated with high-degree atrio-ventricular (AV) conduction abnormalities; these can result in various forms of heart block, including bradycardia and loss of AV synchrony. Management typically consists of temporary right ventricular pacing until the cardiac conduction system recovers function.

10.7.2 Free wall rupture
This usually leads to hemopericardium and death secondary to cardiac tamponade. It occurs most frequently 1–4 days following a transmural myocardial infarction, and is more common in elderly patients, hypertensive patients and patients who have received corticosteroids. It usually involves the anterior and lateral walls of the left ventricle and most commonly occurs at the junction of infarcted and normal muscle. Presenting symptoms include jugular venous distention, hypotension, paradoxical pulse and distant heart sounds. The presentation is generally catastrophic with sudden death from pericardial tamponade. Occasionally the tear may be subacute with the patient complaining of pain (generally pleuritic) with hypotension and often dramatic ST segment elevation on the

electrocardiogram. Prompt recognition leading to surgical repair is mandatory for survival.

10.7.3 Intraventricular septal rupture

This usually occurs 1–4 days following a transmural myocardial infarction. It is more common in elderly patients and patients with hypertension. The size of the septal defect determines the degree of shunting (left to right) and consequently survival. Anterior wall infarction is associated with apical septal rupture whereas inferior wall infarction is associated with a basal septal rupture and has a higher mortality secondary to a more complicated surgical procedure. Intraventricular septal rupture presents with a new loud systolic murmur that generally is holosystolic and can be heard maximally at the left lower sternal border or the apex. Patients frequently are hypotensive and have signs and symptoms of congestive heart failure. Two-dimensional echocardiography will be diagnostic, as will placement of a pulmonary artery balloon catheter with oximetry. A step-up in oxygenation saturation from the right atrium to the pulmonary artery is considered a definitive sign. The treatment is surgical. Stabilization with the use of an intra-aortic balloon pump is usually necessary.

10.7.4 Rupture of papillary muscle

This usually occurs 1–4 days following a transmural myocardial infarction. Inferior wall infarction leads to rupture of the posteriomedial papillary muscle, whereas patients with anterior wall infarction can have ruptures of the anterolateral papillary muscle. The presentation is similar to the rupture of an interventricular septum and can be difficult to distinguish clinically. Two-dimensional echocardiography with color flow Doppler imaging is useful in distinguishing these two entities.

10.8 Subsequent treatment strategies

The use of coronary angiography will differ by clinical presentation.

10.8.1 Unstable angina/NSTEMI

For unstable angina/NSTEMI, the necessity of a routine invasive strategy following admission has been evaluated in four clinical trials. The TIMI 3 trial, which evaluated patients with unstable angina or non-Q wave myocardial infarction, demonstrated no mortality/reinfarction difference between a routine invasive strategy carried out within 48 h versus a conservative strategy with catheterization for breakthrough ischemia or a strongly positive exercise test[29]. In this trial many patients in the 'conservative' group ultimately underwent angiography and there was less rehospitalization in the invasive strategy group. The conclusion was that either strategy was acceptable and in stable patients there was no necessity to transfer patients to a hospital with the facilities to perform coronary intervention. The Vanquish trial of patients with non-Q wave myocardial infarction suggested a mortality benefit for patients randomized to a conservative approach[30]. In this trial, all of the excess mortality was secondary to a high surgical mortality among patients in the invasive group undergoing coronary artery bypass surgery. The FRISC II trial randomized patients to a low molecular weight heparin (Fragmin) or unfractionated heparin with a second randomization to an invasive or conservative strategy. Patients undergoing an invasive procedure did so 4 days following hospital admission and only 10% of the conservative strategy patients underwent coronary angiography. A clinical benefit was observed for patients in the invasive strategy group[31].

The recently completed TACTICS TIMI 18 trial randomized patients with unstable angina and non-Q wave myocardial infarction to an invasive or selective invasive strategy[4]. All patients received the glycoprotein IIb/IIIa inhibitor Tirofiban. Invasive strategy patients underwent coronary angiography 4–48 h following admission. Sixty per cent of the invasive patients underwent revascularization during their initial hospitalization (41% percutaneous coronary intervention, 19% coronary bypass surgery). Fifty-one per cent of the 'selective invasive' patients underwent coronary angiography during their initial hospitalization. By 6 months, 61% of the 'invasive strategy' patients had undergone revascularization, whereas 44% of the 'selective invasive' patients also had revascularization. The primary combined endpoint of death, myocardial infarction and rehospitalization at 6 months was significantly lower in the invasive strategy patients. This improvement was magnified among patients with positive troponin and patients with an intermediate or high TIMI risk score[32]. This would suggest that in the present era of coronary intervention, including the use of stents and glycoprotein IIb/IIIa inhibitors, early coronary angiography is indicated for patients with high-risk features.

10.8.2 Coronary angiography for STEMI
This may be divided into three time periods: rescue angioplasty for those who have an occluded infarct-related artery following thrombolytic therapy, early angioplasty for patients who have a patent (TIMI flow 2 or 3) infarct artery (adjunctive angioplasty), and angiography later in the hospitalization following thrombolytic therapy with possible delayed angioplasty.

The utility of rescue angioplasty has been demonstrated in one randomized trial of patients with anterior wall myocardial infarction, which showed a decrease in 30 day mortality or congestive heart failure[33]. Recent trials have shown improved outcomes in patients undergoing rescue angioplasty. It is likely that patients will benefit from rescue angioplasty if it is carried out as quickly as possible in patients experiencing a large myocardial infarction. Patients should be assessed within 1 h following thrombolytic therapy for signs of reperfusion (pain relief, resolution or marked improvement in ST segments, reperfusion arrhythmia). Should there be a clinical suspicion of thrombolytic therapy failure, clinical consideration should be given to rapid transfer to a catheterization laboratory, particularly if the amount of myocardium in jeopardy appears to be large and a catheterization laboratory is readily available.

Previous studies (TIMI 2A, TAMI (thrombolysis and angioplasty in myocardial infarction), European Cooperative Study Group, ECSG)[34–36] performed in the mid-1980s suggested that patients undergoing immediate percutaneous coronary intervention in association with thrombolytic therapy for acute myocardial infarction were at increased risk for adverse outcomes. In a recent study of patients undergoing early angiography, however, appropriate intervention following half-dose thrombolytic therapy showed no hazard and a shorter time to optimal flow[37]. Observational data from TIMI 10B and TIMI 14[38] also suggest excellent outcomes with reduced hospital length of stay for patients undergoing immediate catheterization and intervention, when appropriate, with TIMI 2 or 3 flow. These improved outcomes may be due, in part, to the availability of stents and better pharmacologic agents. Future trials will be needed to demonstrate the utility of an early invasive strategy among patients treated with pharmacologic therapy for acute myocardial infarction.

The use of a routine invasive strategy a few days following thrombolytic therapy has not demonstrated an advantage over a more conservative strategy. Previous studies were carried out in an era of less advanced interventional and surgical techniques and may not be relevant in the current era. It should be emphasized that patients with recurrent ischemia post-myocardial infarction (either spontaneous or provoked) should undergo coronary angiography.

10.8.3 Stress testing
In patients with unstable angina (NSTEMI) who are admitted with a definite diagnosis of acute coronary syndrome, triage is by their clinical presentation[6]. As previously mentioned, patients with factors associated with increased risk should be considered for early invasive strategy. Stress testing is indicated for those patients who stabilize clinically, appear to be at low risk, and have an ejection fraction greater than 40%. Patients with a 'low-risk'

stress test result can be managed with medical therapy.

Following thrombolytic therapy, patients are considered for a submaximal stress test beginning on day 4 to assess future risk and the need for coronary angiography. Patients with a markedly abnormal test should undergo coronary angiography. Patients with a mildly abnormal test should either undergo an exercise imaging study to further risk stratify or undergo coronary angiography. Patients who undergo a submaximal test that does not suggest an increased risk should undergo a symptom limited test 3–6 weeks following their myocardial infarction.

10.8.4 Echocardiography

The assessment of patients with acute MI and unstable angina is useful when clinical and ECG findings are non-diagnostic. Transient segmental wall motion abnormalities during episodes of chest discomfort are diagnostic of ischemia. A fixed segmental wall motion abnormality can represent an acute myocardial infarction, a remote myocardial infarction, or chronic ischemia (hibernation)[39].

Echocardiography can be used to assess risk. Left ventricular dysfunction, as assessed by echocardiography, predicts early and late complications. It can be used, at the bedside, to demonstrate sequential changes (improvement or deterioration) in left ventricular function[39].

Echocardiography can be used to evaluate complications of myocardial infarction. These complications include acute mitral regurgitation, ventricular septal rupture, infarct expansion and LV remodeling, free wall rupture, intracardiac thrombus, RV infarction (occurring in approximately a third of patients with inferior wall MI) and pericardial effusion[39].

Stress or dobutamine echocardiography is a useful tool to assess risk following myocardial infarction, particularly in those patients in whom baseline abnormalities are expected to compromise interpretation[39].

10.8.5 Indications for hemodynamic monitoring (pulmonary artery catheter)

Insertion of a flow directed catheter into the pulmonary artery may be indicated when there is uncertainty regarding the hemodynamics of a patient following myocardial infarction. Examples include persistent hypotension unresponsive to fluid administration, cardiogenic shock, and suspected mechanical complications such as ventricular septal defect, mitral regurgitation and pericardial tamponade, although these mechanical complications can often be evaluated effectively by physical exam and echocardiography.

10.8.6 Indications for intraaortic balloon counterpulsation

The intraaortic balloon derives its efficacy primarily by reducing left ventricular afterload with rapid balloon deflation in end diastole. In contrast to other methods of afterload reduction, which generally lower arterial pressure, the sequential inflation and deflation of the balloon helps maintain coronary artery perfusion pressure and thus perfusion of the myocardium. The intraaortic balloon pump is recommended for: patients with cardiogenic shock not quickly reversed with pharmacologic therapy, as a stabilizing measure before angiography and prompt revascularization, in patients with acute mitral regurgitation or ventricular septal defect complicating MI as a stabilizing therapy before operative repair, patients with refractory ischemia post-MI as a bridge to angiography and revascularization, and in patients with recurrent ventricular arrhythmias post-MI thought secondary to ischemia or hemodynamic instability. It is probably beneficial in patients with hemodynamic instability, poor LV function or persistent ischemia in the presence of a large myocardial infarction[1].

10.8.7 Standby temporary pacemaker

There are situations post-MI where transcutaneous patches need to be placed to provide standby pacing capability in patients who are felt unlikely to progress to high-grade AV block, and who do not require immediate pacing. As these systems are potentially painful they should not be used if there is a high likelihood that pacing will be required. Transcutaneous pacing does not entail the complications and risks of intravenous pacing, particularly for patients who have recently received thrombolytic therapy. These systems are intended to be prophylactic and temporary, and can be used in an emergency situation as a bridge to temporary transvenous pacing. Patients who are felt to have a high probability of requiring pacing (>30% risk of AV block) should receive a temporary pacing wire. Appropriate situations include those patients with asymptomatic hypotension with sinus bradycardia that is unresponsive or poorly responsive to medical (i.e. atropine) treatment and patients with newly acquired or age-indeterminate left bundle or right bundle branch block with a left fascicular hemiblock. Patients with a new right bundle branch block with a first-degree heart block should also be considered for application of transcutaneous patches.

10.8.8 Indications for temporary transvenous pacing

These include asystole, symptomatic bradycardia (sinus bradycardia or type 1 second-degree AV block, associated with hypotension and unresponsive to atropine), bilateral bundle branch block, new or age indeterminate bifascicular block with first-degree AV block, Mobitz type II second-degree AV block, or third-degree AV block with a wide QRS (generally seen in patients with anterior wall myocardial infarction)[1].

10.8.9 Permanent pacing

Permanent pacing after myocardial infarction is related to the degree and type of AV block present after the myocardial infarction. It is recommended for patients with persistent second-degree AV block in the His–Purkinje system with bilateral bundle branch block or third-degree AV block within or below the His–Purkinje system following AMI. Perma-

nent pacing is also recommended in patients with transient second- or third-degree infranodal AV block and associated bundle branch block. If the site of block is uncertain, an electrophysiological study may be necessary. Permanent pacing is also recommended in patients with persistent symptomatic second- or third-degree AV block[40].

10.8.10 Indications and role for cardiac surgery

A complete description of the indications and role for cardiac surgery in the setting of AMI (non-Q or Q) or unstable angina is beyond the scope of this chapter. In patients with NSTEMI/unstable angina, there are many anatomic, clinical and ventricular function variables that are considered in the decision regarding revascularization following an acute ischemic event. Among patients who have sustained an STEMI, emergent or urgent cardiac surgery is indicated for the repair of post-infarction papillary muscle rupture leading to severe mitral insufficiency, for the repair of a post-infarction ventricular septal defect and for patients with post-infarction ventricular aneurism who are encountering intractable ventricular arrhythmias or pump failure.

10.9 Summary

The treatment of acute coronary syndromes is an ever-evolving field with numerous advances in diagnostic evaluation, medical therapy and interventional (both catheter based and surgical) approaches occurring on a yearly basis. The cardiology community has put a tremendous amount of emphasis on randomized clinical trials that are constantly being conducted and routinely change our approach to caring for different patient subsets. This chapter is meant as an overview and a beginning level of understanding for physicians caring for patients with acute myocardial infarction. Continued attention to the cardiology literature is necessary to update the knowledge obtained from this work.

References

1. Ryan, T.J., Anderson, J.L., Antman, E.M., *et al.* (1996) ACC/AHA guidelines for the management of patients with acute myocardial infarction. *J. Am. Coll. Cardiol.* 1328–1428.

2. Falk, E., Shah, P.K. and Fuster, V. (1994) Coronary plaque disruption. *Circulation* **92:** 657.

3. Tunstall-Pedoe, H., Kuulasmaa, K., Amouyel, P., *et al.* (1994) Myocardial infarction and coronary deaths in the World Health Organization MONICA Project. *Circulation* **90:** 583–612.

4. Cannon, C.P., Weintraub, W.S., Demopoulos, L.A. *et al.* (2001) Comparison of Early Invasive and Conservative Strategies in Patients with Unstable Coronary Syndromes treated with the Glycoprotein IIb/IIIa Inhibitor Tirofiban. *N. Engl. J. Med.* **344:** 1879–87.

5. Antman, E.M., Tansaijevic, M.J., Thompson, B., *et al.* (1996) Cardiac-specific troponin I levels to predict the risk of mortality in patients with acute coronary syndromes. *N. Engl. J. Med.* **335:** 1342–1349.

6. Braunwald, E., Antman, E.M., Beasley, J.W., *et al.* (2000) ACC/AHA guidelines for the management of patients with unstable angina and non-ST-segment elevation myocardial infarction: a report of the American College of Cardiology/American Heart Association Task Force on Practice Guidelines (Committee on the Management of Patients with Unstable Angina). *J. Am. Coll. Cardiol.* **36:** 970–1062.

7. ISIS 2 (Second International Study of Infarct Survival) Collaborative Group (1988) Randomised trial of intravenous streptokinase, oral aspirin, both, or neither among 17,187 cases of suspected acute myocardial infarction: ISIS-2. *Lancet* **2:** 349–360.

8. Antiplatelet Trialists' Collaboration (1994) Collaborative overview of randomised trials of antiplatelet therapy, 1: prevention of death, myocardial infarction, and stroke by prolonged antiplatelet therapy in various categories of patients. *Br. Med. J.* **308:** 81–106.

9. First International Study of Infarct Survival Collaborative Group (1986) Randomised trial of intravenous atenolol among 16,027 cases of suspected acute myocardial infarction. ISIS-1. *Lancet* 57–66.

10. The TIMI Study Group (1989) Comparison of invasive and conservative strategies after treatment with intravenous tissue plasminogen activator in acute myocardial infarction: results of the thrombolysis in myocardial infarction (TIMI) phase II trial. *N. Engl. J. Med.* **320:** 618–627.

11. The Multicenter Diltizem Postinfarction Trial Research Group (1988) The effect of diltizem on mortality and reinfarction after myocardial infarction. *N. Engl. J. Med.* **319:** 385–392.

12. Rutherford, J.D., Pfeffer, M.A., Moye, L.A., *et al.* (1994) Effects of captotril on ischemic events after myocardial infarction: results of the Survival and Ventricular Enlargement trial: SAVE Investigators. *Circulation* **90:** 1731–1738.

13. Yusuf, S., Sleight, P., Pogue, J. *et al.* (2000) Effects of an angiotensin-converting-enzyme inhibitor, ramipril, on cardiovascular events in high-risk patients. The Heart Outcomes Prevention Evaluation Study Investigators. *N. Engl. J. Med.* **342:** 145–153.

14. Eikelboom, J.W., Anand, S.S., Malmberg, K., Weitz, J.I., Ginsberg, J.S. and Yusuf, S. (2000) Unfractionated heparin and low-molecular-weight heparin in acute coronary syndrome without ST elevation: a meta-analysis. *Lancet* **355:** 1936–1942.

15. The PURSUIT Trial Investigators (1998) Inhibition of platelet glycoprotein IIb/IIIa with eptifibatide in patients with acute coronary syndromes. Platelet glycoprotein IIb/IIIa in unstable angina: receptor suppression using integrilin therapy. *N. Engl. J. Med.* **339:** 436–443.

16. Platelet Receptor Inhibition in Ischemic Syndrome Management in Patients Limited by Unstable Signs and Symptoms (PRISM-PLUS) Study Investigators (1998) Inhibition of the platelet glycoprotein IIb/IIIa receptor with tirofiban in unstable angina and non-Q wave myocardial infarction. *N. Engl. J. Med.* **338:** 1488–1497.

17. The GUSTO Investigators (1993) An international randomized trial comparing four thrombolytic strategies for acute myocardial infarction. *N. Engl. J. Med.* **329:** 1616–1622.

18. International Joint Efficacy Comparison of Thrombolytics (1995) Randomised, double-blind comparison of reteplase double-bolus administration with streptokinase in acute myocardial infarction (INJECT): Trial to investigate equivalence. *Lancet* **346:** 329–336.

19. The GUSTO III Investigators (1997) An international, multicenter, randomized comparison of reteplase and tissue plasminogen activator for acute myocardial infarction. *N. Engl. J. Med.* **337:** 1118–1123.

20. The Assessment of the Safety and Efficacy of a New Thrombolytic Investigators (1999) Single-bolus tenecteplase compared with front-loaded alteplase in acute myocardial infarction: the ASSENT-2 double-blind randomised trial. *Lancet* **354:** 716–722.

21. Antman, E.M., Giugliano, R.P., Ribson, C.M., *et al.* for the TIMI 14 Investigators (1999) Abciximab facilitates the rate and extent of thrombolysis: results of the Thrombolysis in Myocardial Infarction (TIMI) 14 trial. *Circulation* 99: 2720–2732.

22 Weaver, W.E., Simes, R.J., Betriu, A., *et al.* (1997) Comparison of primary coronary angioplasty and intravenous thrombolytic therapy for acute mycoardial infarction: a quantitative review. *JAMA* 278: 2093–2098.

23. GUSTO II Angioplasty Substudy Investigators (1997) An international randomized trial of 1138 patients comparing primary coronary angioplasty versus tissue plasminogen activator for acute myocardial infarction. *N. Engl. J. Med.* 336: 1621–1628.

24. Cannon, C.P., Gibson, C.M., Lambrew, C.T., *et al.* (2000) Relationship of symptom-onset-to-balloon time and door-to-balloon time with mortality in patients undergoing angioplasty for acute myocardial infarction. *JAMA* 283: 2941–2947.

25. Hochman, J.S., Sleeper, L.A., Webb, J.G., *et al.* (1999) Early revascularization in acute myocardial infarction complicated by cardiogenic shock. *N. Engl. J. Med.* 341: 625–634.

26. Grines, C.L., Cox, D.A., Stone, G.W., *et al.* (1999) Coronary angioplasty with or without stent implantation for acute myocardial infarction. *N. Engl. J. Med.* 341: 1949–1956.

27. Expert Panel on Detection, Evaluation and Treatment of High Blood Cholesterol in Adults (1993) Summary of the second report of the national cholesterol education program (NCEP) expert panel on detection, evaluation, and treatment of high blood cholesterol in adults (Adult Treatment Panel II). *JAMA* 269: 3015.

28. MIRACL Study (2000) Presented at the annual scientific sessions of the American Heart Association, New Orleans, LA, November 2000.

29. The TIMI IIIB Investigators (1994) Effects of tissue plasminogen activator and a comparison of early invasive and conservative strategies in unstable angina and non-Q-wave myocardial infarction: Results of the TIMI IIIB Trial. *Circulation* 89: 1545–1556.

30. Boden, W.E., O'Rourke, R.A., Crawford, M.H., *et al.* (1998) Outcomes in patients with acute non-Q-wave myocardial infarction randomly assigned to an invasive as compared with a conservative strategy. *N. Engl. J. Med.* 338: 1185–1192.

31. Fragmin and Fast Revascularization during Instability in Coronary Artery Disease Investigators (1999) Invasive compared with non-invasive treatment in unstable coronary-artery disease: FRISC II prospective randomised multi-centre study. *Lancet* 354: 708–715.

32. Antman, E.M., Cohen, M., Bernink, P.J.L., *et al.* (2000) The TIMI risk score for unstable angina/non-ST elevation MI. A method for prognostication and theraputic decision making. *JAMA* 284: 835–842.

33. Ellis, S.G., Ribeiro da Silva, E., *et al.* for the RESCUE Investigators (1994) Randomized comparison of rescue PCI with conservative management of patients with early failure of thrombolysis for acute anterior myocardial infarction. *Circulation* 90: 2280–2284.

34. The TIMI Research Group (1988) Immediate vs delayed catheterization and PCI following thrombolytic therapy for acute myocardial infarction. TIMI IIA results. *JAMA* 260: 2849–2858.

35. Topol, E.J., Califf, R.M., George, K.B.S., *et al.* and the Thrombolysis and Angioplasty in Myocardial Infarction Study Group (1987) A randomized trial of immediate versus delayed elective PCI after intravenous tissue plasminogen activator in acute myocardial infarction. *N. Engl. J. Med.* 317: 581–588.

36. Simoons, M.L., Beitriu, A., Col, J., *et al.* (1988) Thrombolysis with tissue plasminogen activator in acute myocardial infarction: no additional benefit from immediate percutaneous coronary intervention. *Lancet* 1: 197–203.

37. Ross, A.M., Coyne, K.S., Reiner, J.S., *et al.* for the PACT Investigators (1999) A randomized trial comparing primary PCI with a strategy of short-acting thrombolysis and immediate planned rescue PCI in acute myocardial infarction: The PACT Trial. *J. Am. Coll. Cardiol.* 34: 1954–1962.

38. Schweiger, M.J., Cannon, C.P., Murphy, S.A., *et al.* (2000) Percutaneous coronary intervention for TIMI 2 or 3 flow: the combined TIMI 10b/TIMI 14 experience. *Circulation* 102(II): 753.

39. Cheitlin, M.D., Alpert, J.S., Armstrong, J.E., *et al.* (1997) ACC/AHA guidelines for the clinical application of echocardiography: executive summary. A report of the American College of Cardiology/American Heart Association task force on practice guidelines (committee on clinical application of echocardiography). *J. Am. Coll. Cardiol.* 29: 862–870.

40. Cheitlin, M.D., Conill, A., Epstein, A.E., *et al.* (1998) ACC/AHA guidelines for implantation of cardiac pacemakers and antiarrhythmia devices: a report of the American College of Cardiology/American Heart Association task force on practice guidelines (committee on pacemaker implantation). *J. Am. Coll. Cardiol.* 31: 1175–1209.

Chapter 11

Cardiac rhythm disturbances

Magdy Migeed, MD and
Lawrence S. Rosenthal, MD, PhD

Contents

11.1 Introduction

Imagine that you are the most senior physician in the hospital and you are asked at 3 a.m. to evaluate a patient with a wide complex rhythm. The task of making the correct diagnosis and prescribing the best treatment can be a source of fear and apprehension, or can be relatively a straightforward decision, if you know the cues and clues. This chapter will provide a concise approach to the diagnosis and acute management of cardiac arrhythmias.

11.2 ECG analysis and interpretation

The 12-lead ECG analysis plays an integral part in the determination of the arrhythmia and includes:

- identification of P waves and their morphology then determination of atrial rhythm;
- analysis of QRS morphology;
- determination of A–V relationship.

11.2.1 Step I. Determine the atrial rhythm

Knowledge of normal ECG findings makes determination of abnormal findings easier. However, one should interpret ECGs in an algorithmic fashion to avoid missing important findings. The first step in the diagnosis of an arrhythmia is to determine the atrial rhythm. Thus one must carefully inspect the ECG or rhythm strip for P waves. A sinus origin is present if the P waves are upright in leads II, III, and aVF (ecg lead). By convention:

- sinus bradycardia (SB): sinus rate less than 60 beats min^{-1};
- sinus rhythm (SR): sinus rate between 60 and 100 beats min^{-1};
- sinus tachycardia (ST): sinus rate greater than 100 beats min^{-1}.

11.2.2 Step II. Look at the QRS complexes

It now becomes important to differentiate supraventricular tachycardia (SVT) from ven-

tricular tachycardia (VT). Most important in this determination is the evaluation of the hemodynamic status of the patient. Regardless of the underlying mechanism of the arrhythmia, immediate direct electrical cardioversion should be considered in patients with heart failure, acute ischemia, hypotension, hypoxia, or impending cardiovascular collapse. In addition to restoring sinus rhythm, the clinician should look for underlying causes, as many arrhythmias are not primary abnormalities but secondary arrhythmias as a result of other systemic abnormalities such as cardiac ischemia, hypoxia, or electrolyte abnormalities.

11.2.3 Step III. Determine the AV relationship

If P waves always precede QRS complexes by a fixed normal P–R interval (0.12–0.2 s), then AV conduction is normal. Other types of impaired AV conduction include:

- First-degree AV delay: PR interval greater than 200 ms.
- Second-degree heart block:
  Type I (Wenckebach block): Progressive PR lengthening with intermittent dropped QRS complexes;
  Type II: Constant PR intervals with dropped QRS complexes.
- Third-degree heart block: AV dissociation with atrial rate greater than ventricular rate.

11.3 Supraventricular tachycardias

11.3.1 Evaluation of the R–P interval

When confronted with a narrow complex tachycardia, it is often helpful to determine the QRS to P wave relationship. However, at times P waves may be difficult to locate. Thus, the use of vagal maneuvers (see below) or the use of an intravenous AV nodal blocking agent may be helpful in determining the etiology (and even to terminate the tachycardia). Having determined the QRS to P relationship, SVTs can be classified as short R–P tachycardias or long R–P tachycardias (see Figure 11.1). Defining a tachycardia as a short R–P SVT narrows the list of potential arrhythmias. Most SVTs will be short R–P tachycardias consistent with typical atrioventricular nodal reentrant tachycardia (AVNRT). One must still eliminate other possibilities including atrial tachycardia, sinus tachycardia with a first-degree AV delay, and AV reentry or pathway

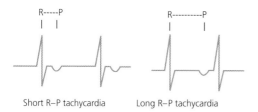

Short R–P tachycardia   Long R–P tachycardia

Figure 11.1 Nomenclature for the classification of SVT. Having determined the QRS to P relationship, SVTs can be classified as short R–P tachycardias or long R–P tachycardias. Defining a tachycardia as a short R–P SVT narrows the list of potential arrhythmias. Most SVTs will be short R–P tachycardias consistent with typical atrioventricular nodal reentrant tachycardia (AVNRT). One must still eliminate other possibilities including atrial tachycardia, sinus tachycardia with a first-degree AV delay, and AV reentry or pathway mediated tachycardias. *Table 11.1* helps with the differential diagnosis of common SVTs.

mediated tachycardias. *Table 11.1* helps with the differential diagnosis of common SVTs.

11.3.2 Diagnostic maneuvers for SVT

Carotid sinus massage (CSM) enhances vagal tone and slows the heart rate, and the response to CSM provides important information (*Table 11.2*). Carotid sinus massage slows the impulse input in to the AV node. If conduction worsens, then this favors block at the level of the AV node or above. If conduction improves, then the site of block is likely below the AV node, ie. His-Purkinje System. CSM should not be performed if a carotid bruit is auscultated. CSM is performed with the patient supine and the head hyperextended and turned away from the side being tested. The carotid impulse can be felt at the angle of the jaw. A gentle touch to carotid sinus to detect hypersensitive response is followed by firm pressure for 5 s first on one side then on the other side with gentle rotating massaging motion. Never test both sides simultaneously. CSM carries the risk of cerebral emboli, particularly in older patients.

Table 11.1 Differential diagnosis of common SVTs

I. Regular supraventricular tachycardias

Short R–P tachycardias (R–P < P–R)	Sinus tachycardia with first-degree AV delay
	Typical AV nodal reentrant tachycardia (common)
	AV reentrant tachycardia
	Atrial tachycardia
Long R–P tachycardias (R–P > P–R)	Sinus tachycardia
	Sinus nodal reentrant tachycardia
	Atypical AV nodal reentrant tachycardia
	AV reentrant tachycardia
	Permanent junctional reciprocating tachycardia

II. Irregular supraventricular tachycardias
Atrial fibrillation
Atrial flutter

Table 11.2 Cardiac response to carotid sinus massage

• Sinus tachycardia	Slowing then return to baseline after massage
• AV node or AV reentry tachycardia (WPW)	Slow, terminate, or no change
• A fib or flutter	Slowing ventricular rate during massage, atrial arrhythmia persists
• second-degree AV block, Type I	Worsens conduction or no change
• second-degree AV block, Type II	Improvement of conduction or no change
• VT (2:1 blocks)	No change, rare conversion

11.4 Treatment of supraventricular arrhythmias

The acute treatment of SVT (*Table 11.3*) is aimed at both arrhythmia diagnosis and termination, but depends on patient hemodynamic stability. If clinically unstable then Advanced Cardiac Life Support (ACLS) guidelines[1] should be followed. In hemodynamically stable patients, it is reasonable to perform vagal maneuvers or administer AV nodal blocking agents in an attempt to terminate their SVT. One should always listen for carotid bruits before carotid sinus massage. In addition, the Valsalva maneuver, splashing cold water on the face, or gently rubbing the upper eyelid have been shown to stimulate the vagus nerve and terminate supraventricular tachycardia. Intravenous use of adenosine, calcium channel blockers, beta blockers, and even digoxin can terminate SVT by causing block at the level of the AV node (see *Table 11.4*). Antiarrhythmic agents can also be used for acute conversion and long-term suppression of SVTs and are listed in *Table 11.5*.

11.4.1 Sinus tachycardia
First determine whether sinus tachycardia is appropriate (i.e. hypovolemia, fever, anemia, hyperthyroidism, CHF). Treat the underlying condition. However, if the sinus tachycardia is causing ischemia, then the preferred drug would be beta adrenergic blockers.

11.4.2 Sinus bradycardia
Treat only if symptomatic (withdrawal of AV nodal agents, temporary or permanent pacemaker, atropine 0.5–2 mg IV).

11.4.3 Atrial premature depolarization (APD)
Usually not clinically symptomatic and requires no therapy. If symptomatic, beta adrenergic blockers may be used.

11.4.4 Multifocal atrial tachycardia
This is often related to underlying lung disease. Treat the underlying cause and optimize cardiopulmonary status. Calcium channel blockers or beta blockers (unless contraindicated) may be used for rate control. Cardioversion has no value.

11.4.5 Atrioventricular nodal reentrant tachycardia (AVNRT)
Acute treatment includes vagal maneuvers (CSM, Valsalva). If no response, IV adenosine, IV verapamil, IV diltiazem, or IV beta blockers may be used. If hemodynamically unstable, electrical cardioversion is warranted. Chronic treat-

---

Table 11.3 Acute and chronic management of SVT

Acute

1. Hemodynamically unstable (CHF, hypoxia, hypotension, impending CV collapse)
- Follow ACLS guidelines

2. Hemodynamically stable
- Carotid sinus massage (see precautions in text)
- Adenosine IV push (doses of 6, repeat 6, then 12 mg if necessary)
- Calcium channel blockers (e.g. verapamil 5 mg IV push)
- Beta adrenergic blockers (e.g. metoprolol 5 mg IV push)
- Digoxin (loading dose necessary)

Chronic

1. Drug therapy
- Calcium channel blockers
- Beta adrenergic blockers
- Digoxin (not very effective)
- Antiarrhythmic agents

2. Catheter ablation

Table 11.4 Intravenous drugs in the acute management of SVT

Drug	Target	IV dosage	Comments
Adenosine (Adenocard)	Adenosine receptors at the level of the AV node and sinus node	6–24 mg	Rapid onset Short half life Reflex sinus tachycardia
Atenolol (Tenormin)	Beta adrenergic receptors	5–10 mg	Bradycardia Hypotension
Diltiazem (Cardizem)	Calcium channels	20–25 mg	Hypotension
Esmolol (Brevibloc)	Beta adrenergic receptors	5–10 mg bolus or infusion	Short half life
Metoprolol (Lopressor)	Beta receptors	5 mg	Longer acting
Verapamil (Calan, Isoptin)	Calcium channels	2.5–5 mg	Hypotension
Digoxin (Lanoxin)	Na^+/K^+ pump inhibitor	0.250 mg	Toxicity Long onset of action
Phenylephrine (Neo-synephrine)	Alpha-1 adrenergic receptors (reflex slowing with increased SVR)	100 µg	May be helpful in hypotension

Table 11.5 Vaughn-Williams classification of antiarrhythmic agents and their site of action

Class Ia	Quinidine, Procainamide, Disopyramide	Na^+ channels
Class Ib	Lidocaine, Mexilitine	
Class Ic	Flecainide, Propafenone	
Class II	Beta blockers	Beta receptors
Class III	Amiodarone, Sotalol, Dofetilide	K^+ channels
Class IV	Calcium channel blockers	Ca^{2+} channels

ment: infrequent, well-tolerated, brief episodes can be treated with vagal maneuvers alone. Patients with frequent symptomatic episodes should consider catheter ablation (>95% success). AV nodal blocking agents such as beta blockers, verapamil, or diltiazem have been used and generally reduce the frequency of episodes.

11.4.6 Atrioventricular reentrant tachycardia (AVRT)

Occurs in patients with accessory pathways (APs). Baseline ECG may show the characteristic delta wave (manifest APs or Wolfe–Parkinson–White (WPW) pattern) or a non-pre-excited ECG as seen in patients with concealed APs (retrograde conduction only). The pathophysiology involves an abnormal muscular network of specialized tissues connecting the atrium and the ventricle (accessory AV pathway). Manifest pathways are found in 0.2–0.4% of population, especially young males. Most patients have no underlying heart disease.

- Asymptomatic patients usually require no therapy.
- Patients with syncope or pre-syncope require electrophysiology (EP) study and consideration for catheter ablation.

Chronic management of SVTs includes oral use of beta blockers, calcium channel blockers, and even the use of antiarrhythmic agents (see *Table 11.6*). However, given the small but ever-present risks of proarrhythmia and drug-related side effects associated with the use of antiarrhythmic agents, most clinicians would favor radiofrequency catheter ablation (>95% success) as an alternative to long-term anti-arrhythmic use.

11.5 Atrial fibrillation

Atrial fibrillation (AF) is the most common arrhythmia. Its prevalence is 5% in patients of 65 years of age or older, and the prevalence increases with advancing age. Data from the Framingham study have shown that AF is associated with a 1.5–1.9-fold higher risk of death,

presumably as a result of thromboembolic stroke. AF is associated with several conditions that should be sought when taking the history (*Table 11.7*).

Overall, about 15–25% of all strokes in the USA (75 000 per year) can be attributed to AF. Known risk factors contributing to the development of AF are male gender, valvular heart disease (rheumatic heart disease), CHF, hypertension and diabetes (*Table 11.8*). Additional risk factors, such as advancing age, prior history of stroke, hypertension, and diabetes place patients with preexisting AF at even higher risk for further comorbidities. Patients with non-valvular AF and with risk factors have a five-fold increased risk for stroke. Patients with rheumatic heart disease have an even higher (17-fold) risk for stroke. Large multicenter clinical trials have clearly demon-

Table 11.6 Oral drugs for long term suppression

Drug	Target	Dosage	Comments
Verapamil	Calcium channel	240–480 mg day^{-1}	Well tolerated
Diltiazem	Calcium channel	120–360 mg day^{-1}	Well tolerated
Atenolol	Beta receptors	25–200 mg day^{-1}	Well tolerated
Metoprolol	Beta receptors	25–200 mg day^{-1}	Well tolerated
Nadolol	Beta receptors	20–160 mg day^{-1}	Well tolerated
Procainamide	Ia antiarrhythmic agent	50 mg kg^{-1} day^{-1}	Long-term side effects
Propafenone	Ic antiarrhythmic agent	150–300 mg t.i.d.	Caution in patients with reduced LVF
Flecainide	Ic antiarrhythmic agent	50–150 mg b.i.d.	Caution in patients with reduced LVF
Sotalol	III antiarrhythmic agent	80–160 mg b.i.d.	Caution in patients with renal dysfunction, CHF
Amiodarone	III antiarrhythmic agent	200–400 mg day^{-1}	Organ toxicity

Table 11.7 Common causes and associated conditions with AF

Advancing age	Hypertension	Diabetes
Cardiomyopathy	Alcohol abuse	Thyrotoxicosis
WPW and sick-sinus syndromes	Thrombosis; particularly pulmonary embolism	Valvular heart disease (e.g. mitral stenosis)

Table 11.8 Risk factors for stroke in non-rheumatic AF

Advancing age	LV dysfunction
Previous TIA, CVA	LA enlargement
Prosthetic valve	Diabetes mellitus
Thyrotoxicosis	Congestive heart failure
Hypertension	

Generally all patients with chronic AF (paroxysmal, persistent, permanent) should receive anticoagulation (see Table 11.9) to an INR between 2 and 3 except patients under 65 years old with no risk factors.

strated that anticoagulation with warfarin reduces the risk of stroke by 50–80%. Anticoagulation, however, carries the risk of bleeding, hemorrhagic stroke, and intracranial bleeding, particularly in elderly patients prone to falls.

AF is classified into acute (<48 h) or chronic (>48 h). Chronic AF is further divided into three groups:

- paroxysmal: intermittent;
- persistent: patient in AF but can be converted to sinus rhythm by chemical or electrical cardioversion;
- permanent: accepted rhythm is AF, goals are anticoagulation and rate control.

The history may reveal symptoms such as palpitations, dizziness, or general malaise. The presence of heart failure suggests concomitant cardiac disease (e.g. valvular heart disease). Persistent SVT can cause a tachycardia-induced cardiomyopathy with LV dysfunction and heart failure. On ECG AF should be distinguished from atrial flutter (AFL) (uniform flutter waves) and from multifocal atrial tachycardia (MAT) (i.e. irregular rhythm with P waves of variable (at least three) morphologies). However, most physicians would anticoagulate patients with AFL in a similar manner to those with AF.

Recommendations for chronic anticoagulation are controversial. Although the risk of bleeding can be minimized with tight control of the INR, the possibility of stroke is frightening to most and can be devastating. Most cli-

nicians generally recommend long-term anticoagulation in any patient with atrial fibrillation or atrial flutter who is not at risk for falls or injury or who cannot determine when they are in atrial fibrillation (*Table 11.9*). Patients with PAF are instructed to call when they have AF lasting more than 12 h, so that prompt cardioversion can be arranged.

11.6 Therapy of AF

Electrical cardioversion is indicated in patients who are clinically unstable (e.g. heart failure, chest pain, hypoxic, hypotensive, impending hemodynamic collapse). Acute AF (<24–48 h) can be cardioverted electrically or chemically regardless of anticoagulation status. For AF (>48 h) cardioversion should be deferred until a minimum of 3 weeks of therapeutic anticoagulation (INR > 2) unless a transesophageal echo (TEE) showed no thrombus. However, if there were any uncertainties about the exact duration of AF, then most clinicians would defer to a more conservative approach, including therapy with warfarin. Treatment of chronic AF includes three goals: control of ventricular rate, maintenance of sinus rhythm, and stroke prophylaxis.

11.6.1 Rate control

Rate control not only alleviates symptoms but also prevents tachycardia-induced cardiomyopathy. In patients who have already developed cardiomyopathy, rate control can dramatically improve ventricular systolic function.

- Pharmacologic rate control can be achieved using three categories of drugs, alone or in combination:

Table 11.9 Anticoagulation of non-rheumatic AF

Age	Risk factors*	Recommend
<65	+	Coumadin, INR 2–3
	–	ASA or nothing
65–75	+	Coumadin, INR 2–3
	–	Coumadin or ASA
>75	+ or –	Coumadin, INR 2.0–2.5

*Risk factors include diabetes, hypertension, prior CVA/TIA.

171

(i) beta adrenergic blockers;
(ii) calcium channel blockers;
(iii) digoxin.

- Non-pharmacologic control of ventricular rate using AV nodal catheter ablation (resulting in complete AV block) with implantation of a pacemaker is indicated if the rate is not well controlled by drugs or the patient has intolerable side effects from these drugs. Improvements in LV size and function, quality of life, and exercise tolerance with AV nodal ablation and permanent pacing have been demonstrated.

11.6.2 Rhythm control

The second goal is maintenance of sinus rhythm after conversion from AF to sinus rhythm (spontaneously or with cardioversion). Note that maintaining sinus rhythm has not been shown to decrease the likelihood of thromboembolism or to increase survival. In fact, some drugs used to prevent AF recurrence can cause new arrhythmias (proarrhythmic effects).

Pharmacologic control of rhythm can be achieved with Class Ia drugs, but these can be associated with Torsades de Pointes (TdP) and increased mortality. Monitor QT interval and initiate these agents with continuous EKG monitoring. These agents also enhance AV nodal conduction, so rate control agents should be given before their use. In patients with structurally normal hearts, Class Ic agents can safely be used. Amiodarone has been proven safe after MI and in systolic dysfunction.

Because of limitations of medical therapy (proarrhythmia, drug side effects, high recurrence rate of AF), there is interest in using nonpharmacologic control of rhythm. These include:

- dual atrial pacing and implantable atrial defibrillators;
- atrial pacing versus ventricular pacing in patients with sick sinus syndrome (SSS) (reduces stroke, CHF and recurrence of AF);
- surgical maze procedure (by creating linear

incisions in the atria that prevent atrial reentry and AF, but requires thoracotomy);
- AF ablation, under development.

11.6.3 Stroke prevention

Because up to 7% of AF patients undergoing cardioversion without anticoagulation experience clinical thromboembolism, patients with AF of longer than 48 h must receive anticoagulation for a minimum of 3 weeks before cardioversion and 4 weeks after cardioversion. Alternatively, TEE may be performed and if no LA or LV thrombus is found, safe cardioversion can be accomplished, followed by 3–4 weeks of anticoagulation. *Table 11.8* lists factors that are known to increase stroke risk.

11.7 Wide complex tachycardias

The diagnosis and treatment of wide complex tachycardias (WCT) (*Table 11.10.*) can be crucial in the care of critically ill patients. When confronted with a WCT, the most important piece of information that one can obtain is whether there is a history of coronary disease, prior heart attack, or heart failure. A 'yes' answer almost certainly means ventricular tachycardia (VT). Unfortunately, the physical exam is of very little clinical utility, as most patients will be hemodynamically compromised. However, there will be patients with wide complex VT who will have heart rates in the low 100s and have sufficient blood pressure to have walked into the emergency room, especially those on antiarrhythmic agents such as amiodarone. Thus the need to identify VT is important because not all patients will present

---

Table 11.10 Differential diagnosis of a regular wide complex rhythm

- VT
- SVT with aberrant conduction
- WPW with antegrade conduction through the accessory pathway (rare)
- Ventricular pacing (usually obvious)

pulseless and hypotensive. In addition, there may be patients with runs of non-sustained wide complex tachycardia, and the ability to distinguish VT from SVT will be critical in the management of such patients. VT is more common in older patients, and in any patient with a history of prior MI, CHF, or reduced LV function from any cause. Thus any person with a history of MI (recent or in the distant past) and reduced LV function, who presents with a wide complex rhythm should be treated as VT until proven otherwise. One should look for signs of AV dissociation such as cannon A waves in the neck as well as signs of CHF, but the initial focus should be on obtaining a 12-lead EKG.

11.7.1 SVT with aberrancy
Distinguishing SVT with aberrancy from VT can be difficult. SVT with aberrancy generally occurs in the setting of atrial fibrillation and variable R–R intervals. Look for long short sequences as the initiating event and the absence of a pause after the arrhythmia terminates. This is more suggestive of aberrant conduction (*Figure 11.2*). After a long R–R interval (that leaves one bundle branch refractory) an early impulse from the atria is conducted aberrantly because the bundle branch has not recovered yet and is still partially refractory. With VT, one often sees a His–Purkinje conduction system that is refractory from retrograde bombardment of ventricular beats. Upon termination of the VT or non-sustained VT, the His–Purkinje system requires extra time to regain normal conduction from the AV node down towards the ventricles (*Figure 11.3*). However, if a wide complex tachycardia is seen in a patient with LV dysfunction, it should be presumed to be VT until proven otherwise.

11.7.2 EKG diagnosis
The nomenclature adopted for the description of a wide complex rhythm begins with the examination of lead V_1. If V_1 is predominantly positive, it is described as a right bundle pattern. If the polarity of V_1 is negative then a left bundle pattern can be diagnosed. The inferior

V1

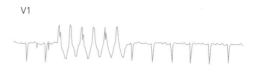

Figure 11.2 SVT with aberrant conduction. Rhythm strip on a 28-year-old women with documented SVT. During her EP study, atrial pacing produced a run of wide complex tachycardia. Note the lack of pause after wide complex tachycardia terminates. Intracardiac electrograms confirmed the diagnosis of SVT.

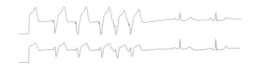

Figure 11.3 Aberrant conduction consistent with VT. Rhythm strip on a 48-year-old male who had suffered an anterior MI and had an LVEF of 35%. Note the pause after termination of wide complex tachycardia. At EP study, the patient was readily inducible for monomorphic VT with a similar configuration.

leads II, III, and AVf help orient the axis of the VT (*Table 11.11*).

Table 11.12 lists the ECG findings favoring the diagnosis of VT. After determining the wide complex tachycardia morphology (right bundle branch block (RBBB) or left bundle branch block (LBBB)), focus on these criteria, which support or refute the diagnosis of VT. With an LBBB tachycardia, first examine lead V_1 (or V_2) and measure the width of the R wave. A broad R wave (>30 ms) or finding of a notch on the downslope of the S wave is consistent with VT. Measurement of the onset of

Table 11.11 Nomenclature for the classification of VT

V_1 positive	Right bundle pattern
V_1 negative	Left bundle pattern
Inferior leads upright	Inferior axis
Inferior leads negative	Superior axis

173

Table 11.12 ECG finding favoring the diagnosis of VT

- QRS > 140 ms (RBBB)
  - (i) V_1 monophasic R, qR, Rr', RS
  - (ii) V_6 R/S < 1
- QRS > 160 ms (LBBB)
  - (i) V_{1-2} R > 30 ms
  - (ii) V_{1-2} notching on the downslope of S wave
  - (iii) V_{1-2} beginning of QRS to nadir of S > 70 ms
  - (iv) V_6 qR
- AV dissociation
- Positive concordance
- Change in axis (from baseline ECG)
- Axis – 90 ± 180
- Fusion beats
- Capture beats

LBBB ECG features in V_1 and V_2 suggestive of VT

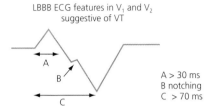

A > 30 ms
B notching
C > 70 ms

Figure 11.4 ECG features of LBBB morphologic VT. A prolonged interval (>70 ms) from the onset of the R wave to the nadir of the S wave or any Q wave in V_6 raises the suspicion of VT. From Wellens, H., and Brugada, P. (1987) Diagnosis of ventricular tachycardia from the 12-lead electrocardiogram. In: *Cardiology Clinics*. Reproduced with permission from W.B. Saunders.

the R wave to the nadir of the S wave (>70 ms) also adds to the mounting evidence pointing to VT (*Figure 11.4*). Finally, any Q wave in V_6 is pathologic and should raise the suspicion of VT. The criteria with RBBB tachycardias are a little more difficult, but making an assessment of the R to S ratio in V_6 is helpful (R/S < 1 is consistent with VT). A comparison of ECG findings is seen in *Figure 11.5*. There will be exceptions, but utilizing this simple algorithm along with patient history should allow the correct diagnosis of VT to be made in most cases.

11.7.3 Treatment of VT

Hemodynamically unstable VT requires immediate action. Remember the time-honored saying, 'Shock early and often'. Studies have shown that the earlier one delivers energy to the heart, the better the chance of success and patient survival. The year 2000 Advanced Cardiac Life Support (ACLS) guidelines have incorporated IV amiodarone into the adult VT/Pulseless VT algorithm. Currently, IV amiodarone is FDA approved for the treatment and prophylaxis of persistent VF as well as hemodynamically unstable VT in patients refractory to other antiarrhythmic agents.

11.8 Approach to the patient with cardiac arrest

The ACLS guidelines have been recently updated; *Figure 11.8* (at the end of this chapter) reproduces the main algorithm. The reader is encouraged to read and study these guidelines in more detail[1].

In the field setting ACLS begins with establishing unresponsiveness, and following ABCD:

A: open Airway by the look, listen, and feel method;
B: assess Breathing and give two slow breaths;
C: assess Circulation and start Chest compressions;
D: attach Defibrillator/monitor and give 200, 300, 360 joules.

If no pulse, continue CPR and assess rhythm.

In the intensive care unit, the situation is usually different (the airway is frequently secured with an endotracheal tube; breathing is monitored on the ventilator or with end-tidal CO_2) and the ACLS flowchart may need to be modified. A quick check of monitoring electrodes should exclude mechanical disconnection as the cause of 'flat-line' EKG. Pulseless conditions (pulseless VT, pulseless electrical activity (PEA)) require immediate institution of chest com-

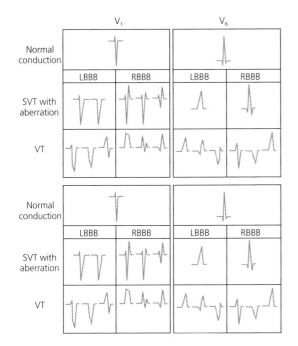

Figure 11.5 Comparison of the bundle branch morphologic criteria in the diagnosis of VT. VT may be difficult to diagnose in the presence of bundle branch block, but interpretation of the QRS complex in leads V_1 and V_6 along with patient history is often helpful. From: Zipes, P. and Jalife, J. (1995) Recognition of VT. In: *Cardiac Electrophysiology: From Cell to Bedside*. Reproduced with permission from W.B. Saunders.

pressions. Rhythms with perfusion pressure (often visible by the arterial line tracing) can usually be dealt with chemically or electrically.

11.8.1 VF/pulseless VT

Give up to three defibrillation shocks. If no response perform CPR for 1 min followed by secondary ABCD survey:

- Airway: place airway device if needed;
- Breathing: secure airway and start ventilation and oxygenation (100% FiO_2 preferred);
- Circulation: gain IV access, identify the rhythm on monitor and administer agents to support blood pressure, such as vasopressin 40 U IV × 1 or epinephrine 1 mg IV q 3–5 min.

If no response:

- Defibrillate: 360 joules within 30–60 s.

If no response:

- consider antiarrhythmic agents (such as amiodarone, lidocaine; *Table 11.13*).

If no response:

- resume attempts to defibrillate.

11.8.2 Asystole or pulseless electrical activity (PEA)

Perform CPR for up to 3 min then proceed to secondary ABC survey as above. Administer epinephrine 1 mg IV q 3–5 min. If no response, administer atropine 1 mg IV q 3– 5 min up to 0.04 mg kg^{-1}.

- For PEA look for a cause:
- Hypovolemia, Hypoxia, Hyper/hypocalcemia, Hypothermia, Hydrogen ion (acidosis);
- Tamponade, Tension pneumothorax, Thrombus (coronary), Thrombus (pulmonary).
- For asystole:
- consider transcutaneous pacing immediately.

11.8.3 Stable ventricular tachycardia

Occasionally, patients will present with hemodynamically stable VT. If the patient is hemodynamically unstable, or if ischemia is suspected, then cardiovert immediately. If hemodynamically stable, one can use any of the following:

Table 11.13 Drugs for the management of ventricular dysrhythmias

Drug	Initial bolus	Secondary infusion(s)	Maintenance infusion
Amiodarone	300 mg IVP (6 cc undiluted, then flush w/NS or D5W)	150 mg IV (3 cc diluted in 100 cc D5W)	1 mg min^{-1} for 6 hours (360 mg) then 0.5 mg min^{-1} for 18 hours (540 mg)
Lidocaine	100 mg IVP (1–1.5 mg kg^{-1})	50–100 mg IVP (0.75–1.5 mg kg^{-1})	1–4 mg min^{-1}
Procainamide	20–30 mg min^{-1} Max 17 mg kg^{-1}	n/a	2–6 mg min^{-1}
Bretylium	5–10 mg kg^{-1}	n/a	0.5–2.5 mg kg^{-1} Max 30 mg kg^{-1} over 24 h

- lidocaine (1 mg kg^{-1} IV push, followed by an IV infusion of 1–4 mg min^{-1}) (*Table 11.13*);
- amiodarone (150 mg IV bolus over 10 min followed by a constant infusion of 1 mg min^{-1} for 6 h and 0.5 mg min^{-1} thereafter, can rebolus with 150 mg for breakthrough VT);
- procainamide IV (18 mg kg^{-1} over 1 h, followed by a constant IV infusion of 2–6 mg min^{-1});
- if the VT does not convert chemically then consider synchronized cardioversion.

11.8.4 Drugs for the management of ventricular dysrhythmias

Table 11.13 provides a quick summary of the initial dose and maintenance infusion for the four commonly used ventricular antidysrhythmics, although most conditions can be managed with either amiodarone or lidocaine. Amiodarone, because of its long half-life, requires a complicated initial dosing scheme. A bolus dose of 300 mg is used to initiate therapy, and a supplemental dose of 150 mg may be given if the patient experiences breakthrough episodes of VT or VF. Once spontaneous circulation is established, an initial maintenance infusion of 360 mg over 6 h (1 mg min^{-1}) is given, followed by an additional 540 mg over 18 h (0.5 mg min^{-1}). Amiodarone is compatible with some other vasoactive agents (isoproterenol, norepinephrine, dopamine, lidocaine,

phenylephrine, dobutamine, nitroglycerin) but compatability is unknown with other agents. The major side effect of amiodarone is hypotension (10–30% of patients when given as a rapid infusion), asystole (1.2%), VT (1.1%), cardiogenic shock (1%) and Torsade de Pointes (<1%)[2]. Pulmonary fibrosis and pneumonitis have been reported a few days following initiation of IV therapy, and can occur any time thereafter[3]. Patients on chronic therapy should be monitored with pulmonary function tests and periodic chest radiographs[4]. After suppression of arrhythmia by IV amiodarone, patients can be switched to an oral formulation, with the dose dependent on the duration of IV treatment.

Lidocaine has been the mainstay of treatment for many years. In contrast to amiodarone, it has a relatively short half life, and no oral equivalent. Serum levels are high after an IV bolus, but drop during the first minutes of continuous infusion, so a second bolus (usually half the initial dose) may be necessary for breakthrough arrhythmias. Lidocaine is metabolized by the liver, and has a tendency to accumulate in elderly patients. The major side effects are central nervous system effects, and can range from tinnitus and confusion at low doses to seizures to CNS depression with severe overdose.

Procainamide is effective against atrial, AV nodal and ventricular arrhythmias, and slows conduction through accessory conduction pathways. It decreases automaticity and conduction in all cardiac tissue, both normal and ischemic. Its toxicity is first manifest on the heart (Torsades des Pointes; AV nodal block, intraventricular conduction delay, myocardial depression) and then the peripheral circulation (vasodilation) and the CNS (excitatory syndrome, confusion, seizures). The lupus-like syndrome with chronic administration is not seen with short-term therapy.

Bretylium is notable for the hypotension it causes with bolus administration, and is now rarely used.

11.8.5 Pacemakers and internal cardiac defibrillators (ICDs)

Patients with pacemakers or ICDs should be treated according to ACLS protocols during episodes of cardiac arrest. If at all possible, avoid delivering shocks directly over such devices as they may shunt energy away from the heart. One should consult a trained expert on the magnet function of such devices. In general, placing a magnet over a pacemaker causes the pacemaker to pace in a preprogrammed, manufacturer-specific, paced mode. Most defibrillators are inhibited from delivering therapy (overdrive pacing protocols and/or shocks) when a magnet is placed over the device. Pacing functions are maintained. Again, not all devices behave similarly and consultation with an expert is advised.

11.8.6 Proarrhythmia

Proarrhythmia refers to the capacity of a drug (cardiac or non-cardiac) to aggravate an existing arrhythmia or provoke a new arrhythmia at therapeutic or sub-therapeutic levels[5]. Risk factors promoting proarrhythmia include having a reduced left ventricular function (LVF), a prolonged QT interval at baseline, electrolyte imbalances, prominent U waves, ischemia, presence of atrial arrhythmias (atrial fibrillation or flutter) or pre-existing ventricular arrhythmias (non-sustained VT)[6] (Table 11.14). Prevention begins with identifying those patients at risk for proarrhythmia, before drug initiation. Electrical instability occurs in the setting of

Table 11.14 Clinical risk factors associated with proarrhythmia

General
- History of VT or VF
- Poor LVEF (<30%)
- CHF
- Female gender
- Metabolic or electrolyte abnormalities
- Diuretic use
- Baseline QT prolongation
- Atrial fibrillation or flutter

Polymorphic VT/VF (Type IA drugs)
- Hypokalemia, hypomagnesemia
- Bradycardia or pauses

Incessant wide complex tachycardia (Type 1C drugs)
- Previous sustained VT
- Prior infarct or scar

hypokalemia, hypomagnesemia, bradycardia, or ischemia. Thus electrolytes should be monitored closely. With the exception of oral amiodarone (long half-life and low incidence of proarrhythmia), antiarrhythmic agents should be started in the inpatient setting. Close monitoring of QT intervals is warranted. The management of proarrhythmia includes eliminating the offending drug, close electrographic monitoring, correcting electrolyte abnormalities, acute treatment, and finally prevention of further episodes. Treatment includes electrical cardioversion of unstable rhythms, overdrive pacing or increasing the heart rate with isoproterenol or atropine, magnesium sulfate infusion (Table 11.15), and even antiarrhythmic agents that do not prolong the QT (lidocaine, beta blockers).

11.8.7 Polymorphic VT/VF (Figure 11.6)

Polymorphic VT/VF suggests ischemia and consideration towards immediate cardiac

Table 11.15 The use of IV magnesium for TdP

- Mg sulfate 2 g bolus over 2 min
- Repeat if necessary
- Infusion of 1–2 mg min^{-1} to 20 mg min^{-1} for the next 24–48 h until QT shortens to <0.5 s

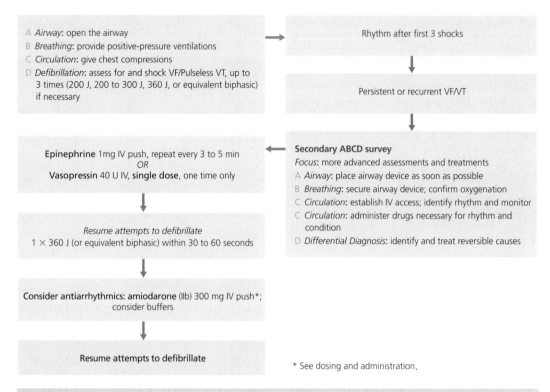

Figure 11.6 Algorithm for treatment of persistent pulseless ventricular tachycardia (VT) and ventricular fibrillation (VF). From: ACC/AHA Guidelines for the management of patients with acute myocardial infarction. *J. Am. Coll. Cardiol.* (1999) **34**: 890–911.

intervention should be considered. After restoration of sinus rhythm one should check the baseline QT interval. If QT interval is normal, consider ischemia or electrolyte imbalance. If cardioversion fails to restore or maintain sinus rhythm, then consider using IV amiodarone or IV lidocaine in addition to cardioversion.

11.8.8 Torsade de Pointes (TdP)

TdP is a pause-dependent form of polymorphic VT with ventricular rates 200–250 beats min^{-1}. The most common form of TdP is iatrogenic or drug induced. Many medications can cause widening of the QT interval, leading to excessive delay in repolarization and the development of early after depolarizations at the cellular level. *Table 11.16* lists drugs that have been associated with TdP. Changes in renal or hepatic function can also affect circulating

drug concentrations, leading to prolongation of the QT interval. Thus one needs to monitor these systems periodically. TdP has also been observed in patients who have undergone AV nodal ablation and permanent pacemaker implantation and have a relatively slow lower rate (e.g. 60 beats min^{-1}). For that reason these

Table 11.16 Drugs associated with TdP

Antiarrhythmics	Antihistamines	Antibiotics
Quinidine	Terfenadine	Pentamidine
Procainamide	Astemizole	Bactrium
Disopyramide		Sparfloxacin
Sotalol	**Antipsychotics**	Erythromycin
Dofetilide	Haloperidol	Clarithromycin
Ibutalinde	Thioridazine	Ketoconazole
Amiodarone		**Other**
Azimilide	**Antireflux**	Terodiline
Tedisimil	Cisapride	Grapefruit juice
Bepridil		ASA

patients are generally paced at relatively high baseline rates (85–95 beats min[-1]) for 1–3 months post-AV node ablation. Additionally, TdP can be seen in patients with CHB with a slow ventricular response (*Figure 11.7*). Correct electrolyte abnormalities and administer IV magnesium (*Table 11.15*). As TdP is pause dependent, consider either IV isoproterenol or temporary overdrive pacing.

11.8.9 Premature ventricular contractions (PVCs)

Asymptomatic PVCs do not require any treatment, as the CAST I and II trials demonstrated[7,8]. Patients with depressed LV function (<40%) and frequent PVCs were given Type Ic antiarrhythmic agents (flecainide and encainide, and later morizicine). PVCs became less frequent at the cost of a higher mortality rate than in patients taking placebo, presumably as a result of ischemic mediated proarrhythmia. This trial underscores the importance of a placebo group. In patients with symptomatic PVCs, a trial of a beta blocker or calcium channel blocker might be warranted.

11.9 Bradyarrhythmias

If there are symptoms (lightheadedness, dizziness, syncope or near syncope, hypotension,

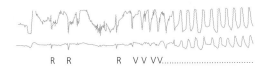

R   R   R   V V VV.................................

Figure 11.7 Pause-dependent Torsades de Pointes (TdP). An elderly woman awaiting pacemaker implantation for complete heart block experienced an episode of TdP. Her cardiac catheterization was unremarkable, and she had preserved left ventricular function. An EP study was also performed and was negative for inducible arrhythmias. TdP is treated with administration of IV magnesium, correction of electrolyte abnormalities, and, if necessary, IV isoproterenol or temporary overdrive pacing.

hypoxia), associated with the bradycardia, consider these options:

* atropine 0.5–1.0 mg IV;
* dopamine 5–20 μg kg[-1] min[-1];
* epinephrine 2–10 μg min[-1];
* transcutaneous pacing or temporary endocardial pacing if available.

If there are no symptoms then evaluate for underlying causes (i.e. an overdose of an AV nodal agent). In general, Type II second-degree or third-degree AV block with heart rates less than 40 beats min[-1] will require transvenous pacing (temporary or permanent).

11.9.1 Temporary pacing

External, transthoracic temporary pacing can be accomplished through most newer external defibrillators. Patches should be positioned in the anterior and lateral positions or in the anterior and posterior positions. As this form of pacing can cause muscle stimulation, it should be reserved for urgent temporary pacing while a temporary endocardial pacemaker is inserted. The preferred venous routes for temporary endocardial pacing leads are via the right internal jugular vein (IJ) or left innominate vein followed by the left IJ and right subclavian vein. Fluoroscopy can make insertion easier (it is necessary when insertion is performed via the femoral veins), but standard techniques can achieve equal success. Most temporary wires have inflatable balloon tips, which allow smooth passage into the RV. By connecting the temporary endocardial pacing wire to an external pacemaker, the operator can visualize ventricular capture. Deflating the balloon and advancing a few millimeters will ensure stable position and serve as a site to measure pacing threshold and sensing parameters. An upright chest X-ray is a must, as it not only eliminates pneumothorax, but also confirms lead position.

11.10 Summary

When faced with any arrhythmia, one should not panic. Knowledge of the underlying rhythm

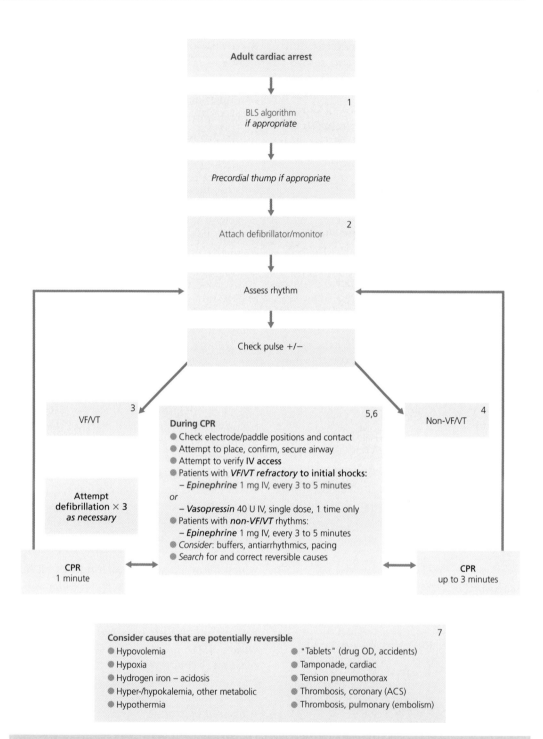

Figure 11.8 Advanced Cardiac Life Support (ACLS) guidelines have been recently updated; vasopressin 40 U IV as a single dose is now recommended as an alternative to epinephrine for VF/VT refractory to initial defibrillation. From: ACC/AHA Guidelines for the management of patients with acute myocardial infarction. *J. Am. Coll. Cardiol.* (1999) **34**: 890–911.

and its cause should be sought. When faced with a wide complex rhythm, remember that VT is more common, especially in older patients and those with a history of infarct or heart failure. A stepwise approach examining first for atrial rhythm, then assessing the QRS complex and finally the AV relationship, will generally disclose the rhythm disturbance and point to the most appropriate therapy (see *Figure 11.8*).

References

1. **The American Heart Association in collaboration with the International Liaison Committee on Resuscitation (ILCOR) (2000)** Guidelines 2000 for cardiopulmonary resuscitation and emergency cardiovascular care. *Circulation* 102(Suppl.): I136–I165.

2. **Gonzalez, E.R., Dannewurf, B.S. and Ornato, J.P.** (1998) Intravenous amiodarone for ventricular arrhythmias: overview and clinical use. *Resuscitation* 39: 33–42.

3. **Dusman, R.E., Stanton, M.S., Miles, W.M., et al.** (1990) Clinical features of amiodarone induced pulmonary toxicity. *Circulation* 82: 51–59.

4. **Hilleman, D., Miller, A.M., Parker, R., et al.** (1998) Optimal management of amiodarone therapy: efficacy and side effects. *Pharmacotherapy* 18: 138S–145S.

5. **Kerin, N.Z. and Somberg, J.** (1994) Proarrhythmia, risk factors, causes, treatment and controversies. *Am. Heart J.* 128: 575–585.

6. **Kerin, N.Z. and Somberg, J.** (1994) Proarrhythmia: Definition, risk factors, causes, treatment and controversies. *Am. Heart J.* 128: 575–585.

7. The CAST investigators: Preliminary report (1989): Effect of encainide and flecainide on mortality in a randomized trial of arrhythmia suppression after myocardial infarction. *NEJM* 321: 406–412.

8. The CAST investigators: (1992) Effect of the antiarrhythmic agent moricizine on survival after myocardial infarction. *NEJM* 327: 227–33.

Chapter 12

Pulmonary embolism in the critically ill patient

Jay S. Steingrub, MD

Contents

12.1 Introduction

Pulmonary embolism (PE) is the third most common cardiovascular disorder in the United States and results in approximately 50 000 deaths per year[1]. It is potentially lethal if not recognized early and aggressively treated. According to autopsy studies and chart reviews, major emboli remain undiagnosed in 60–84% of patients who experience PE[2]. Approximately 11% of patients with pulmonary embolism die within 1 h after the embolic event[3]. Mortality rates in the majority of unsuspected cases who survive longer than 1 h is 30%, but with correct diagnoses and therapy, the mortality rate is reduced to 8%[4]. Our clinical challenge is to improve our ability to diagnose and manage PE more rapidly and more effectively.

12.2 Risk factors

A number of variables place patients at increased risk for venous thromboembolism and hence pulmonary emboli (*Table 12.1*).

- *Surgery and trauma.* Prolonged venous stasis carries the highest risk; causes include venous valvular insufficiency, right heart failure, and prolonged immobility. Type and length of surgery are determinants of deep venous thrombosis (DVT). Abdominal operations requiring general anesthesia for greater than 2 h increase risk for DVT. The risk associated with surgery is higher with pelvic and leg procedures, hip replacement, hip fracture repair or knee replacement[5] (*Table 12.2*). Measures such as perioperative prophylactic therapy with heparin, low molecular weight heparin, or mechanical techniques such as compression stockings or intermittent pneumatic compression can lower the risk. The risk of DVT in trauma patients is related to prolonged immobilization, severe head trauma, paralysis, pelvic and lower extremity fractures, venous trauma, shock and multiple transfusions, with the risk greatest in the first 2 weeks post-injury[6]. With spinal cord injury, the incidence of venous thromboembolism (VTE) is approximately 4% and that of PE about 5%.

- *Age.* Age is an important risk factor for VTE, with the incidence increasing exponentially over the age of 40. The risk of VTE is 46% even for younger patients (<30 years) with multiple trauma. Compared with healthy adults, patients over 30 years of age with any heart disease have a three times higher risk of PE, with this risk increasing with patients in heart failure and arrhythmias, especially atrial fibrillation[7].

- *Indwelling catheters.* Patients with right heart failure and those with indwelling right heart catheters are at increased risk for right ventricular mural thrombi and pulmonary emboli. Central venous catheters are a risk factor for superior vena cava and upper extremity thrombosis.

- *Hypercoagulable states.* Genetic predisposition to thromboembolism is recognized more frequently now. Inherited abnormalities most commonly associated with VTE are the factor V Leiden mutation (resistance to activated protein C), and the prothrombin G20210A mutation[8]. A work-up

Table 12.1 Clinical risk factors for DVT/PE

Age >40 years	• Nephrotic syndrome
• Prolonged immobilization	• Inflammatory bowel disease
• Cancer	• Estrogen use
• Previous DVT or PE	• Acquired or hereditary disorders
• Obesity	• Indwelling femoral catheters
• Varicose veins	• Fractures of pelvis, hip, knee
• CHF	• Major surgery of the abdomen, pelvis, lower extremities
• Stroke	

Table 12.2 Levels of thromboembolism risk in surgical patients without prophylaxis*

Levels of risk examples	Calf DVT, %	Proximal DVT, %	Clinical PE, %	Fatal PE, %	Successful prevention strategies
Low risk Minor surgery in patients <40 years with no additional risk factors	2	0.4	0.2	0.002	No specific measures Aggressive mobilization
Moderate risk Minor surgery in patients with additional risk factors; nonmajor surgery in patients aged 40–60 years with no additional risk factors; major surgery in patients <40 years with no additional risk factors	10–20	2–4	1–2	0.1–0.4	LDUH q 12 h, LMWH, ES or IPC
High risk Nonmajor surgery in patients >60 years or with additional risk factors; major surgery in patients >40 years or with additional risk factors	20–40	4–8	2–4	0.4–1.0	LDUH q 8 h, LMWH or IPC
Highest risk Major surgery in patients >40 years plus prior VTE, cancer or molecular hypercoagulable state, hip or knee arthroplasty, hip fracture surgery; major trauma; spinal cord injury	40–50	10–20	4–10	0.2–5	LMWH, oral anti-coagulants, IPC/ES + LDUH/LMWH or ADH

*Modified from Gallus, A.S., Salzman, E.W. and Hirsh, J. (1994) Prevention of VTE. In: *Hemostasis and Thrombosis: Basic Principles and Clinical Practice*, 3rd Edn (eds R.W. Colman, J. Hirsh, V.J. Marder, *et al.*). Reproduced with permission from Lippincott, Williams & Wilkins.
LDUH, low-dose unfractionated heparin; LMWH, low molecular weight heparin; ES, elastic stockings; IPC, intermittent pneumatic compression; ADH, adjusted dose heparin.

for heritable causes is not indicated after the first episode of VTE particularly in those patients who have clinical risk factors. Hypercoagulability has been implicated as a risk factor and includes inherited abnormalities such as deficiency of antithrombin III, protein C, protein S, hyperhomocysteinemia, and the presence of antiphospholipid syndrome[9].

- *Obesity.* Although obesity alone does not warrant VTE prophylaxis, it increases a patient's potential risk when other clinical factors are present.
- *Varicose veins.* The impact of varicose veins on VTE risk remains controversial. Varicose veins may be an additive risk factor, when

they develop in patients younger than 60 years[10].

- *Malignancy.* Although the association between malignancy and VTE is well known, most patients with pulmonary emboli do not have cancer. Hypercoagulable states secondary to advanced cancer are associated with a higher risk of VTE. The incidence of VTE is 2–3 times higher among patients undergoing surgery for malignant disease than those operated on for non-malignant conditions with other risk factors being equal[11].
- *Estrogen therapy.* Estrogen therapy for prostate cancer may increase the incidence of VTE among men. In women,

estrogen replacement therapy during perimenopausal and postmenopausal periods can be a significant risk factor[12]. Currently, a woman's risk of a VTE-related death from an estrogen-based contraceptive is lower than her risk of death from pregnancy.

- *History of thromboembolism.* A history of thromboembolism is one of the most important risk factors of VTE. The incidence of acute venous thrombosis is nearly eight-fold higher among hospitalized patients with a history of VTE compared with those without a history. Therefore, when undergoing surgery or with periods of prolonged immobility or when in a hospital for serious medical reasons, patients with a history of VTE must receive aggressive prophylactic therapy. The incidence of VTE is 15% among patients who require absolute bed rest for less than 1 week, and is higher among those in bed for longer periods[13]. Recently, an association has been established between VTE and prolonged sitting position as in long automobile or airplane trips[14].

VTE prophylaxis may not be justified by bed rest alone. DVT typically develops in the calf veins and does not typically progress to proximal vein thrombosis, which is more dangerous. Commonly, calf vein thromboses are asymptomatic and usually appear to resolve without clinical sequelae once ambulation is resumed. However, prophylaxis is required if other risk factors, as discussed above are also present.

Postoperative deep venous thromboses are usually clinically silent until they are dislodged to form pulmonary emboli. As venous thrombi can develop despite optimal prophylactic regimens, the question remains whether high-risk patients should undergo postoperative screening tests for DVT. The clinical experience suggests that although venous ultrasonography can actually diagnose proximal vein thrombosis, it appears to be less useful for detecting calf vein thrombosis.

12.3 Pathophysiology of pulmonary embolism

Most pulmonary emboli originate from the deep veins of the lower extremities. Other sites include the iliac and pelvic veins, and less commonly, the inferior vena cava. Two primary pathologic processes explain the typical clinical presentations of PE. Obstruction of the pulmonary circulation can result in circulatory compromise with the extent of the compensation depending on the site and size of the pulmonary embolism, and the previous circulatory reserve of the right heart and pulmonary vasculature. Patients with previously normal pulmonary artery pressures and right heart pressures can withstand moderate or large occlusions of pulmonary arteries caused by PE and still maintain adequate cardiac output. However, in the presence of existing pulmonary hypertension, right heart failure, or extensive clot involvement of vessels, severe elevation of pulmonary artery pressures may result in acute right heart failure and subsequent hemodynamic instability. Furthermore, pulmonary artery obstruction by thromboembolism results in hypoxemia. The mechanism of PE associated hypoxemia can be attributed to a combination of ventilation–perfusion mismatch, atelectasis, redistribution of pulmonary blood flow, and increased blood transit time. Infrequently, acute pulmonary hypertension secondary to PE may lead to the reopening of a patent foramen ovale present in a minority of the population, leading to an intra-atrial right to left shunt and severe refractory hypoxemia.

12.4 Differential diagnosis in the ICU

Making a diagnosis of PE in an ICU is challenging because of obstacles in transporting the patient to radiology for a spiral CT or ventilation perfusion scan. Treatment may be complicated by the underlying or associated illnesses in the critically ill patient. Physical examination may be non-specific, as a result of underlying obstructive pulmonary disease, pneumonia, congestive heart failure or other conditions. Clinical symptoms and signs are non-specific (*Table 12.3*). Except for chest pain and dyspnea, no symptoms are consistently associated with PE. Common physical findings of tachypnea and tachycardia may be suggestive, but again these findings are non-specific. Although the presence of a pleural rub or hemoptysis may be useful diagnostically, these signs are non-specific and frequently absent. The differential diagnosis is extensive, including pneumonia, asthma, myocardial infarction, pleuritis, pericarditis, aortic dissection, cardiac tamponade, and costochondritis. Fixed splitting of the second heart sound, which indicates right ventricular overload and a flow murmur over the lung fields, is of major importance. Rales are heard in approximately 60% of the patients with angiographically proven PE. Chest roentgenographic results, V/Q scanning, and D-dimer assay are less likely to be normal in the absence of a PE, and more difficult to interpret in a critically ill patient in whom PE develops. Unless they can be explained by a more likely diagnosis, dyspnea, tachypnea, and pleural chest pain occurring together in the presence of risk factors for DVT justifies a diagnostic evaluation for PE. Syncope and cyanosis suggest severe massive embolism as signs and symptoms of right heart failure develop.

12.5 Diagnostic tests

Figure 12.1 presents the American Thoracic Society (ATS) algorithm for the evaluation of suspected PE[15].

12.5.1 Arterial blood gas analysis

Respiratory alkalosis as a result of hypoxemia is frequently observed in dyspneic patients with PE. Blood gas analysis will demonstrate an abnormal alveolar arterial oxygen gradient in most patients with PE, with oxygen tension usually less than 80 mmHg. However, patients with PE, especially those with a previously normal cardiopulmonary state, may have a normal alveolar arterial O_2 gradient[16].

12.5.2 D-dimer assay

Recent trials suggest that the D-dimer enzyme-linked immune serum assay (ELISA) may have a role in excluding PE in symptomatic outpatients[17]. The assay detects degradation products of cross-linked fibrin and is very sensitive to activation of the fibrinolytic system. Use of this assay may reduce the use of angiography by 30%, and combining the assay with non-invasive tests for PE might improve the negative predictive values and avoid invasive tests. This test is non-specific, with its negative predictive value for PE is high, but its positive predictive value is low. The assay may be positive even after mild trauma associated with ecchymosis. At this

Table 12.3 Pulmonary embolism manifestations

Symptoms	Signs	ECG	Chest X-ray findings
Dyspnea	Tachypnea	RV strain pattern	Focal oligemia
Cough	Pulmonary rales	Atrial fibrillation	Westermark sign
Hemotysis	Fever	P-wave enlargement	Wedge-shaped density (Hampton hump)
Syncopy	Tachycardia	Q wave deepening (lead III)	
Chest pain (pleuritic)	Phlebitis	T wave inversion (lead V_1, V_5)	
	Edema	Ventricular ectopy	Enlarged descending right pulmonary artery
	Gallop rhythm	S wave enlargement (lead I)	Palla sign

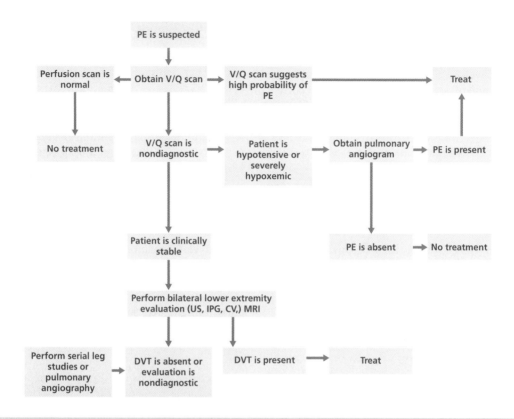

Figure 12.1 Diagnostic algorithm for patients with symptoms suggesting acute pulmonary embolism. As with the approach to acute deep venous thrombosis, the recommended diagnostic approach allows for some flexibility depending upon the resources at a particular institution. PE, pulmonary embolism; V/Q, ventilation–perfusion; US, compression ultrasonography; IPG, impedance plethysmography; CV, contrast venography; MRI, magnetic resonance imaging; DVT, deep venous thrombosis. Adapted from Tapson, V.F., Carroll, B.A., Davidson, B.L., et al. (1999) The diagnostic approach to acute venous thromboembolism. Clinical practice guidelines. Reproduced with permission from American Thoracic Society. *Am. J. Respir. Crit. Care Med.* **160**: 1043–1066.

time, the D-dimer assay may be most useful for ruling out DVT and PE in the emergency department because a negative result is highly reliable. However, routine use as a diagnostic test for PE is not recommended. The combination of a normal dead space ventilation/tidal volume fraction and normal D-dimer concentration was 100% sensitive in excluding PE in a recent trial[18].

12.5.3 Chest roentgenography
Chest X-ray abnormalities include pulmonary infiltrates, pleural effusions, elevated hemi-diaphragm and atelectasis, but may be normal. Hampton's hump, Palla sign or the Wester-mark sign may suggest the diagnosis, but are infrequent and can in no way be taken as evidence that a PE is the cause of the patient's dyspnea.

12.5.4 EKG
Sinus tachycardia is the most common electro-cardiographic abnormality with acute PE. The ECG may reveal P-pulmonale in massive PE. Right heart strain may manifest right bundle branch block. Signs of acute right ventricular strain or the so-called S_1Q_3 (large S wave in lead 1, Q wave in lead 3) pattern are infrequently encountered, and their absence is not reliable evidence that a VE is absent.

12.5.5 V/Q lung scanning

The lung scan is the most commonly used test to diagnose PE. The scanning results is graded on the basis of perfusion defects in relation to lung ventilation as follows.

- *Normal perfusion scan.* Perfusion defect is not observed and effectively rules out clinically significant PE. However, in those cases where there is an overwhelming clinical suspicion of PE with high risk factors and the perfusion scan is normal, one must consider performing pulmonary angiography.
- *High-probability scan.* The presence of more than one large perfusion defect (>75% of the segment) with normal ventilation or ventilatory defect significantly smaller than perfusion defects, or perfusion defects in an area of absent or smaller infiltrates on chest X-ray, strongly suggests PE in a patient with the appropriate clinical profile. A pulmonary angiogram should be considered for patients with a high-probability V/Q scan and low-probability profile, such as absent risk factors for PE. However, a positive compression ultrasonography obtained before the pulmonary angiogram obviates the need for an angiogram for most patients with a high-probability V/Q scan.
- *Indeterminate perfusion scans.* Low- and intermediate-probability scans are sometimes grouped together and called indeterminate or non-diagnostic scans, implying the need for additional studies. Scanning for most patients with suspected PE suggests low or intermediate probability. A low-probability scan does not rule out PE and necessitates further studies, using compression ultrasonography. If the test results are positive, anticoagulation therapy should be initiated if no absolute contraindications exist. With negative lower extremity studies, clinical observation is appropriate for patients with a low-probability V/Q scan. The negative predictive value of a low-probability scan increases when there is no strong clinical impression for a PE.

Intermediate-probability V/Q scans require further evaluation via pulmonary angiogram or other studies to confirm or exclude PE.

The most useful data regarding the utility of V/Q scanning for PE was from the PIOPED trial, the Prospective Investigation of Pulmonary Embolism Diagnosis[19]. This study compared the sensitivity and specificity of V/Q scanning with that of angiography. The researchers also estimated the clinical likelihood of PE before the results of the scanning and angiography were known. Approximately 1000 patients in whom PE was suspected underwent both V/Q lung scanning and pulmonary angiography. In this study, a minority of patients (13%) had a high-probability V/Q scan. The most frequently seen results were intermediate-probability (39%) and low-probability (34%) scans. The findings of the study revealed the following.

- A normal or near-normal perfusion scan made PE very unlikely. A high-probability V/Q scan strongly supports a diagnosis of PE with probability increasing with a high clinical suspicion or in the absence of underlying cardiopulmonary disease.
- V/Q scanning did not yield high-probability findings for most patients with angiographic proven pulmonary emboli. Approximately 41% of patients with angiogram proven PE had high-probability scans.
- More than 50% of documented PEs were in patients with intermediate- or low-probability scans. In patients with low- or intermediate-probability scans the likelihood of PE ranged from 14 to 31%.
- For most patients with suspected PE, the diagnosis cannot be ruled out with scanning alone. Clinical assessments were more accurate in excluding than in identifying PE.

In summary, the PIOPED findings suggest that a high-probability scan has excellent positive predictive value but identifies fewer than half of all pulmonary emboli. If low- and intermediate-probability scans are considered negative, a significant number of cases will not be diagnosed. If every patient with abnormal V/Q scans were treated, many patients would be unnecessarily treated. For most patients with suspected PE, V/Q scans must be complemented by further testing to confirm or rule out the diagnosis of PE.

12.5.6 Pulmonary angiography

Pulmonary angiography has been considered to be the gold standard for the diagnosis of pulmonary embolism. Indications include high clinical suspicion of DVT with non-diagnostic studies, in situations where anticoagulation is considered high risk, and before embolectomy or thrombolytic therapy. The test provides information about the size of the clot in approximately 20–30% of patients with clinically suspected PE and a non-diagnostic scan, and identifies pulmonary artery pressure measurements[20]. The procedure is considered safe and when performed by experienced clinicians carries an estimated mortality of approximately 0.3% and morbidity of 1–4% (arrhythmias, acute right heart failure and right ventricular perforation). The procedure increases the patient risk of bleeding when standard anti-coagulation is given. It also prevents administration of a thrombolytic agent because of the potential for severe bleeding from the puncture site. A study obtained within 1–2 weeks of acute symptoms will reliably diagnose PE. The angiogram has a high sensitivity for emboli in the large central pulmonary arteries and a much lower sensitivity for small peripheral emboli. Risks associated with pulmonary angiography are considerably overrated. Renal failure (creatinine ≥2 mg dl^{-1}) is considered an absolute contraindication, because of the risk of the contrast agent. Recent myocardial infarctions, current arrhythmias, and severe pulmonary hypertension are relative contraindications. Interobserver agreement in the PIOPED study was only 66% for subsegmental PE diagnosis using angiography. Interobserver agreement among radiologists interpreting angiograms deteriorates for subsegmental and smaller PE. For

these reasons, newer non-invasive methods of diagnosing PE are being employed.

12.5.7 Helical (spiral) CT

New generation scanners that employ rapid sequential scanning can reliably identify a clot in the second to fourth division of pulmonary vessels. Sensitivity and specificity of a contrast enhanced helical (spiral) CT scan for the diagnosis of PE vary in the literature, with some studies reporting sensitivities ranging from 53% to 100% and specificities ranging from 81% to 100%[21]. A normal helical CT scan result when the index of suspicion is high should be followed by pulmonary angiography and the careful evaluation of the distal pulmonary vascular bed. Although helical CT may be inadequate to detect subsegmental emboli, it is unclear how often subsegmental emboli occur in the absence of larger emboli. Outcome studies are being carried out to evaluate the use of spiral CT in patients with PE. Current limitations of helical CT angiography include the requirement of an intravenous contrast agent and the unavailability of equipment and personnel needed to perform and interpret the study at every hospital. Performing CT contrast venography in tandem with CT angiography may improve the diagnostic yield. Helical CT is useful in patients with baseline V/Q scan abnormalities and provides information about potentially other disease processes in the lungs.

12.5.8 Compression ultrasonography

Non-invasive lower extremity testing with compression ultrasonography should be considered to evaluate for evidence of DVT when lung testing is non-diagnostic. Although this test does not rule out pulmonary embolus, a large majority of pulmonary emboli arise from the femoral vein, and the treatment for both DVT and PE will be the same. Therefore, a diagnosis of DVT provides grounds for initiating therapy for pulmonary embolus without further investigation. Compression ultrasound has a sensitivity of 89–98% for proximal DVT[22]. The test's accuracy decreases in asymptomatic patients and in those with chronic DVT or pelvic thromboembolic disease. A normal examination does not rule out PE when clinical suspicion is moderately high. In patients at high risk for DVT, including those with pelvic or hip trauma, and critical illness, compression ultrasonography is the most sensitive and specific lower extremity study. Impedance plethysmography test is highly accurate for diagnosing proximal deep vein thrombosis, but it is not widely available. Forms of venous obstruction and congestive heart failure can produce false positive results.

12.5.9 Magnetic resonance angiography

Magnetic resonance angiography is a fast and accurate modality for detecting PE and does not involve nephrotoxic contrast agents. It may also be a non-invasive alternative for venography to detect deep vein thrombosis. It is a promising technique that appears to be highly sensitive to pulmonary embolus. This technique has the added advantage of distinguishing between acute and chronic thrombosis and scanning the lungs and the legs at the same time. The sensitivity of the magnetic resonance technique was 100% in one study and its specificity was 95%[23].

12.6 Treatment

Providing effective therapy for PE in the ICU setting is more complicated than it would be outside the ICU. ICU patients are more likely to have a number of complicating conditions, including stress gastritis, ulcers, thrombocytopenia, anemia, and coagulopathies, or have sustained trauma or undergone a recent surgical procedure.

The decision on whether to treat suspected PE is usually based on the results of the V/Q scan. A high-probability scan is an indication for treatment. A non-diagnostic scan should be followed by pulmonary angiography if the patient is hypotensive or severely hypoxemic or by bilateral leg evaluation (i.e. compression ultrasonography) if the patient's condition is stable. In those patients who have a normal perfusion scan, prophylactic therapy may be given where risk factors for DVT or PE are present.

Specific treatment issues in the management of the PE include:

- anticoagulation therapy;
- low molecular weight heparin (LMWH) in treatment and prophylaxis;
- thrombolytic therapy;
- Inferior vena cava (IVC) filter;
- management of hypotension with pharmacologic support;
- surgical embolectomy.

12.6.1 Heparin

Heparin remains the mainstay of therapy for PE and DVT involving the proximal veins of the thigh or pelvic veins. Heparin inhibits thrombin by activating antithrombin. Therapeutic heparinization will prevent additional clot formation; the body's intrinsic fibrinolytic system should subsequently clear the existing clot. Once the diagnosis of a possible life-threatening PE is considered, heparin should be administered if there are no contraindications, while the patient undergoes further non-invasive evaluations (*Table 12.4*). Weight-adjusted protocols have been employed to enhance rapid and consistent anticoagulation and to minimize the risk of recurrent PE and bleeding (*Table 12.5*)[24]. Patients receive 80 U kg⁻¹ of heparin as a bolus, followed by an infusion of 18 U kg⁻¹ per hour. The dose is then titrated to maintain the activated partial thromboplastin time (APTT) more than 1.5 times control.

The APTT is monitored every 6 h until two consecutive therapeutic results are obtained. Subsequently, the APTT can be checked every morning. Additionally, a platelet count is obtained at baseline and every other day until heparin infusion is stopped.

Heparin-induced thrombocytopenia may cause arterial thrombosis. In those patients without a history of hemorrhagic diathesis, hemorrhagic side effects are rare. Heparin

Table 12.4 Guidelines for anticoagulation: unfractionated heparin*

Indication	Guidelines
VTE suspected	• Obtain baseline APTT, PT, CBC count • Check for contraindications to heparin therapy • Order imaging study, consider giving heparin 5000 IU IV
VTE confirmed	• Rebolus with heparin, 80 IU kg⁻¹ IV; start maintenance infusion at 181 U kg⁻¹ h⁻¹ • Check APTT at 6 h to keep APTT in a range that corresponds to a therapeutic blood heparin level • Check platelet count between days 3 and 5 • Start warfarin therapy on day 1 at 5 mg and adjust subsequent daily dose according to INR • Stop heparin therapy after at least 4–5 days of combined therapy when INR is >2.0 • Anticoagulate with warfarin for 3 months at an INR of 2.5; range: 2.0–3.0

*For subcutaneous treatment with unfractionated heparin, give 250 IU kg⁻¹ SC q 12 h to obtain a therapeutic APTT at 6–8 h.
PT, prothrombin time.

Table 12.5 Body weight-based dosing of IV heparin*

APTT, S†	Dose change, IU kg⁻¹ h⁻¹	Additional action	Next APTT, h
<35 (<1.2 × mean normal)	+4	Rebolus with 80 IU kg⁻¹	6
35–45 (1.2–1.5 × mean normal)	+2	Rebolus with 40 IU kg⁻¹	6
46–70 (1.5–2.3 × mean normal)	0	none	6§
71–90 (2.3–3.0 × mean normal)	−2	none	6
>90 (>3.0 **Q4** × mean normal)	−3	Stop infusion for 1 h	6

*Initial dosing: loading, 80 IU kg⁻¹; maintenance infusion; 18 IU kg⁻¹ h⁻¹ (APTT in 6 h).
†Therapeutic range in seconds.
§During the first 24 h, repeat APTT every 6 h. Thereafter, monitor APTT once every morning unless it is outside the therapeutic range.

should not be given for longer than 5 days. Failing to achieve adequate anticoagulation in the first 24 h of treatment significantly increases the risk of recurrent emboli.

Therapy commonly requires 5 days of heparin and a warfarin-induced prolongation of the international normalized ratio (INR) before discontinuation of heparin. Within the first 24 h of heparin administration, warfarin is started with an initial dose of 5 mg day⁻¹. The therapeutic goal is to reach an INR of 2–3. Warfarin acts by inhibiting the vitamin K dependent factors II, VII, IX and X.

It is important to understand that anticoagulation with heparin and warfarin does not prevent the development of persistent pulmonary hypertension, alleviate embolus-induced hemodynamic instability, or avoid subsequent valvular damage to deep veins of the lower extremities. The optimum duration of anticoagulation therapy for DVT and pulmonary emboli remains debatable, with studies showing that 3–6 months of warfarin

Table 12.6 Duration of therapy*

3–6 months	• First event with reversible† or time-limited risk factor (patient may have underlying factor V Leiden or prothrombin 20210A)
≥6 months	• Idiopathic VTE, first event
12 months to lifetime	• First event, recurrent idiopathic VTE are a continuing risk factor‡

*All recommendations are subject to modification by individual characteristics including patient preference, age, comorbidity, and likelihood of recurrence.
†Reversible or time-limited risk factors: surgery, trauma, immobilization, estrogen use.
‡Proper duration of therapy is unclear in first event with homozygous factor V Leiden, homocystinemia, deficiency of protein C or S, or multiple thrombophilias; and in recurrent events with reversible risk factors.

alone results in an acceptable low (<5%) frequency of DVT recurrence[25]. Patients with recurrent DVTs or high risk factors such as CHF or hypercoagulable states should receive anticoagulation therapy for a longer period of time (*Table 12.6*).

Table 12.7 Bridge therapy protocol

(1) Obtain INR 1 week before procedure
　(a) INR 2–3: discontinue warfarin 5 days before surgery
　(b) INR 3–4.5: discontinue warfarin 6 days before surgery
　(c) Enoxaparin 1 mg kg⁻¹ SC, q 12 h starting 36 h after discontinuing warfarin

(2) Discontinue enoxaparin 12–18 h before surgery

(3) Restart enoxaparin 12–24 h postsurgery or once hemostasis has been achieved

(4) Restart warfarin at the previous maintenance dose. Dosing can be initiated at any time following the surgical procedure, as enoxaparin will provide the necessary anticoagulation during the crossover period

(5) INR 2–3: Stop enoxaparin for 2 consecutive days

INR, international normalized ratio.
In: Merli G.J. (2000) Prophylaxis for deep venous thrombosis and pulmonary embolism in the surgical patient. Reproduced with permission from *Clinical Cornerstone*. **2**: 22.

12.6.2 Low molecular weight heparin (LMWH)

LMWH is as effective as unfractionated heparin for the treatment of hemodynamically stable patients with PE. LMWH has been employed in hip and knee surgery and high-risk abdominal surgery. LMWH binds specifically to antithrombin and has advantages over unfractionated heparin, including its administration of the drug subcutaneously, greater bioavailability in tissue, and more predictable anticoagulation. LMWH use requires no monitoring of APTT. Total costs may thus be lower when laboratory testing over the course of therapy is considered. However, monitoring may be necessary in patients who are morbidly obese, have renal insufficiency, or who weigh less than 50 kg. The incidence of heparin-induced thrombocytopenia is extremely low among patients who receive LMWH compared with unfractionated heparin. The disadvantages of LMWH in certain patients are due to its longer half-life and lesser reversibility with protamine compared with unfractionated heparin. Choosing to use LMWH or unfractionated heparin depends on the clinical setting and the risk factors. In those patients scheduled to undergo invasive procedures, unfractionated heparin may be preferred over LMWH. Protocols for bridging between warfarin and enoxaparin are available (*Table 12.7*)[26].

Table 12.8 Regimens to prevent VTE

Method	Description
LDUH	Heparin 5000 IU SC, given q 8–12 h starting 1–2 h before operation
ADH	Heparin SC, given q 8 h starting at approximately 3500 IU SC and adjusted by ±500 SC, per dose to maintain a mid-interval APTT at high normal values

LMWH and heparinoids	General surgery, moderate risk:
	     Dalteparin, 2500 IU SC, 1–2 h before surgery and once daily postop
	     Enoxaparin, 20 mg IU SC, 1–2 h before surgery and once daily postop
	     Nadroparin, 2850 SC 2–4 h before surgery and once daily postop
	     Tinzaparin, 3500 IU SC 2 h before surgery and once daily postop
	
	 General surgery, high risk:
	     Dalteparin, 5000 IU SC 8–12 h before surgery and once daily postop
	     Danaparoid, 750 IU SC 1–4 h before surgery and q 12 h postop
	     Enoxaparin, 40 mg IU SC, 1–2 h preop and once daily postop
	     Enoxaparin, 30 mg IU SC, q 12 h starting 8–12 h postop
	
	 Orthopedic surgery
	     Dalteparin, 5500 SC 8–12 h preop and once daily starting 12–24 h postop
	     Dalteparin, 2500 SC 6–8 h postop; then 5000 U SC daily
	     Danaparoid, 750 IU SC 1–4 h preop and q 12 h postop
	     Enoxaparin, 30 mg IU SC q 12 h starting 12–24 h postop
	     Enoxaparin, 40 mg SC once daily starting 10–12 h preop
	     Nadroparin, 38 IU kg^{-1} SC 12 h preop, 12 h postop, and once daily on postop days 1, 2 and 3; then increase to 57 IU kg^{-1} SC once daily
	     Tinzaparin, 75 IU kg^{-1} SC once daily starting 12–24 h postop
	     Tinzaparin, 4500 IU SC 12 h preop and once daily postop
	
	 Major trauma
	     Enoxaparin, 30 mg SC q 12 h starting 12–36 h postinjury if hemostatically stable
	
	 Acute spinal cord injury
	     Enoxaparin, 30 mg SC q 12 h
	
	 Medical conditions
	     Dalteparin, 2500 IU SC once daily
	     Danaparoid, 750 IU SC q 12 h
	     Enoxaparin, 40 mg SC once daily
	     Nadroparin, 2850 IU SC once daily

Perioperative warfarin	Start daily dose with approximately 5–10 mg the day after surgery; adjust the dose for a target INR of 2.5 (range 2–3)
IPC/ES	Begin immediately before operation, and continue until fully ambulatory

Postop, postoperative; LDUH, low-dose unfractionated heparin; ADH, adjusted dose heparin; IPC, intermittent pneumatic compression; ES, elastic/graduated compression.

12.6.3 Thrombolytic therapy

Thrombolytics have been utilized most commonly in patients with massive PE and severe hemodynamic compromise. Proven benefits of thrombolytics include improvements in right ventricular hemodynamics and pulmonary perfusion with reversal of right heart failure[27]. For patients with massive pulmonary emboli, right heart failure, or hemodynamic instability, thrombolytic therapy may be potentially life saving. No study to date has shown a reduction in mortality with thrombolytics. In the presence of severe hemodynamic compromise secondary to a PE, and echocardiographic determination of acute pulmonary hypertension, thrombolytic therapy can be employed.

The clearest indication for thrombolytics is hemodynamic instability, in the absence of absolute contraindications. Contraindications to thrombolytic therapy include: current internal bleeding, recent trauma, major surgery or head injury (within the previous 6 weeks), acute cerebrovascular hemorrhage or a cerebrovascular procedure within the previous 2–3 months. Other relative contraindications include: cerebrovascular event within 6 months, a 10 day or shorter post-partum period, recent organ biopsy or puncture of a non-compressible vessel, uncontrolled bleeding diathesis, recent serious internal trauma, pregnancy, cardiopulmonary resuscitation with rib fractures, thoracentesis, paracentesis, lumbar puncture, or any condition that places the patient at an increased risk for bleeding. Most bleeding episodes occur in patients undergoing invasive procedures. Major bleeding complications for PE are approximately 14% in patients undergoing pulmonary angiograms, but only 4% in patients having V/Q scans[28]. If bleeding occurs during therapy, discontinuation of treatment usually is all that is required to control bleeding. However, with ongoing bleeding, cryoprecipitate infusion targeted to attain a fibrinogen level of 100 mg dl^{-1} or more is indicated. If bleeding persists, the administration of fresh frozen plasma should be considered. In the presence of ongoing life-threatening hemorrhage following thrombolytic therapy, antifibrinolytic therapy with ε-aminocaproic acid is indicated.

There is no evidence that any one thrombolytic agent is superior to another. Recommended drugs and dosages are: recombinant tissue type plasminogen activator (rtPA), 100 mg infused over 2 h; urokinase, 4400 IU kg^{-1} given over 10 min as a loading dose, then 4400 IU kg^{-1} h^{-1} infused for 12 h; streptokinase, 250 000 IU loading dose given over 30 min and 100 000 IU h^{-1} infused for 24 h given via a peripheral intravenous site is less cumbersome to employ than the 12–24 h infusion regimen.

12.6.4 IVC filters

Indications for IVC interruption include:

- contraindication to anticoagulant use;
- coagulation-induced hemorrhage;
- hemodynamic instability with absolute contraindication for thrombolytic therapy;
- recurrent thromboemboli owing to anticoagulation failure;
- chronic thromboembolic pulmonary hypertension.

Patients who may survive an initial massive PE must be considered for an IVC filter placement because death in this population may be a result of a relatively small reoccurrence. Employment of an IVC should be based on evidence that thromboemboli are originating from the deep vein of the thigh or pelvic system. The IVC filter can be placed under fluoroscopic guidance in the ICU safely and cost effectively, circumventing the need to transport the critically ill patients to the radiology suite or operating room. Controversy exists on whether to administer anticoagulation therapy to patients with IVC filters in place. Most investigators recommend that if filters are inserted because of recurrent pulmonary emboli during anticoagulation, anticoagulation is usually continued to prevent additional thrombi from forming on the filter. The use of anticoagulation with IVC filters may increase the patency rate of filters over time and facilitate venous drainage. Risk of recurrent PE after IVC interruption is approximately 2–3%.

12.6.5 Surgery and rheolytic thrombectomy

Criteria for pulmonary embolectomy should include patients with severe hemodynamic instability despite heparin and resuscitative efforts, massive PE, and failure of thrombolytic therapy in patients. Emergency surgical thrombectomy is difficult to accomplish unless a cardiac surgical team, including perfusionist, is immediately available. The mortality rate for surgical intervention is reported to be from 10% to 95%[29].

Rheolytic thrombectomy is one of the newest methods for treating massive pulmonary embolus[30]. It involves the use of a catheter that is designed to remove intravascular thrombi from vessels. Direct high-pressure saline jets located at the catheter tip cause mechanical thrombolysis. Dissolving microparticles are aspirated through the same catheter. Larger studies are needed to determine whether this treatment would be an alternative to thrombolysis in a select patient population.

Intra-embolic infusion of thrombolyic therapy has been employed in several institutions where local thrombolysis of massive pulmonary emboli without systemic fibrinogenolysis may be achieved by delivering low-dose thrombolytic therapy (20 mg rtPA) to the site of embolization in the pulmonary artery by means of catheter infusion[31]. Intra-embolic low-dose thrombolysis has been used successfully in critically ill patients with PE in situations where systemic thrombolysis is considered contraindicated, but its efficacy has yet to be demonstrated in randomized, controlled trials.

12.7 Right ventricular function

Right ventricular (RV) dysfunction secondary to right heart failure often causes death in patients with acute massive pulmonary emboli. Therefore, it is important to evaluate the effects of the embolus on RV function. The hemodynamic response to acute PE depends upon embolic size, the presence of pre-existing cardiopulmonary disease and, to a lesser extent, the magnitude of the neurohumoral response to emboli. In the presence of underlying cardiopulmonary disease, a relatively small embolus can have significant consequences. The latter explains why only 50% of fatal emboli are anatomically massive.

The hemodynamic results of acute emboli are a reduction in the cross-sectional area

of the pulmonary circulation resulting in increased resistance to blood flow through the lungs. Physiologically, PE increases right ventricular work or afterload, best measured by assessing mean pulmonary artery pressure or calculating pulmonary vascular resistance with a pulmonary artery catheter. This increase in mean pulmonary artery pressure is directly related to the extent of embolization. In the absence of pre-existing underlying cardiopulmonary disease, patients with emboli have marked levels of pulmonary hypertension when at least 50% of pulmonary vasculature is occluded. Mean pulmonary artery pressure begins to rise at 25% obstruction of the vascular tree, and continues to rise with increased degrees of obstruction to reach a maximum value of about 40 mmHg in the absence of pre-existing pulmonary hypertension. Normally, the RV being a thin-walled chamber cannot accommodate high pulmonary artery pressures (PAP) and increased RV work. Therefore, it predisposes to rapid contractile failure. Right ventricular dysfunction becomes even more apparent when there is an elevation in the mean right atrial pressure. It is usually associated with a mean PAP of 30 mmHg and obstruction of at least 35–40% of the pulmonary vascular tree. As right atrial pressure increases concomitantly with PAP, an initial compensatory cardiovascular response is an increase in heart rate to maintain cardiac output. When the right atrial pressure rises by 10 mmHg and mean PAP is greater than 30–40 mmHg, right ventricular failure occurs and cardiac output will decrease.

In summary, available data suggest that the normal right ventricle is unable to generate a mean PAP greater than 40 mmHg. With excessive resistance to blood flow from PE, this causes the RV to dilate and become hypokinetic, causing a reduction in right ventricular stroke volume. This decline in right ventricular stroke volume contributes to a decrease in LV preload and cardiac output when combined with RV dilation. Echocardiography can determine the degree of pulmonary hypertension in patients with acute PE. Pulsed continuous wave and color Doppler techniques can estimate right ventricular systolic pressure and systolic PAP, demonstrate the presence of tricuspid and pulmonary regurgitation, and determine flow velocities, thereby permitting estimation of right ventricular systolic pressures and systolic PAP[32]. Trans-esophageal echocardiography has been employed to assess for central pulmonary artery thromboemboli in patients with risk factors for PE and right heart strain[33].

12.8 **Other clinical interventions**

12.8.1 Oxygen therapy and mechanical ventilation
Oxygen therapy is administered to augment oxygen saturation and reduce pulmonary vascular resistance caused by hypoxemia. Continuous positive airway pressure may be used in patients with focal atelectasis. Intubation and mechanical ventilation may be required for hypoxemic respiratory failure.

12.8.2 Fluid resuscitation (See Chapter 7)
In the presence of PE-induced hypotension accompanied by impaired right ventricular contractility, initial volume expansion is indicated. However, excessive fluid resuscitation may lead to severe RV dysfunction and high pulmonary artery pressures, subsequently causing right heart failure. The use of volume expansion and vasoactive agents to manage the hemodynamic instability in critically ill patients with PE has not been studied in randomized, controlled trials. Clinical experience suggests that pharmacologic hemodynamic support does improve blood pressure long enough to administer thrombolytic therapy or any other therapy in the acute management of PE. Fluid resuscitation may increase myocardial wall stress, which may decrease the oxygen supply demand ratio, causing ischemia and/or right ventricular infarction. Therefore, it is recommended that volume infusion should be titrated to maintain a systolic blood pressure of 90 mmHg.

12.8.3 Vasoactive agents (See Chapter 8)
Epinephrine or other alpha agents are indicated for therapy of massive PE to reverse significant hypotension from reduced cardiac output. These vasoactive agents attempt to restore normal RV hemodynamics via increased RV coronary blood flow, improved RV contractility and reduced pulmonary vascular resistance. Norepinephrine has been shown to produce consistent hemodynamic improvement and improve cardiac contractility through its beta receptor effect. It can enhance coronary artery blood flow and right ventricular perfusion pressure. Dobutamine may be an adjunct to norepinephrine; it reduces both systemic vascular resistance and pulmonary vascular resistance through vasodilation of respective vascular beds. Dobutamine has been shown to increase cardiac output, decrease pulmonary vascular resistance and improve oxygenation in patients with PE-induced pulmonary hypertension[34]. Combination of norepinephrine and dobutamine may be the best current regimen of vasoactive therapy of hemodynamically unstable patients with pulmonary embolus. Doses should be titrated to preserve organ perfusion.

12.9 **Risk reduction**

12.9.1 DVT prophylaxis
The incidence of DVT in general surgery is approximately 20–70%. Recommended prophylaxis is tailored to the risk classification (see *Table 12.2*). General surgery patients at low risk do not require prophylaxis, except for early ambulation. Low-dose heparin (5000 IU SC every 12 h), LMWH, intermittent pneumatic compression sleeves or gradient elastic stockings are to be given to moderate-risk surgical patients. In high-risk general surgery, low-dose heparin (5000 IU SC every 8 or 12 h) or LMWH is recommended. Placement of a vena caval filter as prophylaxis for major surgery is recommended in patients with significant cardiopulmonary disease and in patients who cannot receive any form of prophylaxis following high-risk surgical procedures. In very

high-risk surgical patients, external pneumatic compression devices and low-dose heparin (5000 U every 8–12 h) or LMWH are recommended.

12.9.2 Bridge therapy

For patients on chronic anticoagulation scheduled for invasive surgical procedures, *Table 12.7* lists the recommendations on the appropriate management of anticoagulants in the perioperative period. A recent study suggests that bridge anticoagulation therapy should depend on the medical condition and the time elapsed since the thromboembolic event[35]. Those with acute venous thromboembolism or acute arterial embolism less than 1 month after the event should receive bridge therapy. Those with acute thromboembolism between 2 and 3 months after the event should be placed on anti-coagulation, postoperatively. All other chronically anticoagulated patients do not require bridge therapy.

12.9.3 Regional anesthesia

Epidural or spinal hematomas have been described following LMWH use. Regional anesthesia should be avoided in patients who are receiving drugs that affect hemostasis, and those having multiple spinal attempts with hemorrhagic aspirates. When DVT/PE prophylaxis is initiated before surgery, spinal needle insertion should be postponed for 10–12 h after the initial LMWH prophylactic dose is administered[36]. In those situations where an epidural anesthesia catheter is in place post-surgery for 24–36 h, LMWH prophylaxis should be delayed for 12 h after catheter removal. Patients should be monitored for early signs of cord compression secondary to epidural bleeding (numbness, weakness, bowel/bladder dysfunction).

12.9.4 Trauma

LMWH is the most efficacious option for most high-risk trauma patients. Current contraindications to early LMWH prophylaxis include intracranial bleeding, incomplete spinal cord injury associated with perispinal hematoma,

ongoing, uncontrolled bleeding, and uncorrected coagulopathy. Lacerations or contusions of the lungs, liver, spleen or kidneys, or the presence of retroperitoneal hematoma associated with pelvic fractures do not by themselves contraindicate the use of LMWH prophylaxis, as long as there is no active bleeding. Mechanical modalities such as elastic stockings and intermittent pneumatic compression can be used in the presence of LMWH contraindications.

12.9.5 Acute spinal cord injury

The highest risk of DVT in hospitalized patients is for patients with acute spinal cord injuries. PE remains the third most common cause of death in this population. LMWH is recommended for prophylaxis; low-dose unfractionated heparin, elastic stockings, and intermittent pneumatic compression are relatively ineffective when used alone.

12.9.6 Non-surgical patients

Although there are a limited number of trials addressing prophylaxis for the non-surgical population, medical patients with risk factors for DVT (cancer, bed rest, heart failure, severe lung disease) should receive LMWH or low-dose unfractionated heparin. For patients with ischemic stroke, LMWH or low-dose unfractionated heparin is recommended.

References

1. **Anderson, F.A., Wheeler, H.B. Goldberg, R.J., *et al*.** (1991) A population-based perspective of the hospital incidence and case-fatality rates of deep vein thrombosis and pulmonary embolism: The Worcester DVT study. *Arch. Intern. Med.* **151:** 933–938.
2. **Dalen, J.E. and Alpert, J.S.** (1975) Natural history of pulmonary embolism. *Prog. Cardiovasc. Dis.* **17:** 259–270.
3. **Tapson, V.F. and Witty, L.A.** (1995) Massive pulmonary embolism. Diagnostic and therapeutic strategies. *Clin. Chest Med.* **16:** 329–340.
4. **Goldhaber, S.Z.** (1998) Pulmonary thromboembolism. *N. Engl. J. Med.* **339:** 93–104.
5. **Gallus, A.S., Salzman, E.W. and Hirsh, J.** (1994) Prevention of VTE. In: *Hemostasis and Thrombosis: Basic Principles and Clinical Practice*, 3rd Edn

(eds R.W. Colman, J. Hirsh, V.J. Marder, *et al.*). J.B. Lippincott, Philadelphia, PA, pp. 1331–1345.

6. **Geerts, W.H., Code, K.I., Jay, R.M., et al.** (1994) A prospective study of venous thromboembolism after major trauma. *N. Engl. J. Med.* **331**: 1601–1604.

7. **Coon, W.W.** (1976) Risk factors in pulmonary embolism. *Surg. Gynecol. Obstet.* **143**: 385–390.

8. **Ridker, P.M., Miletich, J.P., Stampfer, M.J., et al.** (1995) Factor V Leiden and risks of recurrent idiopathic venous thromboembolism. *Circulation* **92**: 2800–2802.

9. **Ridker, P.M., Hennekens, C.H., Selhub, J., et al.** (1997) Interrelation of hyperhomocyst(e)-emia, factor V Leiden, and risk of future venous thromboembolism. *Circulation* **95**: 1777–1782.

10. **Nicolaides, A.N. and Irving, D.** (1975) Clinical factors and the risk of deep venous thrombosis. In: *Thromboembolism Etiology. Advances in Prevention and Management* (ed. A.N. Nicolaides). University Park Press, Baltimore, MD, pp. 193–204.

11. **Rahr, H.B. and Sorenson, J.V.** (1992) Venous thromboembolism and cancer. *Blood Coagul. Fibrinolysis* **3**: 451–460.

12. **Devor, M., Barrett-Connor, E., Renvall, M., et al.** (1992) Estrogen replacement therapy and the risk of venous thrombosis. *Am. J. Med.* **92**: 275–282.

13. **Gibbs, N.M.** (1957) Venous thrombosis of the lower limbs with particular reference to bedrest. *Br. J. Surg.* **45**: 209–236.

14. **Ferrari, E., Chevallier, T., Chapelier, A. and Baudouy, M.** (1999) Travel as a risk factor for venous thromboembolic disease: A case-controlled study. *Chest* **115**: 440–444.

15. **Tapson, V.F., Carroll, B.A., Davidson, B.L., et al.** (1999) The diagnostic approach to acute venous thromboembolism. Clinical practice guideline. American Thoracic Society. *Am. J. Respir. Crit. Care Med.* **160**: 1043–1066.

16. **Tapson, V.F. and Fulkerson, W.J.** (1994) Pulmonary embolism in the intensive care unit. *J. Intensive Care Med.* **9**: 119–131.

17. **Van Beek, E.J., Schenk, B.E., Michel, B.C., et al.** (1996) The role of plasma D-dimers concentration in the exclusion of pulmonary embolism. *Br. J. Haematol.* **92**: 725–732.

18. **Kline, J.A., Meek, S., Boudrow, D., et al.** (1997) Use of the alveolar dead space fraction (V_D/V_T) and plasma D-dimers to exclude acute pulmonary embolism in ambulatory patients. *Acad. Emerg. Med.* **4**: 856–863.

19. **PIOPED Investigators** (1990) Value of the ventilation/perfusion scan in acute pulmonary embolism. Results of the prospective investigation of pulmonary embolism diagnosis (PIOPED). *JAMA* **263**: 2753–2759.

20. **Stein, P.D., Athanasoulis, C., Alavi, A., et al.** (1992) Complications and validity of pulmonary angiography in acute pulmonary embolism. *Circulation* **85**: 462–468.

21. **Rathbun, S.W., Raskob, G.E. and Whitsett, T.L.** (2000) Sensitivity and specificity of helical computed tomography in the diagnosis of pulmonary embolism: a systematic review. *Ann. Intern. Med.* **132**: 227–232.

22. **Lensing, A.W., Prandoni, P., Brandjes, D., et al.** (1989) Detection of deep-vein thrombosis by real-time B-mode ultrasonography. *N. Engl. J. Med.* **320**: 342–345.

23. **Meaney, J.F., Weg, J.G., Chenevert, T.L., et al.** (1997) Diagnosis of pulmonary embolism with magnetic resonance angiography. *N. Engl. J. Med.* **336**: 1422–1427.

24. **Raschke, R.A., Reilly, B.M., Guidry, J.R., et al.** (1993) The weight-based heparin dosing nomogram compared with a 'standard care' nomogram. A randomized, controlled trial. *Ann. Intern. Med.* **119**: 874–881.

25. **Goldhaber, S.Z.** (1999) Treatment of pulmonary thromboembolism. *Intern. Med.* **38**: 620–625.

26. **Spandorfer, J., Lynch, S., Weitz, H., et al.** (1999) Use of enoxaparin for the chronically anticoagulated patient before and after procedures. *Am. J. Cardiol.* **84**: 478–480.

27. **Hyers, T.M., Agnelli, G., Hull, R.D., et al.** (1998) Antithrombotic therapy for venous thromboembolic disease. *Chest* **114**(Suppl.): 561S–578S.

28. **Dalen, J.E., Alpert, J.S. and Hirsch, J.** (1997) Thrombolytic therapy for pulmonary embolism: Is it safe? When is it indicated? *Arch. Intern. Med.* **157**: 2550–2556.

29. **Dalen, J.E. and Hirsch, J. (eds)** (1998) Fifth ACCP Consensus Conference on Antithrombotic Therapy. *Chest* **114**(Suppl.); 439S–769S.

30. **Koning, R., Cribier, A., Gerber, L., et al.** (1997) A new treatment for severe pulmonary embolism: percutaneous rheolytic thrombectomy. *Circulation* **96**: 2498–2500.

31. **Goldhaber, S.Z., Kessler, C.M., Heit, J., et al.** (1992) Recombinant tissue-type plasminogen activator versus a novel dosing regimen of urokinase in acute pulmonary embolism: a randomized, controlled, multicenter trial. *J. Am. Coll. Cardiol.* **20**: 24–30.

32. **Metz, D., Chapoutot, L., Ouzaan, J., et al.** (1991) Doppler echocardiographic assessment of the severity of acute pulmonary embolism: A correlative angiographic study in forty-eight adult patients. *Am. J. Noninvasive Cardiol.* **5**: 223–228.

33. **Ritto, D., Sutherland, G.R., Samuel, L., et al.** (1993) Role of transesophageal echocardiography in diagnosis and management of central pulmonary artery thromboembolism. *Am. J. Cardiol.* **71:** 1115–1118.

34. **Layish, D.T. and Tapson, V.F.** (1997) Pharmacologic hemodynamic support in massive pulmonary embolism. *Chest* **111:** 218–224.

35. **Kearon, C. and Hirsh, J.** (1997) Management of anticoagulation before and after elective surgery. *N. Engl. J. Med.* **336:** 1506–1511.

36. **Horlocker, T. and Heit, J.** (1997) Low molecular weight heparin: biochemistry, pharmacology, perioperative prophylaxis regimens, and guidelines for regional anesthetic management. *Anesth. Analg.* **85:** 874–885.

Chapter 13

Modes of mechanical ventilation

Robert M. Kacmarek, PhD, RRT

Contents

13.1 Introduction

The available modes on mechanical ventilators have markedly expanded over the last 20 years. Before 1980 ICU ventilators provided only volume-targeted modes. Today's newest mechanical ventilators not only incorporate modes that are volume targeted but also provide modes that are pressure targeted as well as a new group of modes most of which are considered combined pressure- and volume-targeted modes. Because with all of these modes feedback regarding the actual ventilatory pattern, they result in automatic adjustment of the way gas is delivered, these modes may more precisely be called closed-loop, computer-controlled modes of ventilation. This

chapter will address global differences between pressure- and volume-targeted modes, all of the standard modes of ventilation and the newest computer-controlled modes of ventilation. Where possible, indications for each mode will be highlighted; however, with many modes few or no data are available to guide the choice of mode.

13.2 Volume versus pressure targeting

With all new generation ICU ventilators the clinician must decide not only on a specific mode but also whether gas delivery is to be pressure or volume targeted[1]. In volume-targeted modes, tidal volume is constant,

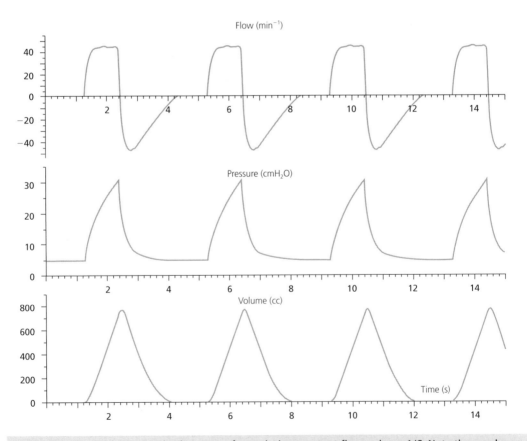

Figure 13.1 Flow, pressure, and volume waveforms during constant flow, volume A/C. Note the nearly square flow waveform, representing a constant flow until the preset volume is delivered.

whereas in pressure-targeted modes, maximum peak alveolar pressure is constant. Volume-targeted modes use a simple, constant flow, whereas pressure-targeted modes require computer-controlled variable flow generators.

13.2.1 Volume ventilation

Figure 13.1 depicts the pressure, flow, and volume waveforms during constant flow, volume ventilation. With the start of each breath, airway pressure increases from baseline in essentially a linear manner, as gas flow is constant. Volume is delivered in a similar linear manner and the total tidal volume is not delivered until the moment inspiration ends. With this approach, V_T, flow rate, and inspiratory time as well as I:E ratio can be adjusted over a wide range. What stays constant is V_T. Peak airway and peak alveolar pressure can vary considerably from breath to breath as impedance to ventilation or ventilatory drive changes. In volume ventilation some ventilators allow a decelerating ('reverse ramp' waveform) flow to be selected (*Figure 13.2*). With a decelerating flow, flow linearly decelerates from a peak level to the terminal level. Many ventilators end the breath when the flow is at a low predetermined level. When changing the inspiratory flow waveform from square to decelerating it is important to consider how a particular model of ventilator responses to the change. Ventilators can either maintain peak flow, and allow the decelerating flow to increase inspiratory time (all else constant), or the ventilator can maintain inspiratory time constant, causing peak flow to increase[2]. During volume ventilation inspiratory time and peak flow are related as follows:

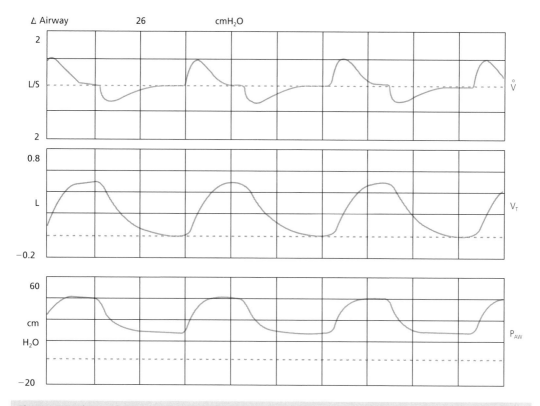

Figure 13.2 Flow, volume, and pressure waveforms during decelerating flow, volume A/C with an end-inspiratory pause. The decelerating (reverse ramp) flow waveform allows a more constant inspiratory pressure waveform.

$$\dot{V}_{pk} = \frac{V_T - (0.5)(\dot{V}_f)(T_I)}{(0.5)(T_I)} \qquad (1)$$

where $\dot{V}_{pk}$ is peak flow, T_I is inspiratory time, and $_f$ is end-inspiratory flow[2].

As discussed in Chapter 1, peak pressure in constant flow, volume ventilation reflects the combined effects of compliance and resistance. In the passively ventilated patient peak alveolar pressure can be determined by setting an inflation hold of 0.5 s or less.

Critical alarms and monitors during volume ventilation differ from those in pressure ventilation. With volume ventilation peak airway pressure is the most critical variable to monitor, whereas with pressure ventilation tidal volume is the most critical monitored variable[2]. The importance of this different approach to monitoring is illustrated during the expansion of a

tension pneumothorax. With volume ventilation, peak pressure increases with every breath, causing the high-pressure alarm to sound and continue to sound with each breath. During pressure ventilation, the airway pressure does not vary but V_T decreases with each breath. The low-V_T alarm begins to sound and continue with each breath. The maximum pressure of the tension pneumothorax is also limited in pressure ventilation to the set ventilatory pressure.

13.2.2 Pressure ventilation

Figure 13.3 depicts the airway pressure, flow, and volume waveforms during pressure ventilation. As noted, these differ considerably from those seen with conventional volume ventilation (*Figure 13.1*). The primary reason for this difference is the pressure target. The ventilator delivers high flow to rapidly drive airway pres-

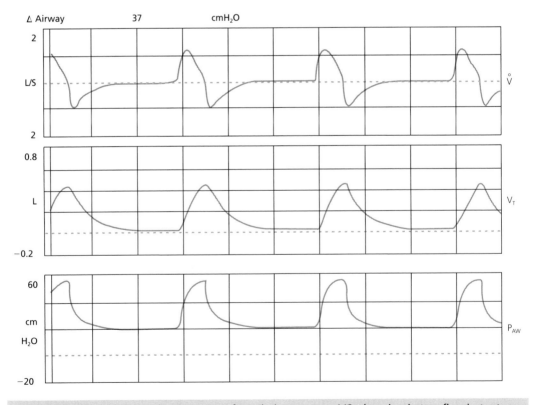

Figure 13.3 Flow, volume, and pressure waveform during pressure A/C where inspiratory flow just returns to zero before the end of inspiration.

sure to the target level. However, once the target is reached flow must decrease to avoid pressure exceeding the target. As a result, flow may decrease in a linear or in an exponential manner. Generally, the greater the impedance to ventilation the more likely flow will decelerate in an exponential manner[3]. As inspiratory time is set in pressure assist/control ventilation, with very stiff lungs or chest wall, flow can decrease to zero before the end of the inspiratory phase, resulting in a plateau appearance of the volume wave (*Figure 13.4*).

Figures 13.3 and *13.4* depict the key characteristics of pressure ventilation. Because flow decreases as inspiratory time progresses, the majority of the tidal volume is delivered early in the inspiratory phase. If flow decreases to zero before the end of inspiration, peak airway pressure is equal to peak alveolar pressure[2]. In addition, with pressure ventilation delivered flow varies with patient demand; thus, as demand increases, flow increases. This is contrary to what happens in volume ventilation, where peak flow and waveform are constant regardless of patient demand.

As demonstrated in *Figures 13.3* and *13.4*, tidal volume during pressure control is affected by inspiratory time[3]. In patients breathing spontaneously, inspiratory time is set to equal the patient's spontaneous inspiratory time. However, during controlled ventilation in ARDS patients, inspiratory time should be set to ensure that flow decreases to zero followed by a short 0.1–0.3 s inspiratory pause. Allowing flow to return to zero ensures that V_T is maximized at the specific pressure setting. *Figure 13.5* demonstrates that increasing inspiratory time increases V_T to a maximum but

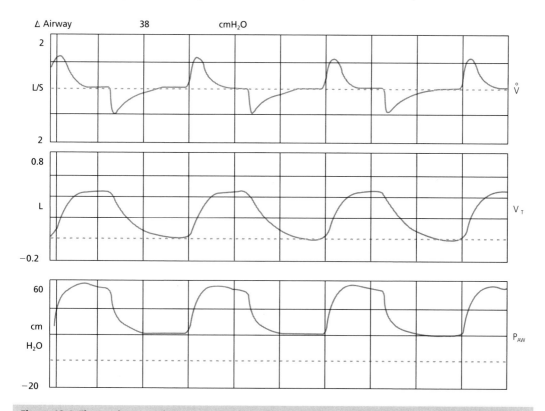

Figure 13.4 Flow, volume, and pressure waveform during pressure A/C ventilation when inspiratory flow returns to zero with an end-inspiratory pause caused by the lengthy inspiratory time. This is the same patient as in *Figure 13.3* but with inspiratory time lengthened.

further increases past a short plateau result in a decreased tidal volume[3]. The actual V_T, and inspiratory time ensuring maximum V_T, is dependent upon compliance, resistance and auto-PEEP. The greater the airway resistance or auto-PEEP and the lower the compliance, the lower the V_T at a set pressure level and inspiratory time. Whenever adjustments are made to the pressure control setting and V_T decreases, auto-PEEP should be considered. As the ventilator does not measure auto-PEEP with each breath it cannot compensate for the level of auto-PEEP[3]. In volume ventilation auto-PEEP increases peak airway and peak alveolar pressure. However, with pressure ventilation, as maximum pressure is targeted, auto-PEEP results in a decreased V_T^2. Airway pressure goes from the set baseline to the auto-PEEP level without any gas delivery. Essentially, auto-PEEP decreases the pressure control level by the auto-PEEP level, thus decreasing driving pressure and V_T.

Few data are available to distinguish the use of pressure and volume ventilation during control ventilation. The decision to use one is based on the clinician's desire to primarily maintain peak alveolar pressure or V_T constant. However, it is possible to maintain peak alveolar pressure constant with volume ventilation or tidal volume constant with pressure ventilation but considerable monitoring and adjustment is required. In ARDS where current data indicate that a 6 ml kg^{-1} V_T should be targeted, either approach can be used[4]. If volume ventilation is used, a decelerating flow pattern does result in better distribution of ventilation[5]. Pressure ventilation, with its variable flow delivery, better meets the changing demand of spontaneously breathing patients than volume ventilation[6,7]. Pressure ventilation is always preferable in the spontaneously breathing patient, especially if demand is rapidly changing. *Table 13.1* compares pressure and volume ventilation.

13.3 Traditional modes of ventilation

Modes of ventilation have traditionally been classified based on the level of patient interaction with the mechanical ventilator: control, assist/control (A/C), and assist ventilation[8]. Synchronized intermittent mandatory ventilation (SIMV), developed in the 1970s, is also considered a traditional ventilatory mode. All

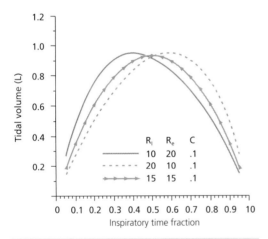

Figure 13.5 Relationship of inspiratory time fraction to tidal volume (pressure target = 20 cmH$_2$O). When inspiratory (R_I) and expiratory (R_E) resistance are equal, optimal duration (D) = 0.5. When $R_I > R_E$, more inspiratory time is required, and optimal D > 0.5. Conversely, when $R_E > R_I$, optimal D < 0.5. From: Marini, J.J., Crooke, P.S. and Truitt, J.P. (1989) Determinants and limits of pressure-preset ventilation: a mathematical model of pressure control. Reproduced with permission from the American Physiological Society. *J. Appl. Physiol.* 67: 1081–1092.

Table 13.1 Pressure vs. volume assist/control ventilation

	Pressure	Volume
Tidal volume	Variable	Constant
Peak alveolar pressure	Constant	Variable
Peak inspiratory pressure	Constant	Variable
Minimum rate	Preset	Preset
Inspiratory time	Preset	Preset
Peak flow	Variable	Constant
Flow pattern	Variable	Constant

of these modes on the newest generation of mechanical ventilators can be set for pressure or volume ventilation.

13.3.1 Control

The control mode implies that the patient does not participate in the process of gas delivery. Today, full support is accomplished by providing appropriate sedation; however, with some older ventilators the control mode prevented the ventilator from responding to the patient's demand. On today's ventilators control has been replaced by assist/control[1].

13.3.2 Assist/control

With assist/control the patient has the opportunity to trigger the mechanical breath. However, if the rate at which the patient triggers the ventilator falls below the set backup rate, a control breath is delivered[8]. When the patient resumes inspiratory effort, he or she can again trigger the ventilator. Pressure control on the newer ventilators is an assist/control mode (PA/C); the patient can trigger each breath as in volume assist/control. As pressure control was introduced in conjunction with inverse ratio ventilation[9,10] many have considered this mode only when inverse ratio was used. More recently, pressure control has been used on all types of patients including those intubated[11] and those receiving noninvasive positive pressure ventilation[12].

With both control and assist/control V_T or pressure level, and flow waveform and flow rate or inspiratory time must be set. In addition, the sensitivity must be set appropriately to allow patient triggering without having to generate excess negative inspiratory pressures.

13.3.3 Assist

True assist ventilation implies that no backup rate is available. Volume-assisted ventilation is not available on any currently manufactured ventilators. Pressure-assisted ventilation is generally termed pressure support (PS). Although most ventilators do not provide a backup rate during pressure support, apnea beyond a set time period converts pressure support to a backup ventilation mode, either pressure or volume targeted[1]. Pressure support is the mode of ventilation that coordinates best with patient demand. Patients control not only initiation of inspiration but also termination of the breath.

With pressure support a breath is terminated by one of three mechanisms: (i) patient inspiratory flow decelerates to a minimal level; (ii) system pressure exceeds set pressure; (iii) a specific time interval is exceeded. The terminal inspiratory flow cycling criterion is either a fixed flow (i.e. 5 l min^{-1}) or a percentage of peak flow (i.e. 25% or 5%)[8]. Peak system pressure, after the first 200–400 ms of inspiration, exceeding the set level by about 2–20 cmH$_2$O (depending on the manufacturer) also causes the breath to cycle to exhalation. With most manufacturers an inspiratory time exceeding 2–3 s results in termination of an assisted breath.

13.3.4 Inspiratory cycling criteria

As illustrated in *Figure 13.6*, problems with pressure support and patient synchrony can occur at the onset and termination of inspiration[13]. Initial flow can be either excessive or inadequate and the criteria to terminate inspiration can be too low or too high a flow. Inspiratory cycling criteria are a potential problem in COPD patients[14,15]. Many COPD patients choose to end inspiration when their peak inspiratory flow is high (*Figure 13.7*). If the flow is higher than the ventilator's cycling criteria, the patient must force airway pressure above the set level by activating accessory muscles of exhalation[15]. If this occurs, patient ventilatory drive is increased and dyssynchrony is common. Some new generation ventilators (Puritan Bennett 840 and Hamilton Galileo) allow for adjustment of the inspiratory termination criteria[1]. However, if the patient's end-inspiratory flow changes the adjustment may again be inadequate. Future generations of ventilators may automatically adjust cycling criteria as the patient's end-inspiratory flow changes. This ongoing adjustment is currently being performed on some of

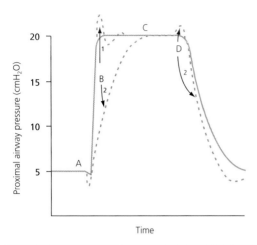

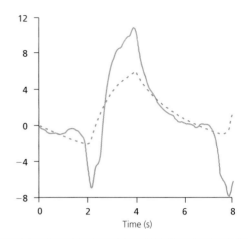

Figure 13.6 Design characteristics of a pressure-supported breath. In this example, baseline pressure (i.e. PEEP) is set at 5 cmH$_2$O and pressure support is set at 15 cmH$_2$O (PIP 20 cmH$_2$O). The inspiratory pressure is triggered at point A by a patient effort resulting in an airway pressure decrease. Demand valve sensitivity and responsiveness are characterized by the depth and duration of this negative pressure. The rise to pressure (line B) is provided by a fixed high initial flow delivery into the airway. Note that if flows exceed patient demand, initial pressure exceeds set level (B, 1), whereas if flows are less than patient demand, a very slow (concave) rise to pressure can occur (B, 2). The plateau of pressure support (line C) is maintained by servo control of flow. A smooth plateau reflects appropriate responsiveness to patient demand; fluctuations would reflect less responsiveness of the servo mechanisms. Termination of pressure support occurs at point D and should coincide with the end of the spontaneous inspiratory effort. If termination is delayed, the patient actively exhales (bump in pressure above plateau) (D, 1); if termination is premature, the patient will have continued inspiratory efforts (D, 2). From: MacIntyre, N., Nishimura, M., Usuada, Y., *et al.* (1990) The Nagoya conference on system design and patient–ventilator interactions during pressure support ventilation. Reproduced with permission from *Chest* 97: 1463–1467.

Figure 13.7 Esophageal pressure (Pes, continuous line) and estimated recoil pressure of the chest wall (Pes$_{CW}$, dashed line) tracings in a patient receiving pressure support ventilation of 20 cmH$_2$O. Pressure tracings have been superimposed so that Pes$_{CW}$ is equal to Pes at the onset of the rapid fall in Pes during late expiration. Times at which the Pes tracing is higher than Pes$_{CW}$ represent lower bound expiratory effort. Note the presence of expiratory muscle activation during late inspiration. From: Jubran, A., van de Graff, W. and Tobin, M.J. (1995) Variability of patient–ventilator interaction with pressure support ventilation in patients with chronic obstructive pulmonary disease. Reproduced with permission from *Am. J. Respir. Crit. Care Med.* **152**: 129–136.

the bilevel pressure ventilators used for non-invasive ventilation. If end-inspiratory pressure exceeds set inspiratory pressure target, the set cycling flow criteria are too low. Inspiratory

termination criteria should be slowly increased until a smooth transition to exhalation occurs.

The other option during end-inspiratory dys-synchrony is to change modes from pressure support to pressure assist/control. As noted from *Table 13.2*, the only difference between pressure support and pressure assist/control is the mechanism used to terminate inspiration, (flow (PS) vs time (PA/C)), otherwise gas delivery is identical[16]. Thus, PA/C set at the same pressure level with inspiratory time set to equal the patient's desired inspiratory time (≤1.0 5) results in better patient comfort and synchrony than PS when the cycling criteria in PS do not match the patient's end-inspiratory flow.

Table 13.2 Pressure A/C vs. PS

	Pressure assist/control	Pressure support
Target	Pressure	Pressure
Inspiratory time	Set	Patient determined
Rise time	Variable	Variable
End inspiration	Set	Variable
Peak flow	Variable	Variable
Rate	Patient determined	Patient determined
Back-up rate	Set	Apnea ventilation

13.3.5 Rise time

The speed with which flow increases driving pressure from baseline to set level during PS or PA/C may not meet patient demand[13]. Many patients in severe respiratory distress demand a rapid rise in pressure to peak levels, whereas other patients not markedly stressed prefer a more gradual rise in pressure[17]. Rise time allows variability in slope of the flow delivery curve. Rise time adjustment is available during both PS and PA/C on most new generation mechanical ventilators. That is, the clinician can match the flow delivery slope to the patient's demand[17–19]. However, as with cycling criteria, rise time setting may need to be changed as patient demand changes[19]. Again, it can be expected that on future generations of ICU ventilators adjustment of rise time will be automated. Proper setting results in a linear increase in the airway pressure curve with pressure not exceeding set level at the onset of inspiration or the pressure curve being concave. Pressure overshoot indicates rise time is too rapid, whereas a concave pressure curve indicates rise time is too slow.

13.3.6 Synchronized intermittent mandatory ventilation (SIMV)

As illustrated in *Figure 13.8*, SIMV is a combination of mechanical breaths and spontaneous unassisted breathing. The mechanical ventilation rate is set, with a window of time based on set rate during which patients can trigger a mechanical breath. If the breath is not triggered during the time window a control breath is delivered. Between time windows, the patient can breath spontaneously without a mechanical breath. As with the other traditional modes, the mandatory breath can be either pressure or volume targeted.

Much concern has been raised regarding patient effort and synchrony during low-rate SIMV[20–22]. Because the respiratory center essentially is programmed by the current breath, patient effort with low rate SIMV (≤ 6 min^{-1}) is no different during the mechanical breaths and spontaneous unassisted breaths[20,21] and patient effort during the mechanical breath increases with decreasing SIMV rate (*Figure 13.9*)[20,21]. It is impossible to distinguish mandatory from spontaneous breaths when observing the diaphragmatic electromyograph (EMG) and esophageal pressure tracings[22]. Leung *et al.* demonstrated that adding pressure support to the spontaneous breaths can markedly modify workloads (*Figure 13.10*)[21]. However, the rationale of adding PS must be questioned, for it would appear that a more appropriate application of ventilatory support would be the use of assist/control or pressure support without SIMV. In general, patient effort during SIMV is equivalent to assist/control or pressure support if the mandatory rate accounts for 80% or more of the patient's minute volume[20].

13.4 Pressure control inverse ratio ventilation (PCIRV)

The use of the pressure assist/control mode in the late 1980s developed in association with

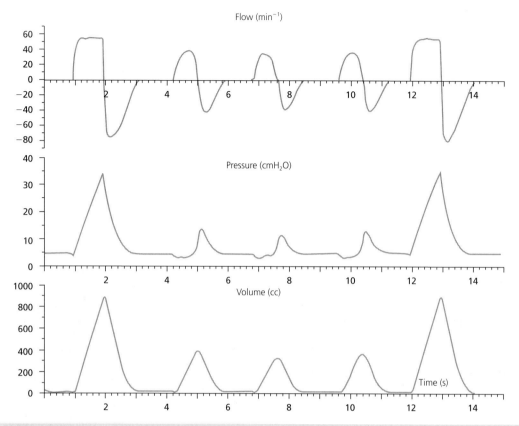

Figure 13.8 Flow, pressure, and volume waveforms during volume-targeted SIMV without pressure support.

PCIRV[9,10]. With PCIRV (*Figure 13.11*) inspiration is lengthened until it exceeds expiration, in some applications establishing an I:E ratio up to 4:1. The goal with PCIRV is to maintain a lengthy inspiratory phase to open collapsed lung and a short expiratory phase to avoid collapse of opened lung. In doing so, high levels of auto-PEEP are established. Proponents of PCIRV argue that high mean airway pressures can be maintained without high peak alveolar pressures[23]. The opponents of PCIRV argue that the auto-PEEP created is maldistributed to units least in need of PEEP and that the high mean airway pressures compromise hemodynamics[24,25]. A number of controlled comparison of PCIRV with normal I:E ratio ventilation in both animal models[25] and humans[26–28] indicate no

benefit from PCIRV in relation to oxygenation but a marginal (about 5%) improvement in PCO_2.

When PCIRV is used progression to an inverse ratio should be gradual. Once the patient is stable in PA/C, assure that the patient is not spontaneously breathing. Fighting the long inspiratory times results in marked hemodynamic compromise and deteriorating gas exchange. Then slowly increase inspiratory time until the oxygenation target is achieved. Generally, increases in inspiratory time of 0.1–0.25 s can be made without hemodynamic compromise; however, a positive fluid balance is commonly needed if the I:E ratio exceeds 1.5:1 or 2:1. In general, the same targeted oxygenation status can be achieved with conven-

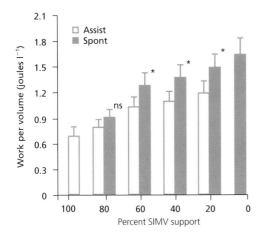

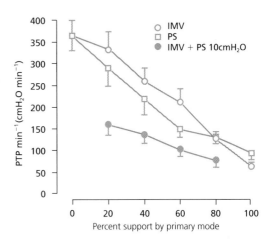

Figure 13.9 Inspiratory work per unit volume (work per liter, W L⁻¹) done by the patient during assisted cycles (open bars) and spontaneous cycles (solid bars). W L⁻¹ increased monotonically with decreasing SIMV percentage for both types of breath. W L⁻¹ for spontaneous breaths tended to exceed that for machine-assisted breaths. Asterisk indicates P < 0.01; ns, not significant. From: Marini, J.J., Smith, T.C. and Lamb, V.J. (1988) External work output and force generation during synchronized intermittent mechanical ventilation. Effect of machine assistance on breathing effort. Reproduced with permission from *Am. Rev. Respir. Dis.* **138**: 1169–1178.

Figure 13.10 Cumulative pressure–time product of both triggering and nontriggering efforts (PTP min⁻¹) increased as the level of pressure support (PS) alone was decreased, as intermittent mandatory ventilation (IMV) alone was decreased, and as IMV was decreased in the presence of PS 10 cmH₂O (P < 0.0005 in each instance). At proportional levels of ventilator assistance, PTP min⁻¹ was not different during IMV alone and PS alone, but both were higher than that of combined IMV and PS 10 cmH₂O. From: Leung, P., Jubran, A. and Tobin, M.J. (1997) Comparison of assisted ventilator modes on triggering, patient effort, and dyspnea. Reproduced with permission from *Am. J. Respir. Crit. Care Med.* **155**: 1940–1947.)

tional I:E ratios (Chapter 15) and appropriately applied PEEP without the problems inherent in lengthy inspiratory times.

13.5 Airway pressure release ventilation (APRV)

APRV is very similar conceptually to PCIRV but differs in respect to the patient's ability to breath spontaneously[8]. As noted in *Figure 13.12*, with APRV two levels of continuous positive airway pressure (CPAP) are set, establishing an inverse I:E ratio as in PCIRV, but as the two airway pressure levels are established by setting alternating levels of CPAP, the patient can breath spontaneously at each CPAP level. In the mechanical ventilators that offer

APRV, the inspiratory (high CPAP) level is set independent of the expiratory (low CPAP) level and the exhalation valve is active throughout the inspiratory and expiratory phases, allowing spontaneous breathing regardless of CPAP level[1]. In some ventilators pressure support can be added to all spontaneous breaths[1].

As with PCIRV, the use of APRV is highly controversial, with limited data in patients with ARDS or acute lung injury indicating a benefit to APRV versus conventional ventilation[29,30]. However, because patients are allowed to breath spontaneously throughout the ventilatory cycles, much less sedation is required during APRV than during conventional mechanical ventilation[30].

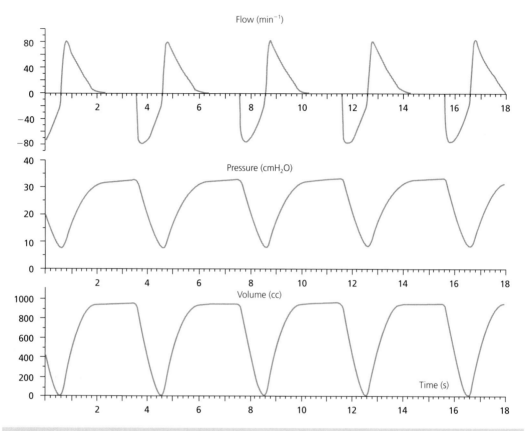

Figure 13.11 Flow, pressure, and volume waveforms during pressure control inverse ratio ventilation (I:E 3:1).

13.6 Combined modes of ventilation

A number of ventilator manufacturers have attempted to develop modes of ventilation that include the beneficial aspects of both pressure and volume ventilation[31], that is, they target both a maximum peak alveolar pressure (allow for variable flow delivery based on patient demand) and a tidal volume. Many of these modes can be considered extensions of the mandatory minute ventilation (MMV) concept of ventilation initially described by Hewlett *et al.* in 1977[32]. During MMV the ventilator insures that minute volume remains at or above a set target. If the patient can maintain minute volume spontaneously no mechanical breaths are applied. However, if

the patient becomes apneic then controlled ventilation at preset levels is applied. Patients can also share the level of ventilation with the ventilator anywhere between these two extremes. The intent is to allow the patient to wean themselves by applying the least amount of ventilatory support required to maintain the target minute volume. Unfortunately, this approach does not work clinically. Patients can assume an inappropriate ventilatory pattern (rapid and shallow), exceeding the target, or simply establish a level of comfort with the provided ventilatory support and not continue to assume a greater percentage of total support.

As listed in *Table 13.3*, these new modes of ventilatory support can be listed as modes that adjust breath delivery within a given breath or adjust breath delivery on the subsequent

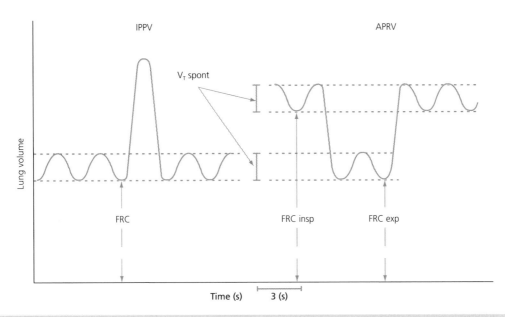

Figure 13.12 Theoretic spirometric tracing depicting change in lung volume that would occur in a patient with SIMV compared with the change that would occur with APRV. Inspiratory lung volume is the lung volume during spontaneous inspiration with CPAP during APRV. Expiratory lung volume is the lung volume during release of Paw during APRV (i.e. lung volume after mechanical expiration). Expiratory lung volume is similar to FRC during APRV. FRC is the passive expiratory lung volume during APRV and is greater than FRC during Intermittent positive pressure ventilation (IPPV). (Used with permission, from Stock, M.C., Downs, J.B. and Frolicher, D.A. (1987) Airway pressure release ventilation. *Crit. Care Med.* **15**: 462–466.)

Table 13.3 Computer controlled modes of ventilation

Within-breath adjustment	Between-breath adjustment
Automatic tube compensation	Volume support
Volume-assured pressure support	Pressure-regulated volume control
	Auto-mode
	Adaptive support ventilation

breath. It should be noted that few data are currently available to support the use of any of these modes of ventilation. As a result, their benefits and risks can be discussed only theoretically. Forms of these modes are currently available on many of the newest generation of mechanical ventilators.

13.6.1 Volume support (VS)

This mode of ventilation can best be described as volume-targeted pressure support[31]. Target V_T and maximum pressure support level are set. The ventilator automatically adjusts the pressure support level up to the maximum pressure setting to insure that the volume target is meet. As noted in *Figure 13.13*, this is accomplished on the Seimens Servo 300 by providing test breaths at 10 cmH$_2$O pressure support, then calculating the pressure support level required to achieve the targeted V_T. Following this, the ventilator delivers three test breaths at 75% of the calculated pressure support level. On subsequent breaths, the ventilator adjusts the pressure support level a maximum of 3 cmH$_2$O per breath to achieve and maintain the targeted tidal volume.

Volume support is intended to insure a specific tidal volume is delivered during changing impedance to ventilation and ventilatory drive,

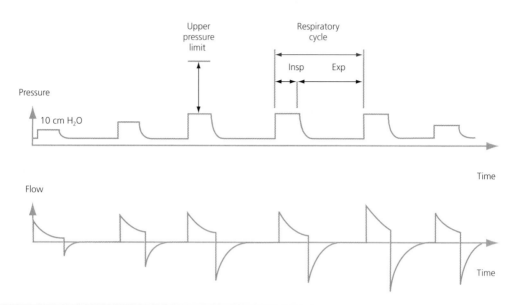

Figure 13.13 Pressure and flow waveforms illustrating volume support mode. See text for details.

or system leaks. This mode does accomplish this task. In small children and neonates with uncuffed endotracheal tubes and variable leak, volume support is able to maintain a constant tidal volume[33]. However, changes in patient demand for ventilation based on developing sepsis, fever, hypoxemia, pain or anxiety may result in diminished levels of pressure support[31,34]. If, because of heightened ventilatory demand, V_T increases at a given pressure support level, the ventilator decreases provided pressure support. As a result, in settings where patients may need more support, VS may provide less[34]. At this time, there are no published papers establishing the benefits of VS. However, it may end up being most clinically indicated in children with uncuffed endotracheal tubes and varying leaks.

13.6.2 Pressure-regulated volume control (PRVC)

PRVC is similar to VS except it is pressure A/C with a volume target[28]. A maximum pressure level and target V_T are set. In addition, a respiratory rate and inspiratory time are set. As with VS, a 10 cmH$_2$O test breath is delivered then pressure control level is adjusted to 75% of max-

imum required. On subsequent breaths, pressure control level is adjusted by up to 3 cmH$_2$O. This mode may be the ideal mode for a lung protective ventilatory strategy in ARDS, as it targets both V_T and peak alveolar pressure. However, as with volume support, there are no data whatsoever to evaluate its effectiveness and to define indications for its use.

13.6.3 Auto-mode

This is a recently introduced mode of ventilatory support on the Seimens Servo 300 ventilator. The mode functions by converting from a controlled mode of ventilatory support to an assisted mode based on the patient's spontaneous breathing capabilities[31]. If the patient triggers the ventilator on two consecutive breaths the ventilator shifts to an assist mode and when the patient fails to trigger a breath for a specified time period the ventilator shifts to a control mode. The Servo 300 can be set in adult, pediatric, and neonatal operating ranges. In the adult range, 12 s of apnea results in a shift to the control mode, whereas 8 s in the pediatric range and 5 s in the neonatal range result in a shift to the control mode. In auto-mode the Servo 300 can be set to shift

214

between 'volume control and volume support', 'pressure control and pressure support', or 'PRVC and volume support'.

It is difficult to conceptualize the benefits of auto-mode over standard modes of ventilation, as each of the 'control modes' is actually an assist/control mode. However, this mode clearly moves the operation of the ventilator further along the continuum of closed-loop controlled ventilation. Unfortunately, as with VS and PRVC, there are no data available to assist our application of this mode or to identify its indications.

13.6.4 Automatic tube compensation (ATC)

This approach to computerized control of ventilation is intended to provide sufficient pressure support during inspiration and sufficient decompression of the ventilator circuit during exhalation to maintain the tracheal pressure at the PEEP level (constant)[31]. This mode is based on the work of Guttmann et al.[35], who showed that tracheal pressure change in intubated patients could be predicted by knowledge of the size of the endotracheal tube and continual measurement of inspiratory flow. Ventilators incorporating this mode (Drager Evita 4, Puritan-Bennett 840) have programmed the resistive properties of various-sized endotracheal tubes and are able to continuously measure flow[1]. As a result, they can vary the level of pressure support applied to maintain tracheal pressure according to the following formula:

$$\text{tracheal } P = \text{proximal airway } P - (\text{tube coeff} \times \text{flow}^2) \quad (2)$$

where P is pressure and tube coeff is the resistance factor of the endotracheal tube. The proposed advantages of ATC are the elimination of the endotracheal tube as a source of imposed work of breathing, improvement in patient–ventilator synchrony, and reduction of air trapping by decompression of the ventilator circuit reducing expiratory resistance. However, the control algorithm prevents expiratory circuit pressure from falling below zero.

A number of groups have demonstrated the efficacy of ATC compared with pressure support[36,37]. ATC results in the use of lower pressure support levels in postoperative patients without COPD but higher pressure support levels in patients with COPD than those set by clinicians.

Secretions and kinks or bends in the endotracheal tube decrease the efficiency of ATC.

Whether the endotracheal tube is a clinical concern for increased work of breathing in adults is hotly debated. Early reports indicated a high imposed endotracheal tube workload[38,39]. However, more recent data suggest this is not the case. Strauss et al.[40] reported that the endotracheal tube accounts for only 10% of the total work of breathing, and Esteban et al.[41] showed no difference between spontaneous breathing trials with 7 cmH$_2$O PS versus a T-piece. However, ATC appears to be a better method of applying PS to a patient requiring ventilatory support. It eliminates the guesswork regarding the level of support required and varies the PS applied based on patient demand not on a fixed V_T target. It should be recalled that spontaneously breathing individuals vary V_T on a breath-to-breath basis based on an integration of all signals received by the respiratory center.

13.6.5 Adaptive pressure support (APS)

This is a mode of ventilation available only on the Hamilton Galileo ventilator. APS is based on the minimal work of breathing concept developed by Otis et al. in 1950[42]. Essentially, APS forces a ventilatory pattern that results in the least patient effort to overcome compliance and airways resistance[31]. As a result, it should be considered a between-breath closed-loop ventilation mode not intended to specifically wean patients but to minimize patient effort while maintaining oxygenation and acid–base balance. This process can be expressed mathematically as

$$\text{respiratory rate} = (1 + 4 \text{ B}^2 \text{ RC} \times (\dot{V}_A/\dot{V}_D) - 1)/2\text{B}^2 \text{ RC} \quad (3)$$

where RC is the respiratory time constant, B is the breathing rate, $\dot{V}_A$ alveolar ventilation, and

$\dot{V}_D$ dead space[31]. APS is set by inputting the patient's ideal body weight. Based on this, the ventilator calculates the patient ideal minute ventilation using 100 ml min^{-1} kg^{-1} for adults and 200 ml min^{-1} kg^{-1} for children. The clinician also selects the percentage of the ideal minute volume the mandatory mechanical breaths provide (20–200% of ideal minute ventilation). Between the mandatory breaths the patient can breathe spontaneously. Once activated, the first few breaths are test breaths measuring compliance, resistance and auto-PEEP using the least-squares fit technique[43]. The ventilator selects a respiratory frequency, inspiratory time, I:E ratio and pressure limit, and measures these variables on a breath-to-breath basis, altering them as required to meet the target ventilatory pattern. The ventilator adjusts inspiratory time and I:E ratio to minimize auto-PEEP, based on the ventilator's calculation of the expiratory time constant. If the patient is not spontaneously breathing the ventilator selects the respiratory rate, V_T, and pressure limit required to deliver the tidal volume, inspiratory time, and I:E ratio. As the patient begins spontaneous breathing the number of mandatory breaths decreases and the ventilator selects a PS setting that establishes a V_T sufficient to insure alveolar ventilation based on a dead space of 2.2 ml kg^{-1}[43].

A number of initial reports indicate that the APS can provide adequate ventilation in both anesthetized and spontaneously breathing patients, and matches the level of gas exchange established by clinician-set parameters[44–46]. Clearly, sufficient data exist to support APS ability to automatically select ventilatory parameters and make changes in response to patient's effects and lung mechanics. However, whether this approach will effect the length of mechanical ventilation is still unknown. It is difficult at this time to identify a clinical role for APS but conceptually it appears sound.

13.6.6 Volume-assured pressure support (VAPS)

The final mode discussed is VAPS (Bird 8400 Sti and T-Bird, Thermo Respiratory Group) or pressure augmentation (PA, Bear 1000 Thermo Respiratory Group)[31]. This mode combines a minimum V_T target with the variable inspiratory flow characteristic of pressure ventilation (*Figure 13.14*)[47]. During VAPS the clinician sets minimum V_T, square-wave flow and a pressure target or pressure support level. A VAPS breath may be either a control or a patient-triggered breath. Once triggered, the ventilator attempts to reach the target pressure as quickly as possible. When the pressure is reached the ventilator determines the volume delivered by the ventilator, compares this with the target volume and determines if the minimum volume can be reached. As noted in *Figure 13.14*, the overall configuration of the pressure and flow waveforms during VAPS can vary markedly dependent on the patient demand. If patient's demand is low, the breath is essentially a volume-targeted square-wave flow breath, except for the potential initial boost of flow to rapidly establish target pressure[31]. If the patient's demand is great, the breath becomes a pressure support breath with the potential of exceeding the target V_T if the patient demands a larger V_T. In this case, inspiration ends like any other pressure support breath. Additionally, anything between these two extremes is also possible.

Choosing the proper flow and pressure setting is critical to successful use of VAPS. If pressure is too high or the volume target is too low, all breaths tend to become PS breaths, negating the volume guarantee. On the other hand, if the set flow is too high all breaths tend to become volume breaths and inspiratory time can be prolonged.

Data from both Amato *et al.*[47] and Haas *et al.*[48] demonstrate less patient effort and better synchrony with VAPS as compared with volume ventilation. This approach to volume targeting during pressure support does not appear to have the inherent problems seen with volume support, and although not necessarily ideal does appear to be a very reasonable approach to providing pressure support with a volume guarantee.

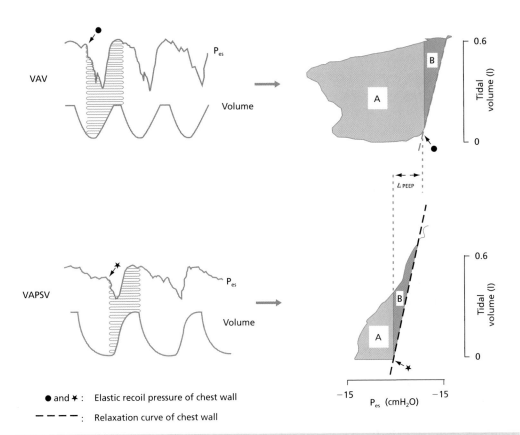

● and ✶ :   Elastic recoil pressure of chest wall

– – – – :   Relaxation curve of chest wall

Figure 13.14 Representative tracings of esophageal pressure (P_{es}) and volume during standard volume-assisted ventilation (VAV) and volume-assured pressure support ventilation (VAPSV) and the corresponding Campbell diagrams. The hatched areas represent the time interval during which the work diagram was plotted (tidal volume versus esophageal pressure, P_{es} versus V_T). Area A presents the work performed to inflate the lung, and area B is the work performed to distend the chest wall. The use of VAPSV resulted in a decreased work of breathing, an increased tidal volume, and a lower end-expiratory P_{es}, indicating less intrinsic PEEP. From: Amato, M.B.P., Barbos, C.S.V., Bonassa, J., et al. (1992) Volume assisted pressure support ventilation (VAPSV): A new approach for reducing muscle workload during acute respiratory failure. Reproduced with permission from *Chest* **102**: 1225–1234.

References

1. **Chatburn, R.L.** (1999) Mechanical ventilation. In: *Respiratory Care Equipment* (eds R.D. Branson, D.R. Hess and R.L. Chatburn). Lippincott, Williams and Wilkens, New York, pp. 395–527.
2. **Hess, D.R. and Kacmarek, R.M.** (1996) *Essentials of Mechanical Ventilation.* McGraw–Hill, New York, pp. 17–25.
3. **Marini, J.J., Crooke, P.S. and Truitt, J.P.** (1989) Determinants and limits of pressure-preset ventilation: a mathematical model of pressure control. *J. Appl. Physiol.* **67**: 1081–1092.
4. **ARDS net** (2000) Ventilation with lower tidal volumes as compared with traditional tidal volumes for acute lung injury and the acute respiratory distress syndrome. *N. Engl. J. Med.* **342**: 1301–1308.
5. **Knelson, J., Howatt, W. and DeMuth, G.** (1970) Effects of respiratory pattern on alveolar gas exchange. *J. Appl. Physiol.* **29**: 328–331.
6. **Cinnella, G., Conti, G., Lofasco, F., Lorino, H., Harf, A., Lemaire, F. and Brochard, L.** (1996) Effect of assisted ventilation on the work of breathing: Volume controlled versus pressure controlled ventilation. *Am. J. Respir. Crit. Care* **153**: 1028–1035.

7. McIntyre, N.R., McConnell, R., Cheng, K.C. and Sane, A. (1997) Patient–ventilator flow dyssynchrony: flow-limited versus pressure-limited breaths. *Crit. Care Med.* 25: 1671–1677.
8. Kacmarek, R.M. and Hess, D. (1994) Basic principles of ventilator machinery. In: *Principles and Practices of Mechanical Ventilation* (ed. M.J. Tobin). McGraw–Hill, New York, pp. 65–110.
9. Tharratt, R.S., Allen, R.P. and Albertson, T.E. (1988) Pressure controlled inverse ratio ventilation in severe adult respiratory failure. *Chest* 94: 755–762.
10. Abraham, E. and Yosihara, G. (1989) Cardiorespiratory effects of pressure controlled inverse ratio ventilation in severe respiratory failure. *Chest* 96: 1356–1359.
11. Amato, M.B.P., Barbas, C.S.V., Medeiros, D.M., *et al.* (1998) Effect of a protective-ventilation strategy on mortality in the acute respiratory distress syndrome. *N. Engl. J. Med.* 338: 347–354.
12. Calderini, E., Confalonieri, M., Puccio, P.G., Francavilla, N., Stella, L. and Gregoretti, C. (1999) Patient–ventilator asynchrony during noninvasive ventilation: the role of expiratory trigger. *Intensive Care Med.* 25: 662–667.
13. MacIntyre, N., Nishimura, M., Usuada, Y., *et al.* (1990) The Nagoya conference on system design and patient–ventilator interactions during pressure support ventilation. *Chest* 97: 1463–1467.
14. Jubran, A., van de Graff, W. and Tobin, M.J. (1995) Variability of patient–ventilator interaction with pressure support ventilation in patients with chronic obstructive pulmonary disease. *Am. J. Respir. Crit. Care Med.* 152: 129–136.
15. Parthasarathy, S., Jubran, A. and Tobin, M.J. (1998) Cycling of inspiratory and expiratory muscle groups with the ventilator in airflow limitation. *Am. J. Respir. Crit. Care Med.* 158: 1471–1478.
16. Williams, P., Muelver, M., Kratohvil, J., Ritz, R., Hess, D.R. and Kacmarek, R.M. (2000) Pressure support and pressure assist/control: are there differences? An evaluation of the newest intensive care unit ventilators. *Respir. Care* 45: 1169–1181.
17. MacIntyre, N.R. and Ho, L. (1991) Effects of initial flow rate and breath termination criteria on pressure support ventilation. *Chest* 99: 134–138.
18. Bonmarchand, G., Chevron, V., Chopin, C., *et al.* (1996) Increased initial flow rate reduces inspiratory work of breathing during pressure support ventilation in patients with exacerbation of chronic obstructive pulmonary disease. *Intensive Care Med.* 22: 1147–1151.
19. Bonmarchand, G., Chevron, V., Menard, J., *et al.* (1999) Effects of pressure ramp slope values on the work of breathing during pressure support ventilation in restrictive patients. *Crit. Care Med.* 27: 715–718.
20. Marini, J.J., Smith, T.C. and Lamb, V.J. (1988) External work output and force generation during synchronized intermittent mechanical ventilation. Effect of machine assistance on breathing effort. *Am. Rev. Respir. Dis.* 138: 1169–1178.
21. Leung, P., Jubran, A. and Tobin, M.J. (1997) Comparison of assisted ventilator modes on triggering, patient effort, and dyspnea. *Am. J. Respir. Crit. Care Med.* 155: 1940–1947.
22. Imsand, C., Feihl, F., Perret, C. and Fitting, J.W. (1994) Regulation of inspiratory neuromuscular output during synchronized intermittent mandatory ventilation. *Anesthesiology* 80: 13–22.
23. Lain, D.C., DiBenedetto, R., Morris, S.L., Van Nguyen, A., Sautlers, R. and Causey, D. (1989) Pressure control inverse ratio ventilation as a method to reduce peak inspiratory pressure and provide adequate ventilation and oxygenation. *Chest* 95: 1081–1088.
24. Kacmarek, R.M., Kirmse, M., Nishimura, M., Mang, H. and Kimball, W.R. (1995) The effects of applied versus auto-PEEP on local lung unit pressure and volume in a four-unit lung model. *Chest* 108: 1073–1079.
25. Mang, H., Kacmarek, R.M., Ritz, R., Wilson, R.S and Kimball, W.R. (1995) Cardiorespiratory effects of volume and pressure controlled ventilation at various I:E ratios in an acute lung injury mode. *Am. J. Respir. Crit. Care Med.* 151: 731–736.
26. Bandolese, R., Broseghini, C., Polese, G., Bernasconi, M., Bandi, G., Milic-Emili, J. and Rossi, A. (1993) Effects of intrinsic PEEP on pulmonary gas exchange in mechanically ventilated patients. *Eur. Respir. J.* 6: 358–363.
27. Mercat, A., Graini, L., Teboul, J.L., Lenique, F. and Richard, C. (1993) Cardiorespiratory effects of pressure controlled ventilation with and without inverse ratio in the adult respiratory distress syndrome. *Chest* 104: 871–875.
28. Lessard, M.R., Guerot, E., Lorino, H., Demaire, F. and Brochard, L. (1994) Effects of pressure-controlled with different I:E ratios versus volume-controlled ventilation on respiratory mechanics, gas exchange, and hemodynamics in patients with adult respiratory distress syndrome. *Anesthesiology* 80: 983–991.
29. Stock, M.C., Downs, J.B. and Frolicher, D.A. (1987) Airway pressure release ventilation. *Crit. Care Med.* 15: 462–466.
30. Sydow, M., Burchardi, H., Ephraim, E., *et al.* (1994) Long term effects of two different ventilatory modes on oxygenation in acute lung

injury. Comparison of airway pressure release ventilation and volume-controlled inverse ratio ventilation. *Am. J. Respir. Crit. Care Med.* **149:** 1550–1556.

31. **Hess, D.R. and Branson, R.D.** (2000) Ventilators and weaning modes. *Respir. Care Clin. N. Am.* **6:** 407–435.

32. **Hewlett, A.M., Platt, A.S. and Terry, V.G.** (1977) Mandatory minute volume. *Anesthesia* **32:** 163–169.

33. **Keenan, H.T. and Martin, L.D.** (1997) Volume support ventilation in infants and children: Analysis of a case series. *Respir. Care* **42:** 281–287.

34. **Sottiaux, T.M.** (2001) Patient–ventilator interactions during volume support ventilation: Asynchrony and tidal volume instability—a report of three cases. *Respir. Care* **46:** 255–262.

35. **Guttmann, J., Eberhard, L., Fabry, B., *et al.*** (1993) Continuous calculation of intratracheal pressure in tracheally intubated patients. *Anesthesiology* **79:** 503–513.

36. **Fabry, B., Haberthur, C., Zappe, D., *et al.*** (1997) Breathing pattern and additional work breathing in spontaneously breathing patients with different ventilatory demands during inspiratory pressure support and automatic tube compensation. *Intensive Care Med.* **23:** 545–552.

37. **Guttmann, J., Bernhard, H., Mols, G., *et al.*** (1997) Respiratory comfort of automatic tube compensation and inspiratory pressure support in conscious humans. *Intensive Care Med.* **23:** 1119–1124.

38. **Shapiro, W., Wilson, R.K., Casar, G. *et al.*** (1986) Work of breathing through different sized endotracheal tubes. *Crit. Care Med.* **14:** 1028–1031.

39. **Wright, P.E., Marini, J.J. and Bernard, G.R.** (1989) *In vitro* versus *in vivo* comparison of endotracheal tube airflow resistance. *Am. Rev. Respir. Dis.* **140:** 10–16.

40. **Strauss, C., Louis, B., Isabey, D., *et al.*** (1998) Contribution of the endotracheal tube and the upper airway to breathing workload. *Am. J. Respir. Crit. Care Med.* **157:** 23–30.

41. **Esteban, A., Alia, I., Gordo, F., *et al.*** (1997) Extubation outcome after spontaneous breathing trials with T-tube or pressure support ventilation. *Am. J. Respir. Crit. Care Med.* **156:** 459–463.

42. **Otis, A.B., Fenn, W.O. and Rahn, H.** (1950) Mechanics of breathing in man. *J. Appl. Physiol.* **2:** 592–603.

43. **Iotti, G.A., Brashi, A., Brunner, J.X., *et al.*** (1998) Respiratory mechanics by least squares fitting in mechanically ventilated patients: Applications during paralysis and during pressure support ventilation. *Intensive Care Med.* **21:** 406–413.

44. **Weiler, N., Eberle, B. and Heinrichs, W.** (1998) Adaptive lung ventilation (AVL) during anesthesia for pulmonary surgery: Automatic response to transitions to and from one-lung ventilation. *J. Clin. Monit.* **14:** 245–252.

45. **Laubscher, T.P., Frutiger, A., Fanconi, S., *et al.*** (1994) Automatic selection of tidal volume, respiratory frequency and minute ventilation in intubated ICU patients as start up procedure for closed-loop controlled ventilation. *Int. J. Clin. Monit. Comput.* **11:** 19–30.

46. **Campbell, R.S., Sinamban, R.P., Johannigman, J.A., *et al.*** (1998) Clinical evaluation of a new closed loop ventilation mode: Adaptive support ventilation (abstract). *Respir. Care* **43:** 856.

47. **Amato, M.B.P., Barbos, C.S.V., Bonassa, J., *et al.*** (1992) Volume assisted pressure support ventilation (VAPSV): A new approach for reducing muscle workload during acute respiratory failure. *Chest* **102:** 1225–1234.

48. **Haas, C.F., Branson, R.D., Folk, L.M., *et al.*** (1995) Patient determined inspiratory flow during assisted mechanical ventilation. *Respir. Care* **40:** 716–721.

Chapter 14

The acute respiratory distress syndrome

C. Allen Bashour, MD
and James K. Stoller, MD

Contents

14.1 Introduction

The acute respiratory distress syndrome (ARDS) is a common clinical condition that affects both medical and surgical patients. It carries a high mortality rate that has changed only modestly since it was first described over 30 years ago. The true incidence of ARDS has been difficult to determine because the definition of the syndrome has only recently been standardized. Promising advances in the treatment of ARDS continue to be evaluated but the benefit of these treatments has not been clearly established, and management strategies have only recently affected mortality. This chapter provides an overview of the definitions, epidemiology, pathogenesis, clinical features, established and evolving treatment, and prognosis in this important clinical syndrome.

14.2 Historical perspective

The acute respiratory distress syndrome was known as 'sudden pulmonary collapse' and 'traumatic wet lung' during World Wars I and II, respectively[1]. The first description of ARDS by Ashbaugh et al. appeared in 1967[2]. Twelve patients described in that report developed acute dyspnea, tachypnea, cyanosis refractory to maximal oxygen therapy, decreased lung compliance, and diffuse bilateral pulmonary infiltrates on chest radiographs, and their mortality rate was 50%.

14.2.1 Definitions
In 1982, Petty provided a definition of the 'adult respiratory distress syndrome'[3]. In 1988,

Murray et al. developed a four-part Lung Injury Score (*Table 14.1*) based on the level of positive end-expiratory pressure (PEEP), the ratio of partial pressure of arterial oxygen (PaO_2) to fraction of inspired oxygen (FiO_2), the static lung compliance, and the extent of pulmonary infiltrates observed on the chest radiograph, to quantify the severity of lung injury[4]. Although this Lung Injury Score cannot be used to predict outcome during the first 3 days[5,6], it has been shown that a score of 2.5 or higher on days 4–7 is associated with prolonged mechanical ventilation[7].

It was not until 1994 that the American–European Consensus Conference on ARDS recommended a new definition, and a new name: 'acute respiratory distress syndrome', to emphasize the acute onset of the syndrome and its occurrence in children[8]. The three new definitional criteria are: a PaO_2 to FiO_2 ratio of 200 or less, bilateral pulmonary infiltrates on the chest radiograph, and a pulmonary artery occlusion pressure of 18 mmHg or less. The third criterion excludes left ventricular failure or a cardiogenic cause of pulmonary edema. Patients with less severe hypoxemia (PaO_2 to FiO_2 ratio ≤300) are considered to have acute lung injury (ALI), a milder functional lung injury resulting from structural changes in the alveolar–capillary unit. The term ARDS is therefore used for the most severe form of ALI.

14.2.2 Epidemiology
The true incidence of ARDS has been difficult to determine because there have been various definitions of the syndrome since it was first described. The incidence has been reported to

Table 14.1 Murray scale for acute lung injury

Points	0	1	2	3	4
Chest X-ray (no. of quadrants)	No infiltrate	one	two	three	four
PaO_2/FiO_2	≥300	225–299	165–224	100–174	<100
PEEP	≤5	6–8	9–11	12–14	≥15
Cs	≥80	60–79	40–59	20	≤19

Final score is aggregate sum divided by number of components: 0 indicates no lung injury; 0.1–2.5 indicates mild to moderate lung injury; 2.5 indicates ARDS. From: Murray, J.F. et al (1988) An expanded definition of the adult respiratory distress syndrome. Reproduced with permission from *Am. Rev. Respir. Dis.* **138**: 720–723.

be as low as 1.5–8.3 cases[9–11] and as high as 75.0–88.6 cases[12,13] per 100 000. A prospective epidemiological study using the 1994 consensus committee definition is currently being undertaken to more accurately determine the incidence of ARDS.

14.3 Pathogenesis

The acute respiratory distress syndrome is a common end-point response to either direct or indirect lung injury. Precipitating factors that directly injure the lung include pneumonia, aspiration of gastric contents, pulmonary contusion, fat emboli, near-drowning, inhalational injury, and reperfusion pulmonary edema after lung transplantation or pulmonary embolectomy. The acute respiratory distress syndrome may occur as a consequence of indirect lung injury in the setting of a systemic process such as sepsis, severe trauma with shock and multiple transfusions, cardiopulmonary bypass, drug overdose, acute pancreatitis, and transfusion of blood products[14]. Of all the ARDS precipitating factors, sepsis has the greatest potential to induce ARDS, and the presence of multiple predisposing factors significantly increases the risk of developing the syndrome[15] (*Table 14.2*).

14.3.1 Early ARDS

The result of direct or indirect lung injury is diffuse alveolar damage with capillary endothelial and alveolar epithelial cell necrosis, proteinacious edema accumulation, and hyaline membrane formation. This process begins within the first 24 h and marks the beginning of the acute or exudative stage of ARDS, which continues for approximately 1 week. During this stage, there is build-up of exudative fluid that moves from the intravascular to the interstitial space, and ultimately into the alveolar unit. The ARDS-induced accumulation of interstitial pulmonary edema is difficult to distinguish radiographically from cardiogenic pulmonary edema and causes a decrease in lung compliance. It is by attempting to maintain adequate oxygenation and ventilation in the setting of decreasing lung compliance and gas exchange that secondary or ventilator-induced lung injury can occur.

The alveolar epithelium and capillary endothelium together form a barrier that prevents crossing of edema fluid from the intravascular space into the alveolus. The alveolar epithelium is composed of flat (type I) and cuboidal (type II) cells. The flat epithelial cells make up 90% of the total alveolar surface and are more susceptible to ventilator-induced

Table 14.2 Prevalence of ARDS with predisposing factors

Clinical condition	n	Prevalence with this factor alone (%)	Prevalence with multiple risk factors
Sepsis syndrome	38	38	47
Gastric aspiration	23	30	31
Pulmonary contusion	29	17	38
Multiple transfusions	17	24	45
Multiple fractures	12	8	44
Near-drowning	3	67	–
Pancreatitis	1	100	–

Reprinted from Pepe et al. (1982) Clinical predictors of the adult respiratory distress syndrome. *Am. J. Surg.* **144**: 124–130. With permission from Excerpta Medica Inc.

lung injury. The more resilient cuboidal cells produce surfactant and participate in ion transport. Injured cuboidal cells differentiate into flat type I alveolar cells and produce either no surfactant or surfactant that has altered lipid content and increased minimal surface tension[16,17]. The alveolar epithelium is normally less permeable than the capillary endothelium and contributes more to overall barrier function. A lung injury that involves the alveolar epithelium will therefore disproportionately increase permeability and allow influx of protein-rich fluid into the alveolus. Barrier loss also allows for alveolar bacterial translocation similar to what can occur in the intestine when gut mucosal integrity is lost. Patients with bacterial pneumonia and loss of the alveolar–capillary barrier may develop bacteremia and septic shock[18]. In addition to barrier loss, alveolar epithelial cell injury results in abnormal fluid transport, and fluid accumulation in the alveolar space[19,20].

The ARDS-precipitating factor may lead to neutrophil activation and sequestration. Eighty per cent of patients who develop ARDS have a transient decrease in neutrophil count because neutrophils adhere to the vascular endothelium[21]. The subsequent release of mediators of the inflammatory response (elastase, proteolytic enzymes, oxygen free radicals, leukotrienes, thromboxane, tumor necrosis factor, and platelet activating factor) directly damages the capillary endothelium, compromises barrier function, and leads to increased interstitial edema.

During the acute stage of ARDS, several factors lead to reduced gas exchange and lung compliance. The normally small interstitial space between capillary and alveolus widens as a result of edema formation, migrating neutrophil accumulation, and procollagen release from fibroblasts. This widened gap impairs gas exchange. On the alveolar side, hyaline membranes form and line the denuded basement membrane, further blocking gas exchange. Alveolar macrophages release macrophage inhibitory factor, tumor necrosis factor-alpha, and interleukins (IL) 1, 6, 8, and 10. Tumor

necrosis factor-alpha and IL-1 activate neutrophils, causing the release of leukotrienes, oxidants, platelet activating factor, and proteases. These factors, as well as inactivated surfactant, necrotic or apoptotic type I cells, fibrin, cellular debris, sloughed bronchial epithelium, red blood cells, and protein-rich edema fluid, flood the alveolus. Swollen and injured capillary endothelial cells and the increased number of neutrophils and platelets in the capillaries impair capillary blood flow and further impede gas exchange.

Oxygen free radical production in ARDS occurs early during sustained exposure to high FiO_2 levels (>0.60) and is generated by neutrophils and macrophages. Naturally occurring antioxidants (glutathione, transferrin, and ceruloplasmin) found in the bronchoalveolar lavage of patients with ARDS offer a defense against oxygen free radical-induced lung injury. The protein-rich fluid itself present within the alveoli as a result of increased permeability may also limit oxidant injury. Plasma levels of the antioxidant vitamin E are low in ARDS, suggesting increased consumption in the setting of increased oxygen free radical production and/or decreased vitamin E absorption as a result of malnutrition[22].

14.3.2 Late ARDS

The initial exudative stage lasts approximately 1 week and is followed either by recovery or progression to a stage characterized by fibroproliferation and subsequent fibrosis. If progression to the fibroproliferative and fibrotic stages occurs, lung compliance continues to decrease and the risk of ventilator-induced lung injury (volutrauma and/or barotrauma) increases as attempts are made to ventilate stiffer lungs with higher pressures. This stage may begin as early as the fifth day when the alveolar space becomes filled with mesenchymal cells. Overstretching of the alveolus stresses the epithelial cells and may cause cell disruption. During the fibroproliferative stage, inflammatory cells accumulate as a result of chemo-attractants released by neutrophils. Normally, inflammatory cells together with alveolar macrophages remove debris and begin repair, but in ARDS epithelial repair is disorganized and may lead to fibrosis and decreased lung compliance[23]. Corticosteroids are thought to be useful during the fibroproliferative (inflammatory) stage, but true benefit has not been established.

14.4 Clinical presentation

Patients with ARDS experience an acute onset of severe dyspnea and respiratory distress and the manifestations of arterial hypoxemia refractory to oxygen therapy: cyanosis, tachypnea, and tachycardia, in the absence of left ventricular failure (pulmonary artery occlusion pressure ≤18 mmHg). A predisposing factor such as sepsis, hypotension, trauma, or multiorgan dysfunction may be present. By definition, the presentation cannot be attributed to congestive heart failure. The key laboratory finding is a PaO$_2$ to FiO$_2$ ratio of 200 or less. The arterial pH relates to the adequacy of ventilation in the setting of decreasing lung compliance and to the presence or absence of sepsis or hypotension that may contribute to metabolic acidemia. If multiorgan failure is present, laboratory investigations may reveal hematologic, coagulation, renal, hepatobiliary, or electrolyte abnormalities. The chest radiograph will show characteristic diffuse bilateral pulmonary infiltrates.

14.5 Treatment

The treatment of ARDS begins with determining and treating the underlying cause. If ARDS is caused by sepsis, the focus should be identified and appropriately treated. If a septic source is identified from blood, respiratory, or urine cultures, or by chest radiography or computed tomography, antibiotics should be directed against the causative organism. Prevention, or early detection and culture-directed treatment of nosocomial infections is essential.

Ventilatory management has been a key aspect of ARDS treatment since the syndrome was first described in 1967. In the initial report, oxygenation was enhanced dramatically in some of the 12 patients by applying an expiratory retard that created PEEP. Since that time, PEEP has been a mainstay of treatment, its benefit mediated by recruiting and maintaining the patency of flooded alveoli. More recently, attention has focused on low-stretch ventilatory strategies as a method to optimize alveolar recruitment while limiting the adverse effects of overdistended alveoli. Results of the NIH ARDS Network trial (comparing low-stretch ventilation (6 ml kg^{-1}) tidal volume versus traditional tidal volumes (12 ml kg^{-1})) show a 32% mortality reduction associated with the low-stretch approach[24].

14.5.1 Recruitment

Optimal ventilatory management of ARDS requires an understanding of the state of the alveoli in ARDS lungs. Indeed, four populations of alveoli exist in ARDS (*Figure 14.1*). The first population is composed of normal alveoli that expand at 20–30 cmH$_2$O. These recruited alveoli participate in gas exchange and can be damaged if overdistended or exposed to end-inspiration plateau pressures greater than 35 cmH$_2$O. The second population of alveoli is composed of atelectatic alveoli that can be re-expanded and are therefore recruitable. These alveolar units can be enlisted to participate in gas exchange if increased PEEP is employed to hold open the units and if sufficient inspiratory time is used. Positive end-expiratory pressure is used to restore functional residual capacity above the closing volume, thereby reducing the risk of derecruitment or alveolar collapse during exhalation. Adhered walls of collapsed terminal bronchi typically require high inflation pressures to separate but will remain open at much lower pressures once opened. The compliance in these alveolar units is normal. The third population is composed of alveolar units that have poor compliance and require increased time and peak inflation pressure to open and keep expanded. Opening these alveoli requires exceeding the critical opening pressure for an adequate time period. These alveolar units may become derecruited and thus excluded from gas exchange

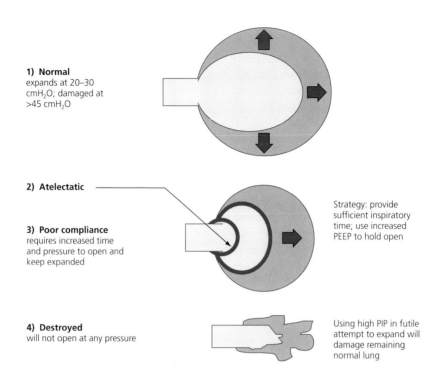

1) Normal
expands at 20–30
cmH$_2$O; damaged at
>45 cmH$_2$O

2) Atelectatic

Strategy: provide
sufficient inspiratory
time; use increased
PEEP to hold open

3) Poor compliance
requires increased time
and pressure to open and
keep expanded

4) Destroyed
will not open at any pressure

Using high PIP in futile
attempt to expand will
damage remaining
normal lung

Figure 14.1 Four populations of alveoli.

if the critical opening pressure is not reached and maintained. The fourth population is made up of destroyed alveolar units that will not open at any pressure. Using high PEEP in a futile attempt to re-expand these units will damage the remaining normal lung.

In the context of this spectrum of alveoli, it has been shown that reduced lung compliance in patients with ARDS is due to a decrease in the number of normally functioning alveoli rather than to a generalized dysfunction that affects all alveolar units equally, as is suggested by the appearance of diffuse bilateral alveolar infiltrates on chest radiography[25]. Computed tomographic scans of lungs in patients with ARDS have demonstrated consolidation and atelectasis in the dependent lung zones, with other areas being relatively spared[26,27].

14.5.2 Positive end-expiratory pressure
Positive end-expiratory pressure redistributes pulmonary edema from the alveolar to the interstitial space and increases functional residual capacity as a result of recruitment of collapsed alveoli, thereby improving gas exchange[28]. During the initial exudative stage, hypoxemia rapidly progresses from mild and FiO$_2$ responsive (meaning that an adequate PaO$_2$ can initially be maintained by increasing the FiO$_2$) to severe in spite of a maximal FiO$_2$. Maintaining adequate oxygenation during this early stage depends on using incrementally higher levels of PEEP. In the later fibroproliferative and fibrotic stages, hypoxemia becomes refractory to both high FiO$_2$ and PEEP levels. Optimal PEEP is the level that allows for adequate tissue oxygenation with an FiO$_2$ of 0.60 or less. The level of PEEP is therefore individualized for each patient. Amato *et al.* have shown benefit by raising PEEP to a level above the lower inflection point on a pressure–volume curve determined for each patient[29]. In general, PEEP should be employed early and increased to a level that maintains an adequate

oxygen saturation ($SpO_2 \geq 90\%$) at the lowest possible FiO_2. Prophylactic PEEP (8 cmH$_2$O) in patients at risk for ARDS has been shown not to confer benefit[30].

The risk of pneumothorax increases with higher PEEP levels. Although prophylactic bilateral chest tubes have been advocated by some to prevent this complication, we do not advocate this practice. Tube thoracostomy carries potential risks including bleeding from an intercostal artery or from the lung parenchyma itself, as well as infection. Therefore, the ARDS patient is closely monitored and a chest tube is inserted only if a pneumothorax occurs.

Once optimal PEEP is reached, it is maintained and weaned gradually only after the patient stabilizes and begins to recover. An improvement in pulmonary compliance (the change in volume for a unit pressure) is an early indicator of recovery and can be calculated daily to determine when recovery is beginning. The change in volume (ΔV) for a unit pressure (ΔP) under conditions of no flow is termed the pulmonary static compliance (Cs) and can be calculated using the following formula:

$$\text{static compliance (Cs)} = \Delta V / \Delta P$$

$$\text{Cs} = V_t/[\text{plateau airway pressure} - (\text{PEEP} + \text{auto PEEP})]$$

(normal Cs is 100 ml per mH$_2$O).

Similarly, pulmonary dynamic compliance can be calculated substituting peak for plateau airway pressure in the formula above. A related early indicator of recovery is decreasing peak inflation pressure. This is followed by improved oxygenation at progressively lower FiO_2 and PEEP levels. The chest radiograph will improve in appearance but this change usually lags by 1 week or more after the earlier indicators of recovery appear.

In ARDS survivors, maximal recovery typically occurs by 6 months after extubation and pulmonary function at 1 year following hospital discharge is normal or only mildly impaired. Poorer outcomes are seen in patients

who have a more severe ARDS course and a longer ventilation period[31]. Long-term pulmonary function sequelae may include tracheal stenosis from long-term intubation and/or tracheotomy, and mild impairment of diffusing capacity.

14.5.3 Secondary lung injury

The main objective in ARDS management is to adequately oxygenate and ventilate the patient while avoiding oxygen toxicity as a result of oxygen free radical production at higher FiO_2 levels, volutrauma caused by overstretching non-compliant alveolar units, and barotrauma from high inflation pressures. These three potential lung injuries are collectively termed secondary or ventilator-induced lung injury. At higher FiO_2 levels (≥ 0.60), oxygen free radicals are produced to an extent that causes lipid peroxidation, neutrophil recruitment, and protein degradation, causing alveolar epithelial and vascular endothelial cell damage and increased permeability. Antioxidant use has been proposed to protect against secondary lung injury as a result of oxygen free radical production. In one trial using the antioxidants N-acetylcysteine and procysteine there was no difference in mortality among study group; however, the number of days of ALI and the incidence of new multiorgan system failure were decreased[32].

14.5.4 Volutrauma

Secondary lung injury caused by overstretching alveoli is referred to as volutrauma. Type II cuboidal cells are susceptible to this type of lung injury, which impairs their ability to produce surfactant. Several recent studies have suggested that avoiding alveolar overdistention during ventilatory support enhances survival in patients with ARDS. In the NIH ARDS Network trial, patients treated with lower tidal volumes of 6 ml kg^{-1} (a normal tidal volume for people breathing at rest) and with plateau pressures less than 35 cmH$_2$O experienced higher survival and fewer non-pulmonary organ failures than did patients treated with conventional tidal volumes[24]. The formulae for calculating the predicted (ideal) body weight (kg), which should be used instead of the measured body weight, to determine the tidal volume setting, are:

> for men: weight (kg) = 50.0 + 0.91 (cm of height – 152.4);
> for women: weight (kg) = 45.5 + 0.91 (cm of height – 152.4).

Given this current evidence, low-stretch ventilation, often achieved using a pressure-controlled ventilatory mode, has become the standard of care in patients with ARDS. Of course, one consequence of the low-stretch approach in patients with stiff lungs is that minute ventilation decreases, which results in hypercapnea and respiratory acidemia. This 'permissive hypercapnea' and the associated acidemia is accepted as a consequence of the benefits of avoiding volutrauma. Recognizing that profound acidemia can have independent adverse effects (e.g. cardiac arrhythmias, refractoriness to inotropic agents), the NIH study accepted acidemia to a pH of 7.30. Lower pH values led to bicarbonate infusion in that trial. As a possible explanation of the survival benefit of a low-stretch ventilatory approach, recent evidence has shown that cyclic opening and closing of alveoli can initiate a cascade of pro-inflammatory cytokine release, which may enter the circulation and cause other organ systems to fail[33]. The enthusiasm for these ventilatory advances reflects the fact that the low-stretch approach is the first ARDS treatment of many studied to confer a survival advantage[24]. Other proposed treatments, including high-frequency ventilation and raising systemic oxygen transport with inotropes, have not been shown to be beneficial. Still, maintaining oxygen delivery, which is the product of cardiac output and arterial oxygen content, is sensible. Although there is no automatic transfusion threshold, blood transfusion to maintain hemoglobin values at 8 mg dl^{-1} or more is often advocated to avoid a decreased arterial oxygen content and consequent reduced systemic oxygen transport. The goal is to maintain oxygen delivery while avoiding ventilator-induced lung injury caused by oxygen toxicity, volutrauma, or barotrauma.

14.5.5 Barotrauma

Barotrauma or pressure-induced lung injury can cause pneumomediastinum, pneumoperitoneum, tension or simple pneumothorax, interstitial emphysema, tension gas cyst, injury to small and terminal bronchi, lung edema, or subcutaneous emphysema, and becomes more likely with higher plateau pressures. This form of lung injury more often appears gradually and may therefore not be obvious. If subcutaneous emphysema extends into the neck, it may compress and thereby completely obstruct the airway. This is critical in both the intubated and non-intubated patient. Although the endotracheally intubated patient with subcutaneous emphysema has a reasonably secure airway, it is important to consider airway patency before extubation. In ARDS patients, as lung compliance decreases, end-inspiration plateau pressures rapidly increase and, if not recognized, will lead to pressure-induced lung injury or barotrauma. Limiting inflation pressures can minimize barotrauma. Although an absolutely safe inflation pressure has not been well defined, maintaining a plateau pressure of 35 cmH$_2$O or less has been traditionally accepted as desirable[34]. In fact, the recent NIH trial suggests that tidal volume may be more important than plateau pressure in determining patient outcome[24].

14.5.6 Prone positioning

Prone positioning is being evaluated as a way of enhancing oxygenation in patients with ARDS. In available studies, patients were shown to have improved oxygenation after prone positioning typically within 2 h, and the improvement was sustained at about 50% beneficial effect when the patient was returned to the supine position[35–38]. The optimal duration of prone position is not defined, alternating between supine and prone position every 6–8 h is common practice. In one study in which 14 ARDS patients were treated for at least 1 h in the prone position, the mortality of the prone positioned patients was 42% (versus 58% in those not turned prone)[38]. The responders (PaO_2 to FiO_2 ratio increase >10%) were treated for at least 6 h. Eleven were primary responders and two of the other three improved with a second prone positioning. Although the mechanism by which prone positioning might confer benefit is not known, the benefits may in part be due to the relatively nonuniform distribution of lung injury in ARDS. A benefit, however, has not been established.

Potential complications of prone positioning include hemodynamic instability, vena caval compression, decreased functional residual capacity, peripheral nerve injury, joint dislocation, corneal damage, decubiti of the face and chest, accidental extubation or central venous or arterial line removal, endotracheal tube obstruction by mucus, and aspiration of enteral nutrition formulas. A specific risk for cardiac surgery patients related to prone positioning is delay in emergency reopening of the sternotomy if required for hemodynamic instability.

14.5.7 Steroids and non-steroidal anti-inflammatory agents

During the fibroproliferative stage of ARDS, pulmonary interstitial inflammation peaks. It is during this stage that glucocorticoid use has been proposed to attenuate the inflammatory response and thereby improve lung compliance. However, large prospective trials have demonstrated that glucocorticoids administered early in the course of established ARDS do not confer benefit[39–41]. Moreover, in early ARDS it is difficult to exclude infection as the precipitating cause, and glucocorticoids can increase mortality if administered in the setting of unrecognized infection. More encouraging results have been reported in studies where glucocorticoids were administered later in the course of ARDS[42,43]. The current recommendation is that high-dose glucocorticoids can be used as rescue therapy in the fibroproliferative stage in patients who have poor lung compliance and non-resolving disease as long as infection has been excluded either as a cause or complication of ARDS. An uncontrolled study reported an 80% survival and an improved Lung Injury Score when a methylprednisolone 200 mg bolus was administered followed by 2–3 mg kg^{-1} day^{-1}, and tapered after extubation. It is important to point out, however, that 60% of the treated patients in this study developed infection[42]. Use of the non-steroidal anti-inflammatory agents pentoxyfylline, a phosphodiesterase inhibitor with anti-inflammatory effects on neutrophils and macrophages, prostacyclin (PgI2) which decreases pulmonary and systemic pressures and intrapulmonary shunt, PgE1, and nitric oxide, which has anti-inflammatory as well as vasodilating activity, in ARDS has been proposed, but there is insufficient evidence of benefit to support their use[44–46].

14.5.8 ECMO, ECO_2R, surfactant, nitric oxide, and partial liquid ventilation

Other techniques that have been tried to improve outcome in ARDS include extracorporeal membrane oxygenation (ECMO), extracorporeal membrane carbon dioxide removal ($ECCO_2R$), exogenous surfactant use, nitric oxide, and partial liquid ventilation. Given the success of ECMO in infant respiratory distress syndrome, the reversibility of alveolar damage in ARDS, and the presence of severe hypoxemia despite maximal ventilator support, ECMO was tried in adults with ARDS in the late 1970s. The NIH ECMO trial that initially planned to recruit 300 patients to evaluate ECMO as a therapy for severe acute respiratory failure was terminated after the first 90 patients because of poor survival (<10%)[47]. In this study, ECMO was intended for short-term use to theoretically rest the lungs while recovery could begin. However, the membrane oxygenators frequently failed, and bleeding and infection complicated the patient's intensive care course. Extracorporeal membrane oxygenation reversed the poor oxygenation and supported respiratory gas exchange in these patients, but it did not improve survival. Studies using $ECCO_2R$ have shown no mortality improvement[48].

Because surfactant levels are low, and because alveolar collapse and reduced lung compliance are features of ARDS, alveolar surfactant replacement has been proposed as a treatment for ARDS. However, in a trial using a 5 day course of nebulized synthetic surfactant in 725 patients, there was no significant effect on 30 day survival or PaO$_2$ to FiO$_2$ ratio[49]. Thus, surfactant is not routinely used in adult patients with ARDS. Some have proposed that alternative surfactant preparations and methods of delivery might be effective, and newer products and methods of delivery are currently being investigated. Nitric oxide (NO), a selective pulmonary vasodilator with rapid onset and reversal, has appeal in ARDS patients because it has been shown to improve ventilation–perfusion matching by dilating vessels only in well-ventilated lung regions. Although NO has been shown to reduce shunt fraction and improve oxygenation[50], a multicenter trial using NO (1.25–80 ppm) in 177 ARDS patients failed to show a change in mortality or ventilator time[51]. Thus, despite its occasional use as short-term salvage therapy to improve oxygenation, NO cannot at present be endorsed in ARDS.

Partial liquid ventilation (PLV) using perfluorocarbons that have a low surface tension and high solubility, and that offer gas exchange and surfactant functions, has been evaluated in patients with ARDS. As the lungs fill with perfluorocarbons, the closed alveoli open and exudates are flushed out. In animal studies, increased lung compliance and oxygenation has been observed, and in 10 adult patients with ARDS on ECMO, partial liquid ventilation was well tolerated with decreased physiologic shunting and increased static lung compliance. However, the overall survival of patients treated with PLV was 50%, equal to that of historic controls[52]. To date, benefit has not been clearly established and research in this area is ongoing.

14.5.9 Fluid balance

The increase in pulmonary edema that occurs during the early exudative stage in ARDS peaks within 24–48 h and subsides by 3–5 days. This observation led to the proposal that a decrease in intravascular volume by aggressive diuresis could decrease pulmonary interstitial edema and thereby improve oxygenation. The risk associated with this strategy is that fluid restriction and aggressive diuresis causes reduced cardiac filling pressures and a low cardiac output. This increases the risk of multiorgan failure and creates the need for inotropic support. Hypotension in spite of inotropic support, and a diuresis-induced pre-renal state, can lead to acute renal failure that converts single organ failure to multisystem failure with a commensurately increased overall mortality. It is important, therefore, to maintain normal intravascular volume so as to optimize oxygen delivery and assure adequate tissue perfusion. Aggressive diuresis will not decrease pulmonary interstitial edema or improve lung compliance, and may lead to renal insufficiency. Once intravascular volume is optimized, vasopressors may be used to increase cardiac output and restore normal oxygen delivery[53]. Two prospective studies of high-risk surgical patients have shown no relationship between positive fluid balance and development of ARDS[54,55].

14.5.10 Nutritional support

Nutritional support should be initiated once the diagnosis of ARDS is established. The patient with ARDS will require prolonged intensive care and therefore there is no reason to delay feeding. Enteral feeding is preferable to parenteral because it helps maintain normal intestinal mucosa integrity and maintains a barrier against Gram-negative bacterial translocation and subsequent sepsis. Additionally, the enteral route has fewer potential complications. Feeding via the enteral route avoids the risks of central venous line insertion, which include hemothorax, pneumothorax, and thoracic duct injury, as well as the risks associated with indwelling central venous lines, which include sepsis, catheter erosion into a vascular structure, and air embolism.

Difficulty can be encountered when placing and maintaining the correct position of a nasoenteric feeding tube. The preferred tip location is in the fourth portion of the duodenum. A nasogastric tube may be used but is not required if the feeding tube tip is in proper position and the head of the bed is maintained at 30° at all times. Correct feeding tube position must be confirmed radiographically after placement, as the tube may be malpositioned in the trachea, bronchus, or beyond. Finally, prevention of gastrointestinal bleeding and venous thromboembolism is critical in these patients.

14.6 Prognosis and outcome

In the majority of patients who survive ARDS, pulmonary function is normal or only slightly impaired within 6–12 months following extubation[31]. Until recently, the mortality rate of ARDS has remained 40–60%[56,57]. However, two recent reports suggest a decreasing mortality rate of approximately 35%[58,59]. The outcome improvement may be related to better critical care and more effective treatment for sepsis syndrome, as well as to the increased use of protective lung ventilation strategies[60]. Features associated with poorer survival in ARDS include failure of the PaO_2 to FiO_2 ratio to improve over the first week of therapy and the

presence of liver disease, non-pulmonary organ dysfunction, sepsis, and advanced age[5,6,61]. In fact, only 16% of deaths from ARDS are caused by respiratory failure (hypoxemia, hypercapnia, and respiratory acidosis)[62]. Most of the attributable mortality is due to multi-organ failure mediated by inflammatory cytokine release from the lungs and spread via the circulation to other organs, and is not related to the length of ventilator time.

14.7 Conclusions

There is significant morbidity associated with ARDS and mortality has only recently been shown to be decreasing from the level first reported by Ashbaugh *et al.* in 1967[2]. The definition of ARDS has now been clarified and this should make future studies more reliable. The etiology is often multifactorial and undetermined. Management remains largely supportive (*Table 14.3*) but with newer strategies such as low-stretch pressure-controlled ventilation, the goal of providing adequate oxygenation and ventilation with the least amount of secondary lung injury is being achieved, and mortality is being reduced. The role of newer

---

Table 14.3 Summary of recommended management strategies for treating acute respiratory distress syndrome

- Identify underlying causes; if infection is identified, treat with appropriate antibiotics
- Increase PEEP to a level that allows for an $FiO_2 \leq 0.60$ (typically 12–18 cmH_2O), to avoid oxygen free radical induced lung injury; once optimal PEEP is reached, wean gradually (to avoid alveolar derecruitment) only when signs of recovery appear
- Use a low-stretch pressure-controlled ventilatory (PCV) approach (6 ml kg^{-1} with end-inspiratory plateau pressure <35 cmH_2O) to avoid volutrauma (kg is predicted or ideal, not measured, body weight)
- Accept hypercapnea as long as the arterial pH can be maintained above 7.25
- Use recruitment maneuvers
- Provide adequate sedation, and neuromuscular blockade if necessary
- Maintain normal intravascular volume
- Although there is no automatic transfusion threshold level, maintain oxygen delivery by keeping hemoglobin levels ≥8 mg dl^{-1}, and by using inotropic support if required to normalize cardiac output
- Initiate prophylaxis against gastrointestinal bleeding and venous thromboembolism
- Initiate nutritional support (enteral is preferable to parenteral) once the diagnosis of ARDS is made
- Consider glucocorticoid use in the fibroproliferative stage only if infection has been excluded (methylprednisolone 2 mg kg^{-1} day^{-1})

interventions is being defined. Acute respiratory distress syndrome survivors generally resume productive lives without pulmonary limitation.

References

1. **Buford, T.H. and Burbank, B.** (1945) Traumatic wet lung: Observations on certain physiologic fundamentals of thoracic trauma. *J. Thorac. Surg.* **14:** 415–424.

2. **Ashbaugh, D.G., Bigelow, D.B., Petty, T.L. and Levine, B.E.** (1967) Acute respiratory distress in adults. *Lancet* **2:** 319–323.

3. **Petty, T.L.** (1982) Adult respiratory distress syndrome: Definition and historical perspective. *Clin. Chest Med.* **3**(1): 3–7.

4. **Murray, J.F., Matthay, M.A., Luce, J.M. and Flick, M.R.** (1988) An expanded definition of the adult respiratory distress syndrome. *Am. Rev. Respir. Dis.* **138:** 720–723.

5. **Doyle, R.L., Szaflarski, N., Modin, G.W., et al.** (1995) Identification of patients with acute lung injury: predictors of mortality. *Am. J. Respir. Crit. Care Med.* **152:** 1818–1824.

6. **Zilberberg, M.D. and Eptein, S.K.** (1998) Acute lung injury in the medical ICU: co-morbid conditions, age, etiology, and hospital outcome. *Am. J. Respir. Crit. Care Med.* **157:** 1159–1164.

7. **Heffner, J.E., Brown, L.K., Barbieri, C.A., Harpel, K.S. and DeLeo, J.** (1995) Prospective validation of an acute respiratory distress syndrome predictive score. *Am. J. Respir. Crit. Care Med.* **152:** 1518–1526.

8. **Bernard, G.R., Artigas, A., Brigham, K.L., et al.** (1994) The American–European Consensus Conference on ARDS. Definitions, mechanisms, relevant outcomes, and clinical trial coordination. *Am. J. Respir. Crit. Care Med.* **149:** 818–824.

9. **Webster, N.R., Cohen, A.T. and Nunn, J.F.** (1988) Adult respiratory distress syndrome—how many cases in the UK? *Anaesthesia* **43:** 923–926.

10. **Villar, J. and Slutsky, A.S.** (1989) The incidence of the adult respiratory distress syndrome. *Am. Rev. Respir. Dis.* **140:** 814–816.

11. **Thomsen, G.E. and Morris, A.H.** (1995) Incidence of the adult respiratory distress syndrome in the state of Utah. *Am. J. Respir. Crit. Care Med.* **152:** 965–971.

12. **Murray, J.F.** (1977) Conference Report: Mechanisms of acute respiratory failure. *Am. Rev. Respir. Dis.* **115:** 1071–1078.

13. **Lewandowski, K., Metz, J., Deutschmann, C., et al.** (1995) Incidence, severity, and mortality of acute respiratory failure in Berlin, Germany. *Am. J. Respir. Crit. Care Med.* **151**(4): 1121–1125.

14. **Ware, L.B. and Matthay, M.A.** (2000) The acute respiratory distress syndrome. *N. Engl. J. Med.* **342:** 1334–1349.

15. **Pepe, P.E., Potkin, R.T., Reus, D.H., Hudson, L.D. and Carrico, C.J.** (1982) Clinical predictors of the adult respiratory distress syndrome. *Am. J. Surg.* **144:** 124–130.

16. **Greene, K.E., Wright, J.R., Steinberg, K.P., et al.** (1999) Serial changes in surfactant-associated proteins in lung and serum before and after onset of ARDS. *Am. J. Respir. Crit. Care Med.* **160:** 1843–1850.

17. **Gregory, T.J., Longmore, W.J., Moxley, M.A., et al.** (1991) Surfactant chemical composition and biophysical activity in acute respiratory distress syndrome. *J. Clin. Invest.* **88:** 1976–1981.

18. **Kurahashi, K., Kajikawa, O., Sawa, T., et al.** (1999) Pathogenesis of septic shock in *Pseudomonas aeruginosa* pneumonia. *J. Clin. Invest.* **104:** 743–750.

19. **Modelska, K., Pittet, J.F., Folkesson, H.G., et al.** (1999) Acid-induced lung injury. Protective effect of anti-interleukin-8 pretreatment on alveolar epithelial barrier function in rabbits. *Am. J. Respir. Crit. Care Med.* **160:** 1450–1456.

20. **Sznajder, J.I.** (1999) Strategies to increase alveolar epithelial fluid removal in the injured lung. *Am. J. Respir. Crit. Care Med.* **160:** 1441–1442.

21. **Thommasen, H.V., Russell, J.A., Boyko, W.J. and Hogg, J.C.** (1984) Transient leucopenia associated with adult respiratory distress syndrome. *Lancet* **1**(8381): 809–812.

22. **Richard, C., Lemonnier, F., Thibault, M., et al.** (1990) Vitamin E deficiency and lipoperoxidation during adult respiratory distress syndrome. *Crit. Care Med.* **18:** 4–9.

23. **Bitterman, P.B.** (1992) Pathogenesis of fibrosis in acute lung injury. *Am. J. Med.* **92:** 39S–43S.

24. **The Acute Respiratory Distress Syndrome Network** (2000) Ventilation with lower tidal volumes as compared with traditional tidal volumes for acute lung injury and the acute respiratory distress syndrome. *N. Engl. J. Med.* **342:** 1301–1308.

25. **Marini, J.J.** (1990) Lung mechanics in the adult respiratory distress syndrome. Recent conceptual advances and implications for management. *Clin. Chest Med.* **11:** 673–690.

26. **Goodman, L.R.** (1996) Congestive heart failure and adult respiratory distress syndrome. New insights using computed tomography. *Radiol. Clin. N. Am.* **34:** 33–46.

27. **Gattinoni, L., Bombino, M., Pelosi, P., et al.** (1994) Lung structure and function in different stages of severe adult respiratory distress syndrome. *JAMA* **271**: 1772–1779.

28. **Falke, K.J., Pontoppidan, H., Kumar, A., et al.** (1972) Ventilation with end-expiratory pressure in acute lung disease. *J. Clin. Invest.* **51**: 2315–2323.

29. **Amato, M.B.P., Barbas, C.S.V., Medeiros, D.M., et al.** (1998) Effect of a protective ventilation strategy on mortality in the acute respiratory distress syndrome. *N. Engl. J. Med.* **338**: 347–354.

30. **Pepe, P.E., Hudson, L.D. and Carrico, C.J.** (1984) Early application of positive end-expiratory pressure in patients at risk for adult respiratory-distress syndrome. *N. Engl. J. Med.* **311**: 281–286.

31. **McHugh, L.G., Milberg, J.A., Whitcomb, M.E., et al.** (1994) Recovery of function in survivors of the acute respiratory distress syndrome. *Am. J. Respir. Crit. Care Med.* **150**: 90–94.

32. **Bernard, G.R., Wheeler, A.P., Arons, M.M., et al.** (1997) A trial of antioxidants N-acetylcysteine and procysteine in ARDS. The Antioxidant in ARDS Study Group. *Chest* **112**: 164–172.

33. **Slutsky, A.S. and Tremblay, L.N.** (1998) Multiple system organ failure: is mechanical ventilation a contributing factor? *Am. J. Respir. Crit. Care Med.* **157**: 1721–1725.

34. **Rappaport, S.H., Shpiner, R., Yoshihara, G., et al.** (1994) Randomized, prospective trial of pressure-limited versus volume-controlled ventilation in severe respiratory failure. *Crit. Care Med.* **22**: 22–32.

35. **Langer, M., Mascheroni, D., Marcolin, R. and Gattinoni, L.** (1988) The prone position in ARDS patients. A clinical study. *Chest* **94**: 103–107.

36. **Pappert, D., Rossaint, R., Slama, K., et al.** (1994) Influence of positioning on ventilation–perfusion relationships in severe adult respiratory distress syndrome. *Chest* **106**: 1511–1516.

37. **Chatte, G., Sab, J.M., Dubois, J.M., et al.** (1997) Prone position in mechanically ventilated patients with severe acute respiratory failure. *Am. J. Respir. Crit. Care Med.* **155**: 473–478.

38. **Flaatten, H., Aardal, S. and Hevroy, O.** (1998) Improved oxygenation using the prone position in patients with ARDS. *Acta Anaesthesiol. Scand.* **42**: 329–334.

39. **Bernard, G.R., Luce, J.M., Sprung, C.L., et al.** (1987) High-dose corticosteroids in patients with the adult respiratory distress syndrome. *N. Engl. J. Med.* **317**: 1565–1570.

40. **Luce, J.M., Montgomery, A.B., Marks, J.D., et al.** (1988) Ineffectiveness of high-dose methylprednisolone in preventing parenchymal lung injury and improving mortality in patients with septic shock. *Am. Rev. Respir. Dis.* **138**: 62–68.

41. **Sprung, C.L., Caralis, P.V., Marcial, E.H., et al.** (1984) The effects of high-dose corticosteroids in patients with septic shock. A prospective, controlled study. *N. Engl. J. Med.* **311**: 1137–1143.

42. **Meduri, G.U., Belenchia, J.M., Estes, R.J., et al.** (1991) Fibroproliferative phase of ARDS. Clinical findings and effects of corticosteroids. *Chest* **100**: 943–952.

43. **Meduri, G.U., Chinn, A.J., Leeper, K.V., et al.** (1994) Corticosteroid rescue treatment of progressive fibroproliferation in late ARDS. Patterns of response and predictors of outcome. *Chest* **105**: 1516–1527.

44. **Walmrath, D., Schneider, T., Schermuly, R., et al.** (1996) Direct comparison of inhaled nitric oxide and aerosolized prostacyclin in acute respiratory distress syndrome. *Am. J. Respir. Crit. Care Med.* **153**: 991–996.

45. **Zwissler, B., Kemming, G., Habler, O., et al.** (1996) Inhaled prostacylin (PgI2) versus inhaled nitric oxide in adult respiratory distress syndrome. *Am. J. Respir. Crit. Care Med.* **154**: 1671–1677.

46. **Bone, R.C., Slotman, G., Maunder, R., et al.** (1989) Randomized double-blind, multicenter study of prostaglandin E1 in patients with the adult respiratory distress syndrome. Prostaglandin E1 Study Group. *Chest* **96**(1): 114–119.

47. **Zapol, W.M., Snider, M.T., Hill, D., et al.** (1979) Extracorporeal membrane oxygenation in severe acute respiratory failure. A randomized progressive study. *JAMA* **242**: 2193–2196.

48. **Morris, A.H., Wallace, C.J., Menlove, R.L., et al.** (1994) Randomized clinical trial of pressure-controlled inverse ratio ventilation and extracorporeal CO_2 removal for adult respiratory distress syndrome. *Am. J. Respir. Crit. Care Med.* **149**: 295–305.

49. **Anzueto, A., Baughman, R.P., Guntupalli, K.K., et al.** (1996) Aerosolized surfactant in adults with sepsis-induced acute respiratory distress syndrome. Exosurf Acute Respiratory Distress Syndrome Sepsis Study Group. *N. Engl. J. Med.* **334**: 1417–1421.

50. **Zapol, W.M., Falke, K.J., Hurford, W.E., et al.** (1994) Inhaling nitric oxide: a selective pulmonary vasodilator and bronchodilator. *Chest* **105**: 87S–91S.

51. **Dellinger, R.P., Zimmerman, J.L., Taylor, R.W., et al.** (1998) Effects of inhaled nitric oxide in patients with acute respiratory distress

syndrome: Results of a randomized phase II trial. Inhaled Nitric Oxide in ARDS Study Group. *Crit. Care Med.* **26:** 15–23.

52. **Hirschl, R.B., Pranikoff, T., Wise, C., et al.** (1996) Initial experience with partial liquid ventilation in adult patients with the acute respiratory distress syndrome. *JAMA* **275:** 383–389.

53. **Matthay, M.A. and Broaddus, V.C.** (1994) Fluid and hemodynamic management in acute lung injury. *Semin. Respir. Crit. Care Med.* **15:** 271–288.

54. **Bishop, M.H., Jorgens, J., Shoemaker, W.C., et al.** (1991) The relationship between ARDS, pulmonary infiltration, fluid balance, and hemodynamics in critically ill surgical patients. *Am. Surg.* **57:** 785–792.

55. **Svensson, L.G., Hess, K.R., Coselli, J.S., et al.** (1991) A prospective study of respiratory failure after high-risk surgery on the thoracoabdominal aorta. *J. Vasc. Surg.* **14:** 271–282.

56. **Fowler, A.A., Hamman, R.F., Good, J.T., et al.** (1983) Adult respiratory distress syndrome: risk with common predispositions. *Ann. Intern. Med.* **98:** 593–597.

57. **Suchyta, M.R., Clemmer, T.P., Elliott, C.G., et al.** (1992) The adult respiratory distress syn-drome. A report of survival and modifying factors. *Chest* **101:** 1074–1079.

58. **Milberg, J.A., Davis, D.R., Steinberg, K.P., et al.** (1995) Improved survival of patients with acute respiratory distress syndrome (ARDS): 1983–1993. *JAMA* **273:** 306–309.

59. **Abel, S.J., Finney, S.T., Brett, S.J., et al.** (1998) Reduced mortality in association with the acute respiratory distress syndrome (ARDS). *Thorax* **53:** 292–294.

60. **Luhr, O.R., Antonsen, K., Karlsson, M., et al.** (1999) Incidence and mortality after acute respiratory failure and acute respiratory distress syndrome in Sweden, Denmark, and Iceland. The ARF Study Group. *Am. J. Respir. Crit. Care Med.* **159:** 1849–1861.

61. **Monchi, M., Bellenfant, F., Cariou, A., et al.** (1998) Early predictive factors of survival in the acute respiratory distress syndrome. A multivariate analysis. *Am. J. Respir. Crit. Care Med.* **158:** 1076–1081.

62. **Montgomery, A.B., Stager, M.A., Carrico, C.J. and Hudson, L.D.** (1985) Causes of mortality in patients with the adult respiratory distress syndrome. *Am. Rev. Respir. Dis.* **132:** 485–489.

Chapter 15

Lung-protective ventilation strategies

Robert M. Kacmarek, PhD, RRT

Contents

Over the last 10 years much of the emphasis regarding mechanical ventilation of critically ill patients with acute lung injury (ALI) or acute respiratory distress syndrome (ARDS) has focused on lung protection, specifically, the establishment of ventilatory settings that avoid the extension of lung injury by the use of lung-protective ventilatory strategies (LPVSs). There clearly is a large quantity of data indicating that specific ventilatory strategies induce injury and affect outcome in animal models[1–10]. In addition, two recent clinical trials have established a link between outcome (death and ventilation-free days) and ventilatory strategy[11,12]. This chapter will address the concept of ventilator-induced lung injury and lung-protective ventilatory strategies.

15.1 Ventilator-induced lung injury (VILI)

Numerous terms are currently used to address specific types or causes of VILI (*Table 15.1*). Barotrauma has been used for years to define the form of VILI manifest by the movement of air out of the lung into a body space or tissue (*Figure 15.1*)[13,14]. Generally, this occurs as a result of rupture of the lung parenchyma and dissection of air via fascial planes into the pleural, mediastinal, or pericardial space[14]. Although not precisely linked to high airway pressure, barotrauma occurs most commonly in settings where severe lung disease exists along with mechanical ventilation using high alveolar pressures and large tidal volumes[13].

15.1.1 Volutrauma

VILI that results in an increase in the permeability of the alveolar capillary membrane, the development of pulmonary edema, the accumulation of neutrophils and protein within

Table 15.1 Terms used to refer to specific types of VILI

Barotrauma – Rupture of lung parenchyma resulting in gas outside the lung
Volutrauma – Injury similar to ARDS caused by overdistention
Atelectrauma – Injury similar to ARDS caused by repetitive opening and closing of unstable lung units
Biotrauma – Pulmonary inflammatory mediator activation by overdistention or inadequate PEEP

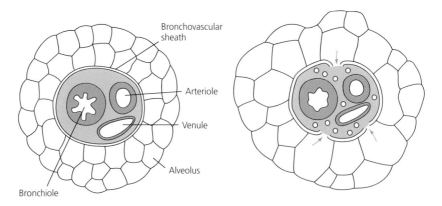

Figure 15.1 Mechanism of alveolar rupture during mechanical ventilation. Pressures between adjacent alveoli equalize rapidly, but especially in the presence of high alveolar volume, increased alveolar pressure in comparison with that in the adjacent bronchovascular sheath establishes a pressure gradient that may result in rupture of the alveolar wall, allowing passage of air into the interstitial tissue of the bronchovascular sheath. From: Maunder, R.J., Pierson, D.J. and Hudson, L.D. (1984) Subcutaneous and mediastenal emphysema: pathophysiology, diagnosis, and management. Reproduced with permission from The American Medical Association. *Arch. Intern. Med.* **144:** 1447–1453.

the lung parenchyma, the disruption of surfactant production, the development of a hyaline membrane and a decrease in compliance of the respiratory system is called volutrauma[15]. The term volutrauma is used because the primary mechanism for the development of VILI proposed by Dreyfuss and Saumon is overdistention of local lung units by high alveolar volumes associated with high alveolar pressure[15]. Webb and Tierney first demonstrated in an intact animal the effects of large tidal volumes (V_T) at high distending pressure on the development of lung injury[4]. They ventilated healthy rats with peak airway pressures of 45 cmH$_2$O and zero positive end-expiratory pressure (PEEP) (V_T of 40 mL kg^{-1}) for 60 min, resulting in gross hemorrhagic edema and decreased compliance. As noted in *Figure 15.2*, Dreyfuss *et al.* observed marked alternations at the alveolar capillary membrane after only 20 min of ventilation in rats ventilated at peak alveolar pressures of 45 cmH$_2$O (V_T 40 mL kg^{-1})

and no PEEP[5]. In fact, they demonstrated that injury was observed in minutes after the onset of the injurious ventilatory pattern. Similar injury was observed by Parker *et al.* in isolated perfused dog lungs[3]. Increasing peak alveolar pressure beyond 30 cmH$_2$O resulted in an exponential increase in capillary filtration pressure. Similar data are now available in a wide variety of animal models confirming the relationship of large distending lung volumes and VILI[15].

The single pressure most responsible for the development of VILI appears to be the transpulmonary pressure gradient[10]. In a now classic experiment, Dreyfuss *et al.* demonstrated that rats with their chest walls strapped were protected from VILI compared with those ventilated with the same peak alveolar pressure but without chest wall binding[10]. In fact, injury was similar regardless of the use of positive or negative pressure ventilation provided high transpulmonary pressures were established. As a result, higher ventilating pressures

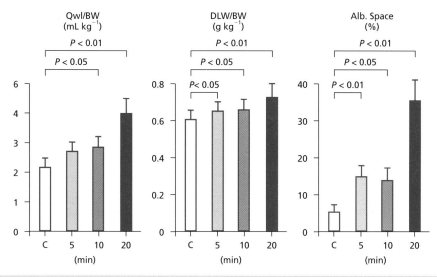

Figure 15.2 Effect of ventilation at a peak airway pressure of 45 cmH$_2$O for 5–20 min in closed-chest rats. Pulmonary edema was assessed by measuring the extravascular lung water content (Qwl/BW) and changes in permeability by determining the bloodless dry lung weight (DLW/BW), and the distribution space of ^{125}I-labeled albumin (Alb. Space) in lungs. Control rats (C) were ventilated at a peak airway pressure of 7 cmH$_2$O. Pulmonary edema developed rapidly (5 min) and was associated with changes in permeability. All the indices increased markedly after 20 min of mechanical ventilation ($P < 0.01$ versus other groups). From: Dreyfuss, D., Basset, G., Soler, P. and Saumon, G. (1985) Intermittent positive-pressure hyperventilation with high inflation pressures produces pulmonary microvascular injury in rats. Reproduced with permission from *Am. Rev. Respir. Dis.* 132: 880–884.

can be used in the presence of a decreased chest wall compliance without the development of VILI, as the decreased chest wall compliance results in lower tidal volumes at a given peak alveolar pressure.

In addition to causing injury in healthy animal models, inappropriate ventilatory patterns can extend injury in animals presenting with lung injury[16]. Again in rats, Dreyfuss *et al.* demonstrated increased extravascular lung water and distribution of albumin within the lung parenchyma within 2 min of ventilation at 45 cmH$_2$O peak alveolar pressure[16].

15.1.2 PEEP effects

As noted in *Figure 15.3*, a PEEP of 10 cmH$_2$O in spite of a peak airway pressure of 45 cmH$_2$O decreased the level of VILI compared with similar animals with the same peak pressure but zero PEEP[4]. Only mild interstitial edema developed in the animal with 10 cmH$_2$O PEEP. Similar findings have been reported by Corbridge *et al.* in dogs with hydrochloric acid-induced lung injury[17]. Dogs ventilated with 12.5 cmH$_2$O PEEP and a V$_T$ of 15 mL kg^{-1} after lung injury had much lower wet lung weight and dry lung weight to body weight ratios at autopsy than dogs ventilated with 3.2 cmH$_2$O PEEP and 30 mL kg^{-1}, in spite of the fact that peak alveolar pressure (33 cmH$_2$O) was the same during the 5 h of ventilation.

Other groups have also shown in various animal models that PEEP has a protective effect on the development or extension of lung injury. Dreyfuss and Saumon, in healthy rats, showed that the beneficial effects of PEEP on reducing the extent of lung injury could be minimized by the administration of dopamine[16]. They argued that part of the reduction of edema formation with PEEP was a direct result of cardiac output reduction and decreased pulmonary perfusion. Recent data from Broccard *et al.* also point to a relationship between pulmonary vascular flow and VILI[18]. This group studied the effect of three levels of constant intravenous infusion and two levels of end-inspiratory plateau pressure (P$_{plat}$) at zero PEEP. Isolated rabbit lungs receiving 900 mL min^{-1} of perfusion at a P$_{plat}$ of 30 cmH$_2$O demonstrated the greatest decrease in lung compliance, the highest level of alveolar hemorrhage, and the greatest weight gain as compared with animals receiving 300 mL min^{-1} perfusion at P$_{plat}$ of 30 cmH$_2$O or 500 mL min^{-1} perfusion at P$_{plat}$ of 15 cmH$_2$O. These data support the suggestion that PEEP protects the lung by decreasing vascular flow.

Although vascular flow may affect the level of VILI, the data from Muscedere *et al.* support the independent effect of PEEP on the development of VILI[19]. This group studied the effect of PEEP in an *ex vivo* rat lung model on the development of VILI. Four groups were compared (*Figure 15.4*): PEEP of 0 cmH$_2$O (peak pressure 30 cmH$_2$O), PEEP less than P$_{flle}$ (4 cmH$_2$O, peak pressure 26 cmH$_2$O), PEEP greater than P$_{flle}$ (15 cmH$_2$O, peak pressure

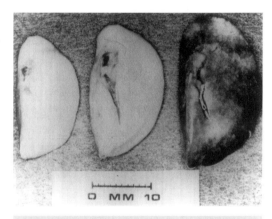

Figure 15.3 Comparison of left lungs excised from rats ventilated with peak pressure of 14 cmH$_2$O, zero positive end-expiratory pressure (PEEP); peak pressure of 45 cmH$_2$O, 10 cmH$_2$O PEEP; and peak pressure 45 cmH$_2$O, zero PEEP (left to right). The perivascular groove is distended with edema in the lungs from rats ventilated with peak pressure of 45 cmH$_2$O and 10 cmH$_2$O PEEP. The lung ventilated at 45 cmH$_2$O and zero PEEP is grossly hemorrhaged.From: Webb, H.H. and Tierney, D. (1974) Experimental pulmonary edema due to intermittent positive pressure ventilation, with high inflation pressures, protection by positive end-expiratory pressure. Reproduced with permission from *Am. Rev. Respir. Dis.* **110**: 556–565.

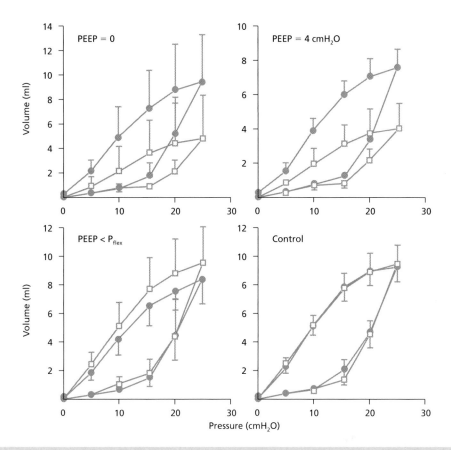

Figure 15.4 Composite pressure–volume curves before (circles) and after (squares) *ex vivo* ventilation with different levels of positive end-expiratory pressure (PEEP). From: Muscedere, J.F., Mullen, B.M., Gan, K. and Slutsky, A.S. (1994) Tidal ventilation at low airway pressures can augment lung injury. Reproduced with permission from *Am. J. Respir. Crit. Care Med.* **149**: 1327–1334.

32 cmH$_2$O), and PEEP of 4 cmH$_2$O (control, no ventilation), where P$_{flle}$ is the inflection point on the inspiratory pressure–volume (P–V) curve of the lung. Following a 2 h ventilation period, animals in the PEEP greater than P$_{flle}$ group demonstrated no change in compliance (similar to control animals), whereas the PEEP of 0 cmH$_2$O and PEEP less than P$_{flle}$ groups showed a marked decrease in compliance.

15.1.3 Mechanism for PEEP protection

Although the precise mechanics by which PEEP attenuates VILI is still unclear, the most plausible cause was described by Mead *et al*. in 1970 using mechanical and mathematical models[20]. Using the formula

$$P_{eff} = P_{appl} (V/V_o)^{2/3}$$

where P$_{eff}$ is the effective stress pressure across the alveolar wall, P$_{appl}$ is applied alveolar pressure, V is final alveolar volume and V$_o$ is initial alveolar volume, they argued that stress pressure much greater than the pressure applied to adjacent alveoli would be experienced by collapsed alveoli. They predicted, on the basis of the above formula and the model in *Figure 15.5*, that an alveolar pressure of 35 cmH$_2$O would result in stress pressure across the wall of a collapsed alveolus greater than 150 cmH$_2$O. As noted in *Figure 15.5*, as the central collapsed alveolus is expanded the pressure within this alveolus is increased but when

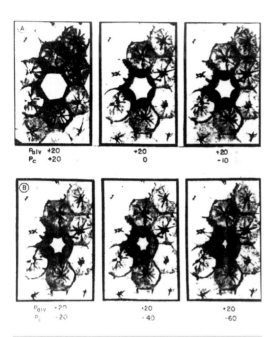

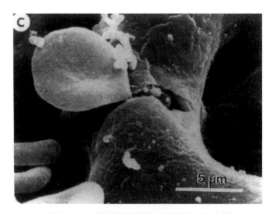

Figure 15.6 Scanning electron micrograph showing disruption of the blood–gas barrier with a red blood cell protruding from the fracture of a rabbit lung perfused at 20 cmH$_2$O transpulmonary pressure and 52.5 cmH$_2$O transmural pressure. From: Fu, Z., Costello, M.L., Tsukimoto, K., *et al.* (1992) High lung volume increases stress failure in pulmonary capillaries. Reproduced with permission from *J. Appl. Physiol.* **73:** 123–133.

Figure 15.5 Cross-sectional configuration and pressure within central unit (P$_c$) of a balloon model of the lung at several central unit balloon volumes, while pressure in surrounding units (P$_{alv}$) is held constant at 20 cmH$_2$O. From: Mead, J., Takishima, T. and Leith, D. (1970) Stress distribution in lungs: a model of pulmonary elasticity. Reproduced with permission from *J. Appl. Physiol.* **28:** 596–608.

totally collapsed a large stress pressure gradient exists across adjacent alveolar walls. It is the repetitive opening and closing of these unstable lung units with each breath that contributes to VILI. This type of VILI is referred to as atelectrauma. PEEP is thus believed to attenuate lung injury by preventing the recruitment and derecruitment of these unstable lung units. Thus, the most appropriate PEEP level is one that maintains lung units open at end exhalation.

15.1.4 Translocation of cells

In addition to the injury already described, data from Fu *et al.* (*Figure 15.6*) clearly indicate that high lung volumes and low PEEP levels in animals result in fractures of the capillary walls.[21] If this is true in humans, cells and other substances can migrate from the

lung into systemic circulation. In fact, two studies in large animal models have clearly demonstrated that animals with their lung inoculated with bacteria and then ventilated with a high V$_T$ and low PEEP developed bacteremia whereas those animals ventilated with a low V$_T$ and high PEEP did not develop bacteremia[22,23].

15.1.5 Inflammatory mediator production

Cytokines and other mediators direct recruitment and activation of neutrophils at the alveolar level. These molecules are associated with inflammation and severe disruption of normal lung function[24]. Increasing data are now available to support the hypothesis that the mechanical stress of inappropriate application of mechanical ventilation activates inflammatory mediators in the lung[25–30]. Tremblay *et al.* in an *ex vivo* healthy and injured rat lung model, demonstrated that both pro- and anti-inflammatory mediators are activated by ventilatory patterns associated with high peak alveolar pressure causing overdistention and zero PEEP (*Figure 15.7*)[29]. In those animals in

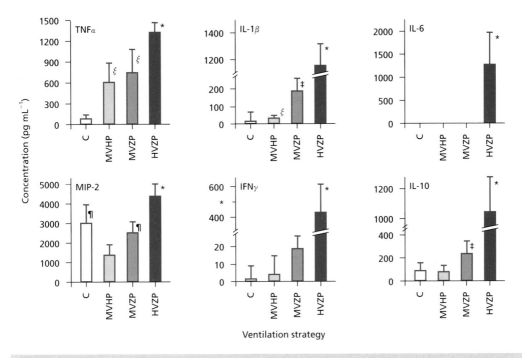

Figure 15.7 Effect of ventilation strategy on absolute lung lavage cytokine concentration for animals previously lung injured with lipopolyaccharide injection. (C, control; MVHP, moderate volume, high PEEP; MVZP, moderate volume, zero PEEP; HVZP, high volume, zero PEEP: TNFα, tumor necrosis factor alpha; IL-1β, interleukin-1β; MIP-2 IFNγ, immune interferon.) The pattern of lavage cytokines seen in response to ventilation strategy was similar to the saline-treated groups except for MIP-2, in which the control group (C) has comparable levels with the MVZP group (both increased significantly versus the MVHP group). *$P < 0.05$ versus C, MVHP, MVHP; ‡$P < 0.05$ versus C, MVHP; ζ$P < 0.05$ versus C; ¶$P < 0.05$ vs MVHP. From: Tremblay, L., Valenza, F., Riberiro, S., *et al.* (1997) Injurious ventilatory strategies increases cytokines and c-fos mRNA expression in an isolated rat lung model. *J. Clin. Invest.* **99:** 944–952.

which PEEP was set greater than P_{flle} and overdistention was avoided, minimal mediator activation was observed. Similar data were reported by Bethmann *et al.* in an *ex vivo* perfused mouse lung model[26]. Hyperventilation at 2.5 times normal transpulmonary pressure using either positive or negative pressure ventilation resulted in a 1.75-fold increased expression of tumor necrosis factor alpha (TNFα) and interleukin-6 messenger RNA (mRNA). Imai *et al.*[28] and Takata *et al.*[30] noted greater TNFα mRNA expression with conventional ventilation at low peak pressures (30 cmH₂O) but low PEEP (5 cmH₂O) as compared with high-frequency oscillation at a mean airway pressure of 15 cmH₂O (same as with

conventional ventilation). Ranieri *et al.* showed the same effect of ventilatory pattern on pulmonary lavage and serum TNFα level in ARDS patients[31]. In a randomized comparison, patients ventilated with PEEP set greater than P_{flle} and peak alveolar pressure kept below the upper inflection point of the pressure–volume curve had a decrease in lung lavage and serum TNFα after 36 h. Patients randomized to PEEP based on oxygenation and V_T set to produce eucapnia increased TNFα levels after 36 h. These data support the contention that inappropriate ventilatory patterns result in increased expression of pro- and anti-inflammatory mediators leading to increasing lung inflammation and dysfunction.

15.1.6 Multiorgan system failure

Both Drefuss and Saumon[32] and Slutsky and Tremblay[33] have proposed that VILI may cause or extend the level of multiple system organ failure (MSOF). As noted in the previous discussion, an inappropriate ventilatory pattern can induce both mechanical failure of the lung and the release of inflammatory mediators. These inflammatory mediators can move from the lung into the systemic circulation via fractures in pulmonary capillaries and affect organ systems external to the lung. Although this is speculative, the evidence in animal models clearly indicates it is plausible. In fact, the lung may be the engine in many settings that drives the extent of MSOF[33].

15.2 Lung-protective ventilatory strategies (LPVSs)

As already defined, an LPVS primarily consists of a ventilatory strategy that avoids over-distention and repetitive collapse of unstable lung units. However, an increasingly important aspect of an LPVS primarily studied in laboratory models is the need to recruit the lung, that is to open collapsed, atelectatic lung units before applying an LPVS.

15.2.1 P–V curve

Much of the approach to an LPVS is based conceptually on the implications of the inflation and deflation P–V curves of the respiratory system. As noted in *Figure 15.8*, two points on the inspiratory P–V curve are commonly referred to during LPVS; the P_{flle} and the upper inflection point (UIP). The P_{flle} is believed to be the airway pressure where significant recruitment begins and the UIP the airway pressure where the rate of recruitment decreases and overdistention of select lung units begins. It should, however, be emphasized that some ARDS patients do not demonstrate a P_{flle} because of markedly nonhomogeneous distribution of lung disease. Generally, LPVSs have focused on ventilating between these two pressures, that is, setting PEEP above P_{flle} and maintaining peak alveolar pressure (end-inspiratory plateau pressure) below the UIP. The point of maximum compliance change (PMC) on the deflation limb has been referred to as the pressure where derecruitment begins. However, the inflation and deflation curves are different, primarily as a result of hysteresis. This means that the lung volume maintained at a given pressure is greater on the deflation than on the inflation limb. If the lung is fully recruited (sufficient airway pressure applied to open collapsed lung units) and PEEP is applied without ventilator circuit discontinuation, the volume maintained at end exhalation is greater following recruitment than without a lung recruitment maneuver (RM) even if the same PEEP level is applied.

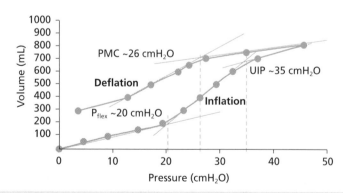

Figure 15.8 Ideal pressure–volume curve of the respiratory system in ARDS, determined with a peak pressure of 45 cmH$_2$O. P_{flex}, lower inflection point; UIP, upper inflection point; PMC, point of maximum curvature on the deflation limb.

15.2.2 Clinical data

There are five prospective, randomized clinical trails comparing conventional ventilatory strategies with LPVSs[11,12,34–36]. In each of these trials a low tidal volume was compared with a larger tidal volume. However, in all trials the strategy for setting PEEP was the same in the control and treatment groups, except for the Amato et al.[11] trial (*Table 15.2*). That trial used the results of a prerandomization P–V curve to identify PEEP level (P_{flle} + 2 cmH_2O) and determine maximum end-inspiratory plateau pressure. In addition, the Amato et al. trial was the only trial that used recruitment maneuvers: 35–40 cmH_2O CPAP for 30–40 s before setting PEEP and whenever the patient was disconnected from the ventilator. All other approaches to ventilator management were similar across both groups in all five studies.

Table 15.3 lists the mortality and number of subjects from each trial. Only two of the five trials were positive, with lower mortality in the treatment (LPVS) group than in the control group. The other three studies demonstrated similar mortality, although a strong trend for better outcome in the control group existed in the Brochard et al. trial[36].

To understand why these differences existed and derive a recommended approach to ventilating ARDS patients from these data, careful comparison of actual data for V_T, plateau pressure (P_{plat}) and PEEP in each trial group (*Figure 15.9*) must be performed and compared with the actual protocols for each trial (*Table 15.3*). As noted in *Table 15.3*, by design large differences in V_T and as a result P_{plat} between groups should have occurred in each trial; however, actual data in *Figure 15.9* would indicate that only in the Amato et al.[11] and NIH (ARD-

Snet)[12] trials were protocolized differences in V_T and P_{plat} between groups maintained. In all three of the other trials only small difference existed in V_T and P_{plat} between control and LPVS groups. As a result, the V_T difference signal may have been insufficient in the Brochard et al.[36], Stewart et al.[35], and Brower et al.[34] trials to produce an effect on outcome, whereas in the NIH[12] and Amato et al.[11] trials much larger difference in V_T and P_{plat} were maintained. In fact, in these trials over the first 7 days V_T values of 6 and 12 mL kg^{-1} were maintained in the two groups. However, the question to be asked is why the NIH[12] trial required about 425 patients in each group to demonstrate a significant difference in mortality between groups when the Amato et al.[11] trial was able to demonstrate a difference in mortality with only 29 patients in the LPVS group and only 24 patients in the control group. The answer to this may be in the approach to setting PEEP.

As noted in *Table 15.3* and *Figure 15.9*, the Amato et al.[11] trial was the only trial that used a different approach to setting PEEP in each group, and maintained the difference throughout the trial. In the Amato LPVS group, initial PEEP was about 16 cmH_2O and tended to decrease over time. In the Amato control group, and in the LPVS and control groups of the other four trials (*Figure 15.9*), a low PEEP level (8–10 cmH_2O) was used throughout the first week of the trial. It appears reasonable to argue that the much smaller number of patients needed in the Amato trial versus the NIH trial to achieve significance was a result of the high PEEP used in the Amato LPVS group. Two additional factors were different in the Amato LPVS group compared with all other

Table 15.2 LPVS trials outcome mortality

	Amato[11]	Stewart[35]	Brochard[36]	Brower[34]	NIH[12]
LPVS	38% (29)*	46% (60)	47% (58)	50% (26)	31% (429)†
Control	71% (24)	48% (60)	38% (58)	46% (26)	40% (432)

*$P < 0.002$; †$P = 0.0054$.
Values are percentages of patient dying, with number of patients in that group given in parentheses.

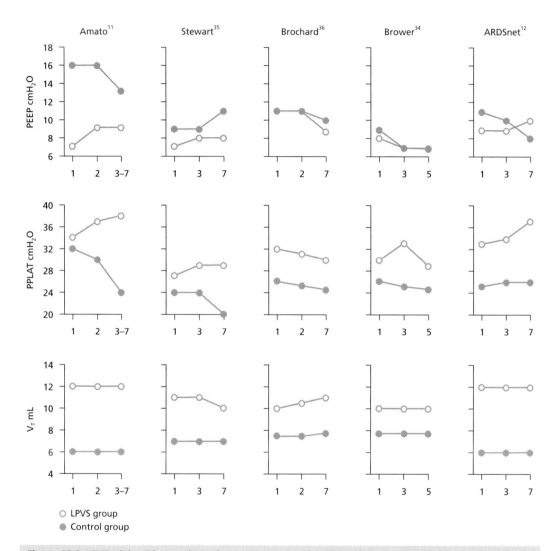

Figure 15.9 LPVS trials with actual V_T, plateau pressure and PEEP levels in the LPVS groups and control groups.

groups in the five trials: lung recruitment and the use of pressure control ventilation. On the basis of other available data, mode of ventilation is unlikely to have had an impact on mortality; however, as discussed in the next section, lung recruitment and high PEEP tend to be most effective when used together.

Much criticism regarding the high mortality in the Amato[11] control group (71%) has been raised. However, as noted in *Table 15.4*, although the patients were younger in the

Amato trial than in any of the other trials they also had a greater number of organ system failures (3.6) compared with the other trials. As a result, on the basis of historical data, one would expect a high rate of mortality in the Amato control groups.

15.2.3 Ventilation guidelines (*Table 15.5*)
On the basis of the above data V_T in ALI or ARDS should be maintained at about 6 mL kg^{-1} (8–4 mL kg^{-1}) with end-inspiratory plateau

Table 15.3 LPVS trials: protocols

	Amato[11]		Stewart[35]		Brochard[36]		Brower[34]		NIH[12]	
	LPVS	Control	LPVS	Control	LPVS	Control	LPVS	Control	LPVS	Control
V_T (mL kg^{-1})	<6	12	<8	10–15	7	10–15	8	10–12	6	12
Pressure Limit (cmH$_2$O)	PIP 40	No limit	PIP 30	PIP 50	P_{plat} 25	PIP 60	P_{plat} 30	P_{plat} 45	P_{plat} 30	P_{plat} 50
PEEP	P_{flex} + 2 cmH$_2$O	Based on oxygenation	Both based on oxygenation		Both based on oxygenation		Both set by F$_i$O$_2$/PEEP Table		Both set by F$_i$O$_2$/PEEP Table	

Table 15.4 LPVS trials: number of organ system failures and age

	Amato[11]		Stewart[35]		Brochard[36]		Brower[34]		NIH[12]	
	LPVS	Control	LPVS	Control	LPVS	Control	LPVS	Control	LPVS	Control
Age	33±13	36±14	59±17	58±19	57±15	56±15	50±14	47±17	51±17	52±18
No.	3.6±1.3	3.6±1.5	1.4±1.0	1.3±1.2	1.3±0.6	1.3±0.7	NA	NA	2.8±1.1	2.8±1.0

No. is total number of organ system failures. Age in years.

Table 15.5 Ventilatory settings in ARDS

V_T	6 mL kg^{-1} (range 4–8 mL kg^{-1})
Rate	25–35 min^{-1} (limit rate based on development of auto PEEP)
Inspiratory time	<1.0 s controlled and assisted ventilation
Mode	Pressure or volume assist/control (my preference pressure A/C)
PEEP	15 cmH$_2$O (10–20 cmH$_2$O) (set to prevent derecruitment after a lung recruitment maneuver)
F$_I$O$_2$	<0.6 if possible (set to achieve target PaO$_2$ 55–80 mmHg)

Recruitment at initiation of ventilation and whenever lung derecruited.

pressure less than 30 cmH$_2$O. To maintain an adequate level of ventilation, respiratory rate must be increased, frequently into the upper twenties per minute (25–35 min^{-1}). Respiratory rate is generally limited to the highest rate that does not cause auto-PEEP. Mode of ventilation is based on clinician preference. With either pressure or volume ventilation a V_T of 6 mL kg^{-1} can be targeted. There are no convincing data supporting extending inspiratory time to establish an inverse I:E ratio[37]. Particularly with high rates inspiratory time needs to be short (≤1.5 s) during controlled ventilation and even shorter (<1.0 s) during assisted ventilation. Sufficient PEEP should be set to prevent end-expiratory collapse of unstable lung units. Generally, in adults with ARDS this is about 15 cmH$_2$O, ranging in most patients between 10 and 20 cmH$_2$O (see later sections). F$_I$O$_2$ is set to maintain the target PaO$_2$ (55–80 mmH$_2$O) after PEEP is set. Ideally, F$_I$O$_2$ should be less than 0.6. I would also recommend the use of recruitment maneuvers at the onset of an LPVS and whenever derecruitment occurs (see later section). It should be remembered that the NIH trial determined that a 6 mL kg^{-1} V_T is better than a 12 mL kg^{-1} V_T but did not test any other aspect of ventilatory support.

15.2.4 Permissive hypercapnia

Because ALI or ARDS patients are ventilated with small V_T values, and as their overall dead space to tidal volume ratio is commonly elevated, maintaining a normal PaCO$_2$ in spite of increased respiratory rates is difficult. In some patients it becomes impossible to maintain the PaCO$_2$ without increasing V_T and P$_{plat}$. As a result, permissive hypercapnia becomes the only option. That is, permissive hypercapnia should not be the desired outcome but the only acceptable outcome considering the pathophysiology of the patient and the need for an LPVS[38].

Generally, problems with permissive hypercapnia are not related to the PaCO$_2$, but to pH and the effect pH has on other organ system function. That is, an otherwise healthy chest trauma patient may easily tolerate a pH of 7.2 as a result of permissive hypercapnia, whereas a patient with sepsis and poor myocardial function may not tolerate a pH of 7.3. Clearly, patients with sepsis and metabolic acidosis, increased intracranial pressure, myocardial dysfunction, and renal failure may not tolerate the acidosis associated with the rapid development of permissive hypercapnia[38]. However, most patients will tolerate moderate permission hypercapnia (PaCO$_2$ 50–60 mmHg) if it is allowed to develop slowly enough to insure the kidneys can compensate for the respiratory acidosis[39]. A PaCO$_2$ rise of 1 mmHg per hour or two in the appropriate patient is usually well tolerated[40].

15.2.5 Lung recruitment

Lung recruitment maneuvers are the application of an airway pressure higher than that used to ventilate patients for a short period of time, to open collapsed lung. Lung recruitment is not new and has been frequently proposed as part of the initial establishment of high-frequency oscillation[41]. The use of lung recruitment maneuvers (RM) during conventional ventilation can be credited to Amato *et al.* in their LPVS trial[11].

Lungs are recruited because the collapsed lung requires greater pressure to ventilate, increases the risk of VILI (repetitive opening and closing), requires a high F_iO_2, depresses surfactant production, and increases the likelihood of nosocomial pneumonia[32,33,41]. Numerous animal studies illustrate the ability of an RM to markedly elevate PaO_2 and to sustain the elevated PaO_2 level over time with appropriate PEEP (*Figure 15.10*)[42–46]. In otherwise healthy, anesthetized, supine individuals 40 cmH_2O CPAP sustained for 7–15 s is required to open atelectasis areas[47], whereas, in alert and healthy individuals, Greaves *et al.* indicated that 30 cmH_2O transpulmonary pressure is required to reverse atelectasis[48]. Upwards to 60 cmH_2O have been required in animal models of ARDS to recruit atelectatic lung[42,43]. In patients, Gattinoni *et al.* reported needing 46 cmH_2O peak airway pressure to fully recruit lung[49], and in a single patient case report Medoff *et al.* reported the need for 60 cmH_2O (PEEP 40 cmH_2O, pressure control 20 cmH_2O, I:E 1:1,

rate 10 min⁻¹ for 2 min) to recruit the lung of a young septic patient[50].

The greatest concerns during a recruitment maneuver are barotrauma, hemodynamic compromise, and arterial desaturation. As a result, very careful monitoring of the cardiopulmonary system during and after the recruitment maneuver is required (*Table 15.6*). Any time a patient becomes unstable or meets monitoring thresholds the recruitment maneuver should be immediately discontinued.

On the basis of available patient data, recruitment maneuvers performed to a maximum pressure of 40 cmH_2O appear to be safe[11,47–51]. However, patients selected for RM should not have an existing pneumothorax or a high probability of developing a pneumothorax (severe COPD, pulmonary cysts or blebs), and should be hemodynamically stable with adequate fluid balance. Ideally, RM should be performed early in the course of ALI or ARDS. Although data are not yet available, it seems reasonable to assume that fibrotic lung in late ARDS is not as recruitable as atelectatic lung in early ARDS.

Recruitment maneuvers should always be performed with the mechanical ventilator, as disconnection of a manual ventilator and reconnection to the ICU ventilator can result in derecruitment. In addition, in CPAP or pressure ventilation the target pressure is maintained, as additional volume is provided to accommodate the recruited lung volume. I would recommend first trying an RM at 30 cmH_2O CPAP for 30–40 s. If this is well tolerated, elevate the CPAP level to 35 then

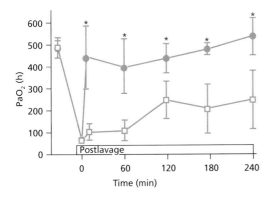

Figure 15.10 Arterial oxygen tension (PaO_2) median ±95% confidence interval for the recruitment maneuver group and control group in lavage injured rabbits. RM consists of 30 cmH_2O CPAP for 30 s. PEEP set above P_{flex} in both groups. *$P < 0.05$. From: Rimensberger, P.C., Cox, P.N., Frndova, H., *et al.* (1999) The open lung during small tidal volume ventilation: concepts of recruitment and optimal PEEP. *Crit. Care Med.* **27**: 1946–1952.

Table 15.6 Monitoring during recruitment maneuvers[47]

Abort RM if:
- Mean arterial pressure <60 mmHg or decreased by >20 mmHg
- SpO_2 <85%
- Heart rate >140 min⁻¹ or <60 min⁻¹
- New arrthythmias develop

40 cmH$_2$O. As indicated, few patient data are available at greater than 40 cmH$_2$O RM pressure[49,50]. However, in many animal models, up to 60 cmH$_2$O is required to recruit the lung[42,43,46] and multiple RM are needed to maximize the recruiting effect[43,46,51]. Finally, before any recruitment maneuver the patient should be stabilized on 100% oxygen.

15.3 Setting of PEEP

In patients with ARDS PEEP should always be set at the minimal level maintaining the PaO$_2$ following recruitment. To determine this level, first maximally recruit the lung. Then set PEEP at a level higher than anticipated (20 cmH$_2$O), after which decrease the F$_I$O$_2$ until the SpO$_2$ is 90–95%. Following stabilization slowly decrease the PEEP in 2 cmH$_2$O increment (every 15–20 min) until the patient desaturates (SpO$_2$ < 90%). The PEEP level just preceding desaturation is the ideal PEEP level: the lowest PEEP maintaining the oxygenation response of the RM. The lung should then again be recruited and PEEP set at the identified level. To insure maximum recruitment is maintained, PEEP should be decreased from a level higher than needed rather than increased from a level lower than required. Whatever the method used for setting PEEP, if the oxygenation benefit of the recruitment maneuver is lost over time the PEEP level is inadequate. Rerecruit the lung and set the PEEP at a high level.

During weaning of F$_I$O$_2$ and PEEP, F$_I$O$_2$ should always be weaned before PEEP and PEEP not weaned until the F$_I$O$_2$ is less than 0.5. If during the weaning of PEEP oxygenation decreases, the PEEP should always be restored. A decreased oxygenation during PEEP decrease always reflects derecruitment and requires reestablishment of PEEP.

15.4 Prone positioning

Prone positioning recruits lung of ALI or ARDS patients, resulting in a PaO$_2$ increase of 20 mmHg or more in 75% or more of patients[52–57]. Although the precise mechanism for improve-

ment in PaO$_2$ is still controversial, the overall benefits of prone position are essentially a result of improved ventilation–perfusion matching in the prone versus the supine position[58–61]. A more uniform transpulmonary pressure gradient exists in the prone versus the supine position, resulting in a greater distribution of ventilation to dependent lung in the prone position and better matching with perfusion[59,61]. Table 15.7 summarizes the mechanisms that contribute to better distribution of ventilation to dependent lung in the prone position.

15.4.1 Clinical response

The most detailed clinical study of prone positioning is that of Chatte *et al.*[52], who presented a case series of 32 consecutive patients with ALI or ARDS and PaO$_2$/F$_I$O$_2$ ratios of less than 150 mmHg. A total of 25 of 32 patients (78%) responded to prone positioning. However, as noted in *Figure 15.11*, the benefit of prone positioning on oxygenation did not persist in all patients. Chatte *et al.* categorized some patients as persistent responders (oxygenation benefit persisted after return to the supine position), non-persistent responders (oxygenation benefit lost after return to the supine position), and non-responders to prone positioning. No data

Table 15.7 Potential mechanisms for improved PaO$_2$ in the prone position

Ventilation effects
- More homogeneous pleural pressure gradient
- Smaller percentage of lung dependent (triangular shape of lung)
- Less gravitational effect from heart or great vessels
- Altered shape of the thorax or decreased thoracic compliance
- Increased functional residual capacity (FRC)
- Mobilization of secretions

Perfusion effect
- Less dependent perfusion in prone position

Overall effect: improved ventilation–perfusion ratio ($\dot{V}/\dot{Q}$)

From: Kacmarek, R.M. and Schwartz, D. (2000) Lung recruitment. *Respir. Clin. N. Am.* **6:** 597–623. Reproduced with permission from W.B. Saunders.

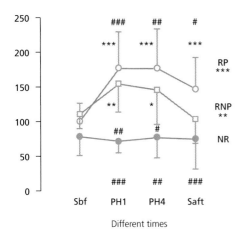

Different times

Figure 15.11 Evolution of PaO$_2$/F$_I$O$_2$ before, during, and after the first 4 h of a prone trial in different groups. Sbf, 1 h before prone; PH1, first hour during prone; PH4, fourth hour during prone; Saft, 1 h after returning to supine; NR, nonresponders; RNP, responders nonpersistent; RP, responders persistent. Results among the four times (ANOVA) are indicated with larger asterisk than results between PH1, PH4, and Saft to Sbf (*t*-test). *$P < 0.05$; **$P < 0.01$; ***$P < 0.001$. From: Chatte, G., Sab, J.M., Dubois, J.M., *et al.* (1997) Prone position in mechanically ventilated patients with severe acute respiratory failure. Reproduced with permission from *Am. J. Respir. Crit. Care Med.* **155**: 473–478.

are available to prospectively differentiate patients into the three categories but it seems most likely that patients with well-defined dependent atelectasis or consolidation in the supine position respond well to prone positioning whereas those with a more generalized pattern of atelectasis or consolidation are least likely to respond. However, data from Pelosi *et al.*[57] indicate that patients whose chest wall compliance decreases with prone positioning are most likely to respond to prone positioning. In some patients a large quantity of secretions is removed when placed prone[58]. As a result, their oxygenation remains improved when returned to the supine position.

15.4.2 Risks of prone positioning
Placing critically ill patients in the prone position is not without risks (*Table 15.8*). The most

Table 15.8 Risks associated with prone positioning

- Hemodynamic instability
- Cardiac arrhythmias
- Arterial desaturation
- Vascular line occlusion or loss
- Inadvertent endotracheal extubation
- Dependent edema (facial edema)
- Apical atelectasis
- Skin breakdown

severe risk is the loss of the artificial airway or vascular lines. Although these are significant risks, they can be avoided by appropriate care during positioning. Hemodynamic instability and desaturation are also potential problems. However, they generally can be avoided by appropriate fluid balance before positioning. Skin breakdown and facial edema are the most distressing concerns of family, and family members should be alerted to these expected sequelae before patients are positioned prone.

15.4.3 Prone positioning and lung protection
At least one animal study indicates that prone positioning results in less VILI than supine positioning[62]. In addition, prone positioning results in less need for F$_I$O$_2$ and PEEP, and lung recruitment maneuvers in animal models work better in the prone than the supine position[63]. The prone position should be an integral part of an LPVS. Prone positioning should be considered in any ALI or ARDS patient requiring greater than 60% O$_2$ after RMs and appropriate adjustment of PEEP. As with other LPVSs, the earlier in the course of the disease they are implemented the greater the likelihood for success.

15.4.4 How long to position prone
Few data on how long to maintain patients prone are available. However, if prone positioning continues to demonstrate a positive response, why move the patient back to the supine position except for nursing care? *Figure 15.12*, from Fridrich *et al.*[64], illustrates the continued benefit of 20 h per day of prone positioning. This appears to be the ideal length of

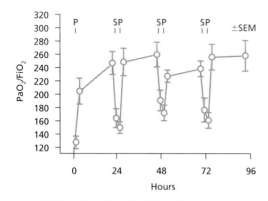

Figure 15.12 Course of PaO_2/F_iO_2 ratios during four consecutive 24 h periods of prone positioning. In each period patients were prone (P) 20 h and supine (S) 4 h. From: Fridrich, P., Krafft, P., Hochleuthner, H., et al. (1996) The effects of long-term prone positioning in patients with trauma-induced adult respiratory distress syndrome. *Anesth. Analg.* **83**: 1206–1211.

time to maintain patients prone. The 4 h supine positioning period is generally sufficient for nursing care.

15.5 Summary

It is increasingly clear that the approach to mechanical ventilation does affect outcome in ARDS. From the onset of mechanical ventilation an LPVS should be employed. This strategy is characterized by low V_T, high PEEP following lung recruitment, and prone positioning. The critical concepts of this approach are to avoid overdistention, opening the lung and keeping it open.

References

1. **Egan, A.** (1982) Lung inflation, lung solute permeability, and alveolar edema. *J. Appl. Physiol.* **53**: 121–125.

2. **Hernandez, L.A., Coker, P.J., May, S., et al.** (1990) Mechanical ventilation increases microvascular permeability in oleic acid-injured lungs. *J. Appl. Physiol.* **69**: 2057–2061.

3. **Parker, J.C., Hernandez, L.A., Longenecker, G.L., et al.** (1990) Lung edema caused by high peak inspiratory pressures in dogs. *Am. Rev. Respir. Dis.* **142**: 321–328.

4. **Webb, H.H. and Tierney, D.** (1974) Experimental pulmonary edema due to intermittent positive pressure ventilation, with high inflation pressures, protection by positive end-expiratory pressure. *Am. Rev. Respir. Dis.* **110**: 556–565.

5. **Dreyfuss, D., Basset, G., Soler, P. and Saumon, G.** (1985) Intermittent positive-pressure hyperventilation with high inflation pressures produces pulmonary microvascular injury in rats. *Am. Rev. Respir. Dis.* **132**: 880–884.

6. **Kolobow, T., Moretti, M.P., Fumagalli, R., et al.** (1987) Severe impairment in lung function induced by high peak airway pressure during mechanical ventilation. *Am. Rev. Respir. Dis.* **135**: 312–315.

7. **Tsuno, K., Miura, K., Takeya, M., et al.** (1991) Histopathologic pulmonary changes from mechanical ventilation at high peak airway pressures. *Am. Rev. Respir. Dis.* **143**: 1115–1120.

8. **Wyszogrodski, I., Kyei-Aboagye, K., Taeusch, H.W. and Avery M.** (1975) Surfactant inactivation by hyperventilation: conservation by end-expiratory pressure. *J. Appl. Physiol.* **38**: 461–466.

9. **Albert, R.K., Lakshminarayan, S., Hilderbandt, J., et al.** (1979) Increased surface tension favors pulmonary edema formation in anesthetized dogs' lung. *J. Clin. Invest.* **63**: 1015–1018.

10. **Dreyfuss, D., Soler, P., Basset, G. and Saumon, G.** (1988) High inflation pressure pulmonary edema: respective effects of high airway pressure, high tidal volume, and positive end-expiratory pressure. *Am. Rev. Respir. Dis.* **137**: 1159–1164.

11. **Amato, M.B.P., Barbas, C.S.V., Medeiros, D.M., et al.** (1998) Effect of protective-ventilation strategy on mortality in the acute respiratory distress syndrome. *N. Engl. J. Med.* **338**: 347–354.

12. **ARDSnet** (2000) Ventilation with lower tidal volume as compared with traditional tidal volume for acute lung injury and the acute respiratory distress syndrome. *N. Engl. J. Med.* **342**: 1301–1308.

13. **Pierson, D.J.** (1995) Barotrauma and bronchopleural fistula. In: *Principles and Practice of Mechanical Ventilation* (ed. M.J. Tobin). McGraw–Hill, New York, pp. 813–836.

14. **Maunder, R.J., Pierson, D.J. and Hudson, L.D.** (1984) Subcutaneous and mediastenal emphysema: pathophysiology, diagnosis, and management. *Arch. Intern. Med.* **144**: 1447–1453.

15. **Dreyfuss, D. and Saumon, G.** (1998) Ventilator induced lung injury: Lessons from experimental studies. *Am. J. Respir. Crit. Care Med.* **157**: 294–323.

16. **Dreyfuss, D., Soler, P. and Saumon, G.** (1995) Mechanical ventilation-induced pulmonary edema: interaction with previous lung alterations. *Am. J. Respir. Crit. Care Med.* **151**: 1568–1575.

17. **Corbridge, T.C., Wood, D.H., Crawford, G.P.** (1990) Adverse effects of large tidal volume and low PEEP in caine acid aspiration. *Am Rev. Respir. Dis.* **142**: 311–315.

18. **Broccard, A.F., Hotchkiss, J.R., Kuwayama, N., et al.** (1998) Consequences of vascular flow on lung injury induced by mechanical ventilation. *Am. J. Respir. Crit. Care Med.* **157**: 1935–1942.

19. **Muscedere, J.F., Mullen, B.M., Gan, K. and Slutsky, A.S.** (1994) Tidal ventilation at low airway pressures can augment lung injury. *Am. J. Respir. Crit. Care Med.* **149**: 1327–1334.

20. **Mead, J., Takishima, T. and Leith, D.** (1970) Stress distribution in lungs: a model of pulmonary elasticity. *J. Appl. Physiol.* **28**: 596–608.

21. **Fu, Z., Costello, M.L., Tsukimoto, K., et al.** (1992) High lung volume increases stress failure in pulmonary capillaries. *J. Appl. Physiol.* **73**: 123–133.

22. **Nahum, A., Hoyt, J., Schmitz, L., et al.** (1997) Effect of mechanical ventilation strategy on dissemination of intratracheally instilled *Escherichia coli* in dogs. *Crit. Care Med.* **25**: 1733–1743.

23. **Verbrugge, S.J.C., Sorm, V., Veen, A., et al.** (1998) Lung overinflation without positive end-expiratory pressure promotes bacteremia after experimental *Klebsiella pneumoniae* inoculation. *Intensive Care Med.* **24**: 172–177.

24. **Christman, J.W. and Blackwell, T.S.** (1998) Mechanical stress and cytokine production: implications for mechanical ventilation. *Intensive Care Med.* **24**: 884–885.

25. **Rimensberger, P.C., Fedorko, L., Cutz, E. and Bohn, D.J.** (1998) Attenuation of ventilator-induced acute lung injury in an animal model by inhibition of neutrophil adhesion by leumedine (NPC 15669). *Crit. Care Med.* **26**: 3548–3555.

26. **Bethmann, A.N., Brasch, F., Nusing, R., et al.** (1998) Hyperventilation induces release of cytokines from perfused mouse lung. *Am. J. Respir. Crit. Care Med.* **157**: 263–272.

27. **Wirtz, H.R.W. and Dobbs, L.G.** (1990) Calcium mobilization and exocytosis after one mechanical stretch of lung epithelial cells. *Science* **250**: 1266–1269.

28. **Imai, Y., Kawano, T., Miyasaka, K., et al.** (1994) Inflammatory chemical mediators during conventional ventilation and during high frequency oscillatory ventilation. *Am. J. Respir. Crit. Care Med.* **150**: 1550–1554.

29. **Tremblay, L., Valenza, F., Riberiro, S., et al.** (1997) Injurious ventilatory strategies increases cytokines and c-fos mRNA expression in an isolated rat lung model. *J. Clin. Invest.* **99**: 944–952.

30. **Takata, M., Abe, J., Tanaka, H., et al.** (1997) Intraalveolar expression of tumor necrosis factor alpha gene during conventional and high-frequency ventilation. *Am. J. Respir. Crit. Care Med.* **156**: 272–279.

31. **Ranieri, V.M., Tortorella, D., DeTullio, R., et al.** (1999) Limitation of mechanical lung stress decreases BAL cytokines in patients with ARDS. *JAMA* **282**: 54–61.

32. **Dreyfuss, D. and Saumon, G.** (1998) From ventilator-induced lung injury to multiple organ dysfunction? *Intensive Care Med.* **24**: 102–104.

33. **Slutsky, A. and Tremblay, L.** (1998) Multiple system organ failure: is mechanical ventilation a contributing factor? *Am. J. Respir. Crit. Care Med.* **157**: 1721–1725.

34. **Brower, R.G., Shanholtz, C.B., Fessler, H.E., et al.** (1999) Prospective, randomized, controlled trial comparing traditional versus reduced tidal volume ventilation in acute respiratory distress syndrome patients. *Crit. Care Med.* **27**: 1492–1496.

35. **Stewart, T.E., Meade, M.O., Cook, D.J., et al.** (1998) Evaluation of a ventilator strategy to prevent barotrauma in patients at high risk for acute respiratory distress syndrome. *N. Engl. J. Med.* **338**: 355–361.

36. **Brochard, L., Roudot-Thoravol, F., Roupie, E., et al.** (1998) Tidal volume reduction for prevention of ventilator-induced lung injury in acute respiratory distress syndrome. *Am. J. Respir. Crit. Care Med.* **158**: 1831–1838.

37. **Froese, A.B.** (1997) High frequency oscillatory ventilation for adult respiratory distress syndrome: Let's get it right. *Crit. Care Med.* **25**: 906–908.

38. **Hickling, K.G., Walsh, J., Henderson, S., et al.** (1994) Low mortality rate in adult respiratory distress syndrome using low-volume, pressure-limited ventilation with permissive hypercapnia. A prospective study. *Crit. Care Med.* **22**: 1568.

39. **Kacmarek, R.M. and Hickling, K.G.** (1993) Permissive hypercapnia. *Respir. Care* **38**: 373.

40. **Feihl, F. and Perret, C.** (1994) Permissive hypercapnia. How permissive should we be? *Am. J. Respir. Crit. Care Med.* **150**: 1722.

41. **Froese, A.B., McCulloch, P.R., Sugiura, M., et al.** (1993) Optimizing alveolar expansion prolongs the effectiveness of exogenous surfactant therapy in the adult rabbit. *Am. Rev. Respir. Dis.* **148**: 569–577.

42. Sjostrand, U.H., Lichtwarck-Aschoff, M., Nielsen, J.B., *et al.* (1995) Different ventilatory approaches to keep the lung open. *Intensive Care Med.* 21: 310–318.

43. Fujino, Y., Goddon, S., Dolhnikoff, M., *et al.* (1999) Repetitive high pressure recruitment maneuvers (RM) required to maximally recruit lung in ARDS sheep model. *Am. J. Respir. Crit. Care Med.* 159: A479.

44. Rimensberger, P.C., Cox, P.N., Frndova, H., *et al.* (1999) The open lung during small tidal volume ventilation: concepts of recruitment and optimal PEEP. *Crit. Care Med.* 27: 1946–1952.

45. Rimensberger, P.C., Pristine, G., Mullen, J.B.M., *et al.* (1999) Lung recruitment during small tidal volume ventilation allows minimal PEEP without augmenting lung injury. *Crit. Care Med.* 27: 1940–1945.

46. Van der Kloot, T.E., Blanch, L. and Youngblood, A.M. (2000) Recruitment maneuvers in three experimental models of acute lung injury. *Am. J. Respir. Crit. Care Med.* 161: 1485–1494.

47. Rothen, J.U., Neuman, P., Berglund, J.E., *et al.* (1999) Dynamics of re-expansion of atelectasis during general anesthesia. *Br. J. Anaesth.* 82: 551–556.

48. Greaves, I.A., Hildebrandt, J. and Hopppin, F.G. (1985) Micromechanics of the lung. In: *Handbook of Physiology* (eds P.T. MacKlem and J. Mead). American Physiologic Society, Bethesda, MD, pp. 217–231.

49. Gattinoni, L., Pelosi, P., Crotti, S., *et al.* (1995) Effects of positive end-expiratory pressure on regional distribution of tidal volume and recruitment in adult respiratory distress syndrome. *Am. J. Respir. Crit. Care Med.* 151: 1807–1995.

50. Medoff, B.D., Harris, R.S., Kesselman, H., *et al.* (2000) Use of recruitment maneuvers and high position end-expiratory pressure in a patient with acute respiratory distress syndrome. *Crit. Care Med.* 18: 1210–1216.

51. Lapinsky, S.F., Aubin, M., Mehta, S., *et al.* (1994) Safety and efficacy of a sustained inflation for alveolar recruitment in adults with respiratory failure. *Intensive Care Med.* 25: 1297–1301.

52. Chatte, G., Sab, J.M., Dubois, J.M., *et al.* (1997) Prone position in mechanically ventilated patients with severe acute respiratory failure. *Am. J. Respir. Crit. Care Med.* 155: 473–478.

53. Blanch, L., Mancebo, J., Perez, M., *et al.* (1997) Short-term effects of prone position in critically ill patients with acute respiratory distress syndrome. *Intensive Care Med.* 23: 1033–1039.

54. Jolliet, P., Bulpa, P., Ritz, M., *et al.* (1997) Additional beneficial effects of prone position, nitric oxide, and almitrine bimesylate on gas exchange and oxygen transport in the acute respiratory distress syndrome. *Crit. Care Med.* 25: 786–794.

55. Langer, M., Mascheroni, D., Marcolin, R., *et al.* (1988) The prone position in ARDS patients. A clinical study. *Chest* 94: 103–107.

56. Mure, M., Martling, C.R. and Lindahl, S.G. (1997) Dramatic effect on oxygenation in patients with severe acute lung insufficiency treated in the prone position. *Crit. Care Med.* 25: 1539–1544.

57. Pelosi, P., Tubiolo, D., Mascheroni, D., *et al.* (1998) Effects of the prone position on respiratory mechanics and gas exchange during acute lung injury. *Am. J. Respir. Crit. Care Med.* 157: 387–393.

58. Kacmarek, R.M. and Schwartz, D. (2000) Lung recruitment. *Respir. Clin. N. Am.* 6: 597–623.

59. Gattinoni, L., Pelosi, P., Vitale, G., *et al.* (1991) Body position changes redistribute lung computed-tomographic density in patients with acute respiratory failure. *Anesthesiology* 74: 15–23.

60. Amis, T.C., Jones, H.A. and Hughes, J.M. (1984) Effect of posture on inter-regional distribution of pulmonary ventilation in man. *Respir. Physiol.* 56: 145–167.

61. Albert, R.K., Leasa, D., Sanderson, M., *et al.* (1987) The prone position improves arterial oxygenation and reduces shunt in oleic-acid-induced acute lung injury. *Am. Rev. Respir. Dis.* 135: 628–633.

62. Broccard, A.F., Shapiro, R.S., Schitz, L.L., *et al.* (1997) Influence of prone position on the extent and distribution of lung injury in a high tidal volume oleic acid model of acute respiratory distress syndrome. *Crit. Care Med.* 25: 16–27.

63. Caker, N., Van der Kloot, T., Youngblood, M., *et al.* (2000) Oxygenation response to a recruitment maneuver during supine and prone positions in an oleic acid-induced lung injury model. *Am. J. Respir. Crit. Care* 161: 1949–1956.

64. Fridrich, P., Krafft, P., Hochleuthner, H., *et al.* (1996) The effects of long-term prone positioning in patients with trauma-induced adult respiratory distress syndrome. *Anesth. Analg.* 83: 1206–1211.

Chapter 16

Nosocomial pneumonia

Thomas L. Higgins, MD

Contents

16.1 Introduction

Nosocomial or hospital-acquired pneumonias are infections of the lung parenchyma occurring more than 48 h after hospital admission and excluding infections incubating at the time of admission[1]. Environmental sources (air, water, food, fomites), medical devices (endotracheal tubes, suction catheters, bronchoscopes, respiratory therapy equipment), other patients, and hospital staff can serve as vectors for nosocomial infection[2]. Pneumonia is the most common nosocomial infection in the ICU and the second most common hospital-acquired infection. Occurrence ranges from 0.4% in unselected hospitalized patients to 23% in the ICU[3]. The risk of ventilator-associated pneumonia (VAP; a subset of nosocomial pneumonia) is estimated to be 1% per day of mechanical ventilation[4]. More than half of patients with ventilator-associated pneumonia die during the same hospitalization, although not all deaths are directly related to pneumonia. The attributable mortality (percentage of deaths that would not have occurred in the absence of infection) is lower. In a case–control study of 41 patients who developed nosocomial pneumonia, 44% of the deaths were attributed to infection[5].

ICU patients with any nosocomial infection have 2½ times the death rate of uninfected patients. Even after adjustment is made for confounding factors such as organ system dysfunction, APACHE II score and intensity of therapy, the mortality risk is at least doubled[6]. Nosocomial infection has its greatest mortality impact in younger, less severely ill patients, where failure to accurately diagnose and treat infection plays a larger role than in elderly patients with multiple mortality risks[6]. Nosocomial pneumonia also prolongs hospital stay by an average of 7–9 days, and increases hospital expenses[7].

16.2 Risk factors for developing nosocomial pneumonia

The risk of developing nosocomial pneumonia depends on the host, the environment and medical interventions (*Table 16.1*). Neurologic failure on the third ICU day[5], witnessed aspiration, exposure to paralytic agents[8], supine position (head of bed <30°)[9], sedative use[10], nasogastric tubes, reintubation, blood transfusion[11] and patient transport from the ICU[12] increase risk. Subsequent mortality, once pneumonia occurs, is related to APACHE II score, the number of dysfunctional organs, nosocomial bacteremia, the presence of an underlying

Table 16.1 Risk factors for development of nosocomial pneumonia

Patient related

Alcoholism
Advanced age
Azotemia
Cigarette smoking
CNS dysfunction
Coma
COPD
Diabetes mellitus
Malnutrition
Number of organ dysfunctions
Physiologic derangement (APACHE score)
Underlying fatal illness

Environment

Condensation in ventilator tubing
Contaminated respiratory equipment
Head of bed in horizontal (<30°) position
Pooling of secretions over endotracheal tube
    cuff
Poor hand-washing practice
Transfer from another ICU

Intervention

Antacids
Corticosteroids
Cytotoxic agents
H2 blockers or gastric overgrowth
Presence of endotracheal or nasogastric tube
Prolonged and inappropriate use of antibiotics
Prolonged or complicated surgery
Sedatives and neuromuscular blocking drugs
Thoracoabdominal procedures

CNS, central nervous system; COPD, chronic obstructive pulmonary disease; H2, histamine type 2. From: Higgins, T.L. (1999) Nosocomial pneumonia: intensive care unit perspective. Reproduced with permission from *Curr. Treatment Options Infect. Dis.* **1**: 159–175.

fatal illness, and admission from another ICU[13].

16.3 Pathogens and routes of entry

Organisms typically associated with community-acquired pneumonia (CAP) plus organisms in the hospital environment likely to colonize the upper airway are responsible for most nosocomial infections. About half of nosocomial pneumonia isolates in mechanically ventilated patients are polymicrobial[14,15]. Viral etiologies must also be considered. Pathogens frequently associated with nosoco-

mial pneumonia (*Table 16.2*) include *S. pneumoniae* and *Haemophilus influenzae* with early onset and aerobic Gram-negative bacilli or *Staphylococcus aureus* as hospital stay lengthens. A growing percentage of nosocomial organisms have become resistant to antibiotics (see Section 16.8.1).

16.4 Diagnosis

16.4.1 Colonization

In clinically unstable patients who might also be febrile with an elevated white blood cell count, it is difficult not to react to a positive culture report from the microbiology laboratory,

Table 16.2 Common pathogens currently associated with nosocomial pneumonia*

Pathogen	Frequency, %	Source of organism
Early onset bacterial pneumonia		
S. pneumoniae	5–20	Endogenous, other patients, respiratory droplet
H. influenzae	<5–15	
Late-onset bacterial pneumonia		
Aerobic Gram-negative bacilli	>20–60	Endogenous, other patients,
P. aeruginosa		environment, enteral
Enterobacter spp.		feeding, health-care workers,
Acinetobacter spp.		equipment or devices
K. pneumoniae		
S. marcescens		
E. coli		
Gram-positive cocci	20–40	Endogenous, health-care
S. aureus		workers, environment
Early and late-onset pneumonia		
Anaerobic bacteria	0–35	Endogenous, potable water, showers,
L. pneumophila	0–10	faucets, cooling towers
M. tuberculosis	<1	Endogenous, other patients or staff
Viruses		
Influenza A and B	<1	Other patients or staff
Respiratory syncytial virus	<1	Other patients or staff, fomites
Fungi or Protozoa		
Aspergillus	<1	Air, construction, endogenous,
Candida spp.	<1	other patients or staff
P. carinii	<1	Endogenous, other patients or staff

*Crude rates of pneumonia may vary by hospital, patient population, and method of diagnosis. Adapted from: Craven, D.E. and Steger, K.A. (1995) Epidemiology of nosocomial pneumonia: New perspectives on an old disease. Reproduced with permission from *Chest* **108**(Suppl.): 1S–16S.

yet it is critical to distinguish colonization of the airway from true pulmonary infection, particularly with conditions that mimic pneumonia on chest X-ray (*Table 16.3*). Organisms such as *Enterobacter, Citrobacter, Flavobacterium, Pseudomonas cepacia*, and *Stentrophomonas* (formerly *Xanthomonas*) *maltophilia* are unusual causes of nosocomial pneumonia, but often appear as colonizers and prompt inappropriate antibiotic 'coverage'. *Staphylococcus aureus*, whether methicillin sensitive or multi-resistant, is a common colonizer but only occasionally the cause of ventilator-associated pneumonia. Colonization alone should not be treated, as inappropriate use of powerful antimicrobials alters the microflora environment and encourages the emergence of highly resistant strains.

16.4.2 Clinical diagnosis

Although invasive strategies offer advantages in establishing the microbiologic cause of nosocomial pneumonia[16], routine clinical practice is more likely to rely on non-invasive diagnosis. Clinical diagnosis of nosocomial pneumonia requires a chest radiographic abnormality that is new, progressive or persistent for more than 24 h, with evidence of infec-

---

Table 16.3 Non-infectious findings on chest X-ray that may mimic nosocomial infection

ARDS (often associated with aspiration, pancreatitis, systemic inflammatory response syndrome, multisystem organ failure)
Atelectasis
Bronchiolitis obliterans organizing pneumonia (BOOP)
Cardiac pulmonary edema
Collagen–vascular disorders
Contusion (trauma)
Drug- or radiation-induced lung disease
Fat embolization
Neoplasm
Neurogenic pulmonary edema
Pulmonary hemorrhage
Pulmonary thromboembolism with infarction

From: Higgins, T.L. (1999) Nosocomial pneumonia: intensive care unit perspective. Reproduced with permission from *Curr. Treatment Options Infect. Dis.* **1**: 159–175..

---

tion. Evidence should include at least two of the following: purulent sputum, temperature below 36°C or above 38°C, and a white cell count less than 5000 mm^{-3}, or 10 000 mm^{-3} or more. The specificity of these findings for nosocomial pneumonia is low. Pneumonia is more likely when the chest radiograph shows rapid, progressive cavitation, an air space process abutting a fissure, an air bronchogram, or infiltrate next to an empyema. Pneumonia is less likely if rapid improvement occurs with serial examination, as can be seen with atelectasis, aspiration, hemorrhage, or congestive heart failure.

16.4.3 Microbiology laboratory results

Microbiology results help determine if infection explains new clinical signs and symptoms; identify the pathogen; and help to define prognosis. Semiquantitative reports are generated by a serial plating technique (*Figure 16.1*). Growth in the first quadrant (1+) will almost always occur, but growth in the fourth quadrant (4+) suggests a significant number of organisms. Unfortunately, processing time and inherent unreliability of bacteriologic sampling mandate a strategy of early empiric treatment. Blood cultures are specific but not sensitive, identifying the pathogen in less than 20% of all patients with hospital-acquired pneumonia (HAP)[17]. If blood cultures are positive, however, they define the organism and identify patients at risk for a complicated course.

Sputum examination and culture have limited value in diagnosing nosocomial pneumonia. In intubated patients, endotracheal aspirates (ETAs) are easily obtained, but non-quantitative ETA specimens do not reliably distinguish infection from colonization. A quantitative ETA of more than 1 million colony forming units (c.f.u.) per ml is highly suggestive of infection, but most laboratories do not perform quantitative cultures on ETAs. Elastin fibers, which can be identified using a 40% KOH stain, suggest necrotizing pneumonia[18]. A negative sputum culture excludes certain pathogens, allowing the clinician to

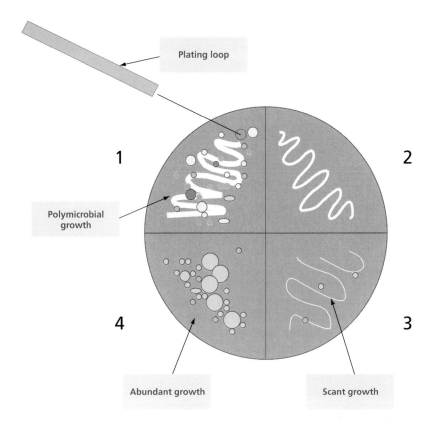

Figure 16.1 Semiquantitative cultures. Microbiology laboratories frequently report semiquantitative results based on organism growth after incubation. The initial specimen is plated in the first quadrant of an agar plate. After flaming the loop, a specimen is drawn from the first quadrant and plated in the second quadrant. The process is repeated from quadrant 2 to 3 and then from 3 to 4. After incubation, the growth is read out as scant (1+), light (2+), moderate (3+) or heavy (4+). Although not as precise as quantitative cultures, this method provides a way to communicate relative abundance to a clinically significant degree. More than one organism may be identified; the relative abundance can help sort out colonizers from true pathogens.

narrow the initially broad empiric antibiotic choices. The antimicrobial sensitivity of isolated organisms can be correctly defined 87% of the time by the endotracheal aspirate[19].

16.4.4 Fiberoptic bronchoscopy and bronchoalveolar lavage

Recent work has confirmed the value of an invasive diagnostic strategy in reducing mortality, organ failure and antibiotic use[16]. Fiberoptic bronchoscopy (FOB) allows acquisition of protected brush specimens (PBSs) and/or broncho-alveolar lavage (BAL) speci-

mens. Bacterial growth can then be quantified, typically using diagnostic thresholds of 1000 c.f.u. ml^{-1} for bronchial brushings and 10 000 c.f.u. ml^{-1} for BAL fluid cultures. These arbitrary thresholds may be too sensitive early in the course of an illness, if the patient has already received antibiotic therapy, or as a result of variation in sampling techniques[20]. The additional risk and cost of FOB is offset in part by improved outcome and lower antibiotic costs[16,21]. A recent study suggests that BAL with 3% infected cells is the only test with sufficient predictive value to guide initial therapy while awaiting culture results[22]. Perhaps the most important contribution of a negative BAL or FOB is to redirect the search for infection in the febrile patient to extrapulmonary sites. FOB and/or BAL should be strongly considered in the patient who fails to respond to therapy or where bronchial obstruction may be present.

16.4.5 Other invasive tests

Thoracentesis is not sensitive, but is highly specific in identifying infection. Thoracentesis is indicated if a parapneumonic effusion is present, particularly when the effusion is large or the patient is seriously ill. Laboratory examination of pleural fluid should include protein, Lactate Dehydrogenase (LDH) and glucose levels, cell count and differential, pH, Gram's stain and acid-fast stain, and bacterial and fungal cultures. Fluoroscopically guided transthoracic needle aspiration is highly specific but subject to sampling false negatives and risks pneumothorax or hemorrhage. Open lung biopsy has a diagnostic yield of 69%, at the cost of additional morbidity and mortality. Transtracheal aspiration of irrigated secretions using a small angiocath through the cricothyroid membrane is highly sensitive and specific, but has a high rate of false positive in patients with COPD, and is not useful if the patient is already intubated.

16.4.6 Serology

Serologic studies are not routinely needed, but can be useful for retrospective confirmation of bacterial, viral and legionella infections. An enzyme-linked immune serum assay (ELISA) is available for rapid detection of legionella serogroup 1 antigen in the urine[23].

16.5 **Antibiotic therapy**

Delay in administration of antibiotics increases mortality[24] so therapy cannot be withheld while studies are pending. Empiric therapy should be initiated as soon as possible, with only minimal delay to obtain pre-therapy sputum samples and/or blood cultures. This chapter focuses on treatment of nosocomial

pneumonia only; treatment for community-acquired pneumonia requires a different strategy[25].

16.5.1 ATS consensus statement

The American Thoracic Society (ATS)[1] produced a consensus statement on hospital-acquired pneumonia in 1995. Although this is still a useful general framework for empiric antibiotic therapy, changes in antibiotic resistance patterns, and the availability of newer agents such as the fluroquinolones modify these recommendations. Treatment decisions are based on the severity of the patient's illness, the presence of risk factors for a specific pathogen, and the time of onset of clinical infection (before versus after day 5)[1] (*Figure 16.2*). The ATS guidelines target empiric therapy based on individual patient risk factors. High-risk patients (as defined in *Table 16.4*) receive broad spectrum coverage (accepting the risk of promoting antimicrobial resistance) whereas low-risk patients receive more focused treatment. Empiric antibiotic choices are

---

Table 16.4 Criteria for severe hospital-acquired pneumonia

Admission to the intensive care unit

Respiratory failure, defined as the need for mechanical ventilation or the need for >35% oxygen to maintain an arterial oxygen saturation >90%

Rapid radiographic progression, multilobar pneumonia, or cavitation of a lung infiltrate

Evidence of severe sepsis with hypotension and/or end-organ dysfunction:
● Shock (systolic blood pressure <90 mmHg or diastolic blood pressure <60 mmHg)
● Requirement for vasopressors for >4 h
● Urine output <20 ml h⁻¹ or total urine output <80 ml in 4 h (unless another explanation is available)
● Acute renal failure requiring dialysis

Adapted from: American Thoracic Society (1995) American Thoracic Society Consensus Statement: Hospital-acquired pneumonia in adults: diagnosis, assessment of severity, initial antimicrobial therapy, and preventative strategies. Reproduced with permission from *Am. J. Respir. Crit. Care Med.* **153**: 1711–1725.

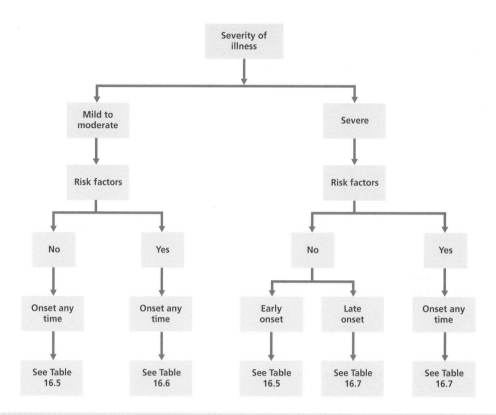

Figure 16.2 Severity of illness. 'Early onset' is before hospital day 5. Adapted from: ATS guidelines American Thoracic Society (1995) American Thoracic Society Consensus Statement: Hospital-acquired pneumonia in adults: diagnosis, assessment of severity, initial antimicrobial therapy, and preventative strategies. Reproduced with permission from *Am. J. Respir. Crit. Care Med.* **153**: 1711–1725).

reassessed once culture and sensitivity information becomes available, generally within 48 h.

16.5.2 Severity of illness

Table 16.5 describes the expected microbiology and initial antibiotic choices for patients having mild-to-moderate nosocomial pneumonia in the absence of significant risk factors. Those criteria are also useful for the patient with early-onset severe pneumonia unless immunosuppression is present. *Table 16.6* addresses the organisms and antibiotic choices in patients with host or therapeutic factors increasing risk for specific pathogens. The ATS guidelines consider patients admitted to the ICU or those with severe organ dysfunction to automatically meet the criteria for severe hospital-

acquired pneumonia. However, intensive care patients with no risk factors and early-onset (before day 5) pneumonia can be treated under the mild-to-moderate guidelines in *Table 16.5*.

16.5.3 Risks for specific pathogens

Risk factors for *Staphylococcus aureus* infection include head trauma, diabetes mellitus, chronic renal failure, age less than 25 years, intravenous drug abuse, and recent influenza infection[26]. Methicillin-resistant *Staphylococcus aureus* (MRSA) is more likely with prior steroid administration, mechanical ventilation for more than 6 days, advancing age, pre-existing COPD, and prior antibiotic therapy. Bacteremia, shock and subsequent mortality are all higher in ventilated patients infected with MRSA than with sensitive strains[27].

Table 16.5 Antibiotic choices for patients with pneumonia

Core organisms	Core antibiotics

Enteric Gram-negative bacilli
(Non-pseudomonal) *Enterobacter* species
    Escherichia coli
    Klebsiella spp.
    Proteus spp.
    Serratia marcescens
    Hemophilus influenzae
Methicillin-sensitive *Staphylococcus aureus*
Streptococcus pneumoniae
	Cephalosporin
	    Second-generation or non-pseudomonal
	    third-generation (e.g. cefotaxime or
	    ceftraxone)
	OR
	β-lactam–β-lactamase inhibitor combination
	OR
	Newer fluoroquinolone

Patients have (a) mild-to-moderate hospital-acquired pneumonia, no unusual risk factors, onset any time; or (b) early-onset, severe hospital-acquired pneumonia (excluding patients with immunosuppression). Adapted from: Higgins T.L. (1999) Nosocomial Pneumonia: Intensive Care Unit Perspective. *Current Treatment in Infectious Disease*. **1**: 159–175.

Table 16.6 Patients with mild-to-moderate hospital-acquired pneumonia with risk factors, onset any time*

Core organisms *Plus*	Core antibiotics *Plus*

Anaerobes
    (recent abdominal surgery, witnessed
    aspiration)
	Clindamycin
	    or β-lactam–β-lactamase inhibitor (alone)

Staphylococcus aureus
    (coma, head trauma, diabetes mellitus,
    renal failure)
	± Vancomycin
	    (until methicillin-resistant
	    Staphylococcus aureus is ruled out)

Legionella (high-dose steroids)	Erythromycin ± rifampin†

Pseudomonas aeruginosa
    (prolonged ICU stay, steroids, antibiotics
    structural lung disease)
	Treat as severe hospital-acquired
	    pneumonia (Table 16.7)

*Excludes patients with immunosuppression.
†Rifampin may be added if *Legionella* sp. is documented. Adapted from: Higgins T.L. (1999) Nosocomial Pneumonia: Intensive Care Unit Perspective. *Current Treatment in Infectious Disease*. **1**: 159–175.

Risk of *Pseudomonas aeruginosa* infection increases with prolonged hospital or ICU stay, prior antibiotics or steroids, the presence of structural lung disease such as bronchiectasis or cystic fibrosis, malnutrition, and mechanical ventilation[28]. Legionella infection is likely with prior steroids, neutropenia, chronic renal failure, chemotherapy, or active cancer.

Anaerobic infection is more likely with recent thoraco-abdominal surgery, a witnessed aspiration, an obstructing foreign body, or poor dentition.

16.6 Choice of antibiotic

No single antibiotic or drug combination is appropriate for all patients. 'Core' antibiotics as defined by the ATS guidelines provide reasonable general empiric coverage, and additional choices or substitutions can be based on the presence of risk factors and severity of illness[1].

16.6.1 Treatment by risk category
Low-risk patients should receive empiric coverage with one of the following: a second or non-pseudomonal third-generation cephalosporin,

or a β-lactam–β-lactamase inhibitor combination. For patients with penicillin allergy, a fluroquinolone or the combination of clindamycin plus aztreonam would be appropriate. The patient with mild-to-moderate hospital-acquired pneumonia with risk factors (*Table 16.6*) should receive the 'core' antibiotics, plus additional risk-specific coverage: clindamycin or a β-lactam–β-lactamase inhibitor for anaerobes, vancomycin for MRSA, and erythromycin or fluroquinolone with or without rifampicin for *Legionella*. Patients at risk for *Pseudomonas* should be treated as having severe hospital-acquired pneumonia. Anaerobes isolated by protected specimen brush usually (63%) produce β-lactamase and thus are not reliably sensitive[29].

The pathogens in patients with severe nosocomial pneumonia are the core organisms plus *Pseudomonas aeruginosa*, *Acinetobacter*, and MRSA. Early-onset, severe pneumonia in a patient without risk factors is likely to be caused by 'core' organisms and can be treated following the recommendations in *Table 16.5*. Late-onset severe nosocomial pneumonia or severe nosocomial pneumonia in the patient with risk factors requires aggressive empiric therapy. Recommendations include an aminoglycoside or a fluroquinolone, plus one of the following: an antipseudomonal penicillin, a cephalosporin such as ceftriaxone or cefoperaxone, a β-lactam– β-lactamase inhibitor combination, a carbapenem, or aztreonam if only Gram-negative coverage is needed. If there is concern for MRSA, vancomycin should be added (*Table 16.6*). Vancomycin should not be used for routine prophylaxis, treatment of colonization, empiric treatment of febrile or neutropenic patients, as first-line therapy for *Clostridium difficile* colitis, or as a topical irrigant. Its use should be restricted to treatment of β-lactam-resistant Gram-positive organisms, serious β-lactam allergy, and failed metronidazole therapy for *C. difficile*. Vancomycin-resistant enterococci are an increasing problem, and may be associated with use of not only vancomycin, but potent β-lactam antibiotics as well[30].

16.6.2 Combination antibiotic therapy versus monotherapy

Antibiotic monotherapy is acceptable for patients with non-pseudomonal mild-to-moderate nosocomial pneumonia. Whether monotherapy is adequate for severely ill patients is less clear. Monotherapy with meropenem versus the combination of ceftazidime plus tobramycin resulted in better clinical response and bacterial eradication[31]. Overall success rate in a randomized trial of 177 patients with nosocomial pneumonia was only marginally improved by adding the aminoglycoside netilmycin to imipenem. Even for patients with *Pseudomonas* infection, monotherapy was equally efficacious[32]. This lack of synergism may reflect a limitation of aminoglycosides owing to poor penetration into the lung or inactivity at an acid pH. Monotherapy with third-generation cephalosporins, however, is associated with emergence of antimicrobial resistance[33].

Combination therapy can be justified by reports of synergistic activity against certain pathogens, especially *Pseudomonas aeruginosa*, the need for broader spectrum coverage than one agent can provide, and concerns about the emergence of resistance during monotherapy. Combination therapy generally employs antibiotics with differing mechanisms of action, such as a β-lactam agent plus an aminoglycoside or fluroquinolone. *Table 16.7* indicates possible combinations for severe nosocomial pneumonia. Combination drug therapy may be needed to cover both 'core' organisms and specific risk factors with lower-grade pneumonia, particularly if the MRSA is a likely pathogen.

16.6.3 Antibiotic dosage and administration (*Table 16.8*)

Bacteriocidal antibiotics are either concentration dependent or time dependent. The aminoglycosides and quinolones are concentration dependent and most effective when high peak concentrations are attained[34]. These drugs also have a post-antibiotic effect, meaning they will suppress bacterial growth even when the serum concentration falls below the minimal inhibitory concentration (MIC) of the infectious

Table 16.7 Patients with severe hospital-acquired pneumonia with risk factors, early onset or patients with severe HAP, late onset*

Core organisms, *Plus*	Therapy

P. aeruginosa
Acinetobacter spp.
	Aminoglycoside or newer fluoroquinolone
	plus one of the following:
	    antipseudomonal penicillin
	    β-lactam–β-lactamase inhibitor
	    Ceftazidime, cefoperazone or cefepime
	    Imipenem or meropenem
	    Aztreonam†

Consider MRSA	± Vancomycin

*Excludes patients with immunosuppression.
†Aztreonam efficacy is limited to enteric Gram-negative bacilli and should not be used in combination with an aminoglycoside if Gram-positive or *Haemophilus influenzae* infection is of concern. Adapted from: Higgins T.L. (1999) Nosocomial Pneumonia: Intensive Care Unit Perspective. *Current Treatment in Infectious Disease*. **1**: 159–175.

agent. Concentration-dependent agents can usually be administered as once-daily therapy, which reduces toxicity and costs without compromising the bacteriologic cure[35].

Penicillins, cephalosporins, aztreonam and vancomycin are time-dependent antibiotics, and rely on keeping the serum level above the MIC threshold for the longest possible time. Multiple daily doses are typically required to achieve adequate therapeutic effect with time-dependent drugs. The carbapenems, unlike most β-lactam antibiotics, have a significant post-antibiotic effect, allowing less frequent dosing intervals. *Table 16.8* provides the specific drugs and usual dosing intervals for agents commonly used in empiric therapy for nosocomial pneumonia.

16.6.4 Duration of therapy
Optimal duration of antibiotic therapy is not well defined and should be individualized based on the organism, severity of illness, and the patient's response to therapy. Infections with lower-grade organisms (*Table 16.5*) are likely to respond adequately to a 7–10 day course of therapy[36]. Patients who are malnourished or debilitated; those with multilobar involvement, or those infected with *Acinetobacter* or *Pseudomonas* species or a necrotizing Gram-negative bacillus usually require 14–21 days of therapy[1]. Whereas initial therapy should be provided with intravenous antibi-

otics, substitution of oral agents is appropriate and economical[37], once the patient demonstrates clinical improvement and the ability to tolerate enteral administration.

16.6.5 Assessing therapeutic response
Radiographic improvement of pneumonia is unlikely to occur in the first 72 h, so the initial antibiotic choice should be maintained unless there is rapid deterioration. Serial cultures are appropriate to document antimicrobial eradication and to identify onset of superinfection. Protected specimen brush sampling yielding more than 10^3 c.f.u. ml^{-1} 72 h after initiation of therapy indicates microbiologic failure to eradicate and better than 50% risk of clinical treatment failure[38]. Further diagnostic work-up including FOB, and, if necessary, open lung biopsy may identify unusual organisms, airway obstruction, or non-infectious processes when pneumonia fails to resolve. Host defense problems may also contribute to non-resolution of infection, particularly in the elderly and patients with chronic obstructive pulmonary disease or diabetes mellitus[39].

16.6.6 Fungal pneumonia
Candida albicans is a frequent colonizer in the ICU setting, but is rarely the cause of pneumonia. Aspiration of *Candida* from the oropharynx will seldom cause a primary pneumonia[40]. More commonly, hematogenously

Table 16.8 Selected antibiotic choices for nosocomial pneumonia

Antibiotics by class	Usual IV dose (adjust as needed for age and renal function)	Notes
Second-generation cephalosporins		
Cefoxitin (Mefoxin)	1 g q 8 h to 2 g q 4 h	*in vitro* induction of β-lactamase
Cefuroxime (Zinacef, Kefurox, Ceftin)	0.75–1 g q 8 h	
Non-pseudomonal third-generation		
Cefotaxime (Claforan)	1 g q 8 h to 2 g q 4 h	(maximum 12 g day^{-1})
Ceftriaxone (Rocephin)	500 mg q 12 h to 2 g q day (q day gives better tissue levels)	'Pseudocholelithiasis' with TPN
Anti-pseudomonal cephalosporins		
Ceftazidime (Fortaz, Ceftaz, Tazidime)	1–2 g q 8–12 h	selection of Vancomycin Resistant Enterococcus (VRE); ESBLs
Cefoperazone (Cefobid)	2 g q 12 h to 4 g q 6 h (max. dose 8 g day^{-1})	Disulfiram-like reactions q 6 h dosage for *Pseudomonas* 'fourth'
Cefepime (Maxipime)	1–2 g q 12 h	generation; less resistance
β-lactam–β-lactamase inhibitor drugs		
Ticarcillin-Clavulanate (Timentin)	3.1 g q 4–6 h	Ticarcillin interferes with platelets; Clavulanate may cause diarrhea
Piperacillin-tazobactam (Zosyn)	3.375 g q 6 h	
Carbapenems and monobactams		
Imipenem-Cilastin (Primaxin)	500 mg q 6 h; decrease in elderly and renal failure	Avoid with Penicillin (PCN) allergy, seizures
Meropenem (Merrem)	1 g q 8 h	False elevation of serum and urine creatinine
Aztreonam (Azactam)	1 g q 8 h to 2 g q 6 h	Gram-negative bacilli (GNB) coverage only; may cross-react with ceftazidime allergy
Aminoglycosides		
Gentamicin (Garamycin)	2 mg kg^{-1} load then 1.7 mg kg^{-1}	Potential ATN, renal failure, deafness, vertigo, augmentation of neuromuscular blockade
Tobramycin (Nebcin)	q 8 h or 5.1 mg kg^{-1} once daily; check trough levels and adjust for renal failure	
Fluroquinolones		
Ciprofloxacin (Cipro IV)	200–400 mg q 12 h	Anaphylaxis; CNS toxicity
Levofloxacin (Levaquin IV)	500 mg q day	enhanced Gram-positive cocci (GPC) and atypical activity
Glycopeptides		
Vancomycin (Vancocin)	15 mg kg^{-1} q 12 h; adjust for renal dysfunction using peak and trough levels	"red man" syndrome; with rapid infusion
Streptogramins		
Quinupristin + dalfopristin (Synercid)	7.5 mg kg^{-1} q 8 h	Reserve for highly resistant organisms including MRSA and some *E. faecium*
Oxazolidinones		
Linezolid (Zyvox)	600 mg q 12 h	Reserve for MRSA, VRE, monitor platelets

Adapted from: Higgins T.L. (1999) Nosocomial Pneumonia: Intensive Care Unit Perspective. *Current Treatment in Infectious Disease*. **1**: 159–175.

disseminated candidiasis will produce a miliary pattern on chest X-ray, along with other organ involvement. Patients who are immunocompromised are at higher risk for fungal infections, but even in this population, diagnosis should not be based on aspirated secretions alone, as benign airway colonization is far more likely than actual pneumonia. Use of antifungal therapy with oral or tracheobronchial colonization is associated with emergence of resistant organisms. Recent practice guidelines recommend histopathological confirmation of the diagnosis of *Candida* pneumonia before treatment[41]. Secondary pneumonia related to hematogenous spread should be treated as disseminated candidiasis.

16.7 Prevention of nosocomial pneumonia

Only a few strategies to prevent nosocomial pneumonia (vaccination, isolation of patients with multiple resistant pathogens, and hand washing) are considered 'probably effective'[1]. Vaccination is effective in preventing pneumonia caused by *Haemophilus influenzae*, pneumococcus, and influenza virus[42]. Although of limited use for the hospitalized patient, vaccination is indicated for those with chronic lung disease or otherwise at risk for hospitalization. Handwashing, although effective, is underutilized[43]. The use of boxed, clean, nonsterile gloves over unwashed hands drastically reduces fingertip colony counts, and there is no additional benefit to prior antiseptic handwashing or the use of individually packaged sterile gloves[44]. Nutritional support, control of gastric pH and volume, respiratory equipment protocols, aspiration of subglottic secretions, and lateral rotation bed therapy are considered of 'promising efficacy' and are easily implemented. Biologic response modifiers, monoclonal antibodies to specific bacterial antigens and manipulation of exogenous sources of bacteria (e.g. manipulation of the bacterial biofilm on endotracheal tubes) are unproven regimens still being evaluated.

16.7.1 Airway issues
Tracheal and gastric intubation bypasses normal defense mechanisms, increasing the likelihood of colonization and aspiration. Routine ventilator tubing changes should occur no more frequently than every 48 h[45]. Re-intubation and nasal intubation (risk of maxillary sinusitis) should be avoided[46]. Microaspiration of secretions occurs commonly, even in healthy patients, and aspiration risk is a function of the amount of time a patient is kept supine. Maintaining the head of the bed at an angle of 30° is effective, no-cost prophylaxis[9,47]. Patients maintained in a semi-recumbent (versus supine) position for the first 24 h in the ICU have a lower rate of ventilator-associated pneumonia, and lower ICU mortality[48]. Specialized endotracheal tubes with an extra lumen above the cuff allow continuous or intermittent aspiration of subglottic secretions. Removing contaminated secretions reduces the incidence of early, but not necessarily late-onset nosocomial pneumonia with more virulent organisms[49].

Specialized ICU beds that provide frequent changes in body position reduce the incidence of early ICU pneumonia in selected patients, but are without significant effect on ventilation or ICU days, or hospital mortality[50,51]. Ventilator-associated sinusitis is a major unrecognized cause of persistent fever, and frequently requires drainage in addition to appropriate antibiotic therapy[52].

16.7.2 Gastric acidity
Normal gastric flora is altered by an alkaline stomach pH[53]. Pneumonia incidence doubles in patients receiving stress-prophylaxis antacids or histamine type 2 antagonists compared with sucralfate, which does not usually alter stomach acidity[54]. Gastric overdistention can precipitate aspiration[53]. Attention to gastric residual volumes, cautious use of opioids, administration of motility agents such as metoclopramide, and use of post-pyloric feeding tubes has experiential if not scientific support.

16.7.3 Selective digestive decontamination

The benefits of topical and systemic antibiotic prophylaxis in critically ill patients are contested. Early studies suggested that selective digestive decontamination (SDD) reduced overall colonization and infection rates without affecting antibiotic resistance[55,56]. Later double-blind, randomized trials, however, failed to document a survival advantage, decreased nosocomial infection rate, reduced mechanical ventilation, or shorter ICU length of stay[57,58]. A recent meta-analysis concludes that antibiotic prophylaxis with combined topical and systemic drugs reduces the rate of respiratory tract infections and overall mortality[59]. Institution of SDD may be effective at controlling outbreaks of nosocomial pneumonia when traditional infection control measures have failed[60].

Prophylactic treatment with aerosolized antibiotics leads to emergence of resistant organisms, and is no longer recommended except for the outpatient cystic fibrosis population[61]. Immunoglobulin has been shown to reduce nosocomial infection, including pneumonia[62], but further studies are needed to demonstrate cost-effectiveness.

16.8 Antimicrobial resistance

The issue of antibiotic resistance should be of great concern to critical care practitioners given that the emergence of resistant organisms in recent years is occurring more rapidly than the pharmaceutical industry can introduce new agents. It is particularly disturbing to note that enterococci (both *Enterococcus faecium* and *Enterococcus faecalis*) resistant to the relatively new antibiotic, quinupristin–dalfopristin (Synercid) have been isolated from livestock where a related antibiotic, virginiamycin, has been used as a growth promoter[63].

16.8.1 Mechanisms of resistance

Bacteria defend themselves through a variety of strategies, including production of β-lactamases and cephalosporinases, alterations of binding sites, changes in porin size and perme-ability, and production of antibiotic-modifying enzymes. Resistance may be transmitted by plasmids or incorporated into the chromosomal structure of the bacteria. The reader is referred to an excellent recent review for a complete description of mechanisms and potential therapeutic strategies[64]. Antibiotics (penicillins, cephalosporins) containing a β-lactam ring are hydrolyzed by β-lactamases; this is the most prevalent mechanism of antibiotic resistance. β-lactamases may be inducible (i.e. encoded by chromosomes) or constitutive (chromosomally or plasma-mediated). Transferable resistance affects β-lactam–β-lactamase combination agents, penicillins, cephalosporins, and monobactams. Plasmids coding for mutant β-lactamases have been recovered from isolates of *Klebsiella*, *E. coli*, and other Enterobacteriaceae. These extended spectrum β-lactamases (ESBLs) cause nosocomial outbreaks. Emergence of resistant strains is encouraged by prolonged and/or inappropriate use of antibiotics[65]. Organisms producing ESBLs can appear to be sensitive on routine susceptibility tests, but can be resistant to therapy in the clinical setting.

Penicillin resistance in *S. pneumoniae* has risen from less than 5% in the 1980s to more than 30% at present[66]. Only half of US isolates of pneumococcus are now fully susceptible to penicillin, resistance to cephalosporin varies from 4% to 92%, and resistance to macrolides ranges from 4% to 14%[66]. At this writing, all *S. pneumoniae* isolates have thus far remained sensitive to vancomycin, although it may only be a matter of time until a case of vancomycin-resistant pneumococcus is reported. Vancomycin-resistant strains of *Staphylococcus aureus* have recently been identified. New agents available to counter these threats include oxazolidinone (Linezolid), streptogramins, such as quinupristin–dalfopristin (Synercid) and next-generation macrolides, fluoroquinolones and glycopeptides currently in development.

16.8.2 Rotation of routine antibiotic choices (crop rotation)

Crop rotation, or scheduled changes in the selection of empiric antibiotic therapy, may diminish the emergence of resistant organisms. In cardiac surgery patients given ceftazidime as usual empiric therapy for 6 months, changing empiric therapy to ciprofloxacin for the next 6 months reduced resistance and the overall rate of ventilator-associated pneumonia[67]. Further study is needed in different ICU patient populations, and using different pairs of antibiotics. Alternatives to third-generation cephalosporins include the β-lactam–β-lactamase inhibitor combinations, carbapenems, fluroquinolones, or fourth-generation cephalosporins which are more resistant to, and have lower affinity for common β-lactamases than the third-generation drugs.

16.9 Summary

Treatment of nosocomial pneumonia requires a thoughtful approach, balancing the need to adequately cover potential pathogens against a risk of fostering antibiotic resistance with inappropriately broad therapy. Prompt administration of antibiotics improves outcome. The spectrum of organisms to be covered is a function of the patient's risk factors, severity of illness, and length of hospitalization. With mild-to-moderate nosocomial pneumonia and no risk factors, monotherapy with the ATS-defined 'core' antibiotics (a second-generation or non-pseudomonal third-generation cephalosporin, a β-lactamase inhibitor combination, or a fluoroquinolone should suffice. Patients with specific risk factors should receive the 'core' antibiotics plus appropriate additional coverage for specific risks including recent abdominal surgery, witnessed aspiration of gastric contents, coma, head trauma, diabetes mellitus, renal failure, chronic high-dose corticosteroid therapy, prior antibiotic treatment, structural lung disease, and prolonged ICU stay. Patients who require intubation and mechanical ventilation need more aggressive coverage, generally consisting of the 'core' antibiotics plus supplemental therapy for virulent pathogens such as *Acinetobacter* species and *Pseudomonas* species. BAL is the only test recognized as having sufficient sensitivity to guide initial antibiotic choices. Initial multi-drug coverage can then be focused based on microbiology results. Invasive diagnostic methods have been shown to reduce mortality and inappropriate antibiotic use, and should also be considered in patients who fail to respond to initial empiric management. Emergence of resistant organisms is of concern, but definitive recommendations regarding crop rotation or other strategies to counter resistance are not yet available.

References

1. **American Thoracic Society** (1995) American Thoracic Society Consensus Statement: Hospital-acquired pneumonia in adults: diagnosis, assessment of severity, initial antimicrobial therapy, and preventative strategies. *Am. J. Respir. Crit. Care Med.* **153:** 1711–1725.

2. **Craven, D.E. and Steger, K.A.** (1995) Epidemiology of nosocomial pneumonia: New perspectives on an old disease. *Chest* **108**(Suppl.): 1S–16S.

3. **Tablan, O.C., Anderson, L.J., Arden, N.H.,** *et al.* (1994) Guideline for prevention of nosocomial pneumonia. *Infect. Control Hosp. Epidemiol.* **15:** 588.

4. **Fagon, J.-Y., Chastre, J., Domart, Y.,** *et al.* (1989) Nosocomial pneumonia in patients receiving continuous mechanical ventilation. *Am. Rev. Respir. Dis.* **139:** 877.

5. **Girou, E., Stephan, F., Novara, A.,** *et al.* (1998) Risk factors and outcome of nosocomial infections: Results of a matched case–control study of ICU patients. *Am. J. Respir. Crit. Care Med.* **157:** 1151–1158.

6. **Bueno-Cavanillas, A., Delgado-Rodriguez, M., Lopez-Luque, A., Schaffino-Cano, S. and Galvez-Vargas, R.** (1994) Influence of nosocomial infection on mortality rate in an intensive care unit. *Crit. Care Med.* **22:** 55–60.

7. **Boyce, J.M., Potter-Bynoe, G., Dziobek, L. and Solomon, S.L.** (1991) Nosocomial pneumonia in Medicare patients. Hospital costs and reimbursement patterns under the prospective payment system. *Arch. Intern. Med.* **151:** 1109–1114.

8. **Cook, D.J., Walter, S.D., Cook, R.J.,** *et al.* (1998) Incidence of and risk factors for ventilator-associated pneumonia in critically ill patients. *Ann. Intern. Med.* **129:** 433–440.

9. **Drakylovic, M.B., Torres, A., Bauer, T,** *et al.* (1999) Supine body position as a risk factor for nosocomial pneumonia in mechanically ventilated patients: A randomized trial. *Lancet* **354:** 1851–1858.

10. **Fernandez-Crehuet, R., Diaz-Molina, C., de Irala, J., *et al.*** (1997) Nosocomial infection in an intensive-care unit: Identification of risk factors. *Infect. Control Hosp. Epidemiol.* **18:** 825–830.

11. **Leal-Noval, S.R., Marquez-Vacaro, J.A., Garcia-Curet, A., *et al.*** (2000) Nosocomial pneumonia in patients undergoing heart surgery. *Crit. Care Med.* **28:** 935–940.

12. **Kollef, M.H., Von Harz, B., Prentice, D., *et al.*** (1997) Patient transport from intensive care increases the risk of developing ventilator-associated pneumonia. *Chest* **112:** 765–773.

13. **Fagon, J.-Y., Chastre, J., Vuagnat, A., *et al.*** (1996) Nosocomial pneumonia and mortality among patients in intensive care units. *JAMA* **175:** 866–869.

14. **Rouby, J.J., DeLassale, E.M., Poete, P., *et al.*** (1992) Nosocomial bronchopneumonia in the critically ill: Histologic and bacteriologic aspects. *Am. Rev. Respir. Dis.* **146:** 1059–1066.

15. **Fagon, J.Y., Chastre, J., Hance, A.J., *et al.*** (1988) Detection of nosocomial lung infection in ventilated patients: Use of a protected specimen brush and quantitative culture techniques in 147 patients. *Am. Rev. Respir. Dis.* **138:** 110–116.

16. **Fagon, J.-Y., Chastre, J., Wolff, M., *et al.*** (2000) Invasive and noninvasive strategies for management of suspected ventilator-associated pneumonia. *Ann. Intern. Med.* **132:** 621–630.

17. **Bryan, C.S. and Reynolds, K.L.** (1984) Bacteremic nosocomial pneumonia. *Am. Rev. Respir. Dis.* **129:** 688–691.

18. **Shales, D.M., Ledeman, M.M., Chmielewski, R., *et al.*** (1983) Elastin fibers in the sputum of patients with necrotizing pneumonia. *Chest* **83:** 885–889.

19. **Kirkland, S.H., Corkey, D.E., Winterbauer, R.H., *et al.*** (1997) The diagnosis of ventilator-associated pneumonia. A comparison of histologic, microbiologic and clinical criteria. *Chest* **112:** 445–457.

20. **Niederman, M.S., Torres, A. and Summer, W.** (1994) Invasive diagnostic testing is not needed routinely to manage suspected ventilator-associated pneumonia. *Am. J. Respir. Crit. Care Med.* **150:** 565–569.

21. **Croce, M.A., Fabian, T.C., Shaw, B., *et al.*** (1994) Analysis of charges associated with diagnosis of nosocomial pneumonia: Can routine bronchoscopy be justified? *J. Trauma* **37:** 721–727.

22. **Veber, B., Souweine, B., Gachot, B., *et al.*** (2000) Comparison of direct examination of three types of bronchoscopy specimens used to diagnose nosocomial pneumonia. *Crit. Care Med.* **28:** 962–968.

23. **Schluger, N.W. and Rom, W.N.** (1995) The polymerase chain reaction in the diagnosis and evaluation of pulmonary infections. *Am. J. Respir. Crit. Care Med.* **142:** 11–16.

24. **Meehan, T.P., Fine, M.J., Krumholz, H.M., *et al.*** (1997) Quality of care, process and outcomes in elderly patients with pneumonia. *JAMA* **278:** 2080–2084.

25. **Heffelfinger, J.D., Dowell, S.F., Jorgensen, J.H., *et al.*** (2000) Management of community-acquired pneumonia in the era of pneumococcal resistance. A report from the Drug-Resistant *Streptococcus pneumoniae* Therapeutic Working Group. *Arch. Intern. Med.* **160:** 1399–1408.

26. **Rello, J., Quintara, E., Ausina, V., *et al.*** (1990) Risk factors for *Staphylococcus aureus* nosocomial pneumonia in critically ill patients. *Am. Rev. Respir. Dis.* **142:** 1320–1324.

27. **Rello, J., Torres, A., Ricart, M., *et al.*** (1994) Ventilator-associated pneumonia by *Staphylococcus aureus*. Comparison of methicillin-resistant and methicillin-sensitive episodes. *Am. J. Respir. Crit. Care Med.* **150:** 1545–1549.

28. **Rello, J., Austina, V. and Ricart, M.** (1993) Impact of previous antimicrobial therapy on the etiology and outcome of ventilator-associated pneumonia. *Chest* **104:** 1230–1235.

29. **Robert, R., Grollier, G., Dore, P., *et al.*** (1999) Nosocomial pneumonia with isolation of anaerobic bacteria in ICU patients: Therapeutic considerations and outcome. *J. Crit Care* **14:** 114–119.

30. **Donskey, C.J., Schreiber, J.R., Jacobs, M.R., *et al.*** (1999) A polyclonal outbreak of predominantly VanB vancomycin-resistant enterococci in Northeast Ohio. *Clin. Infect. Dis.* **29:** 573–579.

31. **Sieger, B., Berman, S.J., Geckler, R.W., *et al.*** (1997) Empiric treatment of hospital-acquired lower respiratory tract infections with meropenem or ceftazidime with tobramycin: A randomized study. *Crit. Care Med.* **25:** 1663–1670.

32. **Cometta, A., Baumgartner, J.D., Lew, D., *et al.*** (1994) Prospective randomized comparison of imipenem monotherapy with imipenem plus netilmicin for treatment of severe infections in nonneutropenic patients. *Antimicrob. Agents Chemother.* **38:** 1309–1313.

33. **Chow, J.W., Fine, M.J., Shlaes, D.M., *et al.*** (1991) Enterobacter bacteremia: Clinical features and emergence of antibiotic resistance during therapy. *Ann. Intern. Med.* **115:** 585–590.

34. **Craig, W.** (1993) Pharmacodynamics of antimicrobial agents as a basis for determining dosage regimens. *Eur. J. Clin. Microbiol. Infect. Dis.* **12:** s6–s8.

35. Hatala, R., Dinh, T. and Cook, D.J. (1996) Once-daily aminoglycoside dosing in immunocompetent adults: A meta-analysis. *Ann. Intern. Med.* **124**: 717–725.

36. Schleupner, C.J. and Cobb, D.K. (1992) A study of the etiologies and treatment of nosocomial pneumonia in a community-based teaching hospital. *Infect. Control Epidemiol.* **13**: 515–525.

37. Paladino, J.A., Sperry, H.E., Backes, J.M., *et al.* (1991) Clinical and economic evaluation of oral ciprofloxacin after an abbreviated course of intravenous antibiotics. *Am. J. Med.* **91**: 462–470.

38. Montravers, P., Fagon, J.Y., Chastre, J., *et al.* (1993) Follow-up protected specimen brushes to assess treatment in nosocomial pneumonia. *Am. Rev. Respir. Dis.* **147**: 38–44.

39. Augustine, G., Fein, A.M., Feinsilver, S.H., *et al.* (1992) When pneumonia fails to resolve: Risk factors and diagnostic options. *J. Crit. Illness* **7**: 213–229.

40. El-Ebiary, M., Torres, A., Fabrega, N., *et al.* (1997) Significance of the isolation of *Candida* species from respiratory samples in critically ill, non-neutropenic patients. *Am. J. Respir. Crit. Care Med.* **156**: 583–590.

41. Rex, J.H., Walsh, T.J., Sobel, J.D., *et al.* (2000) Practice guidelines for the treatment of candidiasis. *Clin. Infect. Dis.* **30**: 662–676.

42. Gross, P.A., Hermogenes, A.W., Sacks, H.S., *et al.* (1995) The efficacy of influenza vaccine in elderly persons: a meta-analysis and review of the literature. *Ann. Intern. Med.* **123**: 518–527.

43. Albert, R.K. and Condie, F. (1981) Handwashing patterns in medical intensive care units. *N. Engl. J. Med.* **304**: 1465–1466.

44. Rossoff, L.J., Borenstein, M. and Isenberg, H.D. (1995) Is hand washing really needed in an intensive care unit? *Crit. Care Med.* **23**: 1211–1216.

45. Craven, D.E., Connolly, M.G., Lichtenberg, D.A., *et al.* (1982) Contamination of mechanical ventilators with tubing changes every 24 or 48 hours. *N. Engl. J. Med.* **306**: 1505–1509.

46. Rouby, J.-J., Laurent, P., Gosnach, M., *et al.* (1994) Risk factors and clinical relevance of nosocomial maxillary sinusitis in the critically ill. *Am. J. Respir. Crit. Care Med.* **150**: 776–783.

47. Torres, A., Serra-Batlles, J., Ros, E., *et al.* (1992) Pulmonary aspiration of gastric contents in patients receiving mechanical ventilation: The effect of body position. *Ann. Intern. Med.* **116**: 540–543.

48. Kollef, M.H. (1993) Ventilator-associated pneumonia. A multivariate analysis. *JAMA* **270**: 1965–1970.

49. Valles, J., Artigas, A., Rello, J., *et al.* (1995) Continuous aspiration of subglottic secretions in preventing ventilator-associated pneumonia. *Ann. Intern. Med.* **122**: 179–186.

50. Fink, M.P., Helsmoortel, C.M., Stein, K.L., *et al.* (1990) The efficacy of an oscillating bed in the prevention of lower respiratory tract infection in critically ill victims of blunt trauma. *Chest* **97**: 132–137.

51. DeBoisblanc, B.P., Castro, M., Everret, B., *et al.* (1993) Effect of air-supported, continuous postural oscillation on the risk of early ICU pneumonia in nontraumatic critical illness. *Chest* **103**: 1543–1547.

52. Souweine, B., Mom, T., Traore, O., *et al.* (2000) Ventilator-associated sinusitis. Microbiological results of sinus aspirates in patients on antibiotics. *Anesthesiology* **93**: 1255–1260.

53. Donowitz, L.G., Page, M.C., Mileur, G.L., *et al.* (1986) Alteration of normal gastric flora in critically ill patients receiving antacid and cimetidine therapy. *Infect. Control Hosp. Epidemiol.* **7**: 23–36.

54. Driks, M.R., Craven, D.E., Celli, B.R., *et al.* (1987) Nosocomial pneumonia in intubated patients given sucralfate as compared with antacids or histamine type 2 blockers. *N. Engl. J. Med.* **317**: 1376–1382.

55. Reidy, J.J. and Ramsey, G. (1990) Clinical trials of selective decontamination of the digestive tract: Review. *Crit. Care Med.* **18**: 1449–1456.

56. Cockerill, F.R., Muller, S.R., Anhalt, J.P., *et al.* (1992) Prevention of infection in critically ill patients by selective decontamination of the digestive tract. *Ann. Intern. Med.* **117**: 545–553.

57. Gastinne, H., Wolff, M., Delatour, F., *et al.* (1992) A controlled trial in intensive care units of selective decontamination of the digestive tract with nonabsorbable antibiotics. *N. Engl. J. Med.* **326**: 594–599.

58. Ferrer, M., Torres, A., Gonzalez, J., *et al.* (1994) Utility of selective digestive decontamination in mechanically ventilated patients. *Ann. Intern. Med.* **120**: 389–395.

59. D'Amico, R., Pifferi, S., Leonetti, C., *et al.* (1998) Effectiveness of antibiotic prophylaxis in critically ill adult patients: Systematic review of randomized controlled trials. *Br. Med. J* **316**: 1275–1285.

60. Nouira, S., Elatrous, S., Boukef, R., *et al.* (1998) Effectiveness of selective digestive tract decontamination to control an outbreak of nosocomial pneumonia caused by *Pseudomonas aeruginosa* in mechanically ventilated patients. *Clin. Int. Care* **9**: 180–184.

61. **Ramsey, B.W., Pepe, M.S., Quan, J.M., et al.** (1999) Intermittent administration of inhaled tobramycin in patients with cystic fibrosis. *N. Engl. J. Med.* **340**: 23–30.

62. **The Intravenous Immunoglobulin Collaborative Study Group** (1992) Prophylactic intravenous administration of standard immune globulin as compared with core-lipopolysaccharide immune globulin in patients at high risk of postsurgical infection. *N. Engl. J. Med.* **327**: 234–240.

63. **Welton, L.A., Thal, L.A., Perri, M.B., et al.** (1998) Antimicrobial resistance in enterococci isolated from turkey flocks fed virginiamycin. *Antimicrob. Agents Chemother.* **42**: 705–708.

64. **Gold, H.S. and Moellering, R.C.** (1996) Antimicrobial drug resistance. *N. Engl. J. Med.* **335**: 1445–1453.

65. **Thomson, K.S., Prevan, A.M. and Sanders, C.C.** (1996) Novel plasmid-mediated β-lactamases in enterobacteriaceae: Emerging problems for new β-lactam antibiotics. *Current Clin. Topics Infect. Dis.* **16**: 151–163.

66. **Doern, G.H., Pfaller, M.A., Kugler, K., et al.** (1998) Prevalence of antimicrobial resistance among respiratory tract isolates of *S. pneumoniae* in North America. *Clin. Infect. Dis.* **27**: 764–780.

67. **Kollef, M.H., Vlasnik, J., Sharpless, L., et al.** (1997) Scheduled change of antibiotic classes. A strategy to decrease the incidence of ventilator-associated pneumonia. *Am. J. Respir. Crit. Care Med.* **156**: 1040–1048.

Chapter 17

Obstructive lung disease: asthma and COPD

Robert M. Kacmarek, PhD, RRT

Contents

17.1 Introduction

Obstructive lung disease, classified largely as chronic obstructive lung disease (COPD) and asthma, is common in the population at large and thus commonly affects patients in the ICU. Although similar in their primary physiologic abnormality 'airway obstruction', the type of obstruction does differ between asthma and COPD. With COPD the obstruction is dynamic, increasing during expiration but not inspiration and not fully reversible. In contrast, the obstruction during an acute asthmatic attack is fixed, making both inspiration and expiration difficult. However, the obstruction is fully reversible; between acute events respiratory mechanics are frequently normal.

In both asthma and COPD, patients present with inflammation, bronchospasm and hypersecretion of mucus caused by a variety of infectious and non-infectious agents. This leads to increased airway narrowing that aggravates ventilation–perfusion matching and causes increased air trapping. Treatment is focused on reversing the cause of the acute problem and reversing the inflammation, bronchospasm, and hypersecretion. However, many of these patients require ventilatory support.

This chapter will discuss the treatment of patients with asthma and COPD in the ICU. Because auto-PEEP is an important development in such patients, auto-PEEP is discussed first, followed by a brief review of pharmacologic management. Because many patients with obstructive lung disease in the ICU may be mechanically ventilated, intensivists must be aware of the unique ventilatory issues associated with airflow obstruction. The remainder of the chapter addresses ventilatory management.

17.2 Auto-PEEP

Air trapping and auto-PEEP as a result of severe airflow limitation are the primary pathophysiologic abnormalities leading to mechanical ventilation of patients presenting in an exacerbation of COPD or severe acute asthma. Auto-PEEP is a primary cause of patient ventilator dyssynchrony but also exerts similar cardiopulmonary effects as applied PEEP[1]. Functional residual capacity is increased, intrathoracic pressure is increased, hemodynamics are compromised and ventilation–perfusion mismatch is increased[1]. In addition, work of breathing is markedly increased and the efficiency of diaphragmatic contraction decreased[2]. Air trapping and auto-PEEP flatten the diaphragm, frequently eliminating its inspiratory muscle capabilities and changing its motion to expiratory in function[2]. The altered pulmonary mechanics observed as auto-PEEP increases frequently leads to the ventilatory muscle dysfunction and blood gas abnormalities that require initiation of mechanical ventilation in COPD and asthma.

The obstruction observed during asthma and COPD does differ. In COPD, the obstruction is primarily expiratory and varies greatly with ventilatory pattern. In asthma, the obstruction is fixed (both inspiratory and expiratory) and frequently so severe that the extent of auto-PEEP is underestimated[3]. As demonstrated by Leatherman and Ravenscraft in severe asthma, at end-expiration some airways are completely closed.[3] As a result, the auto-PEEP behind these obstructions is never measured. As shown in *Figure 17.1*, the measured auto-PEEP is 5 cmH$_2$O but the actual air trapping generates auto-PEEP levels up to 20 cmH$_2$O. This problem is much less likely to occur in COPD; because of the dynamic nature of the auto-PEEP, a relaxed end-expiratory measurement generally results in the true average level of auto-PEEP across lung units.

17.3 Non-ventilatory management

Tables 17.1 and *17.2* summarize the non-ventilatory management of acute exacerbations of COPD and severe asthma[4,5]. Although similar in many respects, there are distinct differences between asthma and COPD that affect management. Frequently, severe exacerbations of COPD are a result of both viral and bacterial infection. Careful identification of the

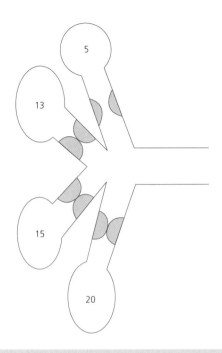

Figure 17.1 Auto-PEEP is the presence of airway closure during exhalation. Using a static end-expiratory occlusion method, the measured level of auto-PEEP is 5 cmH$_2$O. The actual level of auto-PEEP not communicating with the central airway during measurement in some severe asthmatic patients may greatly exceed the measured level. This is a result of complete airway obstruction in these units at end exhalation. From: Leatherman, J.W. and Ravenscraft, S.A. (1996) Low measured auto-positive end-expiratory pressure during mechanical ventilation of patients with severe asthma: Hidden auto-positive end-expiratory pressure. Reproduced with permission from *Crit. Care Med.* **24**: 541–549.

causative organism and appropriate antibiotic therapy are indicated especially in acute purulent COPD exacerbation. *Table 17.3* provides recommendations for antibiotic therapy in an acute exacerbation of COPD[6]. Empirical treatment with antibiotics has become a basic aspect of managing acute exacerbations of COPD characterized by increased volume and purulence of secretions, even if specific organisms cannot be identified. In asthma, antibiotic therapy is normally reserved for those situations where fever is present, the sputum contains neutrophils, or clinical evidence of bacterial pneumonia or sinusitis is present[5]. Most pneumonias in status asthmaticus are viral in origin.

17.3.1 Bronchodilators

In both asthma and COPD, bronchodilators are the mainstay of therapy. In severe asthma, rapid administration of repeated doses of albuterol is recommended[5]. In many situations, continuous or near-continuous initial administration is necessary. In COPD, the norm is standard doses of aerosolized bronchodilators administered every 4 h. However, many also recommend the use of anticholinergics instead of, or in addition to adrenergic agents in managing patients with COPD[4,6]. In addition to bronchodilation, anticholinergics reduce mucous hypersecretion and dyspnea[4]. Many, however, will prefer an adrenergic agent as initial therapy over anticholinergic agents because of more rapid response (5–10 min)[4].

Table 17.1 Medical treatment of an acute exacerbation of COPD

First-line therapies	Example	Dosages
Beta$_2$ agonists	Albuterol (salbutamol)	2.5 mg in NSS via nebulizer or 4 puffs (400 mg) by metered dose inhaler (MDI) with spacer every 4 h
Anticholinergics	Ipratropium bromide	0.5 mg via nebulizer or 2 puffs (18 μg) by MDI with a spacer every 6 h
Corticosteroids	Methylprednisolone	60–125 mg IV every 6 h for 1–3 days, then change to oral prednisone and taper off over 2 weeks
Antibiotics	See *Table 17.3*	See *Table 17.3*
Oxygen	Cannula, ventimask or mask	Titrate to keep SaO$_2$ > 90%

Table 17.2 Medical treatment of status asthmaticus

	Examples	Dosages
First-line therapies		
β_2-agonists	Albuterol (salbutamol)	2.5 mg in normal saline via nebulizer or 4 puffs (400 µg) by MDI with a spacer every 20 min × 3
	Metaproterenol (orciprenaline)	15 mg via nebulizer every 20 min × 3 or 3 puffs (1.95 mg) by MDI with a spacer q 20 min ×3
	Epinephrine (adrenaline)	0.3 ml 1:1000 solution SC every 20 min × 3
Corticosteroids	Prednisone	15–240 mg daily in divided doses
	Methylprednisolone	60–125 mg IV every 6–8 h
Oxygen		Titrate to keep SaO_2 >90%
Second-line therapies		
Methylxanthines	Theophylline	Load: 5–6 mg kg^{-1} IV over 20–30 min (reduced loading dose in patients already taking theophylline preparations) Maintenance: 0.6 mg kg^{-1} h^{-1} IV; titrate to serum theophylline concentration 8–15 µg ml^{-1}
Anticholinergics	Ipratropium bromide	0.5 mg via nebulizer every h × 3

Adapted from: Levy, B.D., Kitch, B. and Fanta, C.H. (1998) Medical and ventilatory management of status asthmaticus. Reproduced with permission from Blackwell Science publishers. *Intens. Care Med.* **24**: 105–117.

17.3.2 Corticosteroids

Systemically administered corticosteroids are a mainstay in the management of severe asthma. Therapy should be initiated upon admission and continued for 7–14 days, then tapered and eventually changed to inhaled preparations for those appropriately responding. In COPD, the use of inhaled steroids is more controversial. The American Thoracic Society recommends steroid use in patients with an asthmatic component to their COPD but also recommends rapid discontinuation in those not responding[7]. The British Thoracic Society also recommends steroid use in COPD patients failing to respond to bronchodilators[8].

17.3.3 Methylxanthines

Although little evidence exists for the beneficial effects of theophylline over beta$_2$ adrenergic agents, these agents are still considered second-line therapy for both acute exacerbations of COPD and status asthmaticus[4,5]. In addition to having a bronchodilator effect, theophylline is an anti-inflammatory agent, improves respiratory muscle endurance and accelerates recovery from fatigue of respiratory muscles[9,10].

17.3.4 Magnesium sulfate

The use of magnesium sulfate in acute asthma is controversial[11,12]. The actual mechanism of action is unknown. Except in patients with renal insufficiency, magnesium sulfate is safe when a dose of less than 2 g is infused intravenously over at least 2 min. This therapy must be considered experimental in asthma and not useful in COPD.

17.3.5 Helium–oxygen mixtures (heliox)

In some severe asthmatics, the use of inhaled helium–oxygen mixtures during spontaneous breathing has lessened the severity of the asthmatic attack[13]. Because of its lower density, helium decreases the pressure gradient required to move inhaled gas past an obstruction. In those patients where heliox is effective, respiratory rate decreases, accessory muscle use diminishes, and intrathoracic pressure change is reduced, resulting in a decrease in pulsus paradoxus and work of breathing[14].

Table 17.3 Recommendations for classification and antibiotic treatment of an acute exacerbation of COPD

Group	Clinical state	Risk factors	Probable pathogens	First choice	Alternatives
I	Acute tracheobronchitis	None	Viral, rarely M. pneumoniae or C. pneumoniae	No antibiotics	Macrolide or tetracycline (for persistent symptoms)
II	Acute exacerbation of chronic bronchitis	None	H. influenzae, Haemophilus spp., M. catarrhalis, S. pneumoniae	Amoxicillin, tetracycline, TMP–SMX	Second-generation cephalosporin, second-generation macrolide, amoxicillin–clavulanate, fluoroquinolone
III	Acute exacerbation of chronic bronchitis with risk factors	Multiple*	Same as above. Also consider Gram-negatives especially in patients with severely impaired lung function	Fluoroquinolone	Amoxicillin–clavulanate, oral second- or third-generation cephalosporin, or second-generation macrolide
IV	Chronic suppurative airway disease	Most have bronchiectasis	Same as group III plus multiresistant Gram-negatives, particularly P. aeruginosa	Antipseudomonal fluoroquinolone (ciprofloxacin)	Consider parenteral therapy with antipseudomonal agents

*FEV1 <50% predicted, frequent exacerbations, significant comorbid conditions, malnutrition, chronic steroid use, mucus hypersecretion, duration of COPD >10 years, previous pneumonia. TMP–SMX, Trimethoprim–sulphamethoxazole.
From: Sherk, P.A. and Grossman, R.E. (2000) The chronic obstructive pulmonary exacerbation. *Clin. Chest Med.* **21**: 705–721

As a result, cardiovascular stress is also reduced.

Not all asthmatics respond to heliox. The reason for the varying response is not clear. However, based on pathophysiology, one can expect patients with primarily small airways involvement and large amounts of retained secretions causing complete airway obstruction to be least likely to respond to heliox[5]. In contrast, patients with primarily large airway obstruction, where gas density determines flow, are most likely to respond. As heliox has no effect on the specific pathology of asthma, its effects are observed only during heliox use. Most responding patients demonstrate improvement within minutes when heliox is applied and demonstrate loss of effect within minutes when heliox is removed.

Heliox is normally administered by partial rebreathing mask (*Figure 17.2*)[15]. The setup used allows the bronchodilator administered to also be powered by heliox if desired. F_IO_2 is generally adjusted by a nasal cannula under the mask or by oxygen titrated into the heliox delivery system. As with all face masks, determination of the precise F_IO_2 is impossible. Delivered oxygen is generally adjusted based on pulse oximetry. The higher the heliox concentration, the greater the likelihood for positive response. Generally, helium concentrations between 60 and 80% are most effective. However, we have noted improvement with even lower helium concentrations. The use of heliox should be continued until the patient's status has improved to the level that removal of the heliox does not cause an increase in cardiopulmonary stress.

No guidelines are established regarding the timing of heliox administration. However, we find it useful to consider heliox use in asthmatic patients who do not demonstrate a positive response after three doses of aerosolized bronchodilator. Few data evaluating the use of heliox in COPD are available and at this time we do not recommend its use in this setting[16]. Limited information on the use of heliox during mechanical ventilation of severe asthmatics is available[17]. Technically, few ventilators are capable of properly operating with this low-density gas. Seimens Servo 900C and 300 ventilators are the two most common ventilators recommended for use with heliox. As with spontaneous breathing, heliox delivers gas past an obstruction requiring a pressure gradient lower than with oxygen–nitrogen mixtures. In volume ventilation, peak pressure tends to decrease whereas with pressure ventilation tidal volumes increase. This frequently allows the F_IO_2 to be decreased because of better $\dot{V}/\dot{Q}$ matching. As with spontaneous breathing, the higher the heliox concentration, the greater the likelihood for success and frequently once heliox is started, F_IO_2 can be lowered. Even with F_IO_2 values of 0.6 or 0.7, we would consider the use of heliox in any mechanically ventilated asthmatic patient. One word of caution: the ventilator display of delivered or exhaled tidal volume is inaccurately low because of the density of the heliox, although airway pressures are accurate. Multiplying the displayed tidal volume by a factor of 1.4–1.8 (depending on helium concentration) provides an estimate of actual delivered V_T[18].

Other than the inability to correctly measure actual tidal volume, the cost of the gas mixture, and therapist's time, there are no side effects or disadvantages of using heliox. Generally, 'H' size tanks need to be changed every 4–6 h.

17.3.6 NIPPV

Published evidence[19] and our clinical experience suggest that noninvasive positive pressure ventilation (NIPPV) is not useful in severe acute asthma. Because of the level of cardiopulmonary distress in severe asthma, patients have a difficult time tolerating NIPPV. The opposite, however, is true in COPD patients. As discussed in Chapter 19, NIPPV must be considered the standard of care for the management of COPD patients in an acute exacerbation[20–22]. This statement is based on data from dozens of case series and at least eight randomized prospective clinical trials demonstrating in COPD patients that NIPPV

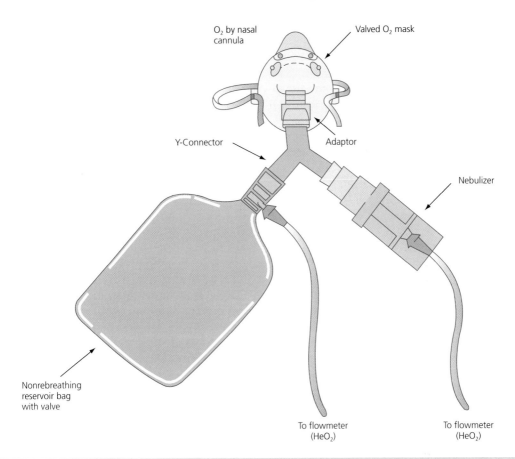

O₂ by nasal cannula

Valved O₂ mask

Y-Connector

Adaptor

Nebulizer

Nonrebreathing reservoir bag with valve

To flowmeter (HeO₂)

To flowmeter (HeO₂)

Figure 17.2 Illustration of a heliox delivery system to spontaneously breathing patients. From: Hess, D. and Chatmongkolchart, S. (2000) Techniques to avoid intubation: Noninvasive positive pressure ventilation and heliox therapy. *Int. Anesth. Clin.* **38**: 161–187.

results in a decrease in endotracheal intubation rate, length of ventilator support and ICU stay, nosocomial pneumonia rate, and mortality (see Chapter 19).

NIPPV is indicated in patients with acute (or acute on chronic) hypercapnic respiratory failure ($PaCO_2 > 45$ mmHg, pH < 7.35)[23]. In the absence of severe gas exchange abnormalities, moderate to severe respiratory distress characterized by respiratory rates >24 min^{-1}, accessory muscle use and paradoxical breathing are also considered indications for NIPPV[23].

Successful application of NIPPV can usually be established within a few hours of initiation. NIPPV should eliminate cardiopulmonary distress and begin to restore blood gas values to baseline. The success of NIPPV depends on a number of factors: the ventilator, the mask, and the personnel at the bedside. In acute respiratory failure either an ICU ventilator or a bilevel pressure ventilator designed for ICU use should be employed. Careful monitoring of patient–ventilator synchrony with appropriate alarms and ability to precisely titrate the F_IO_2 are essential.

The mask is also a crucial aspect of successfully applying NIPPV. In an acute exacerbation of COPD, we favor the use of a full-face mask rather than a nasal mask. Ideally, a mask with exhalation ports as part of the mask is ideal. As recently shown, CO_2 rebreathing can be minimized with masks where the exhalation port is located at the top (nose area) of the mask[24]. This allows for complete flushing of the mask at end exhalation.

Finally, the therapists and nurses caring for the patient must fully understand the principles of NIPPV and the appropriate approach to interacting with the patient. With NIPPV, because sedation is minimized, time must be taken to carefully explain the procedure, gain the trust of the patient and slowly apply the technique. Failure can occur simply as a result of the clinician's approach. (See Chapter 19 for details.)

17.4 Intubation

Many COPD and asthmatic patients require intubation and mechanical ventilation. Although the decision to intubate is often life-saving, intubation may be associated with significant morbidity. Data from NIPPV trials clearly show that intubated COPD patients have a much higher risk of nosocomial pneumonia[25] and a higher mortality than non-intubated patients[26]. The decision to intubate either COPD or asthmatic patients should be made only after exhaustive efforts to manage these patients' respiratory failure more conservatively have failed.

17.5 Mechanical ventilation

Although both COPD and asthma are characterized as bronchospastic or obstructive disease, issues during mechanical ventilation are both similar and very different (*Table 17.4*). With severe asthma, patients can be expected to return to normal baseline function during symptom-free periods. In contrast, COPD patients may be chronically limited and symptomatic. Obstruction is fully reversible with asthma but only partially reversible in COPD. Obstruction in COPD is dynamic, mostly affecting exhalation, whereas in asthma, obstruction is fixed, equally affecting inspiration and expiration. Ventilation is frequently long term in COPD, requiring lengthy weaning, whereas in asthma, ventilation is commonly very short term, with rapid extubation. Similarities are primarily regarding air trapping and auto-PEEP.

17.5.1 Mode of ventilation

As discussed in Chapter 13, two decisions must be made regarding which mode of ventilation should be used. First, should patients be managed with pressure- or volume-targeted ventilation (see *Table 17.5*)? Second, what specific mode of ventilation should be used? In

Table 17.4 Mechanical ventilation of asthma and COPD

	COPD	Asthma
Target	Pressure	Initially volume, pressure when able to assist
Mode	PS, PA/C	Volume A/C then PS or PA/C
PEEP	Improves triggering (5–10 cmH$_2$O)	Not indicated
VT	(6–10 ml kg^{-1})	Initially may be ≤4 ml kg^{-1} up to 10 ml kg^{-1}
P$_{PLAT}$	≤30 cmH$_2$O	≤30 cmH$_2$O
I:E	≤1:3	≤1:3
Inspiratory time	0.6–0.9 s	1.0–1.5 s
Rate	Minimize auto-PEEP	Minimize auto-PEEP
Flow wave	If volume decelerating	If volume decelerating
Peak flow	≥80 l min^{-1}	≥80 l min^{-1}

COPD patients, patient–ventilator synchrony is a major issue, as patients are commonly allowed to continue to interface with the ventilator. As a result, we prefer pressure-targeted ventilation, as gas delivery varies with patient demand and increases the ability of the ventilator to respond in synchrony with the patient[27]. Pressure assist/control or pressure support are the modes of choice. If the patient has control over their ventilatory drive, pressure support is ideal. However, if the patient has periodic breathing because of sedation or exhaustion, pressure assist/control is ideal. Volume assist/control can be used in these patients but it does not allow variability in gas delivery (fixed flow pattern) and therefore increases the likelihood of dyssynchrony and enhanced patient work and effort to breathe.

On the other hand, with asthma volume ventilation, at least at the onset of ventilatory support is essential in most patients. With asthma, high driving pressures are required to move gas into a lung with very high fixed airways resistance. Manually ventilating these patients is a major effort, occasionally requiring 'peak' pressures of 100 cmH$_2$O to deliver tidal volumes of 200 ml. Because of the algorithm governing gas delivery, pressure ventilation cannot sustain the high driving pressures needed to ventilate many asthmatic patients. It should be remembered that lung injury is primarily a result of high distending volumes and high peak alveolar pressures, not high peak airway pressures[28]. In asthma, the driving pressures used to deliver small volumes never affect the distal lung.

With volume ventilation as long as the end-inspiratory plateau pressure is less than 35 cmH$_2$O (ideally <30 cmH$_2$O), the likelihood of ventilator-induced lung injury is limited[28].

During pressure ventilation, the ventilator drives gas flow to rapidly achieve the pressure target. To avoid exceeding the target, flow must be rapidly decreased, frequently in this setting to zero, thereby delivering small or no tidal volume. That is, with a pressure control setting of 30 cmH$_2$O (zero PEEP), driving pressure is 30 cmH$_2$O and peak alveolar pressure is limited to 30 cmH$_2$O. However, gas volume may not be delivered. In volume ventilation at a specific V_T, resulting in an end-inspiratory plateau pressure less than 30 cmH$_2$O, the initial peak pressure may need to increase to 80 cmH$_2$O, providing a driving pressure of 80 cmH$_2$O (zero PEEP) to deliver the desired V_T, but maintaining a safe peak alveolar pressure.

To ventilate asthmatic patients, control ventilation is required. This may be achieved by sedation in some patients; however, many patients require neuromuscular paralysis to achieve successful ventilation. If asthmatics are allowed to continue spontaneous ventilatory efforts, it is frequently impossible to ventilate them. In many asthmatic patients, volume assist/control can be converted to pressure assist/control within a few hours of ventilatory support. However, this is usually unnecessary until spontaneous ventilation resumes. Once the asthmatic patient starts to breathe spontaneously, every effort to insure patient–ventilator synchrony should be made,

Table 17.5 Volume versus pressure ventilation

	Pressure	Volume
Tidal volume	Variable	Constant
Peak inspiratory pressure	Constant	Variable
Peak alveolar pressure	Constant	Variable
Peak flow	Variable	Preset
Flow pattern	Decelerating	Constant
Inspiratory	Preset or variable	Preset

and pressure assist/control or pressure support is indicated.

17.5.2 Tidal volume

In COPD patients, a moderate V_T is frequently desired by the patient (generally between 6 and 10 ml kg^{-1}). In patients with strong ventilatory demand but end-inspiratory plateau pressures less than 30 cmH$_2$O, V_T values up to 10 ml kg^{-1} are not associated with ventilator-induced lung injury[6]. However, avoidance of overdistension and high peak alveolar pressure is always indicated. In asthma, V_T may need to be very small initially ($\leq$4 ml kg^{-1}) because of high airway resistance and air trapping. As airway resistance improves, V_T values can be increased to meet the patient's ventilatory demand. Once pressure support or pressure assist/control is started (provided peak alveolar pressures are <30 cmH$_2$O) V_T values up to 10 ml kg^{-1} maybe necessary to insure patient–ventilatory synchrony[5].

17.5.3 Peak flow, inspiratory time, I:E ratio

Peak flow settings are unnecessary in pressure-targeted ventilation modes but are critical in volume-targeted modes. In general, we recommend the use of a decelerating flow pattern over a square-wave flow pattern in both COPD and asthma when volume ventilation is used. A decelerating flow pattern insures better distribution of inspired gas and distributes the primary effect of airways resistance and compliance to opposite ends of the inspiratory phase, generally decreasing peak airway pressure. At the onset of inspiration, with the flow rate very high but no volume delivered, impedance to gas delivery is primarily a result of airways resistance. In contrast, at the end of the inspiratory phase when the flow rate is very low and tidal volume almost completely delivered, impedance to gas delivery is primarily a result of compliance. A decelerating flow pattern produces a gas delivery pattern similar to pressure ventilation.

Especially in patients breathing spontaneously, initial peak flow should be high in volume ventilation[29]. In the setting of both asthma and COPD, peak flows should be set at 80 l min^{-1} or higher. This insures that flow will better match the patient's inspiratory demand. In pressure ventilation, peak flow automatically varies with demand (generally exceeding 80 l min^{-1}) if the pressure level is set greater than 10 cmH$_2$O[30].

Inspiratory time in spontaneously breathing patients should be set equal to the patient's neuro-inspiratory time. In most COPD patients this is about 0.6–0.9 s. Inspiratory times longer than those desired by the patient tend to increase dyssynchrony. During controlled ventilation in COPD, inspiratory time can be set longer, but considering the problems with air trapping they are generally set at 1.0 s or less.

In asthma, as the impact of airways resistance is fixed and equally affects inspiration and expiration, inspiratory time should not be less than 1.0 s; short inspiratory times prevent gas delivery through the highly obstructed airway. The trade-off is that because of air trapping, expiratory times should also be long. In general, each asthmatic patient defines an experimental setting with inspiratory times adjusted between 1.0 and 1.5 s to insure adequate inspiratory volume and expiratory time lengthened to the level that air trapping is minimized but ventilation (respiratory rate) is adequate[5].

I:E ratio is generally considered a result of the above settings and not a target that is set. However, in both COPD and asthma I:E ratio tends to be small (1:3 to 1:6) with short inspiratory and long expiratory times.

17.5.4 Respiratory rate and auto-PEEP

Respiratory rate is generally set to insure an adequate PaCO$_2$ level. In asthma it may not be possible to achieve normocapnia; permissive hypercapnia is generally the rule early in the ventilatory course, with PaCO$_2$ in the 70s and 80s common. The rate resulting in the best CO$_2$ elimination with minimal air trapping and auto-PEEP is generally patient dependent. In many asthma patients, there is a specific expiratory time that minimizes auto-PEEP;

lengthening expiratory time beyond this level has minimal if any effect on auto-PEEP until the expiratory time becomes unacceptably long. Frequently, patients can be maintained with rates in the mid-to-upper teens if tidal volumes are small. It is overall minute ventilation that has the greatest impact on auto-PEEP[1]. With asthma, care should always be taken when ventilator settings are adjusted to insure that auto-PEEP levels are minimized. Severe asthma is one of the clinical settings in which increasing the level of ventilation can result in increasing CO_2 levels because of decreased cardiac output and increased dead space ventilation as auto-PEEP increases. If an alteration in pressure target, V_T, inspiratory time, or rate does not produce a decrease in CO_2 it was the wrong adjustment and should be reversed. High CO_2 levels may need to be tolerated for days in severe asthma.

With COPD patients, rates should be set to insure minimal auto-PEEP and adequate CO_2 removal during controlled ventilation. This goal is readily achieved in managing patients with COPD. During spontaneous breathing, patients frequently select a rate in the mid-20s. Insurance that peak flow and inspiratory time as well as V_T or pressure target are set appropriately will assist in avoiding dyssynchrony.

17.5.5 PEEP/F_IO_2

In COPD patients, adequate oxygenation can usually easily be managed by administering moderate oxygen levels. With asthma, some patients do require high F_IO_2 values (0.6–0.8) because of both increased shunting (mucous plugging) and $\dot{V}/\dot{Q}$ mismatch.

The use of PEEP in these two clinical settings is controversial. In asthma we have rarely found PEEP to be beneficial. In some patients, it appears that low-level PEEP improves $\dot{V}/\dot{Q}$ matching but in most cases because of the fixed nature of the obstruction applied PEEP is simply additive to auto-PEEP and detrimental.

COPD patients breathing spontaneously (assisted ventilation) frequently benefit greatly from the use of applied PEEP. Appropriately adjusting PEEP can markedly improve patient–ventilator synchrony. Auto-PEEP in COPD is the result of a variable dynamic flow resistor. The pressure difference at end exhalation across the resistor is great; auto-PEEP on one side and end-expiratory ventilator circuit pressure on the other (*Figure 17.3*)[31]. In this setting, applied PEEP less than about 80% of the auto-PEEP level does not increase overall total PEEP, but does reduce the gradient to trigger the ventilator, thereby avoiding missed triggered breaths[32]. It is difficult to measure auto-PEEP during spontaneous breathing, but its presence can easily be identified by observing the expiratory flow waveform (*Figure 17.4*)[33]. In addition, auto-PEEP is normally the cause of the patient's inspiratory efforts failing to trigger an assisted breath. Whenever the patient's respiratory rate exceeds the ventilator response rate, the patient is having difficulty overcoming the auto-PEEP. In this setting slowly increasing PEEP in 1–2 cmH_2O increments and observing the patients ventilatory pattern can dramatically improve synchrony[34]. When every patient effort triggers an assisted breath, the appropriate PEEP level is set. In all COPD patients, 5 cmH_2O applied PEEP is helpful. However, in many patients, levels as high as 12–15 cmH_2O may be necessary because of high auto-PEEP levels. During controlled ventilation there are no data to suggest that the application of PEEP has a beneficial effect. However, PEEP does not appear to be harmful provided its application does not increase total PEEP.

17.6 Weaning from ventilatory support

Details on approaches to weaning are presented in Chapter 18, but special considerations in patients with asthma and COPD deserve mention here. With asthma, patients rarely require prolonged weaning. Because they normally have good ventilatory mechanics once the acute asthma is reversed, they tolerate rapid extubation well. Asthmatic patients who are not heavily sedated rarely tolerate an endotracheal tube without developing bronchospasm. As a result, as soon as airways

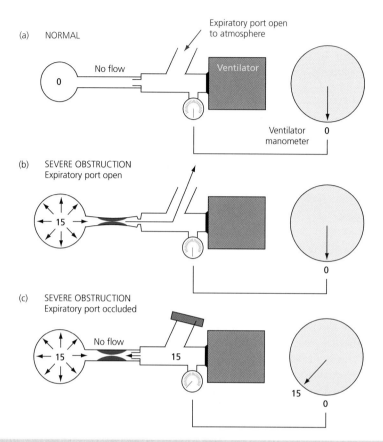

Figure 17.3 Measurement of auto-PEEP by expiratory port occlusion. Normally (see top panel), alveolar pressure is atmospheric at the end of passive exhalation. With severe airflow obstruction (see middle panel) alveolar pressure remains elevated (in this example at 15 cmH$_2$O) and slow flow continues even at the end of the set exhalation period. The ventilator manometer senses negligible pressure because it is open to atmosphere through large-bore tubing and downstream from the site of flow limitation. With gas flow stopped by occlusion of the expiratory port at the end of the set exhalation period (see lower panel), pressure equilibrates throughout the lung–ventilator system and is displayed on the ventilatory manometer. From: Pepe, P.E. and Marini, J.J. (1982) Occult positive end-expiratory pressure in mechanically ventilated patients with airflow obstruction: the auto-PEEP effect. *Am. Rev. Respir. Dis.* **126**: 166–170.

resistance returns to near-normal levels, and ventilation and oxygenation can be maintained at low ventilator settings (F$_I$O$_2$ ≤ 0.4, pressure support or control levels of 10–15 cmH$_2$O and V$_T$ values in the 6–10 ml kg^{-1} range), extubation should be considered[5].

In contrast, COPD patients frequently require a very long weaning period because of chronic airway obstruction, other organ system dysfunction, and a general state of debilitation[35]. These patients require a consistent,

standardized weaning program that incorporates general physical rehabilitation. Some do wean rapidly but most require days to weeks to be successfully liberated from ventilatory support. The use of either a pressure support or spontaneous breathing trial approach to weaning is appropriate. Care should be taken to insure that patients are well rested (particularly at night), well nourished, and that their ventilatory capabilities are challenged daily but are not pushed to the level of fatigue.

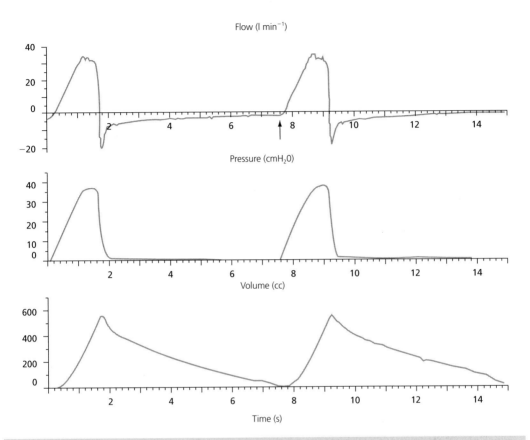

Figure 17.4 Gas flow, airway pressure, and volume waveforms during volume-targeted control ventilation in the presence of auto-PEEP. Expiratory gas flow shows an initial spike that rapidly decreases to a low level throughout the prolonged expiratory time. It should be noted that expiratory gas flow does not return to zero (arrow) indicating the presence of auto-PEEP. From: Kacmarek, R.M. and Hess, D.R. (1993) Airway pressure, flow and volume waveforms, and lung mechanics during mechanical ventilation. In: *Monitoring in Respiratory Care* (eds R.M. Kacmarek, D.R. Hess and J.K. Stoller). Mosby Yearbook, St Louis, MO, pp. 497–543.

References

1. **Pepe, P.E. and Marini, J.J.** (1982) Occult positive end-expiratory pressure in mechanically ventilated patients with airflow obstruction: The auto-PEEP effect. *Am. Rev. Respir. Dis.* **126**: 166–172.

2. **Petrof, B.J., Legare, M., Goldberg, P., et al.** (1990) Continuous positive airway pressure reduces work of breathing and dyspnea during weaning from mechanical ventilation in severe chronic obstructive pulmonary disease. *Am. Rev. Respir. Dis.* **141**: 281–289.

3. **Leatherman, J.W. and Ravenscraft, S.A.** (1996) Low measured auto-positive end-expiratory pressure during mechanical ventila-

tion of patients with severe asthma: Hidden auto-positive end-expiratory pressure. *Crit. Care Med.* **24**: 541–549.

4. **Ferguson, G.T.** (2000) Update on pharmacologic therapy for chronic obstructive pulmonary disease. *Clin. Chest Med.* **21**: 723–738.

5. **Levy, B.D., Kitch, B. and Fanta, C.H.** (1998) Medical and ventilatory management of status asthmaticus. *Intens. Care Med.* **24**: 105–117.

6. **Sherk, P.A. and Grossman, R.E.** (2000) The chronic obstructive pulmonary exacerbation. *Clin. Chest Med.* **21**: 705–721.

7. **American Thoracic Society** (1995) Standards for the diagnosis and care of patients with chronic obstructive pulmonary disease. *Am. J. Respir. Crit. Care Med.* **152**: 584–596.

8. **British Thoracic Society** (1997) Guidelines for the management of chronic obstructive pulmonary disease. *Thorax* **52**: S1–S28.

9. **Weinberger, M. and Hendeles, L.** (1996) Theophylline in asthma. *N. Engl. J. Med.* **334**: 1380–1388.

10. **Ferguson, G.T. and Cherniack, R.M.** (1993) Management of chronic obstructive pulmonary disease. *N. Engl. J. Med.* **328**: 1017–1022.

11. **Skobeloff, E.M., Spivery, W.H., McNamara, R.M. and Greenspan, L.** (1989) Intravenous magnesium sulfate for the treatment of acute asthma in the emergency department. *JAMA* **262**: 1210–1213.

12. **Green, S.M. and Rothrock, S.G.** (1992) Intravenous magnesium for acute asthma: Failure to decrease emergency treatment duration or need for hospitalization. *Ann. Emerg. Med.* **21**: 260–265.

13. **Kass, J.E. and Castriotta, R.J.** (1995) Heliox therapy in acute severe asthma. *Chest* **107**: 757–760.

14. **Manthous, C.A., Hall, J.B., Meled, A., Caputo, M.A., Walter, J., Klocksieben, J.M., Schmidt, G.A. and Wood, L.D.H.** (1995) Heliox improves pulsus paradoxus and peak expiratory flow in non intubated patients with severe asthma. *Am. J. Respir. Crit. Care Med.* **152**: 310–317.

15. **Hess, D. and Chatmongkolchart, S.** (2000) Techniques to avoid intubation: Noninvasive positive pressure ventilation and heliox therapy. *Int. Anesth. Clin.* **38**: 161–187.

16. **Jaber, S., Fodil, R., Carlucci, A., et al.** (2000) Noninvasive ventilation with helium–oxygen in acute exacerbations of chronic obstructive pulmonary disease. *Am. J. Respir. Crit. Care Med.* **161**: 1191–1200.

17. **Gluck, E.H., Onorato, D.J. and Castriotta, R.** (1990) Helium–oxygen mixtures in intubated patients with status asthmaticus and respiratory acidosis. *Chest* **98**: 693–698.

18. **Tassaux, D., Jolliet, P., Thouret, J.M., Roeseler, J., Dorne, R. and Chevrolet, J.C.** (1999) Calibration of seven ICU ventilators for mechanical ventilation with helium–oxygen mixtures. *Am. J. Respir. Care Med.* **160**: 22–32.

19. **Keenen, S.P., Kernerman, P.D., Cook, D.J., Martin, C.M., McCormack, D. and Sibbald, W.J.** (1997) Effect of noninvasive positive pressure ventilation on mortality in patients admitted with acute respiratory failure: A meta-analysis. *Crit. Care Med.* **25**: 1685–1691.

20. **Kramer, N., Meyer, T.J., Meharg, J., Cece, R.D. and Hill, N.S.** (1998) Randomized, prospective trial of noninvasive positive pressure ventilation in acute respiratory failure. *Am. J. Respir. Crit. Care Med.* **151**: 1799–1805.

21. **Brochard, L., Mancebo, J., Wysocki, M., et al.** (1995) Noninvasive ventilation for acute exacerbations of chronic obstructive pulmonary disease. *N. Engl. J. Med.* **338**: 817–822.

22. **Plant, P.K., Owen, J.L. and Elliott, M.W.** (2000) Early use of non-invasive ventilation for acute exacerbation of chronic obstructive pulmonary disease on general respiratory wards: A multicenter randomized controlled trial. *Lancet* **355**: 1931–1936.

23. **Wysocki, M., Tric, L., Wolff, M.A., Millet, H. and Herman, B.** (1995) Noninvasive pressure support ventilation in patients with acute respiratory failure: A randomized comparison with conventional therapy. *Chest* **107**: 761–766.

24. **Schettino, G.P.P., Chatmongkolchart, S., Hess, D. and Kacmarek, R.M.** (2001) CO_2 elimination during B_iPAP ventilation: Effects of mask design and PEEP (abstract). *Am. Rev. Respir. Crit. Care Med.* **163**: A679.

25. **Girou, E., Schortgen, F., Delclaux, C., Brun-Buisson, C., Blot, F., Lefort, Y., Lemaire, F. and Brochard, L.** (2000) Association of noninvasive ventilation with nosocomial infections and survival in critically ill patients. *JAMA* **284**: 2361–2366.

26. **Guerin, C., Girard, R., Chemorin, C., DeVarax, R. and Fournier, G.** (1997) Facial mask noninvasive mechanical ventilation reduces the incidence of nosocomial pneumonia: A prospective epidemiological survey from a single ICU. *Intens. Care Med.* **23**: 1024–1028.

27. **Cinnella, G., Conti, G., Lofaso, F., Lorino, H., Harf, A., Lemaire, F. and Brochard, L.** (1996) Effects of assisted ventilation on the work of breathing: Volume-controlled versus pressure-controlled ventilation. *Am. J. Respir. Crit. Care Med.* **153**: 1025–1033.

28. **Dreyfuss, D. and Saumon, G.** (1993) Role of tidal volume, FRC, and end-inspiratory volume in the development of pulmonary edema following mechanical ventilation. *Am. Rev. Respir. Dis.* **148**: 1194–1203.

29. **Marini, J.J., Rodriquez, M. and Lamb, V.** (1986) The inspiratory workload of patient-initiated mechanical ventilation. *Am. Rev. Resp. Dis.* **134**: 902–906.

30. **Williams, P., Muelver, M., Kratohvil, J., Ritz, R., Hess, D.R. and Kacmarek, R.M.** (2000) Pressure support and pressure assist/control: Are there differences? An evaluation of the newest intensive care unit ventilators. *Respir. Care* **45**: 1169–1181.

31. **Pepe, P.E. and Marini, J.J.** (1982) Occult positive end-expiratory pressure in mechanically ventilated patients with airflow obstruction: the

auto-PEEP effect. *Am. Rev. Respir. Dis.* **126**: 166–170.

32. **Smith, T.C. and Marini, J.J.** (1988) Impact of PEEP on lung mechanics and work of breathing in severe airflow obstruction. *J. Appl. Phys.* **64**: 1488.

33. **Kacmarek, R.M. and Hess, D.R.** (1993) Airway pressure, flow and volume waveforms, and lung mechanics during mechanical ventilation. In: *Monitoring in Respiratory Care* (eds R.M. Kacmarek, D.R. Hess and J.K. Stoller). Mosby Yearbook, St Louis, MO, pp. 497–543.

34. **Petrof, B.J., Legare, M., Goldberg, P., *et al.*** (1990) Continuous positive airway pressure reduces work of breathing end dyspnea during weaning from mechanical ventilation in severe COPD. *Am. Rev. Respir. Dis.* **141**: 281–289.

35. **Vitacca, M., Vianello, A., Colombo, D., *et al.*** (2001) Comparison of two methods for weaning patients with chronic obstructive pulmonary disease requiring mechanical ventilation for more than 15 days. *Am. J. Respir. Crit. Care Med.* **164**: 225–230.

Chapter 18

Weaning from mechanical ventilation

James K. Stoller, MD and
Thomas L. Higgins, MD

Contents

18.1 Introduction

Weaning, the process of freeing the patient from ventilatory dependence, is a common challenge in the ICU and subacute respiratory care units. Weaning encompasses both art and science because measured respiratory parameters alone do not always accurately predict a patient's readiness to breathe without ventilatory assistance. The term 'weaning' must also be distinguished from 'extubation' or removal of the endotracheal tube. For example, patients who cannot protect their upper airway (e.g. in coma) or patients with upper airway obstruction (e.g. with edema or glottic dysfunction) may require placement of an endotracheal tube even though they can breathe spontaneously. Incomplete reversal of neuromuscular blockade can also produce a situation where ventilation is adequate, but airway protection is impaired[1]. This chapter will consider the indications for weaning and extubation, the rationale and clinical utility of weaning predictors, weaning techniques in general and in specific patient subsets, and specific impediments to weaning.

18.2 Who requires gradual withdrawal of mechanical ventilation?

Not all patients require gradual withdrawal of mechanical respiratory support. The majority of patients undergoing surgical procedures can be extubated immediately following surgery, and need to be ventilated only until they have sufficient neurologic function and muscular strength to breathe on their own. Thus, the first important concept in weaning is that the underlying process causing respiratory failure must be improving before weaning can begin. Patients who have undergone uncomplicated operations generally require ventilation only until the effects of anesthetic and neuromuscular blocking drugs have cleared. Even patients undergoing thoracic or upper abdominal operations (those are associated with the greatest impairment of ventilatory function) are usually liberated from mechanical ventilation once acute drug effects resolve, as long as there is no associated cardiovascular instability. Finally, patients for whom intubation is performed for airway protection rather than for ventilatory support can be promptly extubated once the reason for airway compromise resolves.

A subset of complex postoperative patients require ventilatory support for several hours to several days following their surgical procedure. Common reasons for prolonged postoperative ventilatory support include low cardiac output states (where the work of breathing from spontaneous ventilation will impair already tenuous systemic perfusion), unstable hemodynamics, ongoing bleeding and/or the possibility of re-exploration, intravascular volume overload, or a requirement for continued sedation and neuromuscular blockade (as in the neurosurgical patient with elevated intracranial pressure). Although past practice dictated that cardiac surgical patients were ventilated overnight, newer cardiac anesthetic techniques have made it possible to 'fast-track' most patients[2]. Criteria for removing the endotracheal tube in postoperative cardiac patients include hemodynamic stability, normalization of acid–base and electrolyte status, restoration of body temperature to normal, and adequate muscle strength and mental status[3].

Individuals whose respiratory function has been compromised by a serious, protracted insult often require prolonged ventilation and more gradual withdrawal of ventilatory support. Common examples of such conditions include sepsis, the acute respiratory distress syndrome (ARDS), COPD complicated by an acute insult such as pneumonia, and neuromuscular disorders compromising ventilatory function. Such patients require prolonged ICU stays, account for a large proportion of ICU days and attention, and will be the subject of most of the ensuing discussion. Importantly, approaches that have been shown to improve outcomes in such patients have included use of standardized weaning approaches[4,5], protocols that incorporate input from allied health care providers, and teams dedicated to weaning[6].

18.3 Sequelae of prolonged intubation and ventilation

Intubation and prolonged mechanical ventilation are associated with morbidity, including vocal granulomas and ulceration of the true cords, in more than half of patients intubated for more than 24 h[7]. Early tracheal lesions may progress to a circumferential fibrous stenosis that is difficult to later repair. Roughly 20% of patients who survive their ICU stay, and 95% of those dying while intubated, will have significant tracheal lesions[8]. Functional concerns also favor removing the endotracheal tube as early as possible to avert epithelial damage, loss of cilia, and impairment of tracheal mucous clearance[9]. Endotracheal intubation increases the risk of nosocomial pneumonia and often precludes oral feeding, mandating the use of enteral or parenteral nutrition. Iatrogenic malnutrition is thus common in the ventilated patient[10]. Finally, mechanical ventilation elicits an inflammatory response that can be attenuated by minimizing overdistention of the lung[11].

18.4 Overview of the logic of weaning

In approaching the patient on mechanical ventilation for whom weaning is being considered, the clinician must ask:

- Is the patient a candidate to undergo a weaning trial? And, if so,
- Is weaning likely to be successful?

Each question invites several clinical considerations and/or measurements.

18.4.1 Is the patient a candidate to undergo a weaning trial?

For a patient to be considered candidate for a weaning trial, criteria listed in *Table 18.1* must be met. Weaning will not succeed unless the process initially responsible for ventilator dependence has shown improvement. Remediable aspects that can contribute to ongoing ventilator dependence (e.g. bronchospasm,

hypermetabolic state, poor nutrition, cardiac failure) should be optimized.

18.4.2 Is weaning likely to be successful?

Once the patient is deemed a candidate to wean and a weaning trial is planned, predicting the likelihood of weaning success is useful. Weaning prediction is the process of estimating the likelihood that weaning and/or extubation efforts will succeed or fail in a specific patient at a specific time[12]. Although no single respiratory parameter or scoring system performs flawlessly, measuring parameters is helpful as a training device, reduces the dependence on the skills of the individual clinician and helps to guide management.

Many parameters to enhance weaning prediction have been proposed and include both univariate (single variable) measures and multivariate indices whose complexity varies. Multivariate predictors generally utilize measurements of:

- static lung function (e.g. forced vital capacity (FVC));
- ventilatory muscle strength and/or endurance (e.g. maximal inspiratory force, maximal voluntary ventilation);
- gas exchange (e.g. alveolar–arterial gradient or PaO_2/F_IO_2 ratio);
- systemic perfusion (e.g. gastric intramural pH).

The predictive accuracy of most univariate weaning parameters (*Table 18.2*) is low,

---

Table 18.1 Questions to ask in assessing the patient's candidacy to undertake weaning

- Is the process responsible for ventilator dependence improving?
- Is oxygenation adequate?
- Is the patient hemodynamically stable, e.g. free from a requirement for pressors and inotropes?
- Have remediable factors been optimized, e.g. maximum treatment of bronchospasm of metabolic abnormalities that can impair weaning (e.g. hypophosphatemia, hypokalemia), adequate resolution of effects of all sedating and paralytic agents, adequate nutrition?

especially regarding ability to predict weaning failure (i.e. negative predictive value). As a result of this low negative predictive value, slavish adherence to univariate weaning parameters in initiating weaning trials can delay weaning that is actually possible[13]. As shown in *Table 18.3*, some multivariate weaning indices are better predictors of weaning success or failure.

In the sections that follow, we consider several of the multivariate weaning parameters, particularly those regarding the pattern of breathing, work of breathing, measurements of tracheal occlusion pressure, and endurance.

18.5 Evaluation of breathing pattern

Assessing the patient's pattern of breathing provides important insight into the likelihood of weaning outcome, because rapid shallow breathing and paradoxic inward inspiratory motion of the abdominal muscles (so-called 'abdominal paradox') accompany ventilatory failure. Unlike measurements of the maximal inspiratory pressure (MIP), vital capacity (VC), and maximal voluntary ventilation (MVV), the breathing pattern is not highly dependent on patient co-operation.

Table 18.2 Diagnostic performance of selected univariate weaning parameters in predicting weaning

Minute ventilation (VE) <10 L min⁻¹					
Study	n	Sensitivity (%)	Specificity (%)	PPV	NPV
Sahn & Lakshminarayan (1973)[86]	100	92	100	100	71
Tahvanainen et al. (1983)[51]	47	45	78	89	25
Krieger et al. (1989)[13]†	269	NS	NS	93	15
Yang & Tobin (1989)[87]	41	24	69	55	37

*VE < 10 l min⁻¹, MIP < −30 cmH₂O, and MVV > 2 VE.
†VE < 10 l min⁻¹, MIP < −30 cmH₂O, and MVV > 2 VE.
PPV, positive predictive value; NPV, negative predictive value; NS, not stated.

Vital capacity (VC)					
Study	Criterion	n	Sensitivity (%)	Specificity (%)	PPV	NPV
Milbern et al. (1978)[88]	VC > 15 ml kg⁻¹	33	25	0	58	0
Tahvanainen et al. (1983)[51]	VC > 10 ml kg⁻¹	47	97	13	83	50
Pardee et al. (1984)[89]	VC > 17 ml kg⁻¹	133	90	60	88	NS

*VC > 15 ml kg⁻¹ and MIP < −25 cmH₂O.
NS, not stated.

Maximal inspiratory pressure (MIP) ≤ −30 cmH₂O						
Study (date)	n	Patient type	Sensitivity (%)	Specificity (%)	PPV	NPV
Sahn & Lakshminarayan (1973)[86]	100	Mean MV duration 37 h	92	100	100	71
Milbern et al. (1978)[88]†	33	Mean MV 3.1 h	25	0	58	0
Tahvanainen et al. (1983)[51]	47	Mean MV 5 days	68	0	74	0
DeHaven et al. (1986)[90]	48	Mean MV 55 h	49	100	100	12
Krieger et al. (1989)[13]	269	Mean age >70 years MV 71 h	NS	NS	92	21
Yang & Tobin (1989)[87]	41	NS	76	25	61	40

*MIP < −30 cmH₂O, VE < 10 l min⁻¹, and MVV ≥ 2 VE.
†MIP < −30 cmH₂O, and VC ≥ 15 ml kg⁻¹.
PPV, positive predictive value; NPV, negative predictive value; MV, mechanical ventilator; NS, not stated. From: Stoller, J.K. (1991) Establishing clinical unweanability. Reproduced with permission from *Respir. Care* **36**: 186–198.

Table 18.3 Diagnostic performance of selected multivariate indices for weaning prediction

Study	n	Index	Patient type	Positive predictive (%)	Negative predictive (%)
Hilberman et al. (1976)[76]	124	Nurses' assessments	OHS	82	67
Krieger et al. (1984)[12]	269	NIF < −30 cmH$_2$O, VE > 10 l min^{-1}	>70 yr, on MV mean 71 h	93	15
Yang & Tobin (1991)[13]	100	CROP > 13 Freq/V$_T$ ≥ 105	On MV 8.2 ± 1.1 days	71	70
Sheinhorn et al. (1995)[14]	565	P(A-a)O$_2$ BUN, gender	On MV >6 weeks	71	67
Epstein (1995)[15]	184	Freq/VT > 100	MICU on MV, f/VT measured within 8 h of wean onset	83	40
Gluck et al. (1995)[22]	55	Score (5 variables) Points > 3	On MV ≥ 3weeks	58	100

NIF, negative inspiratory force; MV, mechanical ventilator; V$_E$, minute ventilation; CROP, compliance rate oxygenation pressure; OHS, open-heart surgery; NS, not stated; BUN, blood urea nitrogen; MICU, medical intensive care unit; V$_T$, tidal volume. Hypothesis-generating study, not confirmed in a separate dataset; hypothesis-testing dataset included. From: Stoller, J. (2000). Reproduced with permission from *SCCM/ACCP Combined Critical Care Course*[91].

18.5.1 The rapid shallow breathing index

This index, commonly known as the frequency to tidal volume ratio (f/V$_T$), calculates the patient's spontaneous breathing frequency (breaths per minute) divided by the patient's spontaneous tidal volume (in liters) while off mechanical ventilatory assistance. Yang and Tobin proposed that an f/V$_T$ value less than 105 would discriminate between patients who were successfully weaned (defined as maintaining spontaneous breathing for greater than 24 h after extubation) versus those who required ongoing ventilatory support[14]. This index was developed on 36 patients and subsequently validated in 64 different patients. Overall, an f/V$_T$ greater than 105 carried a negative predictive value of 0.95, meaning 95% of patients with a high f/V$_T$ could not be extubated. In contrast, values of f/V$_T$ less than 105 predicted a 78% chance of weaning success. In patients who had received mechanical ventilation for more than 8 days, the negative and positive predictive values were slightly lower

at 0.89 and 0.64 respectively, emphasizing that predicting unweanability in long-term mechanically ventilated patients is more difficult[15]. Subsequent studies[16,17] have confirmed the usefulness of the rapid shallow breathing index, but have also pointed out its shortcomings when non-respiratory factors such as congestive heart failure or upper airway obstruction are present. The diagnostic accuracy of different weaning parameters will vary depending on the underlying cause of respiratory failure. For example, the rapid shallow breathing index has its highest diagnostic accuracy in predicting weaning success in patients with COPD, but does not perform as well in patients with neurologic disease or other causes of acute respiratory failure[18].

18.5.2 The tension–time index of the diaphragm (Tt$_{di}$)

This is derived from the percentage of maximal transdiaphragmatic pressure (P$_{di}$) expended with each breath (P$_{di}$/P$_{di}$max) and the fraction of the breathing cycle time spent in inspiration

$(T_i/T_{TOT})^{19}$. Values of Tt_{di} below 0.15 predict the ability to sustain unassisted respiration for longer than 45 min. Values of Tt_{di} above 0.15 predict eventual ventilatory failure, possibly because of limitation of diaphragmatic blood flow (*Figure 18.1*). Although transdiaphragmatic pressure and inspiratory time are not routinely measured, devices such as the Bicore can provide surrogate measurements that have been advocated by some in enhancing weaning[20].

18.6 Work of breathing (WOB)

Work of breathing is the work expended by the ventilatory muscles in supporting breathing

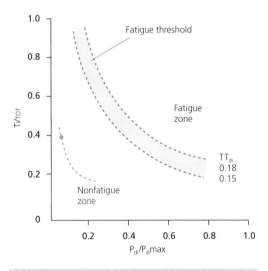

Figure 18.1 Tension–time index for the human diaphragm (TT_{di}). The inspiratory time total ventilatory cycle time (T_i/T_{TOT}) ratio is plotted against transdiaphragmatic pressure during normal breathing/maximum P_{di} possible (P_{di}/P_{di}max) ratio. The fatigue threshold represents a TT_{di} that can be sustained for 1 hour or longer and has a value of 0.15 to 0.18 in the normal human diaphragm. The TT_{di} threshold can be achieved with a large variety of P_{di} and T_i/T_{TOT} values. Patterns in the fatigue zone result in fatigue in less than 1 hour, whereas patterns in the non-fatigue zone can be sustained indefinitely. The circle represents the TT_{di} during resting breathing in normal subjects. From: Grassino, A, Bellemare F, and Laporta D. (1984) Diaphragm fatigue and the strategy of breathing in COPD. Reproduced with permission from *Chest*. **85**: 515–535.

and is measured by integrating the area under a pressure–volume inspiratory curve[21]. Elevated WOB predicts inspiratory muscle fatigue with subsequent weaning failure. Work per minute, defined as the amount of work done per breath multiplied by the respiratory rate, reflects ventilatory requirements. Work per liter is the work per minute divided by V_E and measures efficiency of breathing. In patients requiring prolonged ventilation, work of breathing is a better indicator of successful weaning than standard bedside weaning criteria (i.e. vital capacity, maximum inspiratory pressure, tidal volume, and minute ventilation)[22]. Specifically, as WOB values fall below 1.60 kg-m min^{-1} (16 joules min^{-1}), WOB better discriminates between patients with weaning success versus failure than more conventional measures.

In a study of 23 patients comparing a weaning protocol incorporating WOB and f/V_T versus a clinical approach using conventional weaning criteria (e.g. minute ventilation, negative inspiratory force, tidal volume, and static compliance), the protocol incorporating WOB measurements hastened weaning in at least 41% of instances and shortened the projected mean duration of weaning by 1.68 days[23].

18.6.1 The oxygen cost of breathing
This is a related measure assessed by comparing oxygen (O_2) consumption during complete inspiratory muscle rest (i.e. during paralysis with controlled mechanical ventilation) with O_2 consumption during spontaneous ventilation[24]. In normal individuals, oxygen consumption by the respiratory muscles accounts for approximately 2–5% of total oxygen consumption. In patients who became ventilator dependent, the oxygen cost of breathing was frequently 15% or more of total O_2 consumption. Using a threshold value of 15% as a predictor, the sensitivity of O_2 cost of breathing measurements was 100% and specificity 80%[25]. Despite the physiologic appeal of O_2 cost of breathing measurements in guiding weaning, impediments to clinical use include the needs for metabolic cart measurements and to conduct measurements during complete paralysis.

18.7 Tracheal occlusion pressure

Respiratory center drive is measured by the tracheal occlusion pressure ($P_{0.1}$), the airway pressure generated during the first tenth of a second during an occluded inspiratory effort. Using a threshold value of 6 cmH_2O, the $P_{0.1}$ provides a simple, valid way to assess the likelihood of respiratory muscle fatigue. In one series, $P_{0.1}$ was followed in patients beginning with the first day of acute respiratory failure and was found to decrease before successful extubation[26]. In contrast, in patients in whom $P_{0.1}$ did not change significantly from the initial value, diaphragmatic fatigue eventually developed, and reintubation was necessary within 2–6 days.

18.8 Endurance measurements

Fatigue (lack of ventilatory muscle endurance) is the usual reason for weaning failure. Short of allowing fatigue to develop, it is difficult to predict an individual patient's endurance. Experimentally, the power spectrum of the diaphragmatic electromyogram (EMG) has been used to evaluate endurance[27]. In 12 patients, seven developed EMG evidence of fatigue (i.e. appearance of EMG power spectral shift); in six of these seven, this shift was associated with an abnormal breathing pattern characterized by paradoxical abdominal motion with inspiration. Although EMG is not practical for routine clinical evaluation, it has nicely characterized the clinical sequence of respiratory muscle fatigue (*Table 18.4*) and suggests that the onset of chest wall and abdominal paradox is an early indicator, followed by hypercapnea as a late finding. Notably, later studies suggest that inspiratory paradox indicates respiratory muscle loading and does not distinguish between successful and unsuccessful weaning[28]. However, measurement of the maximal amplitude of diaphragm excursion divided by V_T, and the relationship between rib cage excursion and V_T have been found to be nonspecific but sensitive indicators of respiratory fatigue.

Table 18.4 Clinical sequence of inspiratory muscle fatigue

- Shift of EMG power spectrum
- Tachypnea
- Respiratory alternans
- Paradoxical abdominal motion
- Fall in respiratory rate and minute ventilation
- Elevation of $PaCO_2$
- Arterial acidemia

EMG, diaphragmatic and intercostal electromyogram. Adapted from Cohen *et al.*[27] (1982) Clinical manifestations of inspiratory muscle fatigue. *Am. J. Med.* **73**: 308–316.

18.9 Techniques of weaning

A variety of techniques for weaning patients from mechanical ventilation have been described, including T-piece trials of increasing duration alternating with periods of completely supported breaths, progressive decrease in the intermittent mandatory ventilation (IMV) rate, use of declining levels of pressure support, and combinations of the above (e.g. pressure support weaning with an IMV back-up rate). Strategies in use have changed as new ventilatory modes have became available on newer ventilators. In 1987, before the widespread availability of pressure support ventilation (PSV), IMV was the primary mode of weaning employed by 72% of respondents to a large survey[29]. More recently, a survey of practices in 47 Spanish ICUs[30] showed that in 195 patients undergoing weaning, T-piece trials of increasing duration were used most commonly (24%), followed by synchronized IMV weaning (18%), pressure support weaning (15%), and combined pressure support with an IMV back-up rate (9%). Other combinations applied concurrently or in succession were used in 33%. Each of the weaning techniques is described below, followed by a summary of the evidence supporting specific techniques of weaning. *Figure 18.2* offers an approach to weaning.

18.9.1 T-piece trials

T-piece trials (also known as Briggs trials) allow the patient to breathe spontaneously through the endotracheal tube or tracheostomy connected to a T-piece set-up. CPAP can be applied

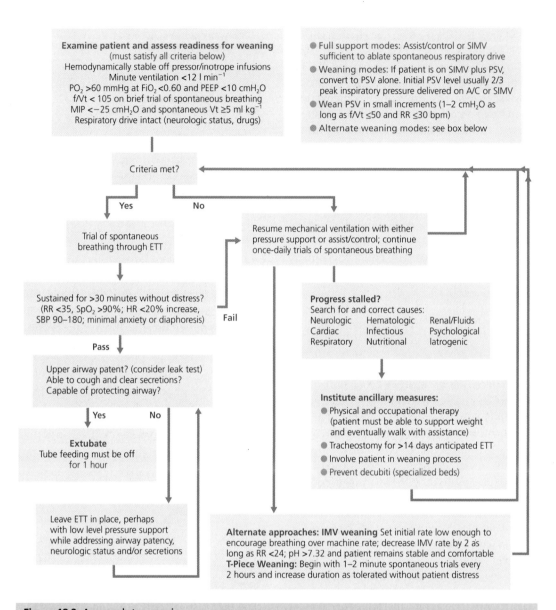

Examine patient and assess readiness for weaning
(must satisfy all criteria below)
Hemodynamically stable off pressor/inotrope infusions
Minute ventilation <12 l min^{-1}
PO$_2$ >60 mmHg at FiO$_2$ <0.60 and PEEP <10 cmH$_2$O
f/Vt < 105 on brief trial of spontaneous breathing
MIP <−25 cmH$_2$O and spontaneous Vt ≥5 ml kg^{-1}
Respiratory drive intact (neurologic status, drugs)

- Full support modes: Assist/control or SIMV sufficient to ablate spontaneous respiratory drive
- Weaning modes: If patient is on SIMV plus PSV, convert to PSV alone. Initial PSV level usually 2/3 peak inspiratory pressure delivered on A/C or SIMV
- Wean PSV in small increments (1–2 cmH$_2$O as long as f/Vt ≤50 and RR ≤30 bpm)
- Alternate weaning modes: see box below

Criteria met?

Yes / No

Trial of spontaneous breathing through ETT

Resume mechanical ventilation with either pressure support or assist/control; continue once-daily trials of spontaneous breathing

Sustained for >30 minutes without distress?
(RR <35, SpO$_2$ >90%; HR <20% increase, SBP 90–180; minimal anxiety or diaphoresis)

Fail

Progress stalled?
Search for and correct causes:
Neurologic   Hematologic   Renal/Fluids
Cardiac   Infectious   Psychological
Respiratory   Nutritional   Iatrogenic

Pass

Upper airway patent? (consider leak test)
Able to cough and clear secretions?
Capable of protecting airway?

Institute ancillary measures:
- Physical and occupational therapy (patient must be able to support weight and eventually walk with assistance)
- Tracheostomy for >14 days anticipated ETT
- Involve patient in weaning process
- Prevent decubiti (specialized beds)

Yes / No

Extubate
Tube feeding must be off for 1 hour

Leave ETT in place, perhaps with low level pressure support while addressing airway patency, neurologic status and/or secretions

Alternate approaches: IMV weaning Set initial rate low enough to encourage breathing over machine rate; decrease IMV rate by 2 as long as RR <24; pH >7.32 and patient remains stable and comfortable
T-Piece Weaning: Begin with 1–2 minute spontaneous trials every 2 hours and increase duration as tolerated without patient distress

Figure 18.2 Approach to weaning.

to the T-piece circuit, although CPAP pressure levels much above 5 cmH$_2$O would be unlikely during T-piece trials, as adequate oxygenation at acceptably low levels of end-expiratory pressure is a criterion for beginning weaning. T-piece trials are labor-intensive, because the patient must be monitored continuously for distress or fatigue. Beginning intervals may be as brief as 2 min each hour and progressively

lengthened by 2 min h^{-1} or more as endurance develops. A reasonable starting point is 5 min of T-piece followed by 60 min of rest. If this first trial is successful, the trial can be increased in 5 min intervals, allowing at least 1 h of rest between attempts. Signs of T-piece weaning failure include a respiratory rate above 35–40, heart rate above 110, and increased blood pressure, diaphoresis, air hunger, and signs of respiratory muscle fatigue. Elevated end-tidal CO_2 is a late sign of decompensation[6]. Optimally, weaning should be stopped just before signs of distress to avoid inducing 'weaning anxiety'. Between weaning periods, full support should be provided with use of assist-control at a rate sufficient to blunt the patient's own respiratory drive.

18.9.2 Intermittent mandatory ventilation weaning

This was first proposed in 1973 as a new and preferred weaning strategy[31]. With IMV weaning, a tidal volume and breathing frequency is set so the ventilator does most, but not all of the work initially, and the intermittent mandatory frequency is then gradually decreased until the patient has assumed most of the minute ventilation. Early studies suggested that IMV was preferable to controlled mechanical ventilation, resulting in less alkalosis, less time on the ventilator, and less increase in O_2 consumption. However, claims that IMV was a preferred weaning mode because it could shorten weaning time have not been supported by later studies. More recent controlled trials comparing time to weaning using this mode versus progressive T-piece or pressure support weaning have shown that IMV is associated with the longest duration of ventilation and is therefore the least attractive initial weaning mode[32]. In our view, IMV weaning remains an option for the versatile clinician, but usually after other modes have proven unsuccessful (*Figure 18.2*).

18.9.3 Pressure support ventilation

Unlike IMV, which is a volume-cycled mode of mechanical ventilation, pressure support ventilation[33] is flow-cycled and delivers gas at a set pressure level for a duration determined by the patient's inspiratory flow demands. Pressure support weaning involves the gradual diminution of the inspiratory pressure level, allowing the patient gradually to assume more of the work of breathing (WOB). In contrast to IMV, in which supported breaths are interspersed with spontaneous ventilation, each PSV breath

is partly supported. Advantages of PSV include increased patient comfort, ability to offset increased work of breathing imposed by the ventilator or the endotracheal tube, and increased efficiency for the clinician overseeing its use[34,35]. The initial pressure level can be set at approximately half the peak fully supported inspiratory pressure, and PEEP is usually set at 5–10 cmH_2O. The level of pressure support may then be adjusted to maintain adequate tidal volume with a respiratory rate between 12 and 24. This allows the patient to perform some respiratory muscle training while minimizing tachypnea and its associated stress. Weaning using inspiratory pressure support can usually be continued for 1 h or more; the patient is placed back on full support if tachypnea or clinical signs of distress develop. Patients will often tolerate PSV for much of the day and require a return to full support only overnight. The pressure–time product, work of breathing, and f/V_t all decrease in a stepwise fashion as PSV is increased, so f/V_t can perhaps be used as an indicator of patient WOB during PSV[36].

18.10 Studies comparing weaning modes

Three recent controlled trials have compared available weaning strategies. Brochard *et al.*[37] randomized 109 patients who failed initial weaning attempts to one of three weaning strategies: (i) T-piece trials, with progressively increasing intervals of spontaneous breathing until the patient tolerated up to three T-piece trials lasting 120 min (n = 35 patients); (ii) synchronized IMV weaning, in which the IMV rate was decreased by 2–4 breaths min^{-1} twice daily until the patient tolerated 24 h at an IMV rate of four or less (n = 43 patients); (iii) pressure support weaning, in which the level of pressure was decreased by 2 or 4 cmH_2O twice daily until the patient could tolerate breathing at pressure support of 8 cmH_2O or less for 24 h (n = 31 patients). The study concluded that pressure support was the preferred weaning mode based on demonstrating that: (i) fewer patients failed to wean with pressure support than with the other modes (23% vs 43% (T-piece) and 42% (IMV), $P < 0.05$); (ii) the probability of requiring continued ventilatory support was lower with pressure support than with the other modes ($P = 0.03$); (iii) weaning duration was shorter with pressure support (mean 5.7 ± 3.7 days) than for the other modes pooled (mean 9.3 ± 8.2 days, $P < 0.05$).

In a second trial of weaning modes, Esteban et al.[38] randomized 130 patients who had failed initial weaning attempts to one of four weaning modes: (i) IMV weaning, in which the rate was decreased by 2–4 breaths min^{-1} at least twice daily until the patient tolerated an IMV rate of five or less for 2 h ($n = 29$ patients); (ii) pressure support weaning, in which the pressure was decreased by 2–4 cmH$_2$O at least twice daily until a pressure support level of 5 cmH$_2$O was tolerated for 2 h ($n = 37$ patients); (iii) intermittent trials of spontaneous breathing, in which T-piece trials of increasing length were undertaken at least twice daily until the patient could tolerate 2 h of spontaneous breathing ($n = 33$ patients); (iv) once-daily T-piece trials, in which a single T-piece trial was undertaken daily until 2 h of spontaneous breathing were tolerated without distress ($n = 31$ patients). In contrast to Brochard et al., Estaban et al. concluded that a once-daily T-piece trial was the preferred strategy, based on a higher rate of success and more rapid weaning with once-daily T-piece trials than with pressure support or IMV modes.

The most recent controlled trial of different weaning strategies, by Ely et al.[39], randomized patients to a once-daily respiratory assessment and trial of spontaneous breathing for up to 2 h with physician notification of a successful trial ($n = 149$ patients) versus usual care by the managing physicians (pulmonologist, cardiologist, or intensivist, $n = 151$ patients). A strategy of conducting daily trials of spontaneous breathing was associated with shorter weaning time (median 1 versus 3 days, $P < 0.001$), shorter duration of mechanical ventilation (median 4.5 versus 6 days, $P < 0.003$), fewer total complications (20% versus 41%, $P < 0.001$), a lower rate of reintubation (4% versus

10%, $P = 0.04$), and lower ICU costs (median \$15 740 versus \$20 890, $P < 0.03$). Taken together, these three studies show that contrary to early views and practices, IMV weaning is the least likely to effect successful extubation and requires longer weaning than other available strategies, and that daily assessment of respiratory status and spontaneous breathing trials was associated with shorter weaning duration than usual practice. Results of a recent meta-analysis of weaning modes confirm these findings[32].

Failure to free the patient from mechanical ventilation using one or more of the above techniques should prompt the clinician to consider special clinical circumstances. These include unsuspectedly high imposed WOB from a small endotracheal tube or auto-PEEP, occult cardiac ischemia, oversedation, and lack of psychological readiness or motivation to wean.

18.11 Non-respiratory impediments to successful weaning

Despite extensive investigation of pulmonary function parameters (e.g. gas exchange and mechanical function) as indicators of weaning, little attention has been given to other, non-respiratory features that may prove equally important. Indeed, failure to consider such factors as nutritional status and non-pulmonary organ dysfunction may contribute to conflicting results obtained in studies of traditional (e.g. pulmonary function) weaning parameters[40,41]. Factors that determine weanability, in addition to pre-existing respiratory status and the reason for mechanical ventilation, include baseline function of other organ systems, complications developing while on the ventilator, duration of critical illness, and the duration of mechanical ventilation. Non-respiratory factors of particular importance include nutritional status, fluid balance, metabolic and acid–base derangements, cardiac and renal function, effects of pharmacologic therapy, and neuropsychiatric factors.

18.11.1 Nutritional status

Patients with acute respiratory failure are often malnourished either on admission or during hospitalization as a result of increased metabolic demands, inadequate nutritional support or inability to utilize provided nutritional support. Malnutrition has adverse effects on the respiratory system, including decreased respiratory muscle strength and function, decreased diaphragmatic mass (both area and thickness) and contractility, and decreased endurance[42].

Malnutrition, particularly amino acid deficiency, decreases the ventilatory response to hypoxemia[43]. The immune system responds to malnutrition with decreased cell-mediated immunity, altered IgG turnover, and impaired macrophage function[44]. In 47 patients who received mechanical ventilation for 3 days or more, 93% of those with adequate nutritional support could be weaned; however, only half of those with inadequate nutritional support could be weaned[45]. Among 14 'unweanable' medical patients, all those who responded with increases in albumin and transferrin during parenteral nutrition were eventually weaned, but those who showed no biochemical response to nutrition remained unweanable[46]. Amino acids are an essential part of parenteral nutrition, and have been shown to restore ventilatory drive and improve both minute ventilation and respiratory rate[43].

Although undernutrition is obviously an impediment to weaning, overnutrition or the wrong kind of nutrition can also frustrate weaning efforts. Excessive carbohydrate intake by increasing the respiratory quotient (ratio of CO_2 produced to O_2 consumed)[47], CO_2 production and work of breathing can increase other causes of increased CO_2 production including fever, sepsis, shivering, seizures, and agitation. Increased CO_2 production may also be caused by inefficient ventilation because of increased dead space; this occurs in the setting of pulmonary embolism without compensatory hyperventilation, obstructive lung disease, late in the course of the acute respiratory distress syndrome (ARDS), and with acute hyper-inflation as a result of a rapid cycling rate and extrinsic PEEP or auto-PEEP.

18.11.2 Metabolic abnormalities

Metabolic causes of weaning failure include hypophosphatemia, hypocalcemia, and hypothyroidism. Hypophosphatemic patients demonstrate increased transdiaphragmatic pressure after repletion to normal levels of phosphate[48]. Hypocalcemia causes decreased diaphragmatic strength[49]. Hypothyroidism can affect weaning, as the hypoxic ventilatory response is markedly blunted with thyroid deficiency[50].

18.11.3 Acid–base disturbances

These are a common problem in patients who develop acute ventilatory failure in the face of chronic CO_2 retention. As the baseline $PaCO_2$ is frequently unknown, these patients may be ventilator-supported during their acute illness to a presumed normal baseline $PaCO_2$ of 40 mmHg, causing acute alkalemia. Three or 4 days later, a new compensatory state develops as the kidneys dump the excess bicarbonate (HCO_3), leaving the patient unable to be weaned in this new steady state. Allowing the $PaCO_2$ to gradually normalize to the patient's pre-morbid baseline over several days may allow weaning to resume. Other acid–base problems that can develop during weaning include respiratory alkalosis, metabolic alkalosis (common as a result of nasogastric drainage and diuretic therapy), and metabolic acidosis (commonly as a result of disease or diabetic ketoacidosis). Complex disorders involving partial compensation and failure of two or more systems frequently confound the issue.

18.11.4 Infection

Infection, particularly sepsis, is a contraindication to weaning because of increased metabolic requirements and the propensity for hemodynamic compromise. The presence of positive blood cultures predicts the need for reintubation in medical patients[51]. Similarly, an active infectious pulmonary process or tracheobronchitis may be an indication for continued mechanical ventilation if secretions are thick or copious, especially in the presence of diminished pulmonary reserve.

18.11.5 Acute left ventricular dysfunction and anemia

In postoperative patients, the transition from controlled ventilation at a rate of 10 or 12 breaths min^{-1} to continuous positive airway pressure (CPAP) is associated with a 10% increase in both O_2 consumption and CO_2 production[52]. Rapid weaning in patients with obstructive lung disease causes marked increases in transmural pulmonary artery pressures[53], which suggests that acute left ventricular dysfunction may occur during the transition from supported to spontaneous ventilation. Anemia, by virtue of decreasing O_2-carrying capacity, interferes with weaning by forcing increases in minute ventilation or cardiac output. The role of erythropoietin in reducing anemia and facilitating ventilation is currently under study.

18.11.6 Renal impairment and volume overload

These can be impediments to successful weaning. Indeed, application of PEEP is used to treat pulmonary edema because increased intrathoracic pressure discourages venous return. Prolonged (10 day) diuretic therapy with reduction of body weight by an average of 5 kg is sometimes necessary to achieve weaning in patients with left ventricular dysfunction[53]. Use of continuous dialysis–ultrafiltration techniques has been shown to reduce fluid overload in patients after coronary artery bypass surgery and to facilitate their weaning from mechanical ventilation[54].

18.11.7 Sleep deprivation

The ICU is frequently noisy, lights are always on, and the constant level of activity makes it difficult for patients to establish a circadian routine. The result may be a state of sleep deprivation and twilight awareness where patients are neither fully awake nor asleep, nap throughout the day, or invert their day–night cycle. One common approach is to give patients sedative-hypnotic drugs at bedtime to promote a good night's sleep and to help restore a normal daily cycle. Because depression is commonly a problem in the long-term ICU patient, antidepressant therapy at bedtime may be useful both for sedative effect and to forestall depression.

18.11.8 Motivation

The attitude of the patient is important, but often difficult to assess or change. Patients who are well informed about what is expected and who strive to meet daily goals seem to progress more rapidly than those who are uninvolved in the process or who are depressed. Weaning goals set by the clinical team should be attainable, should avoid precipitating fatigue or undue discomfort, and should cause each session of weaning to end in success rather than fatigue. From the practical viewpoint, a daily weaning strategy should be developed early in the day and can be canceled if the day is otherwise occupied with laboratory tests or if the patient has a medical setback that makes it impossible to successfully wean that day. Some patients with psychological dependence will hyperventilate at the onset of weaning trials without relation to physiologic need and may have to be weaned surreptitiously. Formal biofeedback can also facilitate weaning by allowing the patient to visualize different breathing patterns[55]. Potential solutions to the problem of dysfunctional breathing patterns include use of opioids to blunt respiratory drive and very slow changes in the level of pressure support or IMV rate to prevent anxiety induced by sudden changes in the response of the lung stretch receptors during the active weaning process.

18.11.9 Other impediments

Upper airway obstruction, as caused by vocal cord paralysis, tracheal mucosal edema, or upper airway compression, can pose an unexpected impediment following extubation, even though the patient has sustained spontaneous breathing well through the endotracheal tube.

Use of the 'leak test', in which the volume of exhaled air is assessed as the endotracheal tube cuff is deflated, has been advocated as a way of predicting the postextubation potency of the upper airway. Exhalation of less than 110 ml with the cuff deflated suggests the possibility of upper airway obstruction, although other studies have challenged the predictive value of the 'leak test'[56]. Interference with the weaning process may also be caused by multiple medications, including narcotics, tranquilizers, sedative hypnotics, paralytic agents, and aminoglycoside antibiotics, which can cause myasthenia-like muscle weakness. Indeed, daily interruption of intravenous sedation, which allows serial reassessment of the patient's immunologic status and need for sedation, has been shown to accelerate liberation from mechanical ventilation[40].

18.12 Respiratory impediments to weaning

18.12.1 Diaphragmatic dysfunction

This can occur secondary to phrenic nerve injury; the incidence is about 1% following coronary artery bypass grafting. Injury to the left phrenic nerve is more common and was once thought to occur as a result of cold injury to the nerve during surgery[57], although more recent experience suggests that phrenic nerve dysfunction following internal mammary dissection may be caused by ischemia or traction on nerves. Bilateral diaphragmatic dysfunction should be considered in the differential diagnosis of orthopnea after extubation and is confirmed if the decrement in vital capacity exceeds 20% on moving from an upright to a supine posture. Atelectasis following coronary artery bypass surgery may also signify phrenic nerve dysfunction[58]. Phrenic nerve recovery may require up to 27 months[59]. When bilateral phrenic nerve dysfunction precludes weaning, long-term management with a rocking bed or nighttime ventilation is required until respiratory muscle strength and endurance improve.

Long-term, low-dose corticosteroids have been shown experimentally to impair diaphragmatic function[60]. Finally, critically ill patients often develop muscle weakness or polyneuropathy with sepsis and multiple organ failure[61,62]. Muscle disuse itself may contribute to weakness as a result of progressive fiber atrophy[63]. These factors, along with residual neuromuscular blockade, can contribute to weaning difficulty.

18.12.2 Patients with chronic obstructive pulmonary disease (COPD)

These pose a special weaning challenge. Rates of failure to wean in such patients may be as high as 24%, and most ventilated COPD patients (58%) require up to 2 weeks of mechanical ventilation[64].

In ventilating and weaning COPD patients, special consideration must be given to the phenomenon of auto-PEEP, also known as intrinsic PEEP. Auto-PEEP is defined as end-expiratory pressure present in the alveoli but not measured at the airway manometer without special maneuvers such as an end-expiratory hold[65]. Auto-PEEP must be distinguished from PEEP purposefully applied and recorded in the proximal airway. Auto-PEEP occurs commonly among mechanically ventilated patients (39–62% of patients assessed) and may produce high alveolar pressures at end expiration (i.e. up to 15 cmH$_2$O)[66]. Auto-PEEP is increased when airflow resistance is increased and when exhalation time is decreased, both of which impair alveolar emptying before the next ventilator breath. Auto-PEEP may frustrate weaning by increasing the work of breathing associated with having to overcome residual alveolar pressure before inhalation can begin[67]. Adding conventional PEEP in COPD patients can offset this inspiratory muscle loading effect of auto-PEEP[68] that is associated with dynamic hyperinflation and airflow limitation. Maneuvers to decrease auto-PEEP also include treating bronchospasm and secretions, slowing the respiratory rate, maximizing the time for expiration, and using low-compliance ventilator tubing to permit rapid gas delivery and to maximize exhalation time.

18.12.3 Perception of breathing

In patients with obstructive lung disease, pulmonary stretch receptors are activated with mechanically delivered volumes much larger than those attained during spontaneous breathing. Failure to recreate these volumes during weaning can lead to agitation[69]. One approach to this problem is to decrease the tidal volume (V_T) during rest periods of mechanical ventilation and increase the supported respiratory rate as necessary to maintain alveolar ventilation. During weaning periods, opioids can be added judiciously to manage anxiety and feelings of respiratory insufficiency.

18.12.4 Endotracheal tube caliber and tracheostomy

Airway resistance increases as endotracheal tube size decreases. To the extent that smaller-caliber tubes (e.g. for nasal intubation) can greatly increase the imposed work of breathing, they can impair weaning[70]. Thus, use of larger caliber (i.e. >7.5 mm inner diameter) endotracheal tubes and avoidance of nasotracheal intubation in patients experiencing weaning difficulty is advised. Tracheotomy is indicated for relief of upper airway obstruction, for access for pulmonary hygiene, and for control of the airway for long-term positive pressure ventilation[71]. Tracheostomy appears to help patients who have trouble clearing secretions, may improve patient comfort, and allows use of a fenestrated tracheostomy tube, which may be occluded to allow the patient to speak during periods of spontaneous breathing. Complications of tracheostomy include pneumothorax, pneumomediastinum, subcutaneous emphysema, incisional hemorrhage, aerophagia, aspiration, and tube displacement[72]. Late complications also include tracheal stenosis, tracheoinnominate artery and tracheoesophageal fistulae, tube obstruction, aspiration, swallowing dysfunction, and stomal infections. In the absence of definitive studies regarding the timing of tracheostomy, we suggest the following indications for tracheotomy during the weaning process:

- anticipation of prolonged (e.g. >2 weeks) intubation and mechanical ventilation;
- absence of a contraindication to tracheostomy (e.g. upper airway burn, mediastinitis);
- copious or tenacious secretions requiring direct access to the airway for suctioning;
- chronic aspiration requiring long-standing airway protection in the absence of other strategies to minimize aspiration (e.g. gastrostomy tubes, jejunostomy tubes, nasogastric feeding).

Clinical predictors for prolonged ventilatory support and eventual tracheostomy include development of nosocomial pneumonia, administration of aerosol treatments, witnessed aspiration event, and requirement for reintubation[73].

18.13 Pharmacologic aids to weaning

Beta-adrenergic agents, aminophylline, and anticholinergics are frequently helpful in the patient with reactive airway disease (see Chapter 17). Aminophylline has also been shown to improve diaphragmatic contractility[74] and to partially mitigate the reduced diaphragmatic activity seen after abdominal surgery[75]. Dopamine improves diaphragmatic strength and blood flow in patients with COPD and acute respiratory failure. An infusion of 10 µg kg^{-1} min^{-1} typically increases heart rate by 17%, cardiac output by 40%, and diaphragmatic blood flow and transdiaphragmatic strength by 30%[76]. Opioids, particularly dihydrocodeine, have been shown to decrease breathlessness and improve exercise tolerance in patients with COPD and may have a role in improving patient comfort during weaning[77]. Respiratory stimulants such as doxapram have been successfully employed in patients with primary alveolar hypoventilation[78] but are not generally recommended in weaning, because respiratory drive should be adequate. Androgens such as oxandrolone decrease net nitrogen loss and improve wound healing[79] and have anecdotally been used to promote weaning, although studies are lacking. Serum testosterone levels decline in elderly men, and replacement therapy may restore body weight and even body mass[80].

18.14 Weaning failure

Despite the best efforts to prepare the patient for weaning and ultimately extubation, some patients will inevitably fail to sustain respiration on their own and will require resumption of ventilatory support. The rate of extubation failure in general surgical patients averaging 65 years of age is approximately 5%[81]. In patients with head injury, approximately 5% require reintubation, primarily for airway protection. Patients undergoing open heart surgery also have an overall reintubation rate of 5–7%, with older patients and those undergoing reoperation, emergency surgery, and valve surgery having a much higher rate of reintubation than those undergoing first-time isolated coronary artery bypass surgery[82]. Predictors of extubation failure include age 65 years or over, preoperative hospitalization, arterial vascular disease, COPD, pulmonary hypertension, severe left ventricular dysfunction, cardiogenic shock, hematocrit of 34% or less, renal insufficiency, malnutrition, reoperation, massive transfusion, prolonged cardiopulmonary bypass time and complex procedures[83]. Reintubation and failure to wean after all issues have been addressed suggests the need for patient placement in a long-term ventilator facility, assuming the patient desires aggressive management.

18.15 Long-term prognosis

The prognosis after successful weaning from mechanical ventilation varies widely, depending on the age of the patient, the underlying disease process, and the presence of other complicating factors. Diseases such as ARDS are associated with high hospital mortality (up to 65%), but similar survival rates at hospital discharge, 1 year, and 3 years[84]. In a study of 100 patients receiving mechanically assisted ventilation in a community hospital, all patients under the age of 50 years who survived the ICU stay survived to leave the hospital and were alive at 1 year[85]. However, in the subset of older patients (i.e. age ≥70 years), hospital survival was only 49% and 1 year survival was only 27%. Patients with COPD who experience acute ventilatory failure have been estimated to have a 57% 1 year and a 51% 2 year survival rate[85]. Although long-term survival prediction helps inform the clinician's understanding of average outcomes, these data must be applied with circumspection to individual patients and with attention to the patient's overall progress to date.

References

1. **Pavlin, E.G., Holle, R.H. and Schoene, R.B.** (1989) Recovery of airway protection compared with ventilation in humans after paralysis with curare. *Anesthesiology* **70**: 381–385.
2. **Engelman, R.M., Rousou, J.A., Flack, J.E., III, et al.** (1994) Fast-track recovery of the coronary bypass patient. *Am. Thorac. Surg.* **58**: 1742–1746.
3. **Higgins, T.L.** (1995) Safety issues regarding early extubation after coronary artery bypass surgery. *J. Cardiothorac. Vasc. Anesth.* **9**(5S1): 24–29.
4. **Horst, H.M., Mouro, D., Hall-Jenssens, R.A. and Pamukov, N.** (1998) Decrease in ventilation time with a standardized weaning process. *Arch. Surg.* **133**: 483–489.
5. **Koleff, M.H., Shapiro, S.D., Silver, P., et al.** (1997) A randomized, controlled trial of protocol-directed versus physician-directed weaning from mechanical ventilation. *Crit. Care Med.* **25**: 567–574.
6. **Cohen, I.L., Bari, N., Strosberg, M.A., et al.** (1991) Reduction of duration and cost of mechanical ventilation in an intensive care unit by use of a ventilatory management team. *Crit. Care Med.* **19**: 1278–1284.
7. **Kastanos, N., Miro, R.E., Perez, A.M., et al.** (1983) Laryngotracheal injury due to endotracheal intubation: Incidence, evolution, and predisposing factors. A prospective long-term study. *Crit. Care Med.* **11**: 362–367.
8. **Stauffer, J.L., Olson, D.E. and Petty, T.L.** (1981) Complications and consequences of endotracheal intubation and tracheostomy. A prospective study of 150 critically ill adult patients. *Am. J. Med.* **70**: 65–76.

9. **Alexopoulos, C., Jansson, B. and Lindholm, C.-E.** (1984) Mucus transport and surface damage after endotracheal intubation and tracheostomy. An experimental study in pigs. *Acta Anaesthesiol. Scand.* **28**: 68–76.

10. **Driver, A.G. and LeBrun, M.** (1980) Iatrogenic malnutrition in patients receiving ventilatory support. *JAMA* **244**: 2195–2196.

11. **Ranieri, V.M., Suter, P.M., Tortorella, C., et al.** (1999) Effect of mechanical ventilation on inflammatory mediators in patients with acute respiratory distress syndrome. *JAMA* **282**: 54–61.

12. **Stoller, J.K.** (1991) Establishing clinical unweanability. *Respir. Care* **36**: 186–198.

13. **Krieger, B.P., Ershowsky, P.F., Becker, D.A., et al.** (1989) Evaluation of conventional criteria for predicting successful weaning from mechanical ventilatory support in elderly patients. *Crit. Care Med.* **17**: 858–861.

14. **Yang, K.L. and Tobin, M.J.** (1991) A prospective study of indexes predicting the outcome of trials of weaning from mechanical ventilation. *N. Engl. J. Med.* **324**: 1445–1450.

15. **Scheinhorn, D., Hassenpflug, M., Artinian, B.M., et al.** (1995) Predictors of weaning after six weeks of mechanical ventilation. *Chest* **107**: 500–505.

16. **Epstein, S.K.** (1995) Etiology of extubation failure and the predictive value of the rapid shallow breathing index. *Am. J. Respir. Crit. Care Med.* **152**: 545–549.

17. **Chatila, W., Jacob, B., Guaglionine, D. and Manthous, C.A.** (1996) The unassisted respiratory rate–tidal volume ratio accurately predicts weaning outcome. *Am. J. Med.* **101**: 61–67.

18. **Valverdu, I., Calaf, N., Subirana, M., et al.** (1998) Clinical characteristics, respiratory functional parameters, and outcomes of a two-hour T-piece trial in patients weaning from mechanical ventilation. *Am. J. Respir. Crit. Care Med.* **158**: 1855–1862.

19. **Bellemare, F. and Grassino, A.** (1982) Effect of pressure and timing of contraction on human diaphragm fatigue. *J. Appl. Physiol.* **53**: 1190–1195.

20. **Petros, A.J., Lamond, C.T. and Bennett, D.** (1993) The Bicore pulmonary monitor. A device to assess the work of breathing while weaning from mechanical ventilation. *Anaesthesia* **48**: 985–988.

21. **Banner, M.J., Kirby, R.R., Gabrielli, A., Blanch, P.B. and Lyon, A.J.** (1994) Partially and totally unleading respiratory muscles based on real-time measurements of work of breathing. *Chest* **106**: 1835–1842.

22. **Fiastro, J.P., Habib, M.P., Shon, B.Y. and Campbell, S.C.** (1988) Comparison of standard weaning parameters and the mechanical work of breathing in mechanically ventilated patients. *Chest* **94**: 223–238.

23. **Gluck, E.H., Barkoviak, M.J., Balk, R.A., et al.** (1995) Medical effectiveness of esophageal balloon pressure manometry in weaning patients from mechanical ventilation. *Crit. Care Med.* **23**: 504–509.

24. **Harpin, R.P., Baker, J.P., Downer, J.P., et al.** (1987) Correlation of the oxygen cost of breathing and length of weaning from mechanical ventilation. *Crit. Care Med.* **15**: 807–812.

25. **Lewis, W.D., Chwals, W. Bennotti, P.N., et al.** (1998) Bedside assessment of the work of breathing. *Crit. Care Med.* **6**: 117–122 Q6.

26. **Murciano, D., Boczkowski, J., Lecocguir, Y., et al.** (1988) Tracheal occlusion pressure: A simple index to monitor respiratory muscle fatigue during acute respiratory failure in patients with chronic obstructive pulmonary disease. *Ann. Intern. Med.* **108**: 800–803.

27. **Cohen, C.A., Zagelbaum, G., Cross, D., et al.** (1982) Clinical manifestations of inspiratory muscle fatigue. *Am. J. Med.* **73**: 308–316.

28. **Tobin, M.J., Guenther, S.M., Peres, W., et al.** (1987) Konno–Mead analysis of rib cage–abdominal motion during successful and unsuccessful trials of weaning from mechanical ventilation. *Am. Rev. Respir. Dis.* **135**: 1320–1328.

29. **Venus, B., Smith, R.A. and Mathru, M.** (1987) National survey of methods and criteria used for weaning from mechanical ventilation. *Crit. Care Med.* **15**: 530–533.

30. **Esteban, A., Alia, I., Ibanez, J., et al.** (1994) Modes of mechanical ventilation and weaning: A national survey of Spanish hospitals. *Chest* **106**: 1188–1193.

31. **Downs, J.B., Klein, E.F., Desautels, D., et al.** (1973) Intermittent mandatory ventilation: A new approach to weaning patients from mechanical ventilation. *Chest* **64**: 331–335.

32. **Butler, R., Keenan, S.P., Inman, K.J., Sibbald, W.J. and Block, G.** (1999) Is there a preferred technique for weaning the difficult-to-wean patients? A systematic review of the literature. *Crit. Care Med.* **27**: 2331–2336.

33. **MacIntyre, N.R.** (1986) Respiratory function during pressure support ventilation. *Chest* **89**: 677–682.

34. **Kacmarek, R.M.** (1988) The role of pressure support ventilation in reducing work of breathing. *Respir. Care* **334**: 99–120.

35. **MacIntyle, N.R.** (1988) Weaning from mechanical ventilatory support: Volume-assisting intermittent breaths versus pressure-assisting every breath. *Respir. Care* **33**: 121–125.

36. **Johannigman, J.A., David, K., Campbell, R.S., et al.** (1997) Use of the rapid/shallow breathing index as an indicator of patient work of breathing during pressure support ventilation. *Surgery* **122:** 737–741.

37. **Brochard, L., Rauss, A., Benito, S., et al.** (1994) Comparison of three methods of gradual withdrawal from ventilatory support during weaning from mechanical ventilation. *Am. J. Respir. Crit. Care Med.* **150:** 896–903.

38. **Esteban, A., Frutoes, F., Tobin, M.J., et al.** (1995) A comparison of four methods of weaning patients from mechanical ventilation. *N. Engl. J. Med.* **332:** 345–350.

39. **Ely, E.W., Baker, A.M., Dunagan, D.P., et al.** (1996) Effect on the duration of mechanical ventilation of identifying patients capable of breathing spontaneously. *N. Engl. J. Med.* **335:** 1864–1869.

40. **Kress, J.P., Pohlman, A.S., O'Connor, M.F. and Hall, J.B.** (2000) Daily interruption of sedative infusions in critically ill patients undergoing mechanical ventilation. *N. Engl. J. Med.* **342:** 1471–1477.

41. **Morganroth, M.L., Morganroth, J.L., Nett, L.M. and Petty, T.L.** (1984) Criteria for weaning from prolonged mechanical ventilation. *Arch. Intern. Med.* **144:** 1012–1016.

42. **Wilson, D.O. and Rogers, R.M.** (1989) The role of nutrition in weaning from mechanical ventilation. *J. Intensive Care* **4:** 124–133.

43. **Weissman, C., Askanazi, J., Rosenbaum, S., et al.** (1983) Amino acids and respiration. *Ann. Intern. Med.* **98:** 41–44.

44. **Pingleton, S.K. and Harmon, G.S.** (1987) Nutritional management in acute respiratory failure. *JAMA* **257:** 3094–3099.

45. **Bassili, H.R. and Deitel, M.** (1981) Effect of nutritional support on weaning patients off mechanical ventilators. *J. Parenter. Enteral Nutr.* **5:** 161–163.

46. **Larca, L. and Greenbaum, D.M.** (1982) Effectiveness of intensive nutritional regimes in patients who fail to wean from mechanical ventilation. *Crit. Care Med.* **10:** 297–300.

47. **Covelli, H.D., Black, J.W., Olsen, M.S. and Beekman, J.F.** (1981) Respiratory failure precipitated by high carbohydrate loads. *Ann. Intern. Med.* **95:** 579–581.

48. **Aubier, M., Murciano, D., Lecocguic, Y., et al.** (1985) Effect of hypophosphatemia on diaphragmatic contractility in patients with acute respiratory failure. *N. Engl. J. Med.* **313:** 420–424.

49. **Aubier, M., Viires, N., Piquet, J., et al.** (1985) Effects of hypocalcemia on diaphragmatic strength generation. *J. Appl. Physiol.* **58:** 2054–2061.

50. **Zwillich, C.W., Pierson, D.J., Hofeldt, F.D., et al.** (1975) Ventilatory control in myxedema and hypothyroidism. *N. Engl. J. Med.* **292:** 662–665.

51. **Tahvanainen, J., Salmenpera, M. and Nikki, P.** (1983) Extubation criteria after weaning from intermittent mandatory ventilation and continuous positive airway pressure. *Crit. Care Med.* **11:** 702–707.

52. **Kemper, M., Weissman, C., Askanazi, J., et al.** (1987) Metabolic and respiratory changes during weaning from mechanical ventilation. *Chest* **92:** 979–983.

53. **Lemaire, F., Teboul, J.-L., Cinotti, L., et al.** (1988) Acute left ventricular dysfunction during unsuccessful weaning from mechanical ventilation. *Anesthesiology* **69:** 171–179.

54. **Coraim, F.J., Coraim, H.P., Ebermann, R. and Stellwag, F.M.** (1986) Acute respiratory failure after cardiac surgery: Clinical experience with the application of continuous arteriovenous hemofiltration. *Crit. Care Med.* **14:** 714–718.

55. **Holliday, J.F. and Hyers, T.M.** (1990) The reduction of weaning time from mechanical ventilation using tidal volume and relaxation biofeedback. *Am. Rev. Respir. Dis.* **141:** 1214–1220.

56. **Engoren, M.** (1999) Evaluation of the cuff-leak test in a cardiac surgery population. *Chest* **116:** 1029–1031.

57. **Wheeler, W.E., Rubis, L.J., Jones, C.W., et al.** (1985) Etiology and prevention of topical cardiac hypothermia-induced phrenic nerve injury and left lower lobe atelectasis during cardiac surgery. *Chest* **88:** 680–683.

58. **Wilcox, P., Baile, E.M., Hards, J., et al.** (1988) Phrenic nerve function and its relationship to atelectasis after coronary artery bypass surgery. *Chest* **93:** 693–698.

59. **Abd, A.G., Braun, N.M.T., Baskin, M.I., et al.** (1989) Diaphragmatic dysfunction after open heart surgery: Treatment with a rocking bed. *Ann. Intern. Med.* **111:** 881–886.

60. **VanBalkom, R.H.H., Dekhuijzen, P.N.R., Folgering, H.T.M., et al.** (1997) Effects of long-term low-dose methylprednisone on rat diaphragm function and structure. *Muscle Nerve* **20:** 983–990.

61. **Latronico, N., Fenzi, F., Recupero, D., et al.** (1996) Critical illness myopathy and neuropathy. *Lancet* **347:** 1579–1582.

62. **Lorin, S., Sivak, M. and Nierman, D.M.** (1998) Critical illness polyneuropathy: What to look for in at-risk patients. Diagnosis requires a high index of suspicion. *J. Crit. Illness* **13:** 608–612.

63. **Ibebunjo, C. and Martyn, J.A.J.** (1999) Fiber atrophy, but not changes in acetylcholine receptor expression, contributes to the muscle dysfunction after immobilization. *Crit. Care Med.* **27**: 275–285.

64. **Menzies, R., Gibbons, W. and Goldberg, P.** (1989) Determinants of weaning and survival among patients with COPD who require mechanical ventilation for acute respiratory failure. *Chest* **95**: 398–405.

65. **Ranieri, V.M., Grasso, S., Fiore, T.,** *et al.* (1996) Auto-positive end-expiratory pressure and dynamic hyperinflation. *Clin. Chest Med.* **17**: 379–394.

66. **Brown, D.G. and Pierson, D.J.** (1986) Auto-PEEP is common in mechanically ventilated patients: A study of incidence, severity, and detection. *Respir. Care* **31**: 1069–1074.

67. **Kirton, O.C., DeHaven, C.B., Morgan, J.P.,** *et al.* (1995) Elevated imposed work of breathing masquerading as ventilator weaning intolerance. *Chest* **108**: 1021–1025.

68. **Petrof, B.J., Legare, M., Goldberg, P.,** *et al.* (1990) Continuous positive airway pressure reduces work of breathing and dyspnea during weaning from mechanical ventilation in severe chronic obstructive pulmonary disease. *Am. Rev. Respir. Dis.* **141**: 281–289.

69. **Wolkove, N., Altose, M.D., Kelsen, S.G.,** *et al.* (1981) Perception of changes in breathing in normal human subjects. *J. Appl. Physiol.* **50**: 78–83.

70. **Habib, M.P.** (1989) Physiologic implication of artificial airways. *Chest* **96**: 180–184.

71. **Heffner, J.E., Scott Miller, K. and Sahn, S.A.** (1986) Tracheostomy in the intensive care unit. Part I: Indications, technique, management. *Chest* **90**: 269–274.

72. **Heffner, J.E., Scott Miller, K. and Sahn, S.A.** (1986) Tracheostomy in the intensive care unit. Part 2: Complications. *Chest* **90**: 430–436.

73. **Kollef, M.H., Ahrens, T.S. and Shannon, W.** (1999) Clinical predictors and outcomes for patients requiring tracheostomy in the intensive care unit. *Crit. Care Med.* **27**(9): 1714–1720.

74. **Aubier, M., De Troyer, A., Sampson, M.,** *et al.* (1981) Aminophylline improves diaphragmatic contractility. *N. Engl. J. Med.* **305**: 249–252.

75. **Dureuil, B., Desmonts, J.M., Mankikian, B. and Prokocimer, P.** (1985) Effects of aminophylline on diaphragmatic dysfunction after upper abdominal surgery. *Anesthesiology* **62**: 242–246.

76. **Aubier, M., Murciano, D., Menu, Y.,** *et al.* (1989) Dopamine effects on diaphragmatic strength during acute respiratory failure in chronic obstructive pulmonary disease. *Ann. Intern. Med.* **110**: 17–23.

77. **Woodcock, A.A., Gross, E.R., Gellert, A.,** *et al.* (1981) Effects of dihydrocodeine, alcohol, and caffeine on breathlessness and exercise tolerance in patients with chronic obstructive lung disease and normal blood gases. *N. Engl. J. Med.* **305**: 1611–1616.

78. **Lugliani, R., Whipp, B.J. and Wasserman, K.** (1979) Doxapram hydrochloride: A respiratory stimulant for patients with primary alveolar hypoventilation. *Chest* **76**: 414–419.

79. **Demling, R.H. and Orgill, D.P.** (2000) The anticatabolic and wound healing effects of the testosterone analog oxandrolone after severe burn injury. *J. Crit. Care* **15**: 12–17.

80. **Bagatell, C.J. and Bremner, W.J.** (1996) Androgens in men—uses and abuses. *N. Engl. J. Med.* **334**: 707–714.

81. **Demling, R.H., Read, T., Lind, L.J. and Flanagan, H.L.** (1988) Incidence and morbidity of extubation failure in surgical intensive care patients. *Crit. Care Med.* **16**: 573–577.

82. **Higgins, T.L.** (1989) Postoperative care of the cardiac surgery patient. *Probl. Anesth.* **3**: 211–227.

83. **Rady, M.Y. and Ryan, T.** (1999) Perioperative predictors of extubation failure and the effect on clinical outcome after cardiac surgery. *Crit. Care Med.* **27**: 340–347.

84. **Schmidt, C.D., Elliott, C.G., Carmelli, D.,** *et al.* (1983) Prolonged mechanical ventilation for respiratory failure: A cost–benefit analysis. *Crit. Care Med.* **11**: 407–411.

85. **Connors, A.F., Jr, Dawson, N.V., Thomas, C.,** *et al.* (1996) Outcomes following acute exacerbation of severe chronic obstructive lung disease. The SUPPORT investigators (Study to Understand Prognoses and Preferences for Outcomes and Risks of Treatment). *Am. J. Respir. Crit. Care Med.* **154**: 959–967.

86. **Sahn, S.A., Lakshminarayan, S.** (1973) Bedside criteria for discontinuation of mechanical ventilation. *Chest* **63**: 1002–1005.

87. **Yang, K.L. and Tobin, M.J.** (1989) Decision analysis of parameters used to predict outcome of a trial of weaning from mechanical ventilation (abstract). *Am. Rev. Respir. Dis.* **139**: (4, part 2) A98.

88. **Milbern, S.M., Downs, J.B., Jumper L.C. and Modell, J.H.** (1978) Evaluation of criteria for discontinuing mechanical ventilatory support. *Arch. Surg.* **113**: 1441–1443.

89. **Pardee, N.E., Winterbauer, R.H. and Allen, J.D.** (1984) Bedside evaluation of respiratory distress. *Chest* **85**: 203–206.

90. **DeHaven, C.B., Hurst, J.M. and Branson, R.D.** (1986) Evaluation of two different extubation criteria; Attributes centributing to success. *Crit. Care Med.* **14:** 92–94.

91. **Stoller, J.K.** (2000) Weaning from mechanical ventilation. **SCCM/ACCP.** Combined Critical Care Course Syllabus: 491–506.

Chapter 19

Noninvasive positive pressure ventilation (NIPPV)

Robert M. Kacmarek, PhD, RRT

Contents

19.1 Introduction

The use of noninvasive applications of ventilatory assistance can be traced to the 1800s where prototypes of the 'Iron Lung' were first used[1]. However, none of these devices were in general use when Drinker in 1928 developed the first electrically powered Iron Lung[2]. Jack Emerson in 1931 greatly improved upon Drinker's original design and marketed a less expensive, lighter, quieter, and easier to operate unit[3]. However, because of the size of negative pressure ventilators and the inability to well coordinate gas delivery with patient demand, the use, in all but the rare neuromuscularly or neurologically diseased patient, has declined since the late 1970s[4].

Noninvasive positive pressure is also not new. Barach *et al.* in the 1930s originally proposed the use of noninvasive continuous positive air pressure (CPAP) for the management of acute pulmonary edema[5]. Intermittent positive pressure breathing (IPPB) by mouthpiece or mask was widely employed in the management of critically ill patients from the 1960s up to the mid-1980s[4]. The use of NIPPV for nocturnal ventilator support dates back to the early 1960s at the Goldwater Rehabilitation Center in New York for the treatment of neuromuscularly diseased patients[6]. However, the use of a face mask to apply NIPPV to patients with Duchenne muscular dystrophy can be credited to Rideau *et al.* in France in 1984[7].

The use of NIPPV to manage acute respiratory failure (ARF) is based on data demonstrating that NIPPV reduced esophageal pressure swings and diaphragmatic electromyogram activity in patients with acute respiratory distress (*Figure 19.1*)[8,9] and three case series that demonstrated that NIPPV could prevent intubation in patients with acute respiratory failure[9–11]. In this chapter the use of NIPPV and noninvasive CPAP for the management of ARF will be discussed.

19.2 NIPPV for acute respiratory failure

Acute respiratory failure is characterized by the inability to eliminate CO_2 and to oxygenate the blood. As illustrated the *Figures 19.2* and *19.3* from a recent consensus conference, there are many points in the mechanisms that induce hypercarbia and hypoxemia where NIPPV or CPAP can reverse the acute failure[12]. In the setting of acute failure noninvasive positive pressure is used to reverse the hypercarbia and hypoxemia by unloading respiratory muscles, augmenting alveolar ventilation and oxygenation, and improving cardiovascular status.

19.3 Indication for noninvasive positive pressure

Table 19.1 lists the clinical settings where noninvasive positive pressure has been used. Although these settings are extensive, outcome data supporting the use of NIPPV are limited to a few of these indications. Overall, as noted in the following sections, more randomized controlled trials demonstrating improved outcome associated with the use of NIPPV exist than in any other aspect of critical respiratory care.

Table 19.1 Settings in which noninvasive positive pressure has been used during acute respiratory failure

- Acute exacerbation of COPD
- Non-COPD hypercarbic acute respiratory failure
- Cardiogenic pulmonary edema
- Hypoxemic respiratory failure
- Immunocompromised patients
- Weaning from ventilatory support
- Community-acquired pneumonia
- Asthma
- Do not resuscitate/do not intubate patients
- Postoperative patients

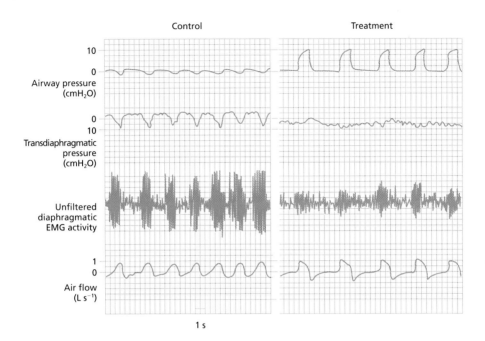

Control   Treatment

Airway pressure
(cmH₂O)

Transdiaphragmatic
pressure
(cmH₂O)

Unfiltered
diaphragmatic
EMG activity

Air flow
(L s⁻¹)

1 s

Figure 19.1 Recording from a representative patient during spontaneous unassisted breathing and after 45 min of treatment with 10 cmH₂O inspiratory positive airway pressure, zero PEEP. From: Brochard, L., Isabey, D., Piquet, J., Amaro, P., Mancebo, J. and Messadi, A.A. (1990) Reversal of acute exacerbations of chronic obstructive lung disease by inspiratory assistance with a face mask. *N. Engl. J. Med.* **95**: 865–870.

19.3.1 COPD

The use of NIPPV in COPD patients with an uncomplicated acute exacerbation is now considered a standard of care. At least seven randomized, controlled prospective trials primarily enrolling COPD patients have demonstrated that NIPPV in this population avoids intubation, decreases mortality, decreases the length of mechanical ventilation, and decreases ICU and hospital stay[13–19]. In addition, a recent meta-analysis by Keenan et al.[20] concluded that NIPPV in COPD decreases frequency of intubation and mortality.

Figure 19.4 from Kramer et al. illustrates the percentage of patients randomized to NIPPV and those randomized to standard medical management without NIPPV who required intubation[14]. Overall a greater percentage in the non-NIPPV group required intubation; however, in those patients with COPD approximately 70% without NIPPV required intubation, whereas only about 10% in the NIPPV group required intubation. Similar data were provided by Brochard et al. in a large European randomized trial of NIPPV[15]. In the NIPPV group 11 of 43 (26%) patients required endotracheal intubation compared with 31 of 42 (74%) patients in the standard therapy group. In addition, significant differences in mortality were observed between these groups. In the NIPPV group four (9%) patients died versus 12

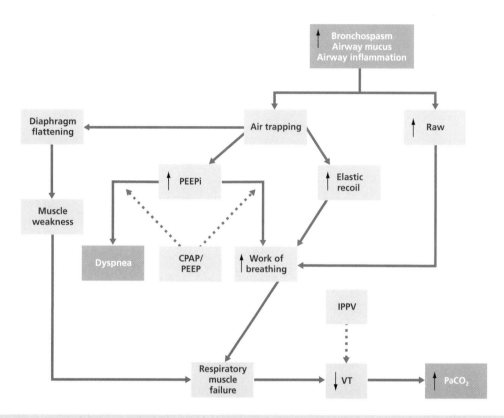

Figure 19.2 When $PaCO_2$ is increased, and minute ventilation is normal or increased, the respiratory muscles are failing to generate sufficient alveolar ventilation to eliminate the CO_2 being produced. Means of correcting this pathophysiology include increasing alveolar ventilation by increasing tidal volume and/or respiratory rate, and reducing CO_2 production ($\dot{V}CO_2$) by decreasing the work of breathing. Respiratory muscle failure can occur when the work of breathing is normal (e.g. numerous acute or chronic neuromuscular problems), or increased (e.g. patients with COPD, asthma, or the obesity hypoventilation syndrome), and presumably because of inadequate delivery of oxygen to the respiratory muscles (e.g. approximately one-third of patients presenting with cardiogenic pulmonary edema). When $PaCO_2$ is increased and minute ventilation is low the level of consciousness is generally impaired. Such patients usually require intubation for airways protection in addition to ventilatory assistance, unless the hypercapnia can be rapidly reversed. From: Consensus statement (2001) International Consensus Conference in Intensive Care Medicine: Noninvasive Positive Pressure Ventilation in Acute Respiratory Failure. Reproduced with permission from *Am. J. Respir. Crit. Care Med.* **163**: 283–291.

(29%) in the standard therapy group. The authors went on to comment that in COPD patients mortality was increased by intubation because of the increased likelihood of nosocomial pneumonia, the high probability of a prolonged ventilator course and the general complications associated with endotracheal intubation in the group of patients.

Two recent studies, one observational[21] and the other using historical controls[22], concluded that endotracheal intubation in COPD increased the likelihood of all types of nosocomial infections. Guerin *et al.*[21] observed in 230 consecutive patients staying 2 days or longer in the ICU and requiring 1 day or more of mechanical ventilation that none of the 60 patients managed only with NIPPV developed nosocomial pneumonia, whereas 18% of the patients first treated with NIPPV then intubated, 22% of the patients first intubated than

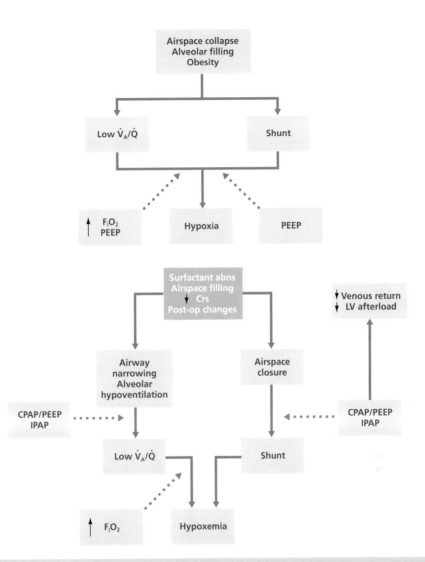

Figure 19.3 Hypoxemia develops as a result of alveolar hypoventilation (which is accompanied by increases in PaCO$_2$ and is addressed in Figure 19.1) and from perfusion going to areas where the ratio of alveolar ventilation ($\dot{V}_A$) to perfusion (Q) is less than 1.0 (i.e. low $\dot{V}_A/\dot{Q}$ or, in the extreme shunt, where perfusion is going to areas of no ventilation). Hypoxemia is treated by augmenting the F$_I$O$_2$ (the lower the $\dot{V}_A/\dot{Q}$ the less the effect), and by recruiting airspaces. Airspace derecruitment occurs when the transpulmonary pressure falls below the airspace collapsing or the closing pressure (as occurs in numerous conditions that alter surfactant or that decrease the lung or the chest wall compliance), and when the transpulmonary pressure applied during inhalation fails to exceed airspace opening pressure. Accordingly, airspace opening can be facilitated by increasing the transpulmonary pressure applied at end exhalation (CPAP) and at end inhalation (i.e. Inspiratory positive airway pressure (IPAP)). An additional beneficial effect of CPAP and IPAP may be seen in patients with cardiogenic pulmonary edema, as they all reduce venous return and functionally reduce left ventricular afterload. abns, abnormalities; Crs, respiratory system compliance. From: Consensus statement (1982) International Consensus Conference in Intensive Care Medicine: Noninvasive Positive Pressure Ventilation in Acute Respiratory Failure. Reproduced with permission from *Am. J. Respir. Crit. Care Med.* **163**: 283–291.

changed to NIPPV, and 28% of the patients intubated only developed nosocomial pneumonia. Girou et al.[22] compared 50 patients with COPD or severe cardiogenetic pulmonary edema who were managed with NIPPV with 50 matched controls endotracheally intubated

and ventilated. They also found that the nosocomial infection rates were significantly lower in the NIPPV group (*Figure 19.5*).

The largest randomized, controlled trial of NIPPV in COPD was conducted by Plant et al. in patients not admitted to the ICU but maintained on medical wards[18]. The results were similar to those of Brochard et al.[15] and Kramer et al.[14]; that is, only 18 of 118 (15%) patients in the NIPPV group required intubation versus 32 of 118 (27%) in the standard therapy group. The single negative study of NIPPV in COPD was reported by Barbe et al.[19], who found no difference in outcome between the NIPPV and control group. However, no patient in either the control or treatment group died or required intubation. On close examination it would appear that none of the patients recruited into this study was sick enough to need any type of ventilatory assistance. In no

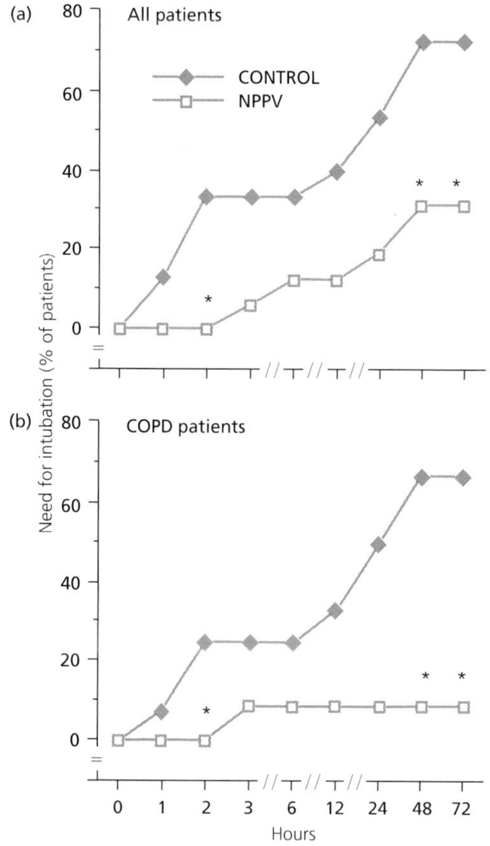

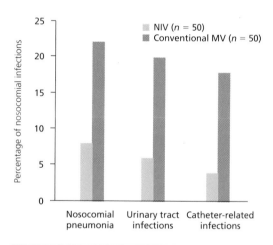

Figure 19.4 Need for intubation (percentage of patients) among all patients (a) and among COPD patients (b) plotted against time in the study. ■, Control patients; □, patients receiving noninvasive positive pressure ventilation (NIPPV). n = 16 NPPV patients (12 with COPD) and 15 control patients (11 with COPD).
*P < 0.05 compared with control patients. From: Kramer, N., Meyer, T.J., Meharg, J., Cece, R.D. and Hill, N.S. (1995) Randomized, prospective trial of noninvasive positive pressure ventilation in acute respiratory failure. Reproduced with permission from *Am. J. Respir. Crit. Care Med.* **151**: 1799–1806.

Figure 19.5 Frequency of nosocomial infections in 50 cases treated with noninvasive ventilation (NIV) and 50 controls treated with intubation and conventional mechanical ventilation (MV). P values between the two groups are 0.04 for nosocomial pneumonia, 0.03 for urinary tract infections and 0.002 for catheter-related infection. From: Girou, E., Schortgen, F., Delclaux, C., Brun-Buisson, C., Blot, F., Lefort, Y., Lemaire, F. and Brochard, L. (2000) Association of noninvasive ventilation with nosocomial infection and survival in critically ill patients. *JAMA* **284**: 2361–2367.

study have patients randomized to the NIPPV group done more poorly on any outcome variable than those randomized to the control group.

Clearly, the data on COPD patients would seem to indicate that NIPPV should be available to all patients with an acute exacerbation of COPD in any institution treating these patients. As noted in *Table 19.2*, NIPPV is indicated in patients with acute hypercarbic respiratory failure that do not have cardiovascular instability to the level requiring immediate intubation. Additional exclusions from NIPPV are facial or airway trauma, inability to protect the airway, and inability to clear secretions in spite of the use of NIPPV. Of course, NIPPV cannot be used in patients who will not tolerate NIPPV. However, patient tolerance may be more a problem with the caregiver and available equipment (see later sections) than with

the patient. Patients most likely to be successfully managed with NIPPV are young (<70 years), with lower acuity of illness scores (APACHE) and better able to co-operate. They also have minimal air leak, have moderate to severe hypercarbia ($PaCO_2$ >45 but <90 mmHg) and moderate to severe acidemia (pH <7.35 but >7.10)[4,23].

19.3.2 Non-COPD hypercapnic respiratory failure

Few systematically acquired data and no randomized controlled trials are available on the use of NIPPV in non-COPD hypercapnic respiratory failure. However, the use of NIPPV in patients with neurologic and neuromuscular disease has been available for acute and chronic management of these patients for over 20 years[24–27]. We would encourage the early use of NIPPV in this group of hypercapnic respiratory failure patients.

There has been interest by a few groups in the use of NIPPV in the management of acute asthma[24,28,29]. Although there have been some isolated successes, we find the use of heliox (see Chapter 17) more suited than NIPPV for the management of these patients. Many asthmatics, in our experience, in severe acute attacks simply will not tolerate NIPPV.

Others have successfully used NIPPV as a bridge to transplantation in cystic fibrosis patients[4,30]. We have also been able to successfully manage some transplantation candidates without endotracheal intubation for days to weeks with NIPPV. NIPPV is also useful in the management of postoperative, hypercapnic respiratory failure[31–33].

19.3.3 Cardiogenic pulmonary edema

Positive pressure has been shown to be beneficial in the management of acute cardiogenic pulmonary edema because the elevated mean intrathoracic pressures decrease venous return, reducing left ventricular preload and afterload, improving cardiac output[34]. In addition, oxygenation is generally improved because of better ventilation–perfusion matching[35]. In fact, four prospective, randomized controlled trials

---

Table 19.2 Selection guidelines: noninvasive ventilation for patients with COPD and acute respiratory failure

Step 1. Identify patients in need of ventilatory assistance:
A. Symptoms and signs of acute respiratory distress:
  (i) moderate to severe dyspnea, increased over usual and
  (ii) RR > 24, accessory muscle use, paradoxical breathing
B. Gas exchange abnormalities:
  (i) $PaCO_2$ > 45 mmHg, pH < 7.35 or
  (ii) $PaCO_2/F_IO_2$ < 200

Step 2. Exclude those at increased risk with noninvasive ventilation:
A. Respiratory arrest
B. Medically unstable (hypotensive shock, uncontrolled cardiac ischemia or arrhythmias)
C. Unable to protect airway (impaired cough or swallowing mechanism)
D. Excessive secretions
E. Agitated or uncooperative
F. Facial trauma, burns, or surgery, or anatomic abnormalities interfering with mask fit

From: Mehta, S. and Hill, N.S. (2001) Noninvasive ventilation. Reproduced with permission from *Am. J. Respir. Crit. Care Med.* **163**: 540–577.

have demonstrated a decrease in endotracheal intubation rate in patients in acute cardiogenic pulmonary edema receiving mask CPAP versus controls without CPAP[34,36–38]. As a result, CPAP has been considered a standard for the management of hypoxemia in acute cardiogenic pulmonary edema[4,12].

As NIPPV became more popular, a number of groups have used NIPPV for the management of cardiogenic pulmonary edema. In the largest case series, Rusterholtz et al.[40] successfully applied (avoided intubation) NIPPV to 21 out of 26 patients. All patients successfully treated were hypercarbic (PaCO$_2$ 54.2 ± 15 mmHg versus 32 ± 2.1 mmHg failures) and had a lower Creatine phosphokinase (CPK) (176 ± 149 versus 1282 ± 2080 IU/I in the failures) than those failing NIPPV. In fact, four of the five failures versus two of the 21 successes had acute myocardial infarctions. Three randomized controlled trials have evaluated NIPPV in acute cardiogenic pulmonary edema[39–42]. In two of these trials the number of patients developing acute myocardial infarctions was higher than the group receiving NIPPV versus CPAP[40] or versus oxygen therapy with high-dose nitrates[41]. In addition, a recent meta-analysis concluded that there was too little evidence to make conclusions regarding the use of NIPPV in acute cardiogenic pulmonary edema[43]. As listed in Table 19.3, CPAP should be used during acute cardiogenic pulmonary edema in all patients presenting with hypoxemia who are eucapnic. NIPPV should be reserved for patients with hypercarbia. Patients presenting with an acute myocardial infarction should be considered for endotracheal intubation.

Table 19.3 Use of positive pressure in acute cardiogenic pulmonary edema

- Hypoxemia but eucapnia, CPAP 8–12 cmH$_2$O
- Hypoxemia and hypercarbia, BIPAP
- Acute cardiogenic pulmonary edema associated with myocardial infarction; consider intubation

19.3.4 Hypoxemic respiratory failure

NIPPV has been most successful during hypercarbic respiratory failure. In fact, Wysocki et al.[44] showed that the lack of hypercarbia was associated with failure of NIPPV (Figure 19.6). This makes intuitive sense; ventilation can be expected to have the most impact on patients who require ventilatory assistance not oxygenation assistance. However, patients with severe hypoxemic experience increased cardiopulmonary work and hypoxemic respiratory failure can be expected over time to show hypercarbic respiratory failure if the hypoxemia is not corrected.

A single prospective randomized trial has evaluated the use of NIPPV in non-hypercarbic, hypoxemic respiratory failure[45]. Antonelli et al.[45] randomized patients to NIPPV or endotracheal intubation. Seventeen patients in the endotracheally intubated group (n = 32) and 23 in the NIPPV group (n = 32) survived. More patients in the endotracheally intubated group experienced serious complication and had a longer hospital stay. However, this was a single-center trial and it is difficult to conclude from the data presented that the patients randomized to conventional mechanical ventilation required endotracheal intubation at the time of randomization.

More recently, Delclaux et al.[46] compared the use of CPAP with oxygen therapy in patients presenting with hypoxemic respiratory failure. They found no differences between groups in the rate of endotracheal intubation, hospital mortality or intensive care length of stay. They did, however, find differences in the number of adverse events. More adverse events occurred in the CPAP group (Table 19.4). Of most concern was the fact that four patients in the CPAP group had cardiac arrests and four other patients developed stress ulcers. No patients in the oxygen-only group developed either complication. They concluded that CPAP, although improving oxygenation, delayed necessary endotracheal intubation and placed patients at greater risk for complications than simply oxygen therapy.

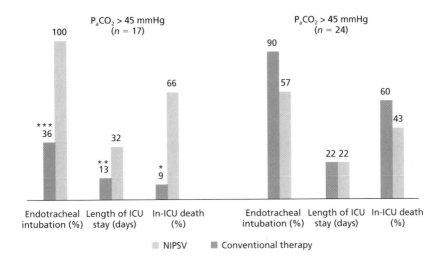

Figure 19.6 Percentage of patients requiring endotracheal intubation, length of ICU stay and in-ICU mortality between patients treated with NIPPV (NIPSV) and those treated with conventional therapy in subgroups of patients with (a) initial P_aCO_2 greater than 45 mmHg ($n = 17$) or (b) initial P_aCO_2 of 45 mmHg or less ($n = 24$). ***$P < 0.02$; **$P < 0.04$; *$P < 0.06$ between NIPSV and conventional therapy. From: Wysocki, M., Tric, L., Wolf, M.A., Millet, H. and Herman, B. (1995) Noninvasive pressure support ventilation in patients with acute respiratory failure: A randomized comparison with conventional therapy. Reproduced with permission from *Chest* **107**: 761–768.

Table 19.4 Adverse events occurring in patients during their intensive care unit stay*

Adverse event	Oxygen alone ($n = 60$)	Oxygen plus CPAP ($n = 62$)	P value between treatment groups
During spontaneous ventilation			
Facial skin necrosis	0	2	0.50
Gastric distention	0	1	0.54
Nosocomial pneumonia	1	0	0.97
Cardiac arrest	0	4*	0.14
During mechanical ventilation			
Nosocomial pneumonia	4	6	0.74
Sinusitis	1	0	0.99
Pneumothorax	0	1	0.54
Stress ulcer	0	4	0.14
Any adverse event, n (%)	6 (10)	18 (29)	0.01
Patients with adverse events, n (%)	5 (8)	14 (23)	0.03

CPAP, continuous positive airway pressure.
*Three patients experienced cardiac arrest at the time of scheduled intubation, in patients receiving CPAP to maintain oxygenation. In another patient, cardiac arrest occurred when CPAP delivered by a face mask was disconnected to allow nursing care, resulting in a rapid worsening of hypoxemia. From: Delclaux, C., L'Her, E., Alberti, C., et al. (2000) Treatment of acute hypoxemic non-hypercapnic respiratory insufficiency with continuous positive airway pressure delivered by a face mask. Reproduced with permission from the American Medical Association. *JAMA* **289**: 2352–2360.

As a result, it is difficult to recommend the use of NIPPV for hypoxemic respiratory failure, and the use of CPAP may need to be restricted to use in patients with acute cardiogenic edema who can maintain eucapnia. When either NIPPV or CPAP is used in these patients careful ongoing assessment is required to avoid delays in endotracheal intubation in those patients where it is required.

19.3.5 Immunocompromised patients

The single group of patients where NIPPV for the management of hypoxemic respiratory failure seems appropriate is immunocompromised patients. The avoidance of endotracheal intubation in these patients reduces the risk of infection and hemorrhagic complications[4]. In a number of case series, endotracheal intubation has been successfully avoided with the use of NIPPV[47,48]. Patients with acute respiratory failure of various etiologies after solid organ transplantation were randomly assigned by Antonelli et al.[49] to receive NIPPV or standard therapy. Patients treated with NIPPV had a reduced need for endotracheal intubation and a lower mortality. There was also a trend toward fewer ventilator-associated pneumonias and a significant reduction in the rate of septic shock. Considering the problems inherent with endotracheal intubation with this group of patients. NIPPV should be considered as first-line therapy.

19.3.6 Community-acquired infection

Patients with community-acquired infections have been included in some of the case series on the use of NIPPV[24,50]. However, only one randomized trial recruiting only patients with community-acquired infections has been performed[47]. Fifty-six patients with severe community-acquired pneumonias were randomized to receive NIPPV plus conventional therapy or conventional therapy alone. Patients receiving NIPPV avoided intubation (21 versus 50%, $P < 0.03$) and had a shorter duration of ICU stay (1.8 versus 6 days, $P < 0.04$). However, closer examination of the data indicates that the beneficial results of NIPPV

occurred only in patients with COPD. As a result, the use of NIPPV for community-acquired pneumonia appears beneficial only in patients with COPD.

19.3.7 Do not resuscitate/do not intubate

This is a controversial indication for NIPPV. However, a number of case series have demonstrated successful use of NIPPV in this setting[51–53]. The central issue is an ethical one, for in patients who choose not to be intubated or resuscitated is NIPPV truly following the wishes of the patient? Patients should fully understand that NIPPV is being used as a form of life support, although noninvasive. On the other hand, for a terminally ill patient NIPPV may relieve dyspnea, preserve the patient's autonomy and permit verbal communication between the patient and family[4]. Indeed, we have seen patients in this category discharged home after successful use of NIPPV. We believe NIPPV is appropriate in many do not intubate/do not resuscitate patients but appropriate communication with the patient and family regarding NIPPV should always occur.

19.3.8 Weaning

A number of case series have indicated that NIPPV is a useful bridge to weaning, especially in patients with COPD[54–57]. Two randomized trials have specifically addressed this issue[58,59]. In both of these trials COPD patients receiving conventional mechanical ventilation were screened 48 h after the initiation of mechanical ventilation. Only those patients failing this initial weaning trial were randomized to either extubation and NIPPV or continued intubation and pressure support weaning. As noted in *Figure 19.7* from the Nava et al. trial[58], patients extubated to NIPPV were weaned more quickly than patients remaining intubated. Mean duration of mechanical ventilation, ICU stay, survival and nosocomial pneumonia rates were all lower in the NIPPV group. In the Girault et al.[59] trial no difference in the number of patients successfully weaned was observed. As expected by protocol, the number of days patients remained intubated was shorter with NIPPV. However, the total days of ventilatory support (7.69 ± 3.79 days versus 16.10 ± 5.24 days NIPPV) was longer in the NIPPV group.

It is difficult to recommend against the use of NIPPV in the patient who is inadvertently extubated or who develops respiratory failure after extubation. But it is also difficult to recommend planned extubation of COPD patients who fail weaning trials to initiate NIPPV, as these patients probably failed NIPPV before intubation. We have attempted to electively extubate COPD patients failing weaning trials but have not been successful maintaining extubation with NIPPV. In our opinion, this is an indication for NIPPV requiring greater research.

19.4 When should NIPPV be initiated for acute respiratory failure?

Table 19.5 summarizes the clinical settings where noninvasive positive pressure is indicated based on data in the literature and our experience. For hypoxemic respiratory failure, asthma, and elective extubation for weaning we believe insufficient data are available to support the unquestioned use of NIPPV.

19.5 Complications or problems with NIPPV

NIPPV is not without complications; however, provided airway pressure is not excessive, the complications are not serious. *Table 19.6* lists the complications observed during NIPPV. Of those listed, gastric distention and subsequent regurgitation are the most potentially dangerous, but, as addressed later in the chapter, if airway pressure is maintained less than 20 cmH$_2$O gastric distention is unlikely. Most of the other problems listed can be corrected with proper equipment (see later discussion). In addition, the use of artificial skin on the bridge of the nose can reduce the likelihood of skin

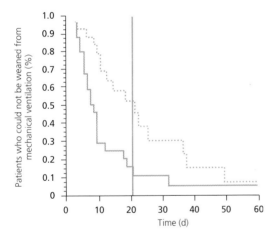

Figure 19.7 Kaplan–Meier curves for patients who could not be weaned from mechanical ventilation (defined as weaning failure or death linked to mechanical ventilation) in two groups. The probability of weaning failure was significantly lower for the noninvasive ventilation group (*P* < 0.01). The vertical line represents day 21. The continuous line represents the NIPPV group; the dashed line the invasive pressure support group. From: Nava, S., Ambrosino, N., Clini, E., Prato, M., Orlando, G., Vitacca, M., Brigada, P., Fraccia, C. and Rubinni, F. (1998) Non-invasive mechanical ventilation in the weaning of patients with respiratory failure due to chronic obstructive pulmonary disease: A randomized study. Reproduced with permission from the American College of Physicians. *Ann. Intern. Med.* **128**: 721–728.

Table 19.5 Clinical setting where NIPPV is indicated

- COPD acute exacerbation
- Community-acquired pneumonia in COPD patients
- Acute cardiogenic pulmonary edema presenting with hypercarbia but no evidence of mycardial infarction
- Acute hypercapnic respiratory failure in:
  - Neuromuscular or neurologic disease
  - Postoperative patients
  - Immunocompromised patients
  - Do not resuscitate/do not intubate patients
  - Inadvertently extubated patients
  - Patients failing extubation

Table 19.6 Complication or problems with NIPPV

Problems	Solutions
• Air leak	Different size or type of mask
• Mask discomfort or facial soreness, skin breakdown	Different size or type of mask; artificial skin; lower mask securing pressure
• Eye irritation	Reposition mask; different size or type of mask
• Sinus congestion or oronasal drying	Humidifier; decongestant
• Epistaxis	Humidifier; petroleum jelly
• Gastric insufflation	Lower peak pressure; nasogastric tube

breakdown. This may especially be useful in the elderly with poor peripheral perfusion.

19.6 The application of NIPPV

Establishing an NIPPV program is not without problems. It is common that initial results are not as successful as those published in randomized, controlled trials. The reason for this difference is multifactorial (*Table 19.7*). Most importantly, all involved in the care of the patient receiving NIPPV must fully understand the benefits and problems associated with NIPPV. If the therapists and nurses caring for these patients do not understand the benefits associated with NIPPV or how to properly manage patients and select equipment during NIPPV, their actions (whether conscious or subconscious) can markedly affect the success rate.

Four major factors affect the efficacy of NIPPV and can influence its success: (i) the ventilator; (ii) the facial interphase; (iii) the interaction between the patient and the clinician applying NIPPV; (iv) the interaction between the patient and the mechanical ventilator.

19.6.1 The mechanical ventilator

Any ventilator ever manufactured can be used for NIPPV. However, for the successful application of NIPPV to patients in acute respiratory failure a number of ventilator features are desirable (*Table 19.8*). First, pressure-targeted ventilation should be available. In patients experiencing marked cardiopulmonary stress

Table 19.7 Successful application of NIPPV requires

• Clinician knowledge of the process
• Proper selection of the ventilator
• Proper selection of the mask
• Interaction between patient and clinician
• Interaction between patient and ventilator

Table 19.8 The ideal ventilator for NIPPV use in acute respiratory failure

• Pressure-targeted ventilation available
• Leak compensation
• CO_2 rebreathing minimal
• Precise, accurate, and high F_IO_2 available
• Pressure, volume, and flow waveforms
• Appropriate alarms and monitors

with varying ventilatory demand it has been clearly demonstrated that pressure ventilation more appropriately responds to patient's flow demand than volume ventilation[60]. This does not mean that volume ventilation is always inappropriate, but it does mean that the likelihood for success is greater with pressure than volume ventilation. Second, in acute respiratory failure visual feedback of patient–ventilatory synchrony is essential. As with invasive ventilation, knowledge of the patient's respiratory rate, tidal volume, and coordination with triggering and cycling helps to insure ventilator settings are appropriate. The ventilator must also be able to provide high and precise F_IO_2. In addition, methods of monitoring the patient's status and notifying staff of problems are essential. The ventilator should be able to compensate for leaks and CO_2 rebreathing should be minimal. Can ventilators without these features provide successful NIPPV? Yes, but the likelihood of success is greatly diminished.

19.6.2 ICU ventilators

There is no question that ICU ventilators meet most of the above requirements. Most provide waveforms and monitors, pressure ventilation, precise F_1O_2 delivery, and alarms. In addition, the newest generation of ICU ventilators are very responsive to patient demand[61]. Some of these ventilators (Puritan Bennett 840 and Hamilton Galileo) allow for adjustment of inspiratory termination criteria during pressure support and most of these new generation ventilators allow for rise time adjustment during both pressure support and pressure assist/control ventilation[62,63]. In addition, CO_2 rebreathing is not a problem with ICU ventilators. However, the major problem with the use of ICU ventilators for NIPPV is their inability to compensate for leaks. None of the current generation of ICU ventilators compensates for leaks; none of them incorporates a NIPPV mode. However, as is obvious from the literature, many trials of NIPPV have been conducted with these ventilators[8,21,22,24,45]. It is also important to note that these ventilators impose very little effort when used in the CPAP mode[64].

19.6.3 Bilevel pressure ventilators

This group of ventilators was developed out of the need to provide pressure ventilation to select patients requiring nasal CPAP for sleep apnea. In this application, a very simple approach to ventilation was all that was required. This approach has been shown to work well during the chronic application of NIPPV in the home. In fact it has been shown that the responsiveness of many of these ventilators is equivalent to or better than that of current ICU ventilators[61,62,65]. However, the vast majority of these ventilators are not designed for use in the ICU (*Figure 19.8*). They

do not include alarms or monitors. They are not capable of delivering high or precise F_1O_2 and it is virtually impossible with most to determine if the patient in acute respiratory failure is in synchrony with the ventilator. Most do not include any indication of phase of ventilation. The only ventilator in this group specifically designed for ICU use is the Respironics Inc. Vision Ventilator (*Figure 19.8*). However, it can be expected that similar type ventilators from other manufacturers will soon be available. The Vision incorporates all of the features for successful application of NIPPV to patients in acute respiratory failure and would have to be considered the model ventilator for application in this setting.

19.6.4 CO_2 rebreathing

A problem with all bilevel pressure ventilators that can affect success in acute respiratory failure is CO_2 rebreathing. All of these units have low internal resistance turbine-driven compressors. In addition, none contains a true exhalation valve. Expiration is via a small orifice near the patient's face. As a result, total patient exhalation into the ventilator circuit has the potential of retrograde movement of exhaled gas all the way up to the ventilator[66]. This can be avoided by setting PEEP equal to or greater than about 5 cmH$_2$O (*Figure 19.9*). PEEP maintains a high flow from the ventilator during exhalation, minimizing the likelihood of CO_2 rebreathing[65]. Furthermore, the use of an isolation (plateau) valve that directs gas out of the circuit prevents rebreathing. In addition, it has been recently demonstrated that full face masks with the exhalation port located in the mask prevent or markedly reduce CO_2 rebreathing[67]. Consideration of CO_2 rebreathing is critical during acute application with a oronasal or full face mask. Modifications to prevent CO_2 rebreathing may be the difference between success and failure in a given patient.

19.6.5 The mask

The most critical factor in the successful application of NIPPV is the mask. If the mask does not fit properly, if the mask is too large, if there

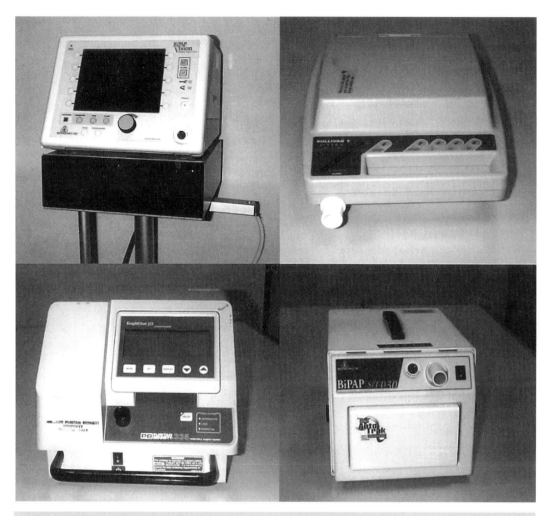

Figure 19.8 Bilevel pressure ventilators.

is a large leak near the patient's eyes, or if the patient finds the mask uncomfortable the likelihood of successful application of NIPPV is markedly diminished. As a general rule, the smaller the mask the better the fit. If gas leaks from the mask into the patient's eyes, the mask is too big. The top of a properly sized and fitted mask should rest about a quarter to a third down from the top of the bridge of the nose and fit snugly along the lateral border of the nose. For nasal masks, the bottom of the mask should sit above the upper lip snug to the nose. With full-face masks the lower border should fit just below the lower lip or down to

the chin depending upon design. In sizing masks, it is useful to use the sizing templates available with many masks (*Figure 19.10*).

Especially with full face masks, the internal volume of the mask should be considered. A large internal volume can result in CO_2 rebreathing. The ResMed oronasal mask avoids this concern by placing the orifice for exhalation at the top of the mask itself[67]. As a result, flow to maintain PEEP flushes the mask during exhalation.

No single type of mask will work on all patients, especially during the acute application of NIPPV. Multiple types of both oronasal

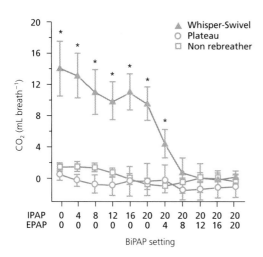

Figure 19.9 Volume of CO_2 inhaled from the ventilator tubing at various IPAP and EPAP settings during B_iPAP ventilatory assistance. Whisper-Swivel—standard BIPAP exhalation valve. Plateau and non-rebreathing valves—prevent retrograde movement of exhaled gas into the ventilator circuit. *$P < 0.05$ compared with other devices at similar B_iPAP settings. From: Ferguson, G.T. and Gilmartin, M. (1995) CO_2 rebreathing during B_iPAP ventilatory assistance. Reproduced with permission from *Am. J. Respir. Crit. Care Med.* **151**: 1126–1132.

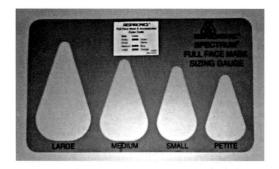

Figure 19.10 Template for sizing masks (Respironics Inc.).

Table 19.9 Nasal versus oronasal masks

	Nasal	Oronasal
Adequacy of ventilation	Low	High
Claustrophobia	Low	High
Ability to speak	Easy	Difficult
Ability to expectorate	Easy	Difficult
Air leak	High	Low
Dead space	Low	High

and nasal masks should be available and taken to the bedside so that the mask that best conforms to the patient's anatomy can be selected (*Figure 19.11*).

During chronic NIPPV either a nasal or oronasal mask can be used. However, when patients are in acute respiratory distress they breathe through their mouths; as a result, oronasal masks are the masks of choice. Although oronasal masks are less comfortable and more claustrophobic, because they prevent mouth leaks they insure better ventilation (*Table 19.9*). A number of companies have chinstraps to prevent mouth leak with nasal masks; however, during acute respiratory failure they do not work. After the first 12–24 h of NIPPV, when acutely distressed patients are stabilized, many can be switched from oronasal to nasal masks for continued NIPPV.

A full-face shield has recently become available from Respironics, Inc. This is a one-size-fits-all mask that covers the whole face. No data are currently available on the use of this mask; however, it appears to be well tolerated by patients in acute failure.

19.6.6 Patient–clinician interaction

Successful application of NIPPV especially in the acute setting requires a clinician who understands what the patient is experiencing, is empathetic to the patient's needs, and is patient and willing to educate and work with the patient during the initial application. Initiation of NIPPV is more difficult than initiation of invasive ventilatory support. The clinician needs to first educate the patient, to explain carefully what is about to happen and why. After the mask has been selected it should be fitted to the patient's face briefly without ventilation to confirm fit. When ventilation is started, PEEP should be set at zero or minimum and inspiratory pressure set at 2–5 cmH$_2$O. The mask should be held to the patient's face by the clinician or patient before it is strapped in place. The mask should never be strapped until

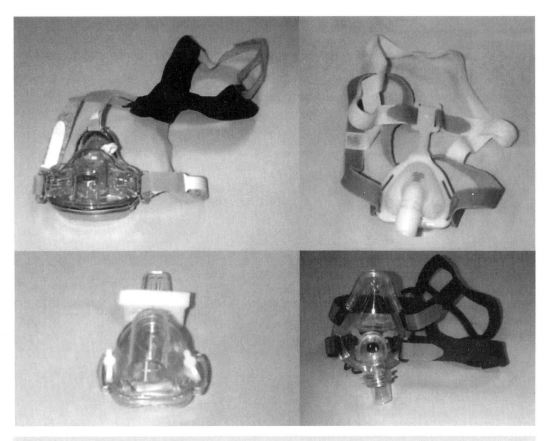

Figure 19.11 Masks used for NIPPV.

the patient is totally accepting and comfortable with the process. The wrong approach is to set the ventilator at 15 cmH$_2$O peak pressure and 5 cmH$_2$O PEEP and on the first breath strap the mask to the patient's face. It is very difficult to rapidly acclimate to these pressures. A gradual buildup of pressure over time insures patient acclimation, elimination of patient's fears and increases the patient's confidence in the process.

Throughout the initial application phase (first 1–2 h) an experienced clinician capable of answering all of the patient's questions and adjusting the ventilator should be immediately available. During this period, the clinician may have to stay at the bedside talking to the patient, eliminating their fears, and insuring the ventilator is set to meet the patient's ventilatory and comfort needs.

19.6.7 Patient–ventilator synchrony

In the acute application of NIPPV it is impossible to insure patient–ventilatory synchrony without visual assessment of the inspiratory and expiratory phase of ventilation. Some of the bilevel pressure ventilators are so quiet and the sound they do make is so similar during inspiration and expiration that it is difficult to tell if the patient is in phase with the ventilator. The most common causes of dyssynchrony are a lack of coordination between the patient and the ventilator during triggering and cycling of inspiration, and the delivery of inadequate or excessive flow at the onset of inspiration[67]. Dyssynchrony during acute respiratory failure is more common with nasal than oronasal masks, as stressed patients breathe through their mouths (*Table 19.10*).

Table 19.10 Patient–ventilator synchrony

Inability to trigger to inspiration
- Improper sensitivity setting
- Auto-PEEP
  - PEEP
  - Reduce peak pressure or VT

System leaks
- Too large a mask
- Use oronasal or full face mask
- Change to pressure assist/control if ICU ventilator

Cycling to exhalation
- Increase cycling criteria if available
- Use pressure assist/control
  - Set inspiratory time 0.6–0.9 s

Gastric distention
- Peak pressure too high
- Cough or dryness of airway or nose
  - Add humidifier

Dyssynchrony with triggering is most commonly a result of auto-PEEP[68]. All of the ICU and bilevel pressure ventilators are very responsive to patient demand and trigger with small pressure changes and short time delays. However, auto-PEEP as with intubated patients can result in an inability of patients to trigger the ventilator with each inspiratory effort. Whenever the patient's respiratory rate is greater then the ventilator response rate auto-PEEP should be considered[69]. Applied PEEP can be adjusted to minimize the difference between central airway and ventilator circuit pressure, and alveolar pressure improving triggering[70]. This works to decrease the gradient to trigger only if the auto-PEEP is a result of dynamic airway obstruction as seen in COPD patients. The auto-PEEP level in COPD patients is increased by excessive airway pressure and large V_T values, particularly if the respiratory rate is high. Dyssynchrony during the transition to exhalation can also increase the level of auto-PEEP.

19.6.8 Transition to exhalation
Termination of the inspiratory phase during pressure support occurs when the patient's inspiratory flow is equal to the inspiratory flow termination criteria of the ventilator[62]. With most bilevel pressure ventilators, the size of the leak is learned and the patient's desire to exhale is well coordinated with the inspiratory flow terminating criteria[69]. This is not true with any other group of currently available ventilators.

During NIPPV lack of coordination between the patient and ventilator during transition from inspiration to expiration with ICU ventilators is common[70]. This problem can be approached in a number of ways. First, only oronasal or full face masks should be used with ICU ventilators. Second, if available the inspiratory termination criteria should be set to a high percentage of the patient's peak flow. Third, the patient can be switched from pressure support to pressure assist/control (*Figure 19.12*)[70]. The use of pressure assist/control is frequently required even with an oronasal mask in ventilators with a low flow inspiratory termination criteria (Puritan–Bennett 7200 5 L min^{-1}; Seimens Servo 300 5% of peak flow). When pressure assist/control is used, a careful assessment of the patient's inspiratory time should be made. In most adults in acute respiratory failure inspiratory time should be set at about 0.6–0.9 s. Spontaneously breathing patients rarely exceed 1.0 s inspiratory time.

19.6.9 Ventilatory pressure
It is rare that high airway pressure is needed during NIPPV. As NIPPV is primarily used in patients with hypercarbic not hypoxemic respiratory failure, peak pressures can easily be kept at 20 cmH$_2$O or less. If airway pressures are allowed to exceed 20 cmH$_2$O gastric distention becomes a concern and may result in dyssynchrony. However, gastric distention of clinical significance is quite rare if peak pressures are kept below 20 cmH$_2$O. Gastric opening pressure is about 20–25 cmH$_2$O. If a nasogastric tube is necessary it is unlikely that NIPPV will be successful. PEEP levels are adjusted to insure inspiratory trigger synchrony. Rarely is more than 7 cmH$_2$O PEEP required. Ventilating pressure (pressure support

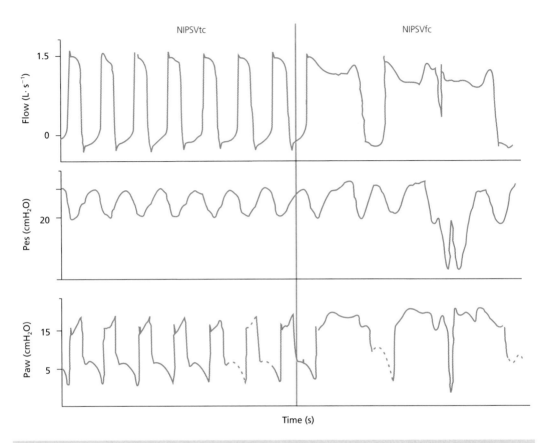

Figure 19.12 Representative flow, esophageal pressure (Pes) and airway pressure (Paw) during NIPPV with pressure assist/control (left side) and during pressure support (right side) using an ICU ventilator. In both, a large mask leak is present. From: Calderini, E., Confalonieri, M., Puccio, P.G., Francavilla, N., Stella, L. and Gregoretti, C. (1999) Patient–ventilator assynchrony during noninvasive ventilation: the role of expiratory trigger. *Intensive Care Med.* **25**: 662–667. Reproduced with permission from Springer-Verlag.

or pressure control level) exceeding 12–15 cmH$_2$O is rarely needed; in fact, many COPD patients can be adequately ventilated with a pressure support level of 8–10 cmH$_2$O.

19.6.10 Humidification

Many patients require humidification during the acute application of NIPPV. This is particularly true if a high concentration of oxygen is required. In most patients an unheated, passover humidifier is sufficient. If a patient persistently coughs after the start of NIPPV, humidify the inspired gas.

19.7 Summary

In acute exacerbations of COPD NIPPV should be considered the treatment of choice. NIPPV has also been shown to be effective in other forms of acute hypercarbic respiratory failure and post-extubation failure (*Table 19.5*). However, NIPPV should only be used cautiously in hypoxemic respiratory failure. In fact, we have found limited success with this application. Numerous factors contribute to a successful NIPPV program. Education of staff and appropriate equipment selection are most important. The learning curve for NIPPV is steep once all the pieces are in place but it does require a defined program be established.

References

1. Woollam, C.H.M. (1976) The development of apparatus for intermittent negative pressure respiration. *Anaesthesia* **31:** 537–547.
2. Drinker, P. and Shaw, L.A. (1929) An apparatus for the prolonged administration of artificial respiration. I. Design for adults and children. *J. Clin. Invest.* **7:** 229–247.
3. Hodes, H.L. (1955) Treatment of respiratory difficulty in poliomyelitis. In: *Poliomielitis Papers and Discussions Presented at the Third International Poliomyeliytis Conference.* Lippincott, Philadelphia, PA, pp. 91–113.
4. Mehta, S. and Hill, N.S. (2001) Noninvasive ventilation. *Am. J. Respir. Crit. Care Med.* **163:** 540–577.
5. Barach, A.L., Martin, J. and Eckman, M. (1938) Positive pressure respiration and its application to the treatment of acute pulmonary edema. *Ann. Intern. Med.* **12:** 754–795.
6. Alba, A., Khan, A. and Lee, M. (1984) Mouth IPPV for sleep. *Rehabil. Gazette* **24:** 47–49.
7. Rideau, Y., Gatin, G., Bach, J. and Gines, G. (1983) Prolongation of life in Ducheme's muscular dystrophy. *Acta Neurol. Belg.* **5:** 118–124.
8. Carrey, Z., Gotfried, S.B. and Levy, R.D. (1990) Ventilatory muscle support in respiratory failure with nasal positive pressure ventilation. *Chest* **97:** 150–158.
9. Brochard, L., Isabey, D., Piquet, J., Amaro, P., Mancebo, J. and Messadi, A.A. (1990) Reversal of acute exacerbations of chronic obstructive lung disease by inspiratory assistance with a face mask. *N. Engl. J. Med.* **95:** 865–870.
10. Meduri, G.U., Conoscenti, C.C., Menashe, P. and Nair, S. (1989) Noninvasive face mask ventilation in patients with acute respiratory failure. *Chest* **95:** 865–870.
11. Elliott, M.W., Steven, M.H., Phillips, G.D. and Branthwaite, M.A. (1990) Noninvasive mechanical ventilation for acute respiratory failure. *Br. Med. J.* **300:** 358–360.
12. International Censensus Conference (2001) International Consensus Conference in Intensive Care Medicine: Noninvasive Positive Pressure Ventilation in Acute Respiratory Failure. *Am. J. Respir. Crit. Care Med.* **163:** 283–291.
13. Bott, J., Carroll, M.P., Conway, J.H., *et al.* (1993) Randomized controlled trial of nasal ventilation in acute ventilatory failure due to chronic obstructive airways disease. *Lancet* **341:** 1555–1557.
14. Kramer, N., Meyer, T.J., Meharg, J., Cece, R.D. and Hill, N.S. (1995) Randomized, prospective trial of noninvasive positive pressure ventilation in acute respiratory failure. *Am. J. Respir. Crit. Care Med.* **151:** 1799–1806.
15. Brochard, L., Mancebo, J., Wysocki, M., *et al.* (1995) Noninvasive ventilation for acute exacerbations of chronic obstructive pulmonary disease. *N. Engl. J. Med.* **333:** 817–819.
16. Angus, R.M., Ahmed, A.A., Fenwick, L.J. and Peacock, A.J. (1996) Comparison of the acute effects on gas exchange of nasal ventilation and doxapram in exacerbations of chronic obstructive pulmonary disease. *Thorax* **51:** 1048–1050.
17. Celikel, T., Sungur, M., Ceyhan, B. and Karakurt, S. (1998) Comparison of noninvasive positive pressure ventilation with standard medical therapy in hypercapnic acute respiratory failure. *Chest* **114:** 1636–1642.
18. Plant, P.K., Owen, J.L. and Elliott, M.W. (2000) Early use of noninvasive ventilation for acute exacerbations of chronic obstructive pulmonary disease on general respiratory wards: A multicenter randomized controlled trial. *Lancet* **355:** 1931–1935.
19. Barbe, F., Togores, B., Rubi, M., Pons, S., Maimo, A. and Agusti, A.G.N. (1996) Noninvasive ventilatory support does not facilitate recovery from acute respiratory failure in chronic obstructive pulmonary disease. *Eur. Respir. J.* **9:** 1240–1245.
20. Keenan, S.P., Kernerman, P.D., Cook, D.J., Martin, C.M., McCormack, D. and Sibbald, W.J. (1997)The effect of noninvasive positive pressure ventilation on mortality in patients admitted with acute respiratory failure: A meta-analysis. *Crit. Care Med.* **25:** 1685–1692.
21. Guerin, C., Giard, R., Chemorin, C., De Varox, R. and Fournier, G. (1997) Facial mask, noninvasive mechanical ventilation reduces the incidence of nosocomial pneumonia; a prospective epidemiological survey from a single ICU. *Intensive Care Med.* **23:** 1024–1032.
22. Girou, E., Schortgen, F., Delclaux, C., Brun-Buisson, C., Blot, F., Lefort, Y., Lemaire, F. and Brochard, L. (2000) Association of noninvasive ventilation with nosocomial infection and survival in critically ill patients. *JAMA* **284:** 2361–2367.
23. Anton, A., Guell, R., Gomez, J., Serrano, J., Castellano, A., Carrasco, J.L. and Sanchis, J.

(2000) Predicting the result of non invasive ventilation in severe acute exacerbations of patients with chronic airflow obstruction. *Chest* **117**: 828–836.

24. **Meduri, G.U., Turner, R.E., Abou-Shala, N., Wunderink, R. and Tolley, E.** (1996) Noninvasive positive pressure ventilation via face mask. *Chest* **109**: 179–193.

25. **Bach, J.R.** (1996) Conventional approaches to managing neuromuscular ventilatory failure. In: *Pulmonary Rehabilitation: the Obstructive and Paralytic Conditions* (ed. J.R. Bach). Henley & Belfus, Philadelphia, PA, pp. 285–301.

26. **Finlay, G., Conconnon, D. and McDonell, T.J.** (1995) Treatment of respiratory failure due to kyphoscoliosis with nasal intermittent positive pressure ventilation (NIPPV). *J. Med. Sci.* **164**: 28–30.

27. **Bach, J.R., Ishikawa, Y. and Kim, H.** (1997) Prevention of pulmonary morbidity for patients with Duchenne muscular dystrophy. *Chest* **112**: 1024–1028.

28. **Meduri, G.U., Cook, T.R., Turner, R.E., Cohen, M. and Leeper, K.V.** (1996) Noninvasive positive pressure ventilation in status asthmaticus. *Chest* **110**: 767–774.

29. **Levy, B.D., Kitch, B. and Fanta, C.H.** (1998) Medical and ventilatory management of status asthmaticus. *Intensive Care Med.* **24**: 105–117.

30. **Hodson, M.E., Madden, B.P., Steven, M.H., Tsang, V.T. and Yacoub, M.H.** (1991) Noninvasive mechanical ventilation for cystic fibrosis patients—a potential bridge to transplantation. *Eur. Respir. J.* **4**: 524–527.

31. **Pennock, B.E., Kaplan, P.D., Carlin, B.W., Sabangan, J.S. and Magovern, J.A.** (1991) Pressure support ventilation with a simplified ventilatory support system administered with a nasal mask in patients with respiratory failure. *Chest* **100**: 1371–1376.

32. **Pennock, B.E., Crawshaw, L. and Kaplan, P.D.** (1994) Noninvasive nasal mask ventilation for acute respiratory failure. *Chest* **105**: 441–444.

33. **Gust, R., Gottschalk, A., Schmide, H., Bottiger, B., Bohrer, H. and Martin, E.** (1996) Effects of continuous (CPAP) and bi-level positive airway pressure (B_iPAP) on extravascular lung water after extubation of the trachea in patients following coronary artery bypass grafting. *Intensive Care Med.* **22**: 1345–1350.

34. **Rasanen, J., Heikkila, J., Downs, J., Nikki, P., Vaisanen, I. and Viitanen, A.** (1985) Continuous positive airway pressure by face mask in acute cardiogenic pulmonary edema. *Am. J. Cardiol.* **55**: 296–300.

35. **Vaisanen, I.T. and Rasanen, J.** (1987) Continuous positive airway pressure and supplemental

oxygen in the treatment of cardiogenic pulmonary edema. *Chest* **92**: 481–485.

36. **Lin, M. and Chiang, H.** (1991) The efficacy of early continuous positive airway pressure therapy in patients with acute cardiogenic pulmonary edema. *J. Formos. Med. Assoc.* **90**: 736–743.

37. **Bersten, A.D., Holt, A.W., Vedig, A.E., Skowronski, G.A. and Baggolery, C.J.** (1991) Treatment of severe cardiogenic pulmonary edema with continuous positive airway pressure delivered by face mask. *N. Engl. J. Med.* **325**: 1825–1830.

38. **Lin, M., Yang, Y., Chiany, H., Chang, M., Chainy, B.N. and Chitlin, M.D.** (1995) Reappraisal of continuous positive airway pressure therapy in acute cardiogenic pulmonary edema: Short-term results and long-term follow-up. *Chest* **107**: 1379–1386.

39. **Mehta, S., Jay, G.D., Woolard, R.H., Hipona, R.A., Connelly, E.M., Cimini, D.M., Drinkwine, J.H. and Hill, N.S.** (1997) Randomized prospective trial of bilevel versus continuous positive airway pressure in acute pulmonary edema. *Crit. Care Med.* **25**: 620–628.

40. **Rusterholtz, T., Kempf, J., Berton, C., Gayol, S., Tournoud, C., Zaehringer, M., Jaeger, A. and Sauder, P.** (1999) Noninvasive pressure support ventilation (NIPSV) with face mask in patients with acute cardiogenic pulmonary edema (ACPE). *Intensive Care Med.* **25**: 21–28.

41. **Masip, J., Betlese, A.J., Vecilla, F., Canizares, R., Padro, J., Paz, M.A., deOtero, J. and Ballus, J.** (2000) Noninvasive pressure-support ventilation versus conventional oxygen therapy in acute pulmonary edema: A randomized trial. *Lancet* **356**: 2126–2132.

42. **Sharon, A., Shpiner, I., Kaluski, E., *et al.*** (2000) High-dose intravenous isosorbide–dinitrate is safer and better than B_iPAP ventilation combined with conventional treatment for severe pulmonary edema. *J. Am. Coll. Cardiol.* **36**: 832–837.

43. **Pang, D., Keenan, S.P., Cook, D.I. and Sibbald, W.J.** (1998) The effect of positive pressure airway support on mortality and the need for intubation in cardiogenic pulmonary edema. *Chest* **114**: 1185–1192.

44. **Wysocki, M., Tric, L., Wolf, M.A., Millet, H. and Herman, B.** (1995) Noninvasive pressure support ventilation in patients with acute respiratory failure: A randomized comparison with conventional therapy. *Chest* **107**: 761–768.

45. **Antonelli, M., Conti, G., Rocco, M., Bufi, M., DeBlasi, R.A., Vivino, G., Gasparetto, A. and Meduri, G.U.** (1998) A comparison of noninvasive positive pressure ventilation and conven-

tional mechanical ventilation in patients with acute respiratory failure. *N. Engl. J. Med.* **339**: 429–435.

46. Delclaux, C., L'Her, E., Alberti, C., *et al.* (2000) Treatment of acute hypoxemic non-hyperapnic respiratory insufficiency with continuous positive airway pressure delivered by a face mask. *JAMA* **289**: 2352–2360.

47. Ambrosino, N., Rubini, F., Callegari, G., Nava, S. and Fracchia, C. (1994) Noninvasive mechanical ventilation in the treatment of acute respiratory failure due to infectious complications of lung transplantation. *Monaldi Arch. Chest Dis.* **49**: 311–314.

48. Conti, G., Marino, P., Cogliati, A., Dell'Utri, D., Lappa, A., Rosa, G. and Gasparetto, A. (1998) Noninvasive ventilation for the treatment of acute respiratory failure in patients with hematologic malignancies: A pilot study. *Intensive Care Med.* **24**: 1283–1288.

49. Antonelli, M., Conti, C., Bufi, M., Costa, M.G., Lappa, A., Rocco, M., Gasparetto, M. and Meduri, G.U. (2000) Noninvasive ventilation for treatment of acute respiratory failure in patients undergoing solid organ transplantation. *JAMA* **283**: 235–241.

50. Confalonieri, M., Potena, A., Carbone, G., Della Porta, R., Tolley, E.A. and Meduri, G.U. (1999) Acute respiratory failure in patients with severe community-acquired pneumonia. *Am. J. Respir. Crit. Care Med.* **160**: 1585–1591.

51. Benhamon, D., Girault, C., Faure, C., Portier, F. and Muir, J.F. (1992) Nasal mask ventilation in acute respiratory failure: Experience in elderly patients. *Chest* **102**: 912–917.

52. Meduri, G.U., Fox, R.C., Abou-Shala, N., Leeper, K.V. and Wunderink, R.G. (1994) Noninvasive mechanical ventilation via face mask in patient with acute respiratory failure who refused endotracheal intubation. *Crit. Care Med.* **22**: 1584–1590.

53. Benhamon, D., Muir, J.F. and Melen, B. (1998) Mechanical ventilation in elderly patients. *Monaldi Arch. Chest Dis.* **53**: 547–551.

54. Udwadia, Z.F., Santis, G.K., Stevan, M.H. and Simonds, A.K. (1992) Nasal ventilation to facilitate weaning in patients with chronic respiratory insufficiency. *Thorax* **47**: 715–718.

55. Goodenberger, D.M., Couser, J. and May, J.J. (1992) Successful discontinuation of ventilation via tracheostomy by substitution of nasal positive pressure ventilation. *Chest* **102**: 1277–1279.

56. Restrick, L.J., Scott, A.D., Ward, E.M., French, R.O., Cornwell, W.E. and Wedjicha, J.A. (1993) Nasal intermittent positive pressure ventilation in weaning intubated patients with chronic respiratory disease from assisted intermittent positive pressure ventilation. *Respir. Med.* **87**: 199–204.

57. Gregoretti, C., Beltrame, F., Lucangelo, U., Burbi, L., Conti, G., Turello, M. and Gregori, D. (1998) Physiologic evaluation of non-invasive pressure support ventilation in trauma patients with acute respiratory failure. *Intensive Care Med.* **24**: 795–790.

58. Nava, S., Ambrosino, N., Clini, E., Prato, M., Orlando, G., Vitacca, M., Brigada, P., Fraccia, C. and Rubinni, F. (1998) Non-invasive mechanical ventilation in the weaning of patients with respiratory failure due to chronic obstructive pulmonary disease: A randomized study. *Ann. Intern. Med.* **128**: 721–728.

59. Girault, C., Daudenthun, I., Chevron, V., Tamion, F., Leroy, J. and Bonmarchand, G. (1999) Noninvasive ventilation as a systematic extubation and weaning technique in acute-on-chronic respiratory failure. *Am. J. Respir. Crit. Care Med.* **160**: 86–92.

60. MacIntyre, N.R., McConnell, R., Cheng, K.C. and Sane, A. (1997) Patient–ventilator flow dyssynchrony: flow-limited versus pressure-limited breaths. *Crit. Care Med.* **25**: 1671–1677.

61. Williams, P., Muelver, M., Kratohvil, J., Ritz, R., Hess, D.R. and Kacmarek, R.M. (2000) Pressure support and pressure assist/control: are there differences? An evaluation of the newest intensive care ventilators. *Respir. Care* **45**: 1169–1181.

62. Chatmongkolchart, S., Williams, P., Hess, D. and Kacmarek, R.M. (2001) Evaluation of inspiratory rise time and inspiratory termination criteria in new generation mechanical ventilators: A lung model study. *Respir. Care.* **46**: 666–678.

63. Chalburn, R.L. (1999) Mechanical ventilation. In: *Respiratory Care Equipment* (eds R.D. Branson, D.R. Hess and R.L. Chatburn). Lippincott, Williams and Wilkins, New York, pp. 395–527.

64. Takeuchi, M., Williams, P., Hess, D. and Kacmarek, R.M. (2002) Continuous positive airway pressure in new generation mechanical ventilation: A lung model study. *Anesthesiology* **96**: 162–172.

65. Bunburaphong, T., Imanaka, H., Nishimura, M., Hess, D. and Kacmarek, R.M. (1997) Performance characteristics of bilevel pressure ventilators. *Chest* **111**: 1050–1058.

66. Ferguson, G.T. and Gilmartin, M. (1995) CO_2 rebreathing during B_iPAP ventilatory assistance. *Am. J. Respir. Crit. Care Med.* **151**: 1126–1132.

67. Schettino, G., Chatmongkolchart, S., Hess, D. and Kacmarek, R.M. (2001) CO_2 elimination during B_iPAP ventilation: Effects of mask design

and PEEP (abstract). *Am. J. Respir. Crit. Care Med.* **163:** A679.

68. **Kacmarek, R.M.** (1999) NIPPV: Patient–ventilator synchrony, the difference between success and failure? *Intensive Care Med.* **25:** 645–647.

69. **Hess, D.R. and Kacmarek, R.M.** (1999) Noninvasive ventilation. In: *Respiratory Care Equipment*, (eds R.D. Branson, D.R. Hess and R.L. Chatburn). Lippincott, Williams and Wilkins, New York, pp. 593–613.

70. **Calderini, E., Confalonieri, M., Puccio, P.G., Francavilla, N., Stella, L. and Gregoretti, C.** (1999) Patient–ventilator assynchrony during noninvasive ventilation: the role of expiratory trigger. *Intensive Care Med.* **25:** 662–667.

Chapter 20

Postoperative care of the cardiac surgical patient

Thomas L. Higgins, MD

Contents

20.1 Introduction

As cardiac surgery is a high-volume procedure, postoperative patients account for a substantial percentage of intensive care admissions at many hospitals. The postoperative care of uncomplicated cardiac surgical patients primarily involves:

- monitoring and control of cardiac output;
- control of high or low blood pressure;
- recovery from anesthesia and hypothermia while controlling the stress response;
- respiratory management and weaning from mechanical ventilation;
- adequate sedation and pain relief to facilitate patient comfort and the above goals;
- monitoring for adverse events that can be prevented or ameliorated.

20.2 Delivery of the patient to the ICU

Transport of a critically ill patient is associated with acute physiologic changes and the potential for mishap[1]. The intensity of monitoring may be inadvertently relaxed while attention is focused on physically moving the patient and associated infusion pumps and monitors. Problems commonly encountered during transport range from sudden hypotension as a result of vasodilation to abrupt awakening with extreme hypertension and the risk for serious bleeding. Marked changes in blood pressure can be minimized with volume loading of the patient, maintaining anesthesia during transport, and assuring all pumps supplying vasoactive medication remain connected and functioning.

The anesthesiologist and surgeon have learned valuable information about a particular patient's response to fluid and vasoactive agents from direct observation and possibly echocardiography in the operating room. This information plus data on the dose and timing of anesthetic agents and antibiotics, blood product and fluid administration, and expected postoperative course should be communicated to the intensive care team. *Table 20.1* gives a list of important concerns at the time of ICU arrival.

20.3 **Respiratory management**

Immediate respiratory system changes include up to a 40% decrease in vital capacity, total lung capacity, inspiratory capacity, and functional residual capacity[2]. Cardiopulmonary bypass (CPB) alters pulmonary function, and the severity of pulmonary edema correlates with the length of bypass[3]. Atelectasis, which occurs in up to 90% of patients, causes increased work of breathing. Maintaining the lungs at 5 cmH$_2$O of CPAP with room air during CBP improves oxygenation and lowers shunt fraction[4]. Direct trauma to the lungs or pleura may occur during surgical retraction or insertion of chest tubes. Pain and splinting cause the patient to limit lung expansion, and reduce the ability to cough and clear secretions. Goals for respiratory management are outlined in *Table 20.2*.

20.3.1 Mechanical ventilation

Conventional practice has been to institute intermittent mandatory ventilation (IMV) at relatively high tidal volumes (8–10 cm^3 kg^{-1}) and a low respiratory rate (8–10) with 60% or higher FiO$_2$ and low levels (5 cm) of PEEP. If the patient is spontaneously breathing at ICU arrival, it may be possible to proceed directly to pressure support ventilation with levels of 5–15 cmH$_2$O. With 'fast-track' protocols, many patients are extubated in the operating room or shortly after ICU arrival. Assist/control or IMV ventilation are more appropriate for heavily narcotized patients, until spontaneous breathing occurs. In the event of difficulty with oxygenation, lung-protective ventilation strategies with lower tidal volumes (6–8 cm^3 kg^{-1}), and higher levels of PEEP may be needed. Higher airway pressures may necessitate fluid loading to maintain cardiac output. In patients with airflow obstruction, occult positive end-expiratory pressure ('Auto-PEEP') is a cause of hypotension and low cardiac output (see Chapters 13 and 17).

Table 20.1 ICU admission concerns

Preparation

Ventilator set to Vt 8–10 cm^3 kg^{-1} with healthy lungs; rate 8–10; FiO_2 0.60; PEEP 2–5 cm

Bedside monitor ready for ECG, CVP, A-line, ± PA or LA pressures

Infusion pumps for inotropes, vasopressors, and vasodilators

Defibrillator, resuscitation cart, surgical 'bleeder' tray available in ICU

On arrival in ICU

Connect monitors and ventilator

Auscultate breath sounds and observe chest excursion

Check pulse oximetry and end-tidal CO_2 if available

Zero pressure transducers, and correlate with cuff pressure

Determine cardiac output if applicable

Check function of IABP and/or assist devices if applicable

Check function of chest tubes and amount of drainage

Order any necessary laboratory studies and CXR

Information to be obtained from operating room team

Patient's name, age, gender, and brief history

Operation performed and any major problems encountered

CPB and circulatory arrest times

Optimum filling pressures as determined in OR

Current drug infusions and titration plans

Pacemaker and antiarrhythmic information

Anesthetics given and plans for awakening ('fast-track')

Fluids and blood products given; urine output

Assessment of hemostasis and heparin reversal

Last hematocrit, potassium, and antibiotic dose in OR

Availability of blood products and surgical salvage

ECG, electrocardiography; CVP, central venous pressure; ICU, intensive care unit; PA, pulmonary artery; LA, left atrial; IABP, intraaortic balloon pump; OR, operating room; CXR, chest radiograph.

Table 20.2 Respiratory management

	Early	**Later**
Goals	Complete O_2 saturation of hemoglobin Normocarbia Minimization of ventilation's hemodynamic effects	Extubation with adequate reserve Restoration of FRC
Assessment	ABGs Cardiac output and filling pressures CXR	Spontaneous tidal volume and f/Vt rate Vital capacity and MIP ABGs, CXR, fluid balance Chest tube output
Interventions	Changes in rate and tidal volume Addition or subtraction of PEEP Sedation and neuromuscular blockade Lung-protective ventilator strategy	Control of secretions Upright position Incentive spirometry Ambulation

ABGs, arterial blood gases; CXR, chest radiograph; FRC, functional residual capacity; MIP, maximal inspiratory pressure. f/Vt, frequency to total volume ratio; PEEP, positive end-expiratory pressure.

20.3.2 Timing of extubation

Factors that enter into the timing of extubation include the total dose and patient's ability to metabolize or eliminate anesthetic agents; whether hypothermia has occurred and has been corrected, hemodynamic stability, and the likelihood of return to the operating room for tamponade or control of bleeding (*Table 20.3*). Until the early 1990s, overnight mechanical ventilation was accepted practice for the cardiac surgical patient, largely because of habit, staffing considerations, and a belief that it was beneficial to the patient's respiratory and cardiovascular function. Shorter-acting anesthetic agents now make it possible to provide a nearly stress-free anesthetic without the need for prolonged postoperative ventilation[5]. Documented advantages of early endotracheal extubation after cardiac surgery include improved left ventricular performance, decreased length of intensive care stay, lower costs, diminished requirement for postoperative medication, lessened cardiopulmonary morbidity, and improved patient comfort[6–8]. In the otherwise stable patient, the ability to maintain arterial pH greater than 7.35 while the IMV rate is decreased to CPAP is a convenient and easily applied test for ability to sustain spontaneous respiration[9].

20.3.3 Long-term ventilation

About 5% of patients will require mechanical ventilation for longer than 72 h following coronary artery bypass grafting (CABG); the corresponding figure for valve surgery patients is only slightly higher. The odds of requiring prolonged ventilation increase with preoperative presence of congestive heart failure, azotemia, valvular heart disease, advanced age, diffuse vascular disease, and with reoperation and emergency procedures[10]. Early enteral feeding or parenteral nutrition should be considered so that malnutrition does not occur as a result of ventilator dependence. Chapter 18 has general advice for the patient with difficulty in weaning.

20.3.4 Common factors limiting removal of mechanical ventilatory support

These factors in the cardiac surgical patient are sepsis, over-feeding[11] renal failure with fluid overload, marked neurologic dysfunction, and unstable hemodynamic status. Acute left ventricular dysfunction occurs in patients with COPD during the shift from mechanical to spontaneous ventilation[12]. Careful attention to fluid balance and aggressive diuresis or use of ultrafiltration[13] ameliorates the abrupt rise in left ventricular filling pressure and allows

Table 20.3 Extubation criteria

Neurologic	Awake, following simple commands, able to protect airway
	Neuromuscular blockade and opiates fully dissipated
Cardiac	Stable; not on IABP, index >2.2 min^{-1} m^{-2}
	MAP >70; no serious arrhythmias
Respiratory	Acceptable CXR, ABGs (pH ≥7.35) on minimal vent support
	Secretions minimal; cough and gag reflexes present
	Comfortable on CPAP or T-piece with spontaneous rate ≤24 and/or f/Vt ratio <100
	Optional: MIP <−25; Vt >5 cm^3 kg^{-1}, Vc >10 cm^3 kg^{-1}
Renal	Diuresing well; not markedly edematous
	Urine output >0.5 cm^3 kg^{-1} min^{-1}
Hematologic	Chest tube drainage <50 cm^3 h^{-1}
Temperature	Temperature >36.0°C

IABP, intraaortic balloon pump; MAP, mean arterial pressure; CXR, chest radiograph; ABGs, arterial blood gases; MIP, maximum inspiratory pressure; F, respiratory rate; Vt, tidal volume; Vc, vital capacity; CPAP, continuous positive airway pressure.

weaning from ventilation to proceed. It is not usual to find patients 'unweanable' until fluid removal reduces body weight to several kilograms below the preoperative value.

20.3.5 Diaphragmatic paralysis

This may complicate any thoracic procedure, but is more common in reoperative patients because of difficulty in identifying the phrenic nerve in fibrotic pericardial tissue. The incidence of diaphragmatic paralysis has not been well characterized; temporary diaphragmatic weakness occurs in about 4% of patients. Diaphragmatic paralysis should be suspected whenever a patient fails to wean from mechanical ventilation, and can be clinically identified by paradoxical movement of the diaphragm during inspiration, and by comparing vital capacity and tidal volumes in the supine and seated positions. Differences in supine and seated vital capacity of more than 10–15% should prompt fluoroscopic examination of the diaphragm ('sniff' test). Measuring gastric pressure during spontaneous breathing also is useful. A negative inspiratory gastric pressure indicates diaphragmatic paralysis. Transient diaphragmatic paralysis may occur secondary to cold injury to the phrenic nerve[14]. Less often, the phrenic nerve is injured or transected during dissection of the internal mammary arteries or in mobilizing the heart in reoperative patients. Other causes of apparent diaphragmatic weakness include noncompliant lung, muscle weakness and wasting, hypophosphatemia, and hypomagnesemia. Long-term management of diaphragmatic paralysis is facilitated by performing a tracheostomy, which allows better secretion control and use of intermittent ventilation.

20.4 Cardiovascular support

There are four immediate cardiovascular goals:

- maintain appropriate perfusion pressure (see Sections 20.4.1–20.4.3);
- deliver adequate oxygen to the brain and other tissues (Sections 20.4.5–20.4.7);

- minimize oxygen demand to the available supply (Sections 20.4.8 and 20.5.3);
- maintain a stable cardiac rhythm (Sections 20.4.9).

20.4.1 Perfusion pressure

This must be adequate to supply the brain, kidney, visceral organs and ultimately all tissues, and also must be high enough that newly placed bypass grafts remain patent, without becoming so high that leaks occur at freshly placed anastamoses. Empirically, a mean arterial pressure of more than 70 mmHg is considered adequate, but elderly patients, and those with renal or cerebrovascular stenoses may require higher pressures.

20.4.2 Postoperative hypotension

This is commonly precipitated by hypovolemia, decreased systemic vascular resistance, or insufficient cardiac output. Hypovolemia can result from diuresis (mannitol in pump prime), release of vasoactive mediators during cardiopulmonary bypass, or blood loss. Volume status is not always easy to assess, even when a pulmonary artery (Swan–Ganz) catheter is available. Ventricular compliance may change during the first several hours after bypass[15], altering the expected relationship between filling pressures and ventricular filling. Observation of the response to fluid challenge is the best measurement of optimal filling pressure for an individual patient. Echocardiography can be used to determine optimal ventricular loading and to help identify new onset cardiac tamponade or outflow obstruction.

Routine use of calcium to treat hypotension and low output following cardiac surgery is controversial. Calcium inhibits the cardiotonic action of beta-adrenergic agonists such as dobutamine, although not the effects of phosphodiesterase inhibitors[16]. Hyperamylasemia, a marker of pancreatic cellular injury, is associated with calcium chloride therapy[17]. Bolus administration of calcium reduces internal mammary artery (IMA) flow and can potentially trigger vasospasm[18]. On the other hand, low ionized calcium affects both cardiac output and systemic resistance, and repletion of hypocalcemia is associated with clinical improvement in these variables.

20.4.3 Postoperative hypertension

In patients with normal or only mild left ventricular impairment and normal volume status, blood pressure changes are influenced more by changes in systemic vascular resistance than by cardiac output[19]. Systemic vascular resistance may initially be low following CPB, but typically rises during the first few postoperative hours, and can later require vasodilator therapy. Nitroglycerine and nitroprusside are the most commonly used vasodilators; however, other agents such as nicardipine, labetalol, hydralazine and prazosin are alternatives (see Chapter 9). The vasodilating properties of propofol may also be useful in this setting[20]. Nitroprusside is widely used because it can be titrated in response to sudden changes in preload and afterload. Labetalol is associated with significant reductions in heart rate and cardiac index, whereas sodium nitroprusside causes significant increases in both[21]. When cardiac output is borderline (<2.3 l min^{-1} m^{-2}) sodium nitroprusside is the agent of choice. Labetalol is preferred in situations where the circulation is hyperdynamic. Esmolol is also effective at reducing blood pressure by depressing a hyperdynamic circulation after cardiac surgery, and its half-life is sufficiently short that stopping the infusion of the drug will quickly reverse any adverse effects.

Other causes of postoperative hypertension include hypoxia, hypercarbia, and hypothermia with shivering, visceral distention, and inadequate sedation, particularly in the presence of residual neuromuscular blockade. In contrast to traditional high-dose opioid anesthesia, 'fast-track' regimens do not automatically provide the patient with residual analgesia, requiring specific attention to pain and discomfort. Cardiopulmonary bypass results in variable increases in circulating epinephrine and norepinephrine levels, which correlate with blood pressure changes and may be the result of sympathetic overdrive.

20.4.4 Assessing cardiac output

Acute myocardial dysfunction occurs in nearly all patients, with the nadir of cardiac function occurring 2–6 h after cardiopulmonary bypass[15]. Clinical indicators such as capillary refill and pedal pulses are unreliable markers for peripheral perfusion after cardiac surgery. Better evidence of adequate perfusion can be obtained by monitoring mixed venous oxygenation, and the generation of lactic acid. Even these markers may be misleading, particularly in the 'wash-out' period following cardiopulmonary bypass, where elevated lactic acid may represent improved perfusion and clearance of lactate from the periphery. A measured cardiac index of more than 2.2 l min^{-1} m^{-2} is generally acceptable; higher cardiac outputs are preferred.

20.4.5 Causes of low cardiac output

In the early postoperative period these include hypovolemia, myocardial dysfunction, and cardiac tamponade. Unless specific blood component therapy is indicated, volume expansion can be achieved with electrolyte solutions. Albumin and hetastarch are more expensive than electrolyte solutions, but will remain in the intravascular compartment longer than crystalloids. If ventricular filling pressures appear adequate (CVP or PCWP between 10 and 18 cmH$_2$O), further increases in cardiac output will require inotropic agents, reductions in afterload, or a combination of the two (see Chapter 8). Right heart failure may occur as the result of prolonged ischemic arrest, and is more common following mitral valve replacement and cardiac transplantation than post-CABG. Pulmonary hypertension and right ventricular failure will limit left ventricular filling and cardiac output. Unfortunately, there are no intravenous agents that specifically dilate the pulmonary vasculature without causing systemic vasodilation. Agents that are frequently helpful with right ventricular failure include catecholamines with dilating action (dobutamine, isoproterenol) and phosphodiesterase inhibitors such as milrirone. Diastolic dysfunction (failure of the heart to relax and fill properly) frequently responds to milrinone.

20.4.6 Mechanical cardiac support

This is needed when low cardiac output persists despite adequate volume loading and administration of inotropes and dilators. Intraaortic balloon counterpulsation is indicated for low cardiac output states, cardiogenic shock, failure to wean from cardiopulmonary bypass, and prophylactic perioperative support in the high-risk patient. The intraaortic balloon pump (IABP) is capable of increasing cardiac output by about 0.7 l min^{-1}, and works best when the cardiac rhythm is stable, preferably sinus. Severe cardiac dysfunction occasionally requires a true pump capable of replacing the function of the heart until recovery occurs. A number of left and right ventricular assist devices are available, and fall into two major categories: pulsatile (e.g. Abiomed, Heartmate) and nonpulsatile (e.g. Biomedicus centrifugal pump). Generally, ventricular assist is used to achieve a cardiac index greater than 2.2 l min^{-1} for a minimum of 24 h. Weaning involves decreasing the pump's contribution while watching for sustained cardiac output without a significant increase in atrial pressures. If adequate systemic flows can be sustained with the device providing minimal support (<500 ml min^{-1} augmentation), the device can usually be removed while maintaining inotropic and/or IABP support.

20.4.7 Myocardial oxygen supply and demand

Myocardial oxygen supply and demand must be balanced. Loss of blood supply can be acute (early graft occlusion or coronary artery spasm) and subacute (IMA hypoperfusion syndrome, systemic hypotension). Myocardial oxygen demand increases with tachycardia, shivering, and agitation. Inadequate myocardial oxygen supply may present as electrocardiographic ST-segment changes, ventricular dyssynergy on echocardiographic examination, and increased left- or right-sided filling pressures, but can be difficult to recognize clinically.

20.4.8 Maintaining a stable cardiac rhythm

Maintenance of a stable cardiac rhythm, optimally normal sinus rhythm at a rate of 70–100 beats min^{-1}, is the final hemodynamic goal. Perioperative heart rates above 100 beats min^{-1} are associated with ischemia and postoperative myocardial infarction; bradycardia may depress cardiac output. If pacing wires have been placed, bradycardia can be treated electrically, and the pacing wires may also be used for arrhythmia detection. Arrhythmias may result from electrolyte imbalance, myocardial ischemia, acid–base abnormalities, and excess catecholamines. Supraventricular tachycardias associated with hemodynamic instability should be treated with synchronous cardioversion at 50–150 joules. Adenosine (initial dose 6 mg IV) is the drug of choice for reentry supraventricular tachycardias[22].

Atrial arrhythmias are common; and occur in about one out of five CABG patients and one out of two valve patients. Magnesium prophylaxis can lessen the incidence of atrial fibrillation following CABG. Rate control can be accomplished with beta-adrenergic blockade, calcium-channel blockers (typically diltiazem), amiodarone, or electrical cardioversion. Aggressive treatment and control of atrial arrhythmias shorten total hospital length of stay.

Ventricular arrhythmias are also common, and frequently can be caused by pulmonary artery (PA) catheter placement and electrolytes. Initial treatment of hemodynamically significant ventricular dysrhythmias is immediate defibrillation and administration of intravenous lidocaine (1 mg kg^{-1} bolus) followed by a continuous infusion of 2–4 mg min^{-1}. Amiodarone, despite higher cost and the potential for pulmonary toxicity, is also considered first-line therapy for ventricular dysrhythmias. Other agents such as ibutalide, bretylium, procainamide, quinidine, and diphenylhydantoin may occasionally be useful. (See Chapter 11 for a complete discussion of arrhythmia management.) Torsades de pointes, a special form of ventricular tachycardia associated with a long QT interval, are commonly seen in patients with ongoing ischemia. Torsades may be precipitated or worsened by type 1A antiarrhythmic drugs and therapy of torsades in the post-CPB setting should first address repletion of Mg^{2+} and control of heart rate and ischemia.

20.5 Postoperative complications

20.5.1 Cardiac tamponade

This presents differently in the postoperative cardiac patient as compared with the trauma patient or in those with constrictive diseases of the pericardium. Because the pericardial sac is generally left open, the compliance of the cavity is altered, and classic equalization of pressures may not be seen. Tamponade may be caused by acute cardiac dilation without hemopericardium or by a small clot strategically placed so that it compresses a vital structure and decreases venous return. The diagnosis of tamponade should always be suspected when hemodynamic status deteriorates, and the etiology of mediastinal tamponade following heart surgery is almost always excessive postoperative bleeding with accumulated clot producing compression of one or more chambers of the heart. Although pericardiocentesis is lifesaving in non-surgical tamponade, it is rarely useful in the post-bypass patient as clot cannot be aspirated, and the procedure risks disrupting newly placed grafts.

Transesophageal echocardiogram (TEE) can be helpful if the time course of deterioration is not rapid. With a high index of suspicion, the usual course is to transport the patient back to the operating room, open the chest and evacuate the clot, at which point hemodynamic improvement is usually dramatic. If immediate return to the operating room is not possible, the lower end of the sternotomy incision can be opened in the intensive care unit, and clot evacuated manually or with a suction catheter.

20.5.2 Perioperative myocardial infarction

This can be difficult to diagnose, as conventional criteria (new electrocardiographic changes; enzyme elevation) can result from surgery itself. Using the criteria of creatinine kinase MB fraction (CPK-MB) greater than 8% and aspartate aminotransferase greater than 80 units dl^{-1}, the rate of infarction is in the range of 3–6%. Reinfusion of shed mediastinal and chest tube drainage also complicates enzyme diagnosis of infarction, as autotransfusion raises the serum levels of creatinine kinase, aspartate aminotransferase, and lactic dehydrogenases[23]. The criteria proposed by the Society of Thoracic Surgeons (STS) (*Table 20.4*) provide a reasonable benchmark for quality assurance[24].

20.5.3 Postoperative shivering

This occurs commonly following CPB, and the ability to abate shivering with steroid pretreatment suggests cytokine or mediator release rather than rewarming as the major instigator[25]. Shivering increases oxygen consumption

---

Table 20.4 STS criteria for myocardial infarction (Adapted from reference 24)

A perioperative myocardial infarction (MI) is diagnosed by finding at least two of the following four criteria:

- Prolonged (<20 min) typical chest pain not relieved by rest and/or nitrates
- Enzyme level elevation; one of: (i) CK-MB >5% of total CPK; (ii) CK greater than 2× normal; (iii) LDH subtype 1 > LDH subtype 2; or (iv) troponin >0.2 μg ml^{-1}
- New wall motion abnormalities
- Serial ECG (at least two) showing changes from baseline or serially in ST-T and/or Q waves that are 0.03 s in width and/or > or + one-third of the total QRS complex in two or more contiguous leads

beyond the level a stressed heart can deliver, and results in lactic acidosis. Patients may also develop acute respiratory acidosis as a result of the inability to increase spontaneous minute ventilation appropriately because of residual opioids and neuromuscular blocking drugs. Shivering responds to radiant heat and/or small doses (12.5–25 mg IV) of meperidine. Full ventilation and neuromuscular blockade may be needed if shivering is severe and cannot be controlled by other methods.

20.5.4 Oliguric or anuric renal failure

This occurs in 1–4% post open heart surgery patients; a rise in serum creatinine can be documented in 2–30% of patients[26,27]. Univariate predictors of renal dysfunction include low cardiac output at the end of CPB, advanced age, preoperative cardiac failure, need for postoperative circulatory support, blood transfusions, and prolonged time on CPB[28]. Despite aggressive ICU care and the availability of dialysis and hemofiltration, mortality from postoperative renal failure may exceed 80%, particularly if other organ system failure occurs simultaneously[29].

When renal failure occurs, it generally follows one of three well-defined patterns (*Figure 20.1*)[30]. Abbreviated acute renal failure occurs after an isolated insult, results in a peak in serum creatinine around the fourth postoperative day, and generally has a favorable prognosis if no other events occur. The second pattern is similar to the first, except that the acute insult is accompanied by prolonged circulatory failure. This pattern runs a longer course, with recovery typically occurring in the second or third week after injury, in tandem with improvements in cardiac output. The final pattern begins like the second, but recovery is complicated by a second insult such as sepsis, massive gastrointestinal bleeding or myocardial infarction. As fluid overload with renal failure may precipitate respiratory and cardiac failure, there has been a trend towards early application of continuous arteriovenous hemofiltration (CAVH) and related techniques to remove excess fluid[13]. There is speculation that aggressive fluid removal may reduce tissue edema and intraabdominal pressure, thus improving renal perfusion pressure and consequently renal function. Other speculation involves the role of renal replacement techniques in removing circulating cytokines, but there are few data proving that cytokine removal results in better outcome.

20.5.5 Neurologic complications

Neurologic complications following open-heart surgery are varied, and findings depend partly on how aggressively they are sought. Minor neuropsychiatric changes can be demonstrated in over half of CPB patients, but gross sensory–motor abnormalities such as hemiparesis, aphasias, and global encephalopathy are relatively uncommon. Despite anticoagulation, subarachnoid hemorrhage is also an uncommon event. Peripheral nerve injury, phrenic nerve injury, and delirium requiring treatment are more common. Major neurologic disability occurs in just over 1% of patients, and can almost always be identified very early in the postoperative period. ICU care of these patients is generally concerned with maintaining reasonable brain perfusion pressure, and ensuring continued protection of the airway, as aspiration is a major risk. Management of the patient who fails to awaken includes withholding all sedatives, narcotics and muscle relaxants, and assessing peripheral neuromuscular function by nerve stimulations. CT or MRI scanning is indicated to rule out structural lesions such as multiple emboli or cerebral edema. EEG and evoked potential monitoring can assess brain electrical activity and rule out seizure activity, but only when other tests have failed to deliver a diagnosis.

Transient postoperative delirium occurs in about 7% of patients, resolving spontaneously or with reassurance and pharmacologic intervention in almost all patients by the sixth postoperative day[31]. Initial management of agitation consists of reassurance and orientation of the patient, and control of pain and anxiety with opioids and benzodiazepines respectively. Additional agents may worsen agitation accompanied by disorientation, and careful

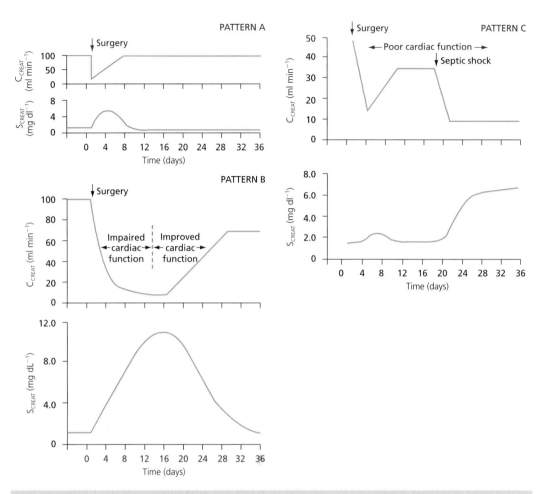

Figure 20.1 Postoperative renal dysfunction typically follows one of three patterns. In Pattern A, an acute insult at the time of surgery results in an abrupt drop in creatinine clearance, which resolves over several days. The patient's serum creatinine peaks around day 4, and returns to normal. If the acute insult is accompanied by impaired cardiac function, the rise in creatinine will be higher and the duration longer. Dialysis may be needed temporarily. If septic shock or other instability occurs during the period of poor cardiac function, Pattern C will occur, and is likely to be associated with a need for chronic dialysis if the patient survives. Modified from Myers, B.D. and Moran, S.M. (1987) Hemodynamically mediated acute renal failure. *N. Engl. J. Med.* **314**: 97. Copyright (1987) Massachusetts Medical Society. All rights reserved.

observation off medication and ample reassurance and reorientation may suffice. If the patient remains agitated and discontented, haloperidol is often useful.

20.5.6 Postoperative bleeding

This can result from numerous causes, including inadequate heparin neutralization, fibrinolysis, complement activation, quantita-tive or qualitative platelet defects, and less often, consumption and decreased levels of factors V, VIII, XIII, fibrinogen and plasminogen. No single test of hemostasis is sufficient. The activated clotting time (ACT) is a good screen for adequate heparin reversal. D-dimer or fibrin split products may be ordered if there is suspicion of disseminated intravascular coagulation as the result of low cardiac output and hypoperfusion. Prothrombin time (PT) and international normalized ratio (INR) are almost always abnormally elevated in any patient undergoing cardiopulmonary bypass in the immediate postoperative period, even without excessive bleeding[32]. Platelet function can be depressed despite sufficient platelet quantity. One approach to postoperative bleeding is to obtain an ACT, and, if elevated, administer protamine 50 mg intravenously, and then recheck the ACT. If bleeding persists and the ACT is normal, then a clotting profile (PT, INR, platelet count) is drawn. At this point, platelets may be indicated even in the presence of a normal count, as function may be impaired. Desmopressin[33], Amicar[34] and aprotinin[35] have all been recommended either for prophylaxis or treatment. Substantial bleeding (more than 300 ml in the first hour, 250 ml in the second hour, or 150 ml h^{-1} thereafter) will probably require surgical exploration[36], although the decision must be individualized based on the surgeon's knowledge of operating room events and the stability of the patient. Surgical exploration is also indicated if a large hemothorax or pericardial tamponade occurs.

20.5.7 Infectious complications
These range from simple wound infections through mediastinitis to sternal dehiscence, the latter occurring in about 1%, but associated with a 13% mortality rate[37]. Predisposing factors for wound complications after open heart surgery include diabetes, low cardiac output, use of bilateral internal mammary grafts, and reoperation for control of bleeding. Mediastinal infection can present as failure to wean, unexplained fever, and an unstable sternum. Management of mediastinitis requires selective antibiotic therapy, debridement, irrigation, drainage, and reclosure. In cases of severe sternal necrosis, early debridement and plastic surgical reconstruction using omental and/or myocutaneous flaps may be required.

Pneumonia, tracheobronchitis, line sepsis, and urinary tract infections are frequently seen in the ventilator-dependent long-term ICU patient (see Chapter 16). As routine antibiotic prophylaxis for cardiac surgery typically 'covers' for staphylococci and enteric Gram-negative rods, postoperative infections commonly involve relatively resistant organisms such as *Candida albicans*, and Gram-negative rods such as *Pseudomonas aeruginosa*, *Klebsiella* and *Providencia* species, and *Serratia marcesans*. Methicillin-resistant *Staphylococcus aureus* (MRSA) and vancomycin-resistant enterococci (VRE) are of increasing concern. Reintubation, nasogastric tubing, prior broad-spectrum antibiotic therapy and blood transfusion are risk factors for acquisition of nosocomial pneumonia[38].

20.5.8 Gastrointestinal complications
Gastrointestinal complications requiring intervention occur in only 1–3% of patients, but are associated with morbidity and mortality[39]. Postoperative ileus and upper gastrointestinal bleeding are the most common complications. Pancreatitis, intestinal ischemia, perforation, or bleeding elsewhere in the gastrointestinal tract tend to occur in complicated patients who have an initial low cardiac output syndrome resulting in ventilator dependence, renal dysfunction, or multiorgan failure. Mesenteric ischemia can occur as a result of low perfusion or embolization of atheroma from large-vessel manipulation. The incidence of gastrointestinal bleeding can be minimized with antacid therapy, histamine blockers, or barrier protection agents such as sucralfate. Enteral nutritional support also appears to protect the gastric mucosa[40].

Jaundice occurs in approximately 20% of patients post cardiopulmonary bypass, and increases risk of subsequent mortality[41]. Acute pancreatitis is less common, but carries a poor prognosis, especially in the setting of multisystem organ failure. Transient elevation of amylase may occur following CPB and be unrelated to pancreatic injury, making hyperamylasemia less valuable as a diagnostic test, unless it is combined with serum lipase assay.

20.6 Discharge criteria

Patients recovering from cardiac surgery are typically monitored and treated for several hours to overnight in a traditional intensive care unit. Increasingly, some centers are using specialized recovery areas, post-anesthesia care units (PACU), or high-dependence nursing units as substitutes for the ICU. In many hospitals, what the ward is called is less important than the nurse-to-patient ratio. The nurse-to-patient ratio for a fresh postoperative patient may well be greater than 1:1 if the patient is hemodynamically unstable, requiring an IABP or other assist device, or actively bleeding. A 1:1 nurse-to-patient ratio is reasonable for the first few hours of instability, and a 1:2 ratio is typically required for the first 6–24 h, depending on the type of anesthesia utilized and rapidity of extubation. Once the patient meets the criteria in *Table 20.5*, less nursing attention will be needed, and the patient can typically be moved to a lower-dependence area. The risks of premature ICU discharge include respiratory compromise, particularly aspiration as a result of residual sedation and/or neurologic changes, and unrecognized renal or metabolic problems, plus continued bleeding. Cardiac arrhythmias are more difficult to predict, and may not occur until the third or fourth postoperative day, so continued electrocardiographic monitoring is appropriate after ICU discharge. ICU readmission rates are typically in the 5–9% range, and are most often precipitated by pulmonary and cardiac complica-

---

Table 20.5 Criteria for ICU discharge following open heart surgery

Neurologic and psychological
Able to protect airway (adequate gag reflex; or tracheostomized)
Able to signal distress (verbal or using call button)

Cardiac
Stable MAP ≥70 without pressor support
Adequate perfusion (CI ≥2.2; warm extremities; satisfactory urine output)
No inotropic support other than low-dose dopamine ($\leq 3 \ \mu g \ kg^{-1} \ min^{-1}$)
Heart rhythm: sinus with few or no PVCs; or atrial fibrillation with controlled rate
Not pacer dependent (unless suitable junctional-ventricular escape rate)

Respiratory
Maintaining pH >7.35 and PCO_2 within 8 mmHg of baseline value
Oxygen saturation ≥92% on nasal cannula or simple mask (<50% F_iO_2)
Coughing well and clearing secretions; suctioned twice per shift or less
No pneumothorax, large effusions, or pulmonary edema on CXR

Renal or metabolic
Urine output at least 0.5 $cm^3 \ kg^{-1} \ h^{-1}$
Weight within 5 kg of preoperative value
Renal function (creatinine) near baseline (or known problem followed by consultant)
Serum potassium ≥3.5 mequiv
Blood glucose adequately controlled

Hematologic
Hematocrit ≥6%
Chest tube output <50 $cm^3 \ h^{-1}$
Clotting parameters within normal range unless deliberately anticoagulated

Infectious
SIRS resolving (temperature ≤38.0°C, WBC <18 000)

The above criteria may be liberalized if nursing and monitoring facilities on a 'step-down' ward are available to meet patient needs.
MAP, mean arterial pressure; CI, cardiac index; PVC, premature ventricular contraction; CXR, chest radiograph.

tions; less often by infection, gastrointestinal bleeding, or neurologic events.

20.7 **Prognosis and outcome**

Several different systems are available for retrospective analysis of outcome in a cardiac surgical program[42]. In general, the risk for morbidity and mortality in an individual patient is increased with emergency procedures, poor left ventricular function (ejection fraction <35%), complex surgery, reoperation, advanced age, low body weight, diabetes, peripheral or carotid vascular disease, and chronic obstructive pulmonary disease[43]. Severity-adjustment tools such as the Acute Physiology and Chronic Health Evaluation (APACHE) and the Mortality Probability Model (MPM) are generally not appropriate for evaluating the cardiac surgical patient whose physiology is deliberately altered in the operating room.

Patients presenting for CABG surgery are older and more seriously ill now than a decade ago. Risk-adjusted mortality has not changed substantially, although complications have diminished, possibly as the result of better intraoperative and postoperative care[44]. The risk of subsequent morbidity and mortality can be predicted based on a patient's condition on arrival in the ICU[45] (*Table 20.6, Figure 20.2*) but all risk predictions are based on population averages and do not necessarily apply to the individual. Patients with single-organ failure have a reasonable chance of functional recovery, although they may require chronic hemodialysis, or tracheostomy and long-term weaning from ventilatory support. Multiple organ failure is a poor prognostic sign[29,37], and mortality correlates with the number of failed organs[45,46]. Physiologic insults (upper gastrointestinal bleeding, aspiration, sepsis) that occur during recovery from the initial bout of organ failure are frequently fatal. Deciding when further care approaches futility is difficult and open to challenge, but should be addressed with the patient's family and the health care

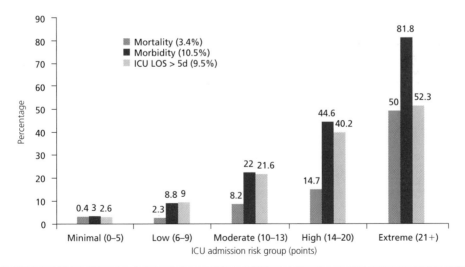

Figure 20.2 The risk of mortality, serious morbidity and prolonged ICU length of stay is a function of condition at ICU admission, calculated by adding the point values in *Table 20.6*. Patients with five points or less have excellent outcomes, whereas those with high scores are likely to have complicated, lengthy postoperative courses. Mortality is included within the definition of morbidity, as patients who die early in the postoperative course may not have time to manifest ventilator dependence, sepsis, renal or neurologic failure. It should be noted, however, that a small percentage of patients with the highest score may still have a good outcome. From: Higgins, T.L., Estafanous, F.G., Loop, F.D., *et al*. (1997) ICU admission score for predicting morbidity and mortality risk after coronary artery bypass grafting. Reproduced with permission from Elsevier Science. *Ann. Thorac. Surg.* **64**: 1050–1058.

Table 20.6 ICU risk-assessment score for cardiac surgical patients

Preoperative factors		ICU admission factors	
Preop albumin <3.5 mg %	5	IABP post CPB	7
Preop creatinine ≥1.9 mg %	4	CPB time ≥160 min	3
Age ≥70 years	3	Arterial bicarb <21	4
History PVD or vasc surg	3	CVP ≥17 mmHg	4
≥2 prior heart operations	2	Cardiac index <2.1	3
One prior heart operation	1	Heart rate ≥100	3
Small size (BSA <1.72 m²)	1	(A–a)PO$_2$ gradient ≥250 torr	2

From: Higgins, T.L., Estafanous, F.G., Loop, F.D., *et al.* (1997) ICU admission score for predicting morbidity and mortality risk after coronary artery bypass grafting. Reproduced with permission from Elsevier Science. *Ann. Thorac. Surg.* **64**: 1050–1058.

team if the patient is not improving by the second or third postoperative week. Characteristics of patients who survive multi-organ failure and prolonged ICU stay are younger age (<70 years), awake neurologic status with a will to live, and unambiguous signs of recovery such as less ventilator or pressor support over time. However, there are no good studies to quantify these impressions.

20.8 Summary

Management of the cardiac surgery patient is becoming ever more complex with changes in demographics and extent of surgery. Successful ICU outcome following cardiac surgery requires constant vigilance and attention to details. Most post-CABG patients are relatively healthy, and will recover nicely on their own as long as important complications are avoided. Statistically, certain patients are more likely to suffer postoperative complications, and it is in this high-risk group that greater attention and interventions can be directed. By understanding the risk factors for catastrophic deterioration, and undertaking preventive measures, outcome can be improved.

References

1. Smith, I., Fleming, S. and Cernaianu, A. (1990) Mishaps during transport from the intensive care unit. *Crit. Care Med.* **18**: 278–281.
2. Braun, S.R., Brinbaum, M.L. and Chopra, P.S. (1978) Pre- and postoperative pulmonary function abnormalities in coronary artery revascularization surgery. *Chest* **73**: 316–320.
3. Ratliff, N.B., Young, G., Jr, Hackel, D.B., Mikat, E. and Wilson, J.W. (1973) Pulmonary injury secondary to extracorporeal circulation. *J. Thorac. Cardiovasc. Surg.* **65**: 425–432.
4. Michalopoulos, A., Anthi, A., Rellos, K., *et al.* (1998) Effects of positive end-expiratory pressure (PEEP) in cardiac surgery patients. *Respir. Med.* **92**: 858–862.
5. Higgins, T.L. (1992) Early endotracheal extubation is preferable to late extubation in patients following coronary artery surgery. *J. Cardiothorac. Vasc. Anesth.* **6**: 488–493.
6. Cheng, C.H., Karski, J., Peniston, C., Raveendran, G., Asokumar, B., Carroll, J., David, T. and Sandler, A. (1996) Early tracheal extubation after coronary artery bypass graft surgery reduces costs and improves resource use. A prospective, randomized, controlled trial. *Anesthesiology* **85**: 1300–1310.
7. Higgins, T.L. (1995) Safety issues regarding early extubation after coronary artery bypass surgery. *J. Cardiothorac. Vasc. Anesth.* **9**: 24–29.
8. Engelman, R.M., Rousou, J.A., Flack, J.E., *et al.* (1994) Fast-track recovery of the coronary bypass patient. *Ann. Thorac. Surg.* **58**: 1742–1746.
9. Millbern, S.M., Downs, J.B., Jumper, L.C. and Modell, J.H. (1978) Evaluation of criteria for discontinuing mechanical ventilatory support. *Arch. Surg.* **113**: 1441–1443.
10. Higgins, T.L., Yared, J.P., Paranandi, L., Baldyga, A. and Starr, N.J. (1991) Risk factors for respiratory complications after cardiac surgery. *Anesthesiology* **75**: 3A.
11. Covelli, H.D., Black, J.W., Olsen, M.S. and Beekman, J.F. (1981) Respiratory failure precipitated by high carbohydrate loads. *Ann. Intern. Med.* **95**: 579–581.
12. Lemaire, F., Teboul, J.L., Cinotti, L., Giotto, G., Abrouk, F., Steg, G., Macquin-Mavier, I. and Zapol, W.M. (1988) Acute left ventricular dysfunction during unsuccessful weaning from mechanical ventilation. *Anesthesiology* **69**: 171–179.

13. **Coraim, F.J., Coraim, H.P., Ebermann, R. and Stellwag, F.M.** (1986) Acute respiratory failure after cardiac surgery: clinical experience with the application of continuous arteriovenous hemofiltration. *Crit. Care Med.* **14**: 714–718.

14. **Wilcox, P., Baile, E.M., Hards, J., Muller, N.L., Dunn, L., Pardy, R.L. and Pare, P.D.** (1988) Phrenic nerve function and its relationship to atelectasis after coronary artery bypass surgery. *Chest* **93**: 693–698.

15. **Breisblatt, W.M., Stein, K.L., Wolfe, C.J., *et al.*** (1990) Acute myocardial dysfunction and recovery: a common occurrence after coronary artery bypass. *J. Am. Coll. Cardiol.* **15**: 1261–1269.

16. **Butterworth, J.F., Zaloga, G.P., Prielipp, R.C., Tucker, W.Y., Jr and Royster, R.L.** (1992) Calcium inhibits the cardiac stimulating properties of dobutamine but not of amrinone. *Chest* **101**: 174–180.

17. **Fernandez-Del Castillo, C., Harringer, W., Warshaw, A.L., Vlahakes, G.J., Koski, G., Zaslavsky, A.M. and Rattner, D.W.** (1991) Risk factors for pancreatic cellular injury after cardiopulmonary bypass. *N. Engl. J. Med.* **325**: 382–387.

18. **Janelle, G.M., Urdaneta, F., Martin, T.D. and Lobato, E.B.** (2000) Effects of calcium chloride on grafting internal mammary artery flow after cardiopulmonary bypass. *J. Cardiothorac. Vasc. Anesth.* **14**: 4–8.

19. **Estafanous, F.G., Urzua, J., Yared, J.P., Zurick, A.M., Loop, F.D. and Tarazi, R.C.** (1984) Pattern of hemodynamic alterations during coronary artery operations. *J. Thorac. Cardiovasc. Surg.* **87**: 175–182.

20. **Higgins, T.L., Yared, J.P., Estafanous, F.G., *et al.*** (1994) Propofol versus midazolam for intensive care unit sedation after coronary artery bypass grafting. *Crit. Care Med.* **22**: 1415–1423.

21. **Chauvin, M., Deriaz, H. and Viars, P.** (1987) Continuous IV infusion of labetalol for postoperative hypertension. *Br. J. Anesth.* **59**: 1250–1256.

22. **Pinski, S.L. and Maloney, J.D.** (1990) Adenosine: a new drug for acute termination of supraventricular tachycardia. *Clev. Clin. J. Med.* **57**: 383–388.

23. **Wahl, G.W., Feins, R.H., Alfieres, G. and Bixby, K.** (1992) Reinfusion of shed blood after coronary operation causes elevation of cardiac enzyme levels. *Ann. Thorac. Surg.* **53**: 625–627.

24. **Society of Thoracic Surgeons** (1999) *Definition of Terms.* STS, National Cardiac Database, Chicago, IL, p. 25.

25. **Yared, J.-P., Starr, N.J., Hoffman-Hogg, L., Bashour, C.A., Insler, S.R., O'Connor, M., Piedmonte, M. and Cosgrove, D.M.** (1998) Dexamethasone decreases the incidence of shivering after cardiac surgery: A randomized, double-blind, placebo-controlled study. *Anesth. Analg.* **87**: 795–799.

26. **Bhat, J.G., Gluck, M.C., Lowenstein, J. and Baldwin, D.S.** (1976) Renal failure after open heart surgery. *Ann. Intern. Med.* **84**: 677–682.

27. **Hilberman, M., Myers, B.D., Carrie, B.J., Derby, G., Jamison, R.L. and Stinson, E.B.** (1979) Acute renal failure following cardiac surgery. *J. Thorac. Cardiovasc. Surg.* **77**: 880.

28. **Koning, H.M., Koning, A.J. and Leusink, J.A.** (1985) Serious acute renal failure following open heart surgery. *Thorac. Cardiovasc. Surg.* **33**: 283–287.

29. **Higgins, T.L., Blum, J.M. and Lytle, B.W.** (1992) Postoperative complications following coronary bypass grafting: implications of elevated bilirubin and elevated creatinine. *Abstracts of Society of Cardiovascular Anesthesiologists Meeting.* Society of Cardiovascular Anesthesiologists, Richmond, Virginia, p. 27.

30. **Myers, B.D. and Moran, S.M.** (1987) Hemodynamically mediated acute renal failure. *N. Engl. J. Med.* **314**: 97.

31. **Calabrese, J.R., Skwerer, R.G., Gulledge, A.D., *et al.*** (1987) Incidence of postoperative delirium following myocardial revascularization. *Clev. Clin. J. Med.* **54**: 29–32.

32. **Milam, J.D., Austin, S.F., Martin, R.F., Keats, A.S. and Cooley, D.A.** (1981) Alteration of coagulation and selected clinical chemistry parameters in patients undergoing open heart surgery without transfusions. *Am. Soc. Clin. Pathol.* **76**: 155–162.

33. **Salzman, E.W., Weinstein, M.J., Weintraub, R.M., *et al.*** (1986) Treatment with desmopressin acetate to reduce blood loss after cardiac surgery: a double-blind randomized trial. *N. Engl. J. Med.* **314**: 1402–1406.

34. **DelRossi, A.J., Cernaiann, A.C., Botros, S., Lemole, G.M. and Moore, R.** (1989) Prophylactic treatment of postperfusion bleeding using EACA. *Chest* **96**: 27–30.

35. **Royston, D., Taylor, K.M., Bidstrup, B.P. and Sapsford, R.N.** (1987) Effect of aprotinin on need for blood transfusion after repeat open-heart surgery. *Lancet* **2**: 1289–1291.

36. **Michelson, E.L., Torosian, M., Morganroth, J. and MacVaugh, H., III** (1980) Early recognition of surgically correctable causes of excessive mediastinal bleeding after coronary artery bypass graft surgery. *Am. J. Surg.* **139**: 313–317.

37. **Mahfood, S.S., Higgins, T.L. and Loop, F.D.** (1991) Management of complications related to

perioperative care in cardiothoracic surgery. In: *Management of Complications Related to Coronary Artery Bypass Surgery* (eds J.A Waldhausen and M.B. Orringer). Mosby-Year Book, St. Louis, MO, pp. 265–280.

38. **Leal-Noval, S.R., Marquez-Varcaro, J.A., Garcia-Curiel, A., Camacho-Larana, P., Rincon-Ferrari, M.D., Ordonez-Fernandez, A., Flores-Cordero, J.M. and Loscertales-Abril, J.** (2000) Nosocomial pneumonia in patients undergoing heart surgery. *Crit. Care Med.* **28:** 935–940.

39. **Krasna, M.J., Flanchbaum, L., Trooskin, Z.S., et al.** (1988) Gastrointestinal complications after cardiac surgery. *Surgery* **104:** 733.

40. **Ephgrave, K.S., Kleinman-Wexler, R.L. and Adar, C.G.** (1990) Enteral nutrients prevent stress ulceration and increase intragastric volume. *Crit. Care Med.* **18:** 621.

41. **Sanderson, R.G., Ellison, J.H., Benson, J.A. and Starr, A.** (1967) Jaundice following open-heart surgery. *Ann. Surg.* **165:** 217.

42. **Peterson, E.D., DeLong, E.R., Muhlbaier, L.H., Rosen, A.B., Buell, H.E., Kiefe, C.I. and Kresowik, T.F.** (2000) Challenges in comparing risk-adjusted bypass surgery mortality results. *J. Am. Coll. Cardiol.* **36:** 2174–2184.

43. **Higgins, T.L.** (1998) Quantifying risk and assessing outcome in cardiac surgery. *J. Cardiothorac. Vasc. Anesth.* **12:** 330–340.

44. **Estafanous, F.G., Loop, F.D., Higgins, T.L., Tekyi-Mensah, S., Lytle, B.W., Cosgrove, D.M., Roberts-Brown, M. and Starr, N.J.** (1998) Increased risk and decreased morbidity of coronary artery bypass grafting between 1986 and 1994. *Ann. Thorac. Surg.* **65:** 383–389.

45. **Higgins, T.L., Estafanous, F.G., Loop, F.D., et al.** (1997) ICU admission score for predicting morbidity and mortality risk after coronary artery bypass grafting. *Ann. Thorac. Surg.* **64:** 1050–1058.

46. **Vincent, J.L., de Mendoca, A., Cantraine, F., et al.** (1998) Use of the SOFA score to assess the incidence of organ dysfunction/failure in intensive care units: results of a multicenter, prospective study. *Crit. Care Med.* **26:** 1793–1800.

Chapter 21

Postoperative care of the thoracic surgical patient

Thomas L. Higgins, MD

Contents

21.1 Introduction

The thoracic surgery patient is typically older, has concurrent medical problems, may be debilitated as a result of cancer and/or malnutrition, and often has significant abnormalities of lung function. Pulmonary abnormalities may have arisen from tobacco use, occupational exposure, or a primary disease process. A history of asthma, wheezing, or allergic airway responses is important, both as a risk factor, and to identify patients in whom bronchodilator management may be needed in the postoperative period.

21.2 Identifying the high-risk patient

Forced vital capacity (FVC) alone is insufficiently sensitive and specific as the sole physiologic predictor of postoperative pulmonary function. Forced expiratory volume in 1 s (FEV_1), is determined by inspiratory muscle strength, elastic recoil and degree of obstructive air trapping, and provides a good indicator of the patient's postoperative ability to cough effectively and clear secretions. The decrease in FEV_1 after lung resection for cancer is not necessarily a simple proportional relationship, as lesser decreases in FEV_1 than calculated will be noted if an obstructed lobar or mainstem bronchus is present. A cutoff value for postpneumonectomy FEV_1 of 800 ml is commonly used as a criterion of resectability.

Lung surgery affects postoperative lung function, and entering the chest cavity, even without resection of tissue, produces substantial changes. Posterior-lateral thoracotomy is associated with greater postoperative impairment than median sternotomy. FVC and functional residual capacity (FRC) can fall to less than 60% of their preoperative values on the first postoperative day. Subsequent return to baseline can take up to 14 days. The decline in FRC is especially important, because the resulting atelectasis causes physiologic shunting and hypoxemia. In patients with severe chronic obstruction, the best predictors of postopera-

tive ventilation requirements were arterial pO_2 less than 70% of predicted for age and the presence of dyspnea at rest[1]. For elective thoracic or abdominal surgery, the risk of postoperative pneumonia increases with:

- low serum albumin concentration on admission;
- high American Society of Anesthesiologists (ASA) physical status classification;
- history of smoking;
- longer preoperative stay;
- longer operative procedure;
- thoracic or upper abdominal surgical site[2].

Numerous studies implicate advanced age, particularly age over 80 years[3] as a risk factor. Elderly patients have a number of age-related changes in pulmonary function, including decreased elastic recoil and progressive stiffening of the chest wall, increase in the ratio of FRC to total lung capacity, and diminished vital capacity and FEV_1[4]. The activity of upper airway reflexes is blunted, which may result in impaired clearance of secretions and ability to protect the airway. In patients over the age of 70 undergoing thoracotomy, hospital mortality can be 7.5%, with a complication rate of 17%[5].

Obesity results in decreases in FRC and expiratory reserve volume (ERV), to the point that ERV may drop below closing volume, resulting in perfused, unventilated segments of lung and a widened (A–a)pO_2 gradient. Obese patients are more likely to cough poorly, retain secretions and develop basilar atelectasis.

Cigarette smoking is well recognized for its contribution to perioperative morbidity via effects on the cardiovascular system, mucus secretion and clearance, and small airway narrowing. The benefit of smoking cessation before elective surgery is well recognized, although data in coronary artery bypass patients suggests that cessation of smoking within 8 weeks of surgery may actually increase the risk of postoperative pulmonary complications[6], possibly as a result of a transient increase in sputum volume.

A system for classification of the risk of pulmonary complications following thoracic and abdominal procedures was developed by Shapiro et al.[7] (Table 21.1). By applying 0–3 points for spirometric valves, cardiovascular history, arterial blood gases, central nervous system, and expected postoperative ambulation, patients can be classified as low risk, moderate risk, or high risk. Low-risk patients do not generally require oxygen therapy after recovery room discharge. Moderate-risk patients require several days' observation. The high-risk patient often requires postoperative intensive care and significant prophylactic interventions.

21.3 Operating room events affecting ICU care

21.3.1 Anesthetic agents

The speed of postoperative recovery will depend in part on the amount and types of anesthetic agents given as premedication and during the operative procedure. Considerations for the anesthesiologist involve the need to use high inspired oxygen concentrations, particularly during one-lung anesthesia (limiting the use of nitrous oxide) and the goal of early extubation (limiting the use of opioids). Regional techniques alone (spinal, epidural) are generally not applicable to operative anesthesia in thoracic procedures because of the difficulty in providing a high enough spinal level to allow surgery without affecting the brainstem or muscles of respiration. Controlled ventilation is necessary to sustain respiration during open-thorax procedures. The usual plan is to have the patient awake, comfortable and extubated at the end of the procedure, particularly in volume reduction surgery for emphysema where stress on fresh suture lines is undesirable.

Table 21.1 Calculating the risk of pulmonary complication of thoracic and abdominal procedures

Category	Points*
Expiratory spirogram	
Normal (%FVC + %FEV$_1$/FVC >150)	0
%FVC + %FEV$_1$/FVC = 100–150	1
%FVC + %FEV$_1$/FVC < 100	2
Preoperative FVC <20 ml kg^{-1}	3
Postbronchodilator FEV$_1$/FVC <50%	3
Cardiovascular system	
Normal	0
Controlled hypertension, myocardial infarction without sequelae for more than 2 years	0
Dyspnea on exertion, orthopnea, paroxysmal nocturnal dyspnea, dependent edema, congestive heart failure, angina	1
Arterial blood gases	
Acceptable	0
PaCO$_2$ >50 mmHg or PaO$_2$ <60 mmHg on room air	1
Metabolic pH abnormality >7.50 or <7.30	1
Nervous system	
Normal	0
Confusion, obtundation, agitation, spasticity, discoordination, bulbar malfunction	1
Significant muscular weakness	1
Postoperative ambulation	
Expected ambulation (minimum, sitting at bedside) within 36 h	0
Expected complete bed confinement for at least 36 h	1

*Zero points indicate low risk; 1–2 points, moderate risk, 3 points, high risk. From: Shapiro, B.A., Harrison, R.A., Kacmarek, R.M. and Can, R.D. (1985). Reproduced with permission from *Clinical Application of Respiratory Care*, 3rd Edn. Year Book, Chicago, IL.

21.3.2 Selective endobronchial intubation

This allows isolation of the right and left lung, permitting the surgeon to operate on a quiet, collapsed lung, while ventilating on the opposite side. Disposable polyvinyl double-lumen tubes are available in odd sizes between 35 and 41 French in both right-sided and left-sided configurations. Single lumen tubes with a retractable blocker (such as the Uni-Vent tube) can also be used to achieve lung isolation. The nonoperative bronchus is usually chosen for selective intubation in lobectomies and pneumonectomies, so that surgical manipulation does not displace the tube and disrupt lung isolation, and to allow resection of the main-stem bronchus if necessary. When selective endobronchial intubation is impossible (pediatric patients, very small adults, laryngectomy patients), a bronchial blocker can be placed under fiberoptic guidance to selectively occlude a bronchus (*Figure 21.1*).

One-lung ventilation alters the ventilation–perfusion relationship, and blood passing through the unventilated lung effectively causes a right-to-left shunt and reduces arterial oxygenation. Perfusion of the unventilated lung will be reduced by physical collapse of the lung and hypoxic pulmonary vasoconstriction. As the double-lumen endotracheal tube is large with the potential to cause airway trauma and edema, prone to shifts in position, and more difficult to suction through, it is generally removed at the end of the operation and replaced by a single-lumen tube if continued mechanical ventilation is required. Specific indications for continued selective endobronchial intubation would include the need to protect against soilage (pus or blood) and provision of different levels of positive end-expiratory pressure to lung of different compliance (*Table 21.2*). The need for differential levels of PEEP frequently occurs in emphysematous patients undergoing single-lung transplantation. A fiberglass resin tube-changer or a pediatric fiberoptic bronchoscope are essential tools, which should be available for placement and adjustment of double-lumen tubes.

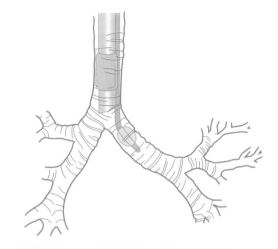

Figure 21.1 Fogarty embolectomy catheter used as a bronchial blocker. From: Rice, T.W., Higgins, T.L., Kirby, T.J. (1995): Mangement of the General Thoracic Surgical Patient. In: Sivak, G.D., Higgins, T.L., Seiver, A. (eds) *The high risk patient: Management of the critically ill.* Reproduced with permission from Lippincott, Williams and Wilkins, Baltimore.

21.3.3 ICU versus PACU versus step-down for recovery

The choice of recovery area following operation will depend primarily on the degree of patient illness, and the ability of a particular unit to deal with postoperative ventilation

Table 21.2 Indication for use of endobronchial intubation

Absolute
  To prevent soilage of contralateral lung with pus, blood or secretions
  To control distribution of ventilation
    Bronchopleural fistula
    Cystic lesions
    Differential lung compliance
  For unilateral bronchopulmonary lavage
  For unilateral lung transplantation

Relative
  Surgical exposure—pneumonectomy and thoracic aneurysm
  Surgical convenience—esophageal resection and lobectomy

From: Shapiro, B.A., Harrison, R.A., Kacmarek, R.M. and Can, R.D. (1985). Reproduced with permission from *Clinical Application of Respiratory Care*, 3rd Edn. Year Book, Chicago, IL.

and/or hemodynamic monitoring. At many hospitals, patients undergoing bronchoscopy, mediastinoscopy, esophageal dilation, esophagoscopy, gastrostomy, jejunostomy, laryngoscopy, video thoracoscopy, or scalene node biopsy can spend a short time in the postanesthesia recovery unit (PACU) and then be transferred to a regular nursing floor, or even sent home. Patients undergoing lobectomy, segmental or wedge pulmonary resections, or hiatal hernia repair (trans-abdominal Nissen repairs) can generally be recovered in PACU and then sent to a step-down unit if there are no complications. Patients undergoing esophagectomy, esophagogastrectomy, and pneumonectomy, may have ongoing monitoring needs or require postoperative ventilation, and thus require management in an intensive care setting.

21.4 Immediate postoperative issues

21.4.1 Usual ICU monitoring

This includes intermittent blood pressure determinations, continuous electrocardiography, and pulse oximetry to detect hypotension, dysrrhythmia and arterial desaturation, respectively. In selected patients, assessing intravascular volume status and cardiopulmonary function may require use of central venous pressure or pulmonary artery catheters.

21.4.2 Chest tubes

These are usually inserted to drain the surgical site at the end of the procedure, except with pneumonectomy patients where standard practice is to avoid a chest tube unless there is an infected pleural space. Chest tubes should never be clamped, even during patient transport, because of the dangers of unrecognized bleeding and tension pneumothorax. Immediately upon arrival in the PACU or ICU, patients should have a quick but comprehensive examination including vital signs, auscultation of breath sounds, and visual inspection of monitoring lines and chest tube connections. Chest tubes, except for tubes in pneumonectomy spaces which require a 'balanced' drainage system, are usually connected to a vacuum regulator to provide –20 cmH$_2$O of suction (*Figure 21.2*). A chest

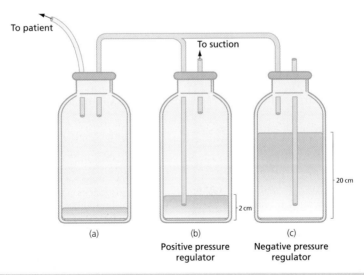

To patient

To suction

(a) (b) (c)

Positive pressure regulator   Negative pressure regulator

2 cm   20 cm

Figure 21.2 The workings of a chest tube drainage system can be best understood when simplified to a three-bottle system. Bottle (a) is the collection chamber; bottle (b) provides a water seal and escape mechanism for extrapleural or intrathoracic air; bottle (c) is a safety device to limit the amount of negative pressure that can be applied. From: Rice, T.W., Higgins, T.L., Kirby, T.J. (1995): Mangement of the General Thoracic Surgical Patient. In: Sivak, G.D., Higgins, T.L., Seiver, A. (eds) *The high risk patient: Management of the critically ill*. Reproduced with permission from Lippincott, Williams and Wilkins, Baltimore.

radiograph should be ordered immediately for confirmation of endotracheal, nasogastric and chest tube placement, and identification of pneumothorax, mediastinal shift or significant atelectasis. Routine chest X-rays are not necessary after uncomplicated removal of chest tubes and the decision to reinsert a chest tube is usually based on clinical appearance rather than radiologic findings[8].

21.4.3 Commercially available chest tube systems

These vary in their appearance, but all provide calibrated drainage chambers, a method to release excess positive pressure, and regulated amounts of negative pressure. The mechanics of these systems can best be understood as a three-bottle system (*Figure 21.2*). Air bubbles are normally expected in the chamber that limits the amount of applied suction; air bubbles in the water seal chamber represent an active leak.

Hourly output from chest tubes should be recorded, and the surgeon notified if drainage is more than 100 cm³ h⁻¹ for more than 4 h, or if more than 200 cm³ of drainage is recorded in any 1 h observation period. Expected chest tube drainage in the first 24 h is 300–600 cm³, tapering to less than 200 cm³ by the second day. The level of fluid in the water seal chamber should fluctuate with each respiration (assuming no air leak) and should be checked frequently to assure chest tube patency. Most pulmonary resection patients will return with mild to moderate air leaks, which become problematic only if the underlying lung parenchyma does not completely expand to fill the pleural space, or when the patient loses a significant percentage of tidal volume out of the chest tubes. In such circumstances, additional pleural drainage may be required, or changes in ventilation made to minimize the air leak and optimize ventilation. Frequently, leaks occur only above a given inflation pressure, and ventilation techniques such as smaller volumes at higher rates or pressure-controlled inverse ratio ventilation can minimize leaking and allow a seal to develop. Once

all air leaks have resolved and drainage is minimal (less than 100 cm³ per 24 h), chest tubes may be removed during the expiratory phase of ventilation or while the patient performs a Valsalva maneuver.

21.5 Endotracheal extubation and airway concerns

Extubation can often be accomplished in the operating room, but specific considerations (concurrent cardiac illness, inability to protect airway, malnutrition, coexisting lung disease) may mandate continued intubation. Silent aspiration of gastric contents is an important complication following pulmonary resections, and maintenance of endotracheal intubation for 24 h postoperatively has been shown to decrease the occurrence of pneumonia and the operative mortality rate[9] in high-risk patients.

Measurement of maximal inspiratory pressure (MIP, often called negative inspiratory force, NIF is helpful in determining respiratory muscle strength, particularly in patients recovering from thymectomy for myasthenia gravis, and in those who have received long-acting neuromuscular blocking agents in the operating room. Residual neuromuscular blockade can be assessed using a train-of-four monitor and reversed, if necessary, with small doses of neostigmine plus vagolytic agents such as atropine or glycopyrrolate. Criteria for extubation include:

- awake and following instructions;
- presence of gag reflex (airway protection) and cough (secretion clearance);
- respiratory rate to tidal volume (f/Vt) ratio of less than 100 (no rapid/shallow breathing);
- MIP of greater than 25 cmH₂O;
- adequate oxygen saturation (92% or more) on FiO₂ of 50% or less at PEEP of five or less.

Although many patients will not strictly meet these criteria for extubation, it is usually best to attempt weaning and extubation rather than risk the complications of continued ventilation in this group of patients. Specific indications for delaying extubation include:

- airway compromise as a result of edema or bleeding (see below);
- inadequate pulmonary reserve post surgery;
- compromised myocardial function especially with perioperative infarction;
- expected large fluid shifts with thoracoabdominal procedures;
- severe neurologic impairment;
- continued bleeding with likelihood of return to operating room;
- esophageal surgery patients (at risk for reflux and aspiration—delay extubation until airway reflexes have fully recovered as for 'full-stomach' intubation).

Considerations for long-term ventilator support, weaning and tracheostomy are covered in Chapter 18.

21.5.1 Laryngeal and glottic edema

This may occur after airway manipulation or intubation with a large double-lumen endotracheal tube. The presence of serious laryngeal edema can be detected by deflating the endotracheal tube cuff (after first suctioning the posterior pharynx), and occluding the endotracheal tube and watching for evidence of airway obstruction. Endotracheal intubation may need to be maintained while edema resolves. Racemic epinephrine and corticosteroids are useful adjuncts. If there is any doubt about airway patency, the endotracheal tube should be removed only under direct laryngoscopic or fiberoptic observation, with a thyrocricoidotomy set immediately at hand to facilitate airway access should reintubation be impossible because of airway swelling.

21.6 Postoperative fluid management

Fluid administration must be individualized based on patient condition, and a 'cookbook' approach is impossible. In patients where pulmonary capillary integrity is likely to be a problem (significant lung retraction, pneu-monectomy, lung transplant recipients, post-aspiration) fluids should be minimized. On the other hand, patients who have had considerable dissection and mobilization of tissue planes where 'third space' losses are likely (esophagectomy, esophagogastrectomy, excision of large mediastinal tumors) will require large volumes (typically 2 l or more) of fluid replacement. This fluid is generally spontaneously mobilized beginning on the second to third postoperative day, which may pose a problem if the patient has cardiac or renal compromise. In some cases, continued ICU care with invasive monitoring and aggressive intervention with inotropes, pressors, fluid boluses or diuretics will be necessary.

Urinary output more than $0.5 \text{ cm}^3 \text{ kg}^{-1} \text{ h}^{-1}$ is considered acceptable. If intravascular fluid volume is required, the usual considerations apply relative to hemodilution and translocation of fluid (see Chapter 7). Because colloid (albumin, hetastarch, plasma) tends to remain in the intravascular compartment longer than crystalloid, administration of colloid will reduce the total amount of volume required by up to 66%. This can be an important consideration in the patient with pre-existing cardiac compromise, or when pulmonary edema is likely (post-transplant, post-pneumonectomy). To maintain oxygen-carrying capacity, the patient's hematocrit should be followed, and transfusions given when necessary (generally if the hematocrit drops below 25% in a healthy patient or below 30% in a patient with coronary disease or severe organ system compromise).

Most patients who have undergone routine pulmonary resections can begin oral intake within the first 24 h. Patients who have undergone a pneumonectomy can develop mediastinal shift, diaphragmatic elevation or alteration of the esophageal hiatus, and are at higher risk for aspiration. As aspiration is a life-threatening complication (in any patient, but particularly in the pneumonectomy patient), it is helpful to assess swallowing and the gag reflex before the resumption of oral intake. Consideration should be given to early institution of enteral or parenteral nutrition in patients with complex clinical problems, particularly those expected to be nil per os (NPO) for more than 48 h, those expected to require long-term ventilation and those with preoperative cachexia. Patients who suffered from dysphagia preoperatively are often severely malnourished and parenteral or enteral support via jejunostomy tube should be employed until recovery is complete[10].

21.7 Prolonged ventilator support

Only a small minority of thoracic surgery patients requires postoperative ventilation. The goals in these patients are to provide enough ventilation (air movement) to prevent CO_2 retention and consequent respiratory acidosis, and distend the parenchyma sufficiently to prevent hypoxemia. In patients with otherwise healthy lungs, a tidal volume of 8–10 ml kg^{-1} delivered at a rate of 8–10 breaths min^{-1} with 3–5 cmH_2O of PEEP will accomplish these goals. In thoracic surgery patients, reduction of barotrauma becomes an additional consideration, which limits both total inflation volume and PEEP. Low tidal volumes (6 ml kg^{-1}) are recommended in the population at risk for ARDS, but this approach has not been well studied in routine thoracotomy patients. The normal inspiratory to expiratory ratio is about 1:2, and inspiratory times longer than 1 s are poorly tolerated in awake patients. Longer inspiratory times will reduce peak airway pressure, but require addition of sedative agents, and in patients with significant airway obstruction may not allow sufficient time for exhalation, resulting in auto-PEEP with consequent hemodynamic compromise.

Intermittent mandatory ventilation or CPAP with pressure support are commonly employed for early postoperative management, as patients can breathe spontaneously with some support as they awaken from anesthesia and metabolize residual neuromuscular blockers. The FiO_2 in the early postoperative period is generally set at 50–60%, and then adjusted as clinically appropriate. The combination of pulse oximetry and end-tidal carbon dioxide

monitoring may obviate the need for frequent arterial blood gas sampling. Controversy still exists as to the optimal level of PEEP in the thoracic surgery patient. Low levels of PEEP (3–5 cm) may be helpful in restoring functional residual capacity and substituting for the 'physiologic PEEP' of the glottis.

21.7.1 High-frequency jet ventilation (HFJV)

This has a role in the operating room during laryngoscopy, bronchoscopy, microlaryngeal procedures, and airway surgery. The role of HFJV in the intensive care unit, particularly for management of hypoxemic respiratory failure, is poorly defined. With bronchopleural fistulae, required ventilation can sometimes be attained with HFJV at lower airway pressures than when using conventional ventilation. The reduction in ventilation pressure will ideally minimize the amount of air passing through the fistula and may promote healing by allowing adjacent tissues to approximate and possibly seal the fistula. In the face of decreased pulmonary compliance, the beneficial effect of HFJV in lowering airway pressure may be lost[11].

21.7.2 Independent lung ventilation

With adequate separation of the right and left lungs, it is possible to ventilate each lung independently. Some commercially available ventilators (such as the Siemens Servo 900-C) can be linked together in a master–slave combination allowing a synchronized respiratory cycle, with independent control of CPAP, tidal volume, and pressure limits for each lung. A single ventilator may also be used to ventilate one lung while a small amount of CPAP is applied to the other lung. These systems allow the establishment of differential airway pressures. This is beneficial in the setting of bronchopleural fistula, or other unilateral lung pathology, where application of sufficient pressure to ventilate the diseased lung could produce overdistention and $\dot{V}/\dot{Q}$ mismatching in the healthy lung. Disadvantages of this technique include the difficulty of placing and maintaining the double-lumen endotracheal tube, and the limitations of suctioning and bronchoscopy through the narrower individual lumens of the double-lumen endotracheal tube. This technique should be utilized for the shortest time possible, usually only when the differential level of pressure between the lungs is greater than 10 cmH$_2$O. Ventilation techniques such as pressure-controlled inverse ratio ventilation (PCIRV) can sometimes achieve re-expansion of atelectatic segments even when there is substantial inhomogeneity of lung tissue.

21.7.3 Respiratory therapy

Patients presenting for general thoracic procedures often have significant underlying COPD, impairment of mucociliary clearance, excessive secretions, and increased closing volumes, all of which predispose to atelectasis. The respiratory therapist plays an important role in providing intensive care with secretion management and chest physiotherapy (percussion and vibration). Other modalities supporting recovery include humidified oxygen, adequate hydration, aerosolized bronchodilators, and early identification and treatment of infection of the tracheobronchial tree. Instruction for chest physiotherapy should begin preoperatively and treatment started as soon as possible postoperatively. Many patients will be unable to cough effectively, unless provided with adequate analgesia. Mucolytic agents (such as N-acetylcysteine) are helpful in solubilizing thick secretions, but may cause bronchospasm. Oral or nasotracheal suctioning is reserved for selected patients because of discomfort and the possibility of complications (hypoxemia, vagal-mediated bradycardia or cardiac arrest). The minitracheostomy (bedside percutaneous cricothyroidotomy for suctioning) can occasionally be utilized for access to the lower airway in patients with thick secretions. Inadequate clearance of secretions occasionally requires flexible bronchoscopy, which is of greatest benefit in the extubated patient who cannot adequately be suctioned. When pulmonary parenchymal involvement is confined to one lung, altering body position can improve gas exchange, by changing the relationships between ventilation and perfusion. The lateral decubitus position, with the uninvolved lung down, allows maximal blood flow to ventilated areas during spontaneous ventilation. This relationship may be altered with mechanical breaths and application of PEEP. In postoperative pneumonectomy patients, placing the operative side down may improve ventilation of the remaining lung. Specialized beds can be set to supine, lateral or rotating modes to optimize oxygenation[12].

When possible, patients should be positioned in a semi-Fowler's position to maximize efficiency of cough and clearance of secretions[13].

21.7.4 Postoperative analgesia

The majority of patients undergoing a lateral thoracotomy will require medication for adequate pain relief, and to minimize the splinting and atelectasis that will otherwise result. Patients undergoing median sternotomy appear to require substantially lower amounts of postoperative narcotics than those undergoing lateral thoracotomy, partly as a result of the nature of the incision and more secure bony closure. Systemic pain relief may be accomplished with intravenous opiates such as morphine and meperidine; however, the potential for respiratory depression exists. Non-opiate agents, such as the parenteral prostaglandin inhibitor ketorolac[14], or selective cyclo-oxygenase (COX) inhibitors such as roficoxib or celecoxib offer a viable alternative to opioids.

Epidural analgesia is highly effective compared with systemic morphine in post-thoracotomy patients and improves respiratory function[15]. Epidural catheters may be placed at either the lumbar or thoracic level, although locations above the cauda equina require an added degree of operator experience. Although a single bolus injection of preservative-free morphine provides 6 h or more of effective analgesia, continuous epidural infusions of opiates with or without local anesthetics can provide superior control for up to several days. Disadvantages to epidural analgesia are the potential for inadvertent entry of the needle or catheter into the subarachnoid space ('wet tap') with subsequent spinal headache, urinary retention, pruritus (common), and delayed respiratory depression as the result of circulation of opiates from the epidural space to the brainstem respiratory center.

Intrathecal administration of morphine has also been used extensively in the thoracotomy population, and offers the advantage of ease of administration. Like epidural administration, intrathecal administration carries the risk of delayed respiratory depression. Typical doses in the thoracotomy patient are 0.25–0.5 mg of preservative-free morphine in normal saline given at the l3 or l4 interspace[16].

Intercostal nerve blocks effectively relieve postoperative pain and muscle spasm. These may be performed intraoperatively (often upon opening as 'preemptive analgesia') or in the ICU. Percutaneous intercostal block (*Figure 21.3*) is generally performed in the posterior lateral area at the level of the surgical incision, and at interspace; above and below the site. If pain occurs at the chest tube insertion site(s), these may also be treated. Intercostal nerve blocks are relatively contraindicated in the post-pneumonectomy patient, because of the risks of entering or contaminating the empty chest cavity, and also because splinting on the side of the pneumonectomy may actually be beneficial in reducing atelectasis in the remaining lung. With a properly performed intercostal block, analgesia will generally last 6–12 h, and in some patients a single procedure is all that is required. Contraindications to intercostal block include chest wall resection with loss of appropriate landmarks, infection or tumor at the injection site and pneumonectomy.

Intrapleural catheters (*Figure 21.4*) have been used to administer local anesthetics following thoracic, breast, renal and upper abdominal surgery and in the treatment of multiple rib fractures. A catheter is inserted in the posterior

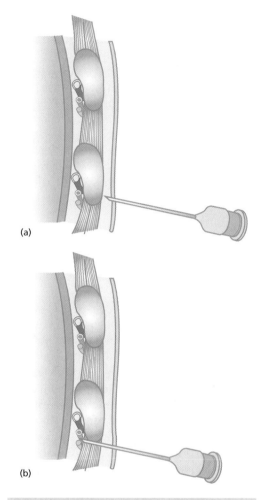

(a)

(b)

Figure 21.3 (a) The intercostal bundle is located by first identifying the inferior border of the adjacent rib. (b) The needle is then advanced below and deep to the inferior rib border. From: *Contemp. Surg.* (1992) front cover, June.

pleural cavity and threaded towards the apex of the lung, and local anesthetics (commonly bupivacaine or lidocaine) are supplied by intermittent bolus or continuous infusion. A single 20 ml injection of 0.5% bupivacaine with epinephrine can be expected to supply between 3 and 10 h of pain relief[17]. Complications include difficulty in placement, pneumothorax, toxicity to the local anesthetic (often in patients with abnormal pleura), and tachyphyl-

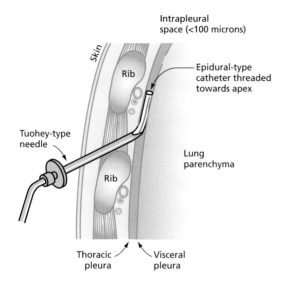

Intrapleural space (<100 microns)

Skin

Rib

Epidural-type catheter threaded towards apex

Tuohey-type needle

Lung parenchyma

Rib

Thoracic pleura   Visceral pleura

Figure 21.4 Placement of intrapleural catheter. Blind percutaneous placement is associated with a high incidence of lung puncture, so preferred placement is under direct vision in the operating room prior to full lung re-expansion. The Tuohey-type needle, available in epidural anesthesia kits, must be placed over the top of the rib to avoid damage to the neurovascular bundle. From: Rice, T.W., Higgins, T.L., Kirby, J.J. (1995) Management of the general thoracic surgical patient. In: Sivak, E.D., Higgins, T.L., Seiver, A. (eds). *The high risk patient: Management of the critically ill.* Reproduced with permission from Lippincott, Williams and Wilkins, Baltimore.

Table 21.3 Postoperative complications following any thoracic procedure

Airway edema or stridor
Arrhythmias (especially atrial fibrillation, multifocal atrial tachycardia)
Arytenoid dislocation
Aspiration of gastric contents
Atelectasis
Bronchospasm
Bronchopleural fistula
Chylothorax
Congestive heart failure
Deep venous thrombosis
Empyema
Hemorrhage
Hemothorax
Infection (superficial, deep)
Lobar collapse
Lobar torsion
Myocardial infarction
Pain and splinting
Pleural effusion
Pneumothorax
Pulmonary embolus
Re-expansion pulmonary edema
Respiratory failure
Retaining secretions
Subcutaneous emphysema
Tension pneumothorax

From: Higgins, T.L. and Chernow, B. (1995) Receptor physiology and pharmacology in circulatory shock. In: Sivak, E.D., Higgins, T.L. and Seiver, A. *The High Risk Patient: Management of the Critically Ill.* Lippincott, Williams and Wilkins, Baltimore.

axis to the local anesthetic with time. Contraindications to interpleural catheters include pleural effusion (which will dilute the local anesthetic), and pleural fibrosis.

21.8 Specific postoperative complications

General and specific complications are listed in *Tables 21.3* and *21.4*.

21.8.1 Airway complications
These occur with prolonged intubation using large or double-lumen endotracheal tubes, the passage of bronchial blockers, rigid bronchoscopes, or frequent reintubation. All can result in trauma or edema of the larynx or trachea. Routinely assessing the patient for an air leak around an occluded endotracheal tube just before extubation can help identify laryngeal and supraglottic edema. Upright or sitting position, intravenous corticosteroids and racemic epinephrine respiratory treatments are the mainstay of edema reduction. A critical airway may be converted to an adequate airway by the administration of heliox, a helium and oxygen mixture[18]. Helium, being denser and less viscous than nitrogen, allows maintenance of laminar flow through the critically swollen upper airway. Prolonged endotracheal intubation or temporary tracheostomy may be required to allow resolution of airway edema.

Table 21.4 Complications of specific thoracic procedures

Procedure	Complications
Anterior mediastinotomy (Chamberlain)	Damage to recurrent laryngeal nerve (particularly left)
Bronchoscopy or mediastinoscopy	Bleeding from major vessels if torn, air leak (rare)
Bronchopleural fistula repair	Persistent leak, dehiscence
Bronchopulmonary lavage	Respiratory distress or contralateral spillage
Bullectomy	Tension pneumothorax; air leak
Chest wall reconstruction	Blood loss, altered chest wall compliance, unstable chest, infection of prosthetic material
Collis–Belsey hiatal hernia repair	Gastric leak
Decortication	Blood loss, air leak(s)
Esophageal dilation	Esophageal perforation, pleural effusion, elevated CPK
Esophagoscopy	Esophageal perforation
Esophagogastrectomy	'Third-spacing' of fluids, anastomotic leak, gastric devascularization, splenic injury, gastric torsion, elevated CPK
Heller myotomy	Esophageal tear
Lobectomy	Bronchial leak, lobar collapse, lobar torsion
Mediastinal tumor excision	Airway obstruction with sedation or anesthesia; damage to recurrent laryngeal nerve
Nissen fundoplication	Esophageal obstruction (with tight wrap), splenic injury
Pectus repair	Costrochondritis, unstable sternum
Pneumonectomy	Atrial arrhythmias (atrial fibrillation, MAT), mediastinal shift, cardiac torsion, air embolism, disrupted bronchus)
Thoracic aortic aneurysm	Paraplegia, bleeding, aortobronchial fistula, esophageal injury
Thymectomy	In myasthenics, possible weakness and respiratory failure
Lung transplant	Rejection (day 5), reperfusion injury, infection, overdistention of native lung, dehiscence
Tracheal resection	Fixed neck flexion postoperatively; dehiscence, air leak

From: Higgins, T.L. and Chernow, B. (1995) Receptor physiology and pharmacology in circulatory shock. In: Sivak, E.D., Higgins, T.L. and Seiver, A. *The High Risk Patient: Management of the Critically Ill*. Lippincott, Williams and Wilkins.

21.8.2 Damage to recurrent laryngeal nerves

The recurrent laryngeal nerves originate from the vagus nerves as they enter the chest. The right recurrent laryngeal nerve arises high in the apex of the right chest and loops around the right subclavian artery to travel back to the larynx in the tracheoesophageal groove. The left recurrent laryngeal nerve, which is more susceptible to injury, wraps around the aortic arch in the left chest before it enters the tracheoesophageal groove. Excessive traction, aggressive dissection about these nerves, or the possible sacrifice of these nerves can result in postoperative palsy. Mediastinoscopy, anterior mediastinotomy, left pulmonary resection with subaortic exenteration and resections of mediastinal tumors are common operations in which the recurrent laryngeal nerve may be damaged. Associated airway and laryngeal edema may allow for adequate coaptation of the vocal cords for the first days post-extubation preventing identification of cord injury until after discharge from the ICU, resulting in ineffective cough or aspiration of secretions. If there is permanent damage or division of the recurrent laryngeal nerve then augmentation of the vocal cord with a long-lasting substance such as Teflon may be considered. In many instances, aggressive chest physiotherapy, careful airway management, and temporary avoidance of oral feeding may eliminate the need for any intervention until recovery of the nerve function has occurred. Intermittent noisy inspiration and painful swallowing characterize arytenoid dislocation, an uncommon cause of post-extubation respiratory failure[19]. Treatment consists of surgical reduction, using gentle pressure with a laryngeal spatula, and must be accomplished before the crico-arytenoid joint becomes fibrosed in poor position.

21.8.3 Retained secretions and blood in the airway

These are especially common if the airway was opened, as during a bronchoplastic procedure or closure of a bronchial stump. If there have been excessive or bloody secretions in the airway, flexible fiberoptic bronchoscopy with clearance of secretions is wise before extubation. The mechanical airway obstruction secondary to secretions may be aggravated by bronchospasm. Many patients have reactive airways and their preoperative bronchodilators should be continued in the perioperative and postoperative course, as secretions can precipitate coughing and bronchospams.

21.8.4 Postoperative air leaks

Most postoperative air leaks are the result of very distal fistulae between tiny bronchioles or respiratory units and the pleural cavity.

One of the main functions of the chest tube is to evacuate air from these small air leaks and assure complete expansion of the lung and coaption of the cut surface of the lung to the parietal pleura. With complete expansion of the lung, these small air leaks will seal. Careful examination of the chest X-ray, insertion of additional chest tubes into undrained spaces, adequate suction applied to the pleural cavity, and full expansion of the lung with vigorous chest physiotherapy help to close these small distal fistulae. If there is a substantial persistent air leak from the chest tube, or there is incomplete or no expansion of the lung in the pleural cavity, a significant bronchopleural fistula should be suspected. Major proximal airway problems such as failure of the anastomosis, disruption of a bronchial closure, or retained secretions or foreign bodies should be excluded early in the postoperative course by bronchoscopy. Within the first seven postoperative days, the fistula is usually secondary to a technical problem. In the subacute phase, usually more than 1 week after the operation but usually within the first 6 weeks, the fistula is often associated with an empyema or local peribronchial abscess.

Occurrence of a bronchopleural fistula in the early postoperative course of a pneumonectomy patient is a surgical emergency. The typical presentation is the sudden expectoration of copious amounts of pink, frothy sputum. Rather than assume that this is pulmonary edema, a bronchopleural fistula should be suspected. The patient should be positioned with the operated or pneumonectomy side down, to trap remaining fluid in the pneumonectomy space and protect the patient from drowning. A chest X-ray will show loss of fluid from the pneumonectomy space. A chest tube should be placed into the pneumonectomy cavity, remembering that there may be significant shift in the mediastinum and diaphragm; the tube should be placed high in the mid-axillary line. Further management, by the thoracic surgeon, will probably include bronchoscopy to assess the stump closure, and probably reoperation.

21.8.5 Empyema

This is initially treated with closed tube drainage and antibiotic therapy. Once the patient has been stabilized and any bronchopleural fistula identified and treated, drainage of the empyema cavity is converted from closed tube drainage to open tube drainage. A chest X-ray is then taken to determine if the mediastinum is fixed or has shifted and compressed the contralateral remaining lung. If the mediastinum is stable, then the drainage of the cavity may be permanently converted to open drainage. This may take the form of rib resection and marsupialization of the pneumonectomy cavity with later closure as the pneumonectomy cavity shrinks in size, using either the Clagett procedure or obliteration of the space with a muscle flap.

21.8.6 Pulmonary or systemic tumor emboli

In the postoperative period, pulmonary emboli are sometimes difficult to diagnose as hypoxemia may be due to sepsis, ARDS or pneumonia. If pulmonary emboli are suspected, ventilation–perfusion scanning, spiral computed tomography, or pulmonary angiography should be performed. Treatment is anticoagulation or lytic therapy (Chapter 12). If these are contraindicated, then an inferior vena caval filter should be placed. Systemic tumor emboli, although uncommon, may be seen after pulmonary resections for primary bronchogenic carcinomas or metastatic sarcomas.

21.8.7 Massive postoperative hemorrhage

This can be a lethal complication, and can manifest as significant shock, and generally requires emergent reoperation. Slower postoperative hemorrhage is more commonly the result of small bleeding arteries or veins in the mediastinum or chest wall. Reoperation may be required for control of bleeding. Failure of the hemothorax to resolve can necessitate later decortication to prevent fibrothorax and restrictive lung disease in the future.

21.9 Pulmonary parenchymal complications

21.9.1 Atelectasis

This is the most common complication following thoracic surgery, and can occur as a result of splinting, hypoventilation, bronchospasm, inadequate cough, retained secretions, and intraoperative trauma to the lung. The increased work of breathing and impaired gas exchange, as a result of the inherent ventilation–perfusion mismatch, may precipitate respiratory failure in a patient with marginal pulmonary reserve. Retained bronchial secretions and the frequent colonization of the airway in patients with COPD facilitates the progression of atelectasis to postoperative pneumonia. With clinically significant atelectasis, the patient may demonstrate tachypnea, tachycardia, arrhythmias, hypoxia, or respiratory failure. Atelectasis alone, however, is unlikely to be the source of postoperative fever[20]. Percussion and auscultation may reveal the signs of a consolidated portion of lung. The chest X-ray may show patterns of platelike atelectatic collapse, to segmental, lobar, or total atelectasis of the lung. Although the operative side is more frequently involved, contralateral lung and bilateral involvement may be seen. Treatment (incentive respirometry, chest physiotherapy, inhalation therapy) is directed at expanding the collapsed lung and clearing the airway of retained secretions. Routine bronchoscopy has been shown not to be advantageous; however, it has a role in established atelectasis[21].

21.9.2 Lobar collapse

This is most commonly seen following right upper lobectomy or right upper plus right middle bilobectomy, because of altered bronchial geometry. Following right upper lobectomy, the horizontal fissure rises and rotates to lie perpendicularly along the mediastinal pleura, and the resultant twisting and kinking of the long and narrow middle lobe bronchus renders it susceptible to occlusion. This complication should prompt early bronchoscopy to rule out torsion and repeated bronchoscopy to remove retained secretions.

21.9.3 Lobar torsion

This is an uncommon complication, which results from the twisting of a mobile piece of pulmonary parenchyma about its hilar structures with resultant bronchial, arterial, and venous occlusion. Torsion also occurs most commonly following right upper lobectomy when the middle lobe has no anchoring attachments save the middle lobe bronchus, artery, and vein. This one-point fixation and the absence of the upper lobe allow the middle lobe to freely rotate. Lobar torsion may also be seen after bilobectomy on the right with torsion of the remaining upper or lower lobe, or after lobectomy on the left with torsion of the remaining lobe. The patient may be asymptomatic, or may present with atelectasis often radiographically more than expected in the early postoperative period. Later in the course, the X-ray may show complete 'white out' of the involved segment or lobe. If ischemia progresses to infarction, biochemical signs of tissue necrosis may be seen, and the patient may cough up bloody, purulent, malodorous secretions. Similar chest tube drainage may be found[22]. Bronchoscopy will demonstrate abrupt occlusion of the involved airway; however, it may be possible to pass the bronchoscope distally into the twisted airway. Pulmonary angiography and perfusion scans will demonstrate lack of flow to the involved portion of lung; however, these tests are not diagnostic. Once diagnosed, urgent thoracotomy with detorsion and likely resection of necrotic tissue is required.

21.9.4 Re-expansion pulmonary edema

This may occur following rapid removal of a large pleural effusion or after re-expansion of a pneumothorax. It is characterized by unilateral alveolar pulmonary edema, which resolves rapidly[23].

21.9.5 Respiratory insufficiency

This may be irreversible and due to inadequate pulmonary reserve, as the result of too aggressive a resection, either from preoperative assessment or technical problems that required a larger than predicted resection. If there is failure to wean from the ventilator and to extubate, arrangements must be made for tracheostomy, feeding tube, and long-term ventilator support (see Chapter 18).

Respiratory failure may be reversible, the result of superimposed treatable complication, such as infection, fluid overload, aspiration, pulmonary edema, pulmonary embolus or pneumothorax.

21.10 Pleural complications

Fluid and air may collect in the pleural space and require correct positioning of a sufficient number of appropriately sized chest tubes. It is often difficult to adequately place the tube with only two-dimensional imaging as with a portable chest X-ray. CT scanning with placement after or during the scan is beneficial, as is drainage with surface ultrasound guidance.

Pneumothorax post thoracic surgery can occur with or without an air leak. The drainage system should be checked to guarantee it is closed with an adequate underwater seal. Chest tube patency should next be ascertained. If the chest tube and drainage system are functioning properly, then a loculated pneumothorax with no communication with the drainage system or large bullae are likely explanations. A persistent pneumothorax not associated with an air leak or signs of sepsis is generally not a problem, but may respond to increased suction on the present system. A persistent pneumothorax associated with an air leak indicates an established bronchopleural fistula.

Significant persistent pleural fluid drainage should prompt analysis of the fluid. A transudative pleural effusion can be drained by thoracentesis, with attention to treatment of the extrathoracic cause. An exudative pleural effusion leads to consideration of an empyema even if cultures of the fluid are negative.

Chylothorax can complicate operations in the chest about the aorta, esophagus or lung.

Any dissection in the posterior mediastinum may result in an injury to the thoracic duct. If there is a suspected injury to the thoracic duct, and this injury cannot be found, then supradiaphragmatic ligation of the thoracic duct is an acceptable approach. Damage to the thoracic duct noted can present as high-output fistula with volumes of 1–3 l day[-1], but diagnosis can be delayed as volume will be minimal while the patient remains NPO. The diagnosis should be confirmed by analysis of the fluid, which will have a high protein content, a large proportion of lymphocytes, and elevated concentrations of fat and chylomicrons. A contrast lymphangiogram or nuclear lymphangiogram using technetium-99m antimony colloid is usually not necessary, but may be used to locate the site of injury[24]. Initial management consists of placing the thoracic duct at rest (patient NPO) and complete drainage of the pleural space to promote full expansion of the lung. Nutrition is provided with either intravenous hyperalimentation or feedings through the GI tract using medium-chain triglyceride (MCT) formulas. If the chylothorax does not resolve, then thoracotomy with ligation of the thoracic duct is indicated.

21.11 **Other considerations**

21.11.1 Infection of thoracic incisions
This is uncommon. The incidence increases following operations where there is a septic complication, operations for empyema, lung abscess and mediastinitis, or if the GI tract is opened as for a perforated esophagus.

21.11.2 Subcutaneous emphysema
This is the result of tracking of air into the subcutaneous space and dissecting along the path of least resistance. Positive pressure ventilation and the positive pressure generated on expiration or coughing generate the driving pressure. Although alarming, subcutaneous emphysema does not generally adversely affect the patient's outcome. Treatment consists of the placement of a properly functioning chest tube into the pleural space, and suction drainage. Rarely,

massive emphysema in a non-intubated patient will compromise the airway and require urgent intubation or possibly tracheostomy for control of the upper airway. Release of paratracheal air will often permit emergent endotracheal intubation. The patient with subcutaneous emphysema should be assured this temporary problem would resolve.

21.11.3 Patients with myasthenia gravis
These patients may be safely extubated in the operating room or shortly after arrival in the ICU if neuromuscular blockade is monitored and adequately reversed. Less than 9% require prolonged mechanical ventilation, which may range from 15 h to 3 days[25]; with routine preoperative plasmapheresis, the incidence of postoperative problems may be even smaller. The need for postoperative mechanical ventilation can be predicted by:

- duration of myasthenia gravis greater than 6 years;
- history of chronic respiratory disease not related to myasthenia;
- pyridostigmine dose greater than 750 mg day[-1];
- preoperative vital capacity less than 2.9 l.

21.11.4 Esophageal surgery
The major complication following esophageal surgery includes leakage of esophageal contents from the surgical site. In 138 patients undergoing gastric interposition following transhiatal esophagectomy, the leak rate was 11%, with aspiration occurring in 4%, and gastric perforation in 1.5%[26]. More recent literature quotes even lower rates of leakage[27].

Early esophageal perforation is usually managed with thoracotomy, reinforced closure with a pedicle wrap and drainage. Manipulation of the esophagus generates release of all three isoenzymes of creatine kinase (CPK), limiting the use of CPK for diagnosis of perioperative myocardial infarction.

21.11.5 Reasons for ICU readmission
The major reason for ICU readmission is respiratory decompensation, as a result of fluid

overload, aspiration, or failure to cough and breathe well enough to prevent atelectasis and retained secretions. Atelectasis is a continuing threat, and can be reduced with the use of incentive spirometry. Bronchodilators and mucolytics are added as needed. More intensive intervention, in the form of percussion, postural drainage, and nasotracheal suctioning, may be needed when secretions are thick or atelectasis persistent. Follow-up care should include periodic chest radiographs, and at least daily physical examination.

References

1. **Nunn, J.F., Miledge, S., Chen, D. and Dore, C.** (1988) Respiratory criteria for fitness for surgery and anesthesia. *Anaesthesia* **43**: 543–611.

2. **Garibaldi, R.A., Britt, M.R., Coleman, M.L., Reading, J.C. and Pace, N.L.** (1981) Risk factors for postoperative pneumonia. *JAMA* **70**: 677–680.

3. **Stein, M. and Cassara, E.L.** (1970) Preoperative pulmonary evaluation and therapy for surgery patients. *JAMA* **211**: 787–790.

4. **Wahba, W.M.** (1983) Influence of aging on lung function—clinical significance of changes from age twenty. *Anesth. Analg.* **62**: 764–776.

5. **Edner, H., Sudkamp, N., Wex, P. and Dragojevic, D.** (1985) Selection and preoperative treatment of over-seventy-year-old patients undergoing thoracotomy. *Thorac. Cardiovasc. Surg.* **33**: 268–271.

6. **Warner, M.A., Offord, K.P., Warner, M.E., Lennon, R.L., Conover, M.A. and Jansson-Schumacher, U.** (1989) Role of preoperative cessation of smoking and other factors in postoperative pulmonary complications: A blinded, prospective study of coronary artery bypass patients. *Mayo Clin. Proc.* **64**: 609–616.

7. **Shapiro, B.A., Harrison, R.A., Kacmarek, R.M. and Can, R.D.** (1985) *Clinical Application of Respiratory Care*, 3rd Edn. Year Book, Chicago, IL.

8. **Palesty, J.A., McKelvey, A.A. and Dudrick, S.J.** (2000) The efficacy of x-rays after chest tube removal. *Am. J. Surg.* **179**: 13–16.

9. **DeHaven, C.B., Hurst, J.M. and Branson, R.D.** (1986) Evaluation of two different extubation criteria: Attributes contributing to success. *Crit. Care Med.* **14**: 92.

10. **Stizman, J.V.** (1990) Nutritional support of the dysphagic patient: Methods, risks, and complications of therapy. *Parent. Enternal Nutr.* **14**: 60–63.

11. **Baumann, M.H. and Sahn, S.A.** (1990) Medical management and therapy of bronchopleural fistulas in the mechanically ventilated patient. *Chest* **97**: 721.

12. **Nelson, L.D. and Anderson, H.B.** (1989) Physiologic effects of steep positioning in the surgical intensive care unit. *Arch. Surg.* **124**: 352–355.

13. **Brandi, L.S., Bertolini, R., Janni, A. *et al.*** (1996) Energy metabolism of thoracic surgical patients in the early post-operative period: Effects of posture. *Chest* **109**: 630–637.

14. **Yee, J.P., Koshiver, J.E., Allbon, C. and Brown, C.R.** (1986) Comparison of intramuscular ketorolac tromethamine and morphine sulfate for analgesia of pain after major surgery. *Pharmacotherapy* **6**(5): 253–261.

15. **Shulman, M., Sandler, A.N., Bradley, J.W., Young, P.S. and Brebner, J.** (1984) Postthoracotomy pain and pulmonary function following epidural and systemic morphine. *Anesthesiology* **61**: 569–575.

16. **Nordberg, G., Hedner, T., Mellstrand, T. and Dahlstrom, B.** (1985) Pharmacokinetic aspects of intrathecal morphine analgesia. *Anesthesiology* **60**: 448–454.

17. **Reiestad, F. and Stromskag, K.E.** (1986) Interpleural catheter in the management of postoperative pain—A preliminary report. *Reg. Anesth.* **11**: 89–91.

18. **Skrinskas, G.J., Hyland, R.H. and Hutcheon, M.A.** (1983) Using helium–oxygen mixtures in the management of acute upper airway obstruction. *Can. Med. Assoc. J.* **128**: 555–558.

19. **Castella, X., Gilabert, J. and Perez, C.** (1991) Arytenoid dislocation after tracheal intubation: An unusual cause of acute respiratory failure? *Anesthesiology* **74**: 613–615.

20. **Marik, P.E.** (2000) Fever in the ICU. *Chest* **117**: 855–869.

21. **Marini, J.J., Pierson, D.J. and Hudson, L.D.** (1979) Acute lobar atelectasis: A prospective comparison of fiberoptic bronchoscopy and respiratory therapy. *Am. Rev. Respir. Dis.* **119**: 971–978.

22. **Mulin, M.J., Zumbro, G.L., Fishback, M.E., *et al.*** (1972) Pulmonary lobar gangrene complicating lobectomy. *Ann. Surg.* **175**: 62–66.

23. **Hymphreys, R.L. and Berne, A.S.** (1970) Rapid re-expansion of pneumothorax: a cause of unilateral pulmonary edema. *Radiology* **96**: 509–512.

24. **Rice, T.W., Kirsh, J.C., Schacter, I.B. and Goldberg, M.** (1987) Simultaneous occurrence of chylothorax and subarachnoid pleural fistula after thoracotomy. *Can. J. Surg.* **30**: 256–258.

25. **Eisenkraft, J.B., Papatestas, A.E., Kahn, C.H., *et al.*** (1986) Predicting the need for postoperative mechanical ventilation in myasthenia gravis. *Anesthesiology* **65**: 79–82.

26. **Agha, E.P., Orringer, M.B. and Amendola, M.A.** (1985) Gastric interposition following transhiatal esophagectomy: radiographic evaluation. *Gastrointest. Radiol.* **10:** 17–21.

27. **Adoumie, R., Shennib, H., Brown, R., Slinger, P. and Chiu, R.C.** (1993) Differential lung ventilation. Application beyond the operating room. *J. Thorac. Cardiovasc. Surg.* **105:** 229–233.

Chapter 22

Thoracic trauma

Imtiaz A. Munshi, MD

Contents

22.1 Introduction

Thoracic injuries are directly responsible for over 25% of trauma-related deaths in the United States each year. Complications from thoracic trauma can contribute another 20% to overall trauma-related deaths[1]. The mechanism of injury and type of death are related (*Table 22.1*). Prompt diagnosis and treatment can prevent the early deaths and reduce the rates of complications and late deaths.

The most common type of thoracic trauma is injury to the ribs. Over 85% of patients with thoracic injuries can be successfully managed 'conservatively' with adequate analgesia, tube thoracostomy, judicious fluid management and ventilatory support. The remaining 15% of patients with blunt and penetrating trauma require thoracotomy to treat injuries[2,3].

22.2 Anatomy[4]

With suspected thoracic injury, it is helpful to think of the thorax as being composed of three units: the chest wall, the lungs and the mediastinum. The bony chest wall is bounded anteriorly by the sternum, laterally by the ribs and the costal cartilages, and posteriorly by the vertebral column (*Figure 22.1*). The wall of the chest is made up of layers of muscle and fascia supported by the thoracic skeleton. The

---

Table 22.1 Time sequence of mortality from chest trauma

Immediate death
- Disruption of the heart or aorta

Early death (minutes–hours)
- Cardiac tamponade
- Tension pneumothorax
- Airway obstruction
- Uncontrolled hemorrhage

Late death (days–weeks)
- Infections (empyema, pneumonia)
- Missed tracheobronchial or esophageal injuries
- Multisystem organ failure (MSOF)
- Acute respiratory distress syndrome (ARDS)

---

nerves, blood vessels and lymphatics of the chest wall pass within these layers. The chest or thoracic cavity is separated into two hemithoraces by a broad median septum called the mediastinum (*Figure 22.2*). The mediastinum is divided into superior, anterior, middle and posterior regions and contains numerous vital structures including the heart, great vessels, esophagus and the tracheobronchial tree. The inferior thoracic aperture is bounded by the diaphragm, a muscle that separates the thoracic and abdominal cavities. The position of the diaphragm is dynamic; upon exhalation the right leaflet rises to the fourth intercostal space and the left to the fifth intercostal space; during inhalation both expand to reach the eight intercostal space.

22.3 Pathophysiology

22.3.1 Blunt injury

One factor common to blunt injuries to the bony thorax is pain, aggravated by movement. Pain by itself can lead to a decrease in vital capacity and the inability to clear secretions, which ultimately manifest as hypoxia and hypercarbia. From the mechanical standpoint bony thoracic injuries such as rib fractures and flail chest result in ventilation–perfusion abnormalities, increase respiratory work and decrease functional residual capacity. Untreated pain thus contributes to worsening hypoxia, hypercarbia and respiratory insufficiency. Lung contusion, hemothorax or pneumothorax also cause ventilation–perfusion mismatching and decrease in lung compliance. Associated hypovolemia secondary to hemothorax can compromise oxygen delivery to tissues, resulting in metabolic acidosis. Methods of pain relief including intercostal nerve block and epidural medications for thoracic surgical patients are discussed in Chapter 21.

22.3.2 Penetrating injury

Penetrating injuries to the chest are divided into stab wounds and gunshot wounds. The gunshot wounds are further classified into low-

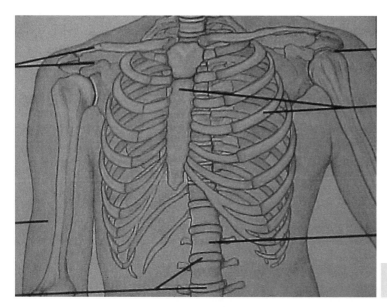

Figure 22.1 Anatomy of the chest wall.

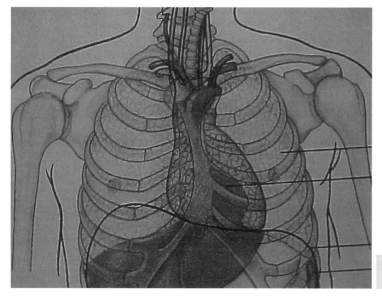

Figure 22.2 Anatomy of the thoracic cavity.

and high-energy injuries based on the velocities of the missiles. High-velocity missiles travel at more than 1500 ft s^{-1} and cause significant tissue destruction secondary to blast effect. Patients with injuries from these weapons often require early operative intervention with debridement and resection of devitalized tissues. Patients with low-velocity wounds and stab wounds have little blast effect and primarily local tissue damage, which may be managed conservatively. Like blunt injury, penetrating injuries can cause lung contusion, pneumothorax and hemothorax, resulting in hypoxia, ventilation–perfusion mismatching and decrease in lung compliance.

22.4 Initial evaluation—ABCs

Initial management of all trauma patients follows the guidelines outlined by the American

College of Surgeons–Committee on Trauma (ACS–COT) in the *Advanced Trauma Life Support (ATLS) Manual*[5]. Assessment of a trauma patient begins with the ABCs (airway, breathing and circulation), securing a patent airway while simultaneously ensuring adequate ventilation; insertion of large-bore intravenous catheters; administration of crystalloid solutions; control of obvious sources of hemorrhage; maintenance of cardiac output and evaluation of the patient for life-threatening injuries such as tension pneumothorax, cardiac tamponade, hemothorax, and pneumothorax. Subsequently, a complete, rapid physical examination is performed. Physical examination findings of chest trauma include crepitus, jugular venous distention, abnormal chest wall movement, diminished or absent breath sounds, diminished heart sounds or new heart murmurs, dullness to percussion of the chest wall or percussion tympany, and identification and localization of wounds or bruises on the chest wall.

22.5 **Injuries to the chest wall**

22.5.1 Soft tissue injuries
The diagnosis of chest wall wounds is often obvious. Patients present with symptoms of pain from the wound and may exhibit respiratory insufficiency secondary to an associated pneumothorax or hemothorax. Chest wall wounds must never be probed because of the risk of causing further injury to underlying structures, resulting in bleeding or pneumothorax. Small open chest wounds can act as one-way valves with air entering during inspiration and not exiting during exhalation, thus creating a pneumothorax ('open pneumothorax'). A resultant decrease in tidal volume and venous return to the heart occurs, leading to further compromise in cardiopulmonary status. Chest wounds exceeding two-thirds the diameter of the trachea result in ineffective ventilation as air preferentially moves across the chest wall defect rather than through the trachea. Open sucking or hissing wounds should be covered with a sterile, airtight dressing while a chest tube is inserted at a separate site on the side of the injury to avoid development of a tension pneumothorax. Chest tubes must never be inserted through existing wounds for fear of following the wound tract and injuring underlying organs. Chest wall wounds will often require surgical debridement and irrigation, allowing the wound to heal secondarily or by delayed primary closure on the fifth postinjury day. Large or complex wounds, particularly from shotgun blasts, require operative debridement with removal of all foreign bodies, including the wadding from the shell. If the wound is extensive enough that closure is not possible a plastic surgical consultation for coverage with a myocutaneous flap is indicated. Myocutaneous flaps can be fashioned from the pectoralis, latissimus dorsi, and rectus abdominus muscles[6].

22.5.2 Subcutaneous emphysema
This is a manifestation of thoracic injury. It results when air from the lung or the tracheobronchial tree communicates with the soft tissues of the chest wall through an opening in the parietal pleura. Injuries to the larynx, pharynx or esophagus may also cause subcutaneous emphysema. The air often tracks through the planes of the soft tissues into the neck, face, back and abdomen. Swelling can reach massive proportions but is rarely life threatening and resolves without intervention. Patients with subcutaneous emphysema should be assumed to have an underlying pneumothorax. Consequently, such patients should have a chest tube(s) placed before operation or placement on positive pressure ventilation.

22.5.3 Traumatic asphyxia
This is caused by an acute increase in the intravascular pressure within the superior vena cava as a result of sudden compression of the chest, usually by a heavy weight. Venous hypertension produces capillary engorgement, resulting in edema and cyanosis of the head, neck and upper torso. Diffuse reddening above the site of compression is characteristic and is secondary to extravasation of blood from

ruptured vessels. Subconjunctival hemorrhage and increased intracranial pressures can also be present. Treatment is administration of supplemental oxygen with elevation of the head of the bed to 30°. Prognosis is good, and the skin, ocular and neurologic manifestations resolve over a period of several weeks[7,8].

22.6 Injuries to the bony thorax

22.6.1 Simple rib fractures

These are the most common injuries seen in blunt chest trauma and are present in 25% of all injured patients. Although rarely life threatening in themselves, rib fractures are an indicator of possible underlying intrathoracic or intraabdominal injury. In addition, patients with rib fractures have significant pain and muscle splinting, which interferes with respiratory mechanics, leading to pulmonary complications. These complications further compromise oxygenation and ventilation. The bony thorax in children is relatively more elastic or compliant than that of the adult. The presence of rib fractures in children should raise suspicion that the mechanism involved a significant transfer of kinetic energy and potential child abuse. In the elderly population, rib fractures significantly increase overall morbidity and mortality, often warranting hospital admission in an otherwise stable and uninjured patient. Each additional rib fractured in an elderly person increases mortality by 19% and the pneumonia risk by 27%[9]. The presence of hypotension in a patient with low rib fractures (ribs 9–11), without hemothorax or tension pneumothorax, should raise suspicion for intraabdominal sources of hemorrhage. Low rib fractures on the right side may injure the liver and those on the left may injure the spleen with resultant hemorrhage.

Diagnosis of rib fractures is largely on clinical grounds and should be suspected in any patient with localized chest wall tenderness following blunt thoracic trauma. A negative chest radiograph does not rule out rib fracture, as up to 50% of rib fractures are *not* visualized on anterior-posterior (AP) chest radiographs[10].

Chest radiographs in patients with suspected rib fractures are obtained to search for hemo- or pneumothorax, lung contusion or other injuries. Treatment of rib fractures is largely supportive, emphasizing adequate analgesia and chest physiotherapy. Intercostal nerve blocks or epidural analgesia may be appropriate in patients with severe pain from multiple fractures or in the elderly. Epidural catheters provide the most effective pain control with minimal adverse effects. This method is the treatment of choice in patients with significant pain from multiple fractures and who are at high risk for respiratory complications. Strapping of the chest is not advocated because it can promote atelectasis and reduce vital capacity. Operative repair of rib fractures with plates and wires is indicated only if the bony chest wall injury is the primary reason for prolonged mechanical ventilation. Repair would be of no benefit if the mechanical ventilation were used to support the underlying pulmonary parenchymal contusion.

22.6.2 Fractures of the first and/or second ribs

These usually indicate that a significant transfer of kinetic energy to the thoracic cage has occurred, as considerable force is needed to fracture these bones. Fractures of these ribs are associated with mortality rates between 15 and 36%, higher than with any other rib fracture pattern[11]. Also, 40% of patients with first and/or second rib fractures have other significant injuries such as aortic rupture, severe head injuries and cervical spine fractures[12,13]. Local trauma to the brachial plexus and subclavian vessels can occur[14]. Operative repair of first and second rib fractures is not required.

22.6.3 Flail chest

This is defined as fracture of three or more consecutive ribs, which are each fractured in two or more areas (*Figure 22.3*). Mechanical malfunction of the injured chest wall is manifested by paradoxical movement (inward collapse) of the affected segment during inspiration. Although this paradoxical motion of

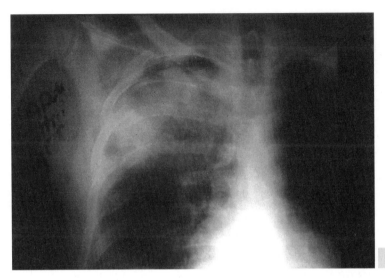

Figure 22.3 Left flail chest.

the chest wall contributes to an increase in work of breathing, the primary cause of hypoxia in these patients is the underlying pulmonary contusion[15]. ICU admission is warranted for initial monitoring with flail chest. As with other bony injuries of the thorax, adequate analgesia, judicious fluid administration and chest physiotherapy are of paramount importance.

22.6.4 Sternal fractures

These are most often the result of a direct blow, classically by impact with the steering column of an automobile or secondary to seat belt use[16,17]. Sternal fractures occur with an incidence of 1.5–4%[18], most often at the junction between the body and manubrium. The manubrium is the densest part of the sternum and is rarely fractured. A fracture of the manubrium requires tremendous force and is associated with more severe underlying injuries and with higher mortality than are fractures of the body[18]. Indirect forces can cause sternal fractures as a consequence of hyperflexion of the spine. Wedge compression fractures of the cervical or thoracic spine are present in 9.6% of patients with sternal fractures[19]. Associated rib fractures occur in 21% of cases[20].

Clinically, these patients may exhibit anterior chest wall pain, point tenderness, swelling and crepitus. Diagnosis is best confirmed with lateral chest radiograph, although deformity may be present on AP films as well. Suspicion or presence of a sternal fracture should direct focus to the diagnosis of underlying cardiac or great vessel injuries. Associated blunt cardiac injury can occur in up to 70% of these patients[17]. Cardiac work-up should include serial electrocardiograms and cardiac enzyme studies whereas echocardiography and angiography are indicated in a select few patients. Treatment of sternal fractures consists of effective analgesia. Surgical repair is indicated in patients with severe displacement, associated costochondral disruptions, or associated flail segments in which operative fixation may permit earlier withdrawal of mechanical ventilation[21].

22.6.5 Clavicular fractures

These are a relatively common injury and are suspected in those with obvious deformity, crepitus or point tenderness (*Figure 22.4*). These fractures rarely result in significant pathophysiologic respiratory changes. However, injury to the brachial plexus or subclavian vessels, although rare, can occur. Diagnosis is usually made on AP chest radiographs. Treatment largely consists of immobilization with an arm sling and adequate analgesia. Surgical repair is unnecessary but

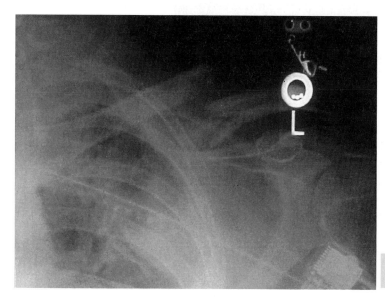

Figure 22.4 Left clavicle fracture.

sometimes indicated in patients with significantly displaced fractures.

22.6.6 Scapular fracture

This, like sternal and first and second rib fractures, is often an indicator that a significant force has been inflicted upon the bony thoracic cavity. The scapulae are well protected by surrounding musculature and are rarely injured. Clinically, pain and swelling are often the only indicators of the injury. Diagnosis is usually made on chest radiography. However, 28% of these injuries will show little or no radiographic evidence of fracture and as many as 43% are missed on initial chest radiographs[22]. Specific oblique radiographic views are necessary to confirm the diagnosis (*Figure 22.5*). Treatment consists of immobilization with arm sling but with early range of motion activity.

22.7 Injuries to the lung

22.7.1 Pulmonary contusions

These are a frequent sequela of blunt and penetrating injury to the thorax. It is believed that the blunt force results in compression of the chest wall with underlying compression of the lung parenchyma; subsequently, a rapid over-expansion with recoil of the lung tissue against the chest wall occurs, damaging the alveoli. Interestingly, the impact can be transmitted across the mediastinum to the contralateral lung resulting in a counter-coup type injury (analogous to cerebral contusions). The pathophysiologic mechanism for the development of contusions is not well characterized. However, it is known that capillary disruption with resulting interstitial and intraalveolar edema decrease lung compliance and increase physiologic shunt, leading to hypoxemia. The hypoxemia usually lasts between 24 and 48 h[23,24]. During this time period it is imperative that chest physiotherapy and adequate analgesia be provided to prevent atelectasis.

Diagnosis of pulmonary contusion can be made by chest radiography (*Figure 22.6*). Approximately two-thirds of patients exhibit patchy infiltration or consolidation on radiographs as early as 6 h after injury, which then develop over the next 24 h[16]. The remaining one-third of patients often have evidence of contusion on X-ray by 24 h after injury[25]. As a general rule, chest X-ray findings often lag by hours behind the typical blood gas changes of respiratory alkalosis and hypoxia. Pulmonary contusions are generally much larger than evidenced by chest radiographic findings. Poor

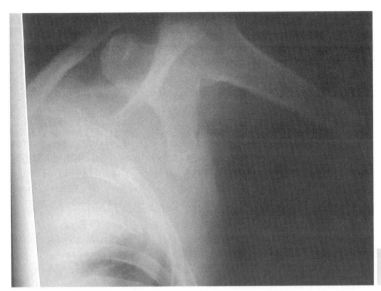

Figure 22.5 Left scapular fracture.

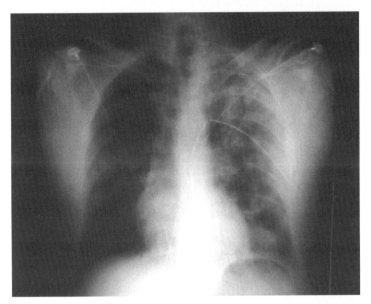

Figure 22.6 Left pulmonary contusion.

outcomes have been noted in patients with: (i) contusions apparent on admission chest X-ray; (ii) presence of three or more rib fractures; (iii) a PaO_2/FiO_2 ratio on admission of less than 250 mmHg[25]. The initial treatment of pulmonary contusions is chest physiotherapy, analgesia, and judicious fluid replacement. Ventilatory support is rarely required if the initial therapy is effective. Ventilatory support using intermittent mandatory ventilation (IMV) or pressure support ventilation (PSV) and posi-

tive end-expiratory pressures (PEEP) provide improved ventilation–perfusion matching and better venous return. Administration of excessive amounts of crystalloid solution can aggravate the pathophysiologic changes that occur with pulmonary contusions[25,26]. In general, enough fluid should be provided to maintain the urine output at 0.5 ml kg^{-1} h^{-1} or more. Central venous pressure or pulmonary arterial catheter monitoring systems are indicated in patients with severe injuries or those with significant cardiac comorbidities that may affect the resuscitation. Patients with unilateral lung injury may benefit from synchronous independent lung ventilation (SILV) provided through a double-lumen endotracheal tube[27]. The SILV technique helps prevent overinflation of the normal lung and underinflation of the damaged lung.

22.7.2 Hemothorax

Hemothorax is blood accumulating within the pleural space and is most frequently caused by blunt or penetrating injury to the lung parenchyma. Other sources of bleeding may include the chest wall, intercostal or internal mammary arteries, great vessels, heart, or diaphragm. The combination of high concentrations of thromboplastin and low arterial pressures within the lung along with the compressive effect of the hematoma help reduce the bleeding from the injured lung parenchyma in most cases. The presence of clot within the thoracic cavity results in the release of substances causing ongoing fibrinolysis, thus continued bleeding may occur until the clot is evacuated. Large blood clots may impede ventilation and affect venous return to the heart. Often, once the blood and blood clot are removed from the chest bleeding from small vessels will stop. Severe hemorrhage is frequently seen with penetrating injuries to the chest. Injuries to the great vessels or even significant amounts of the lung parenchymal damage can result in massive hemothorax.

Knowledge of the mechanism of injury in combination with the physical examination findings and a chest radiograph allow the diagnosis of hemothorax to be made readily. Physical examination findings include decreased breath sounds with dullness to percussion on the affected side. Diagnostic work-up with an upright or decubitus chest X-ray can usually reveal amounts greater than 200 ml of fluid or blood within the pleural space (*Figure 22.7*). Interestingly, as much as 1 l of fluid or blood may be unappreciated on a supine chest radiograph. Ultrasonography can also be useful in diagnosing fluid within the pleural cavity; this can be performed as an extension of the focused abdominal sonogram for trauma (FAST) exam.

General principles of treatment of a hemothorax are to restore blood volume, to provide drainage of the blood within the pleural space using closed tube thoracostomy and to control bleeding. Hemothorax following blunt trauma to the thorax does not often result in massive hemorrhage in contrast to penetrating thoracic injuries. Small collections of blood are resorbed by the body and thus can be

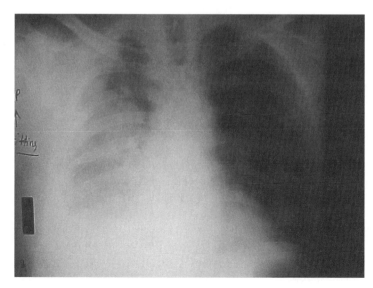

Figure 22.7 Right hemothorax.

observed. Thoracentesis is not indicated in the treatment of every hemothorax. Large collections of blood, however, must be drained as quickly and efficiently as possible using closed tube thoracostomy. A 32–40 French chest tube is ideal for the evacuation of blood from the pleural space with the tube positioned posteriorly. Antibiotic prophylaxis is beneficial in reducing the incidence of empyema in patients having chest tubes placed after penetrating trauma[28]. Most clinicians provide at least 24 h of antibiotic coverage against *Staphylococcus aureus*. Patients with associated intraabdominal injuries or esophageal injuries, patients with AIDS, or with high-velocity gunshot wounds should also receive prophylactic antibiotics with coverage for anerobic and Gram-negative contamination as needed. If blood accumulates after initial chest tube placement and cannot be removed, another chest tube should be inserted and positioned appropriately.

Significant hemorrhage is defined as more than 1500 ml of blood output after initial placement of a chest tube or continuous hemorrhage at 250 ml h^{-1} for 4 h. Significant hemorrhage and/or an associated adverse change in the patients' vital signs are indications for thoracotomy, preferably under controlled conditions in the operating room. Delay in performing a thoracotomy in such patients can result in sudden cardiac arrest. Blood drained from the pleural space is defibrinated and thus can be collected and rapidly reinfused for resuscitation. Significant hemorrhage from chest tubes can be autotransfused to reduce the need for donor blood. Caution should be used in regulating the amount of autotransfused blood replaced, as reinfusion of greater than 2500 ml of blood can lead to coagulopathy[29].

Thoracoscopy is an important tool that can be utilized for diagnosis and treatment in the patient with hemothorax. Diagnostic thoracoscopy allows direct visualization of the lung, chest wall, heart and great vessels. Most hemothoraces resorb spontaneously within 3–4 weeks, but retained or clotted hemothorax, most often after a penetrating injury, can occur as a result of failure of adequate tube thoracostomy drainage. CT scan can differentiate between hemothorax, atelectasis and contusion. Enzymatic liquefaction of the clot by instilling lytic enzymes has not proven satisfactory and is not advocated. Operative intervention with either thoracoscopy or limited thoracotomy is necessary if the hemothorax (i) causes greater than one-third of lung volume loss in one hemithorax, (ii) causes significant atelectasis, or (iii) is associated with infection. Delay of operative intervention beyond 4 weeks usually results in the development of fibrous adhesions along with increased capillary ingrowth from the pleura into the clot. Fibrothorax may result in significant permanent loss of functional residual capacity.

Posttraumatic empyema is a significant problem that can occur after blunt or penetrating thoracic trauma. Causes of empyema include iatrogenic introduction of contaminants, direct infection by penetrating missiles, secondary infection from an abdominal source (via hematogenous or transdiaphragmatic lymphatic routes), or infection secondary to postpneumonic pneumonia. The organisms responsible vary greatly, but are commonly *Staphylococcus aureus* or *Streptococcus* species. Secondary contamination often involves Gram-negative or mixed organisms. Appropriate cultures of the fluid drained from the chest cavity (by thoracentesis, chest tube or CT–ultrasound guided aspiration) should be obtained and broad-spectrum intravenous antibiotic therapy begun until therapy can be narrowed by culture results. Well-established empyemas often require formal thoracotomy and decortication, in which all infected debris is removed, the lung is freed from adhesions and the inflammatory peel is removed. Thoracoscopy may also provide definitive management of empyemas[30].

22.7.3 Pneumothorax

Pneumothorax is the most common intrathoracic injury following blunt and penetrating trauma. A pneumothorax occurs when air originating from the lung parenchyma is trapped between the parietal and visceral pleura. In blunt trauma a pneumothorax may occur secondary to rib fractures, crush injury with damage to alveoli, or from sudden increases in intrathoracic pressure. In penetrating wounds to the chest, particularly with gunshot wounds, a hemothorax often accompanies the pneumothorax, whereas with stab wounds one often sees only a pneumothorax. Large pneumothoraces can easily be detected on physical examination of the chest. Small pneumothoraces are more difficult to diagnose; diagnostic evaluation includes chest radiography with upright films at end expiration. In the supine position, pleural air does not collect at the lung apex, but rather in the basilar and subpulmonic areas. Pneumothoraces are often expressed as a percentage relating the distance across which the lung is collapsed from the chest wall compared with the total lung size, determined on the AP film. The treatment for pneumothorax is tube thoracostomy. For patients with blunt thoracic injury, who often have a simple pneumothorax, a 22–28 French chest tube can be inserted in the third or fourth intercostal space in the midclavicular line. If an associated hemothorax is present, as with penetrating trauma, a larger 32–40 French tube is recommended positioned optimally for both fluid and air evacuation in the fifth or sixth intercostal space in the anterior axillary line. The tube is then connected to an underwater seal with negative suction (usually –20 cmH$_2$O) to facilitate drainage. A chest X-ray is obtained to check the position of the tube and to determine the amount of air or fluid remaining within the chest cavity.

A subset of pneumothorax patients may not require chest tube insertion. These patients, who are hemodynamically stable and have isolated, small pneumothoraces (<20%) and no other injuries, can be followed with a chest radiograph at 6 and 24 h. Resorption of the air within the pleural space often occurs within days and can be facilitated by the administration of supplemental oxygen. However, all patients with a pneumothorax, regardless of size, should have a chest tube inserted before being placed on positive pressure ventilation.

After resolution of the pneumothorax, chest tubes are ready to be removed when no air leak has been present for 24 h and/or when serous drainage from the tube is less than 250 ml day^{-1}. Chest tubes may be removed while on suction. A chest X-ray is obtained within 6 h after removal of the tube. Complications of removal include a recurrent pneumothorax, for which a chest tube is reinserted, if necessary.

A continued pneumothorax is a complication that may be due to improper connections in the external tubing or to the water seal device, improper position of the tube, obstruction of or tear in the bronchi, or a large tear in the lung parenchyma. When the lung is not expanded and a large air leak is present bronchoscopy should be performed to clear the bronchi and to attempt to identify a tracheobronchial injury. Continued large air leak for 24–48 h along with a pneumothorax, with failure of the described measures above, is an indication for thoracotomy. In these patients the incidence of empyema and bronchopleural fistula is very high. A posterior lateral thoracotomy is performed and the patient will require stapling of the lung parenchyma, a limited pulmonary resection or repair of a tracheobronchial injury. Some success in sealing air leaks is possible when autologous blood ('blood patch') or fibrin gel is administered in patients with persistent air leaks via a closed chest tube system[31].

22.7.4 Tension pneumothorax

This is an immediately life-threatening condition in which air at supra-atmospheric pressure accumulates in a hemithorax. The air results in an elevation of the intrapleural pressure that leads to impairment in venous return and a decrease in cardiac output. The underlying pathophysiology is very similar to that seen with cardiac tamponade except that in tamponade the increased pressure is within the pericardium not the pleural space. Elevated intrapleural pressure also causes a shift in the mediastinum to the opposite side manifested by tracheal deviation. Respiration is adversely affected along with circulatory compromise. Physical examination findings include absent breath sounds and hyperresonance to percussion on the affected side. Immediate diagnosis and treatment must be instituted for this life-threatening emergency. Once suspected, time must not be wasted in obtaining a chest X-ray. Rather a large bore (14–16 French) intravenous catheter should be inserted into the second intercostal space in the midclavicular line on the affected side to relieve the tension component. Subsequently, a tube thoracostomy is performed to treat the pneumothorax.

22.7.5 Inhalation injuries

These occur when hot gases, usually secondary to fires in closed spaces, are inhaled. A high index of suspicion based on mechanism necessitates investigation. The pathophysiology of inhalation injury involves: (i) direct thermal injury from heat exposure, usually limited to the supraglottic area; (ii) carbon monoxide poisoning—a byproduct of organic combustion, carbon monoxide binds avidly to hemoglobin (300 times greater affinity than oxygen) decreasing the oxygen-carrying capacity of hemoglobin, decreasing oxygen delivery and leading to hypoxia; (iii) chemical injury to the mucosa (tracheobronchitis) and alveoli (pneumonitis) from corrosive gases and irritants. The last of these results in damage to type 2 pneumocytes, leading to decreased surfactant production and decreased alveolar volume.

Evaluation and control of the airway is essential in management of these patients and should be performed as early as possible. Diagnosis of inhalation injury requires direct laryngoscopy or flexible bronchoscopy to evaluate the glottic region for supraglottic edema, erythema, ulceration, hemorrhage or soot particles. Presence of these findings implies upper airway injury and usually necessitates prophylactic endotracheal intubation to prevent eventual loss of the airway as a result of edema. Other physical findings include tachypnea, hoarseness, labored breathing, altered phona-

tion, stridor, and cyanosis. Flexible bronchoscopy allows the evaluation of the distal tracheobronchial tree and the ability to irrigate and suction the distal airways. Injuries to the distal bronchioles and alveoli are best evaluated by xenon-133 ventilation–perfusion scanning[32]. Arterial blood should be sent for determination of carbon monoxide levels along with the oxygen and acid–base status of the patient. Management involves airway control, postural drainage and treatment of bronchospasm. Prophylactic intravenous antibiotics or steroids are not indicated in the management of patients with inhalation injury. Intravenous antibiotics are initiated only when an organism is identified from cultures.

Physical manifestations of carbon monoxide poisoning are related to the carboxyhemoglobin level in the blood. Normal carboxyhemoglobin is less than 2%, but may approach 8% in smokers. Carboxyhemoglobin levels between 20 and 40% result in headaches and nausea, levels of 40–60% cause neurologic dysfunction, and levels greater than 60% are often fatal. The treatment of carbon monoxide poisoning requires the administration of 100% oxygen via a non-rebreather mask or an endotracheal tube, which decreases the half-life of carbon monoxide from 270 min to 50 min. Treatment is continued until the carboxyhemoglobin level is less than 5% (normal values 0–5%). Hyperbaric oxygen, if available, can reduce the carboxyhemoglobin levels faster and can reverse the neurologic symptoms of carbon monoxide poisoning. Indications for hyperbaric treatment are given in *Table 22.2*.

22.8 Tracheobronchial injury

Traumatic injuries to the trachea or major bronchi are rare. Bronchial injuries occur predominantly on the right side[33,34]. When present they are often life threatening, with the majority of patients presenting with severe respiratory distress or in extremis. Autopsy studies have revealed that the majority of patients with major airway injuries die at the scene

Table 22.2 Indications for hyperbaric oxygen treatment

Air or gas embolism
Complications of uncontrolled decompression during diving
Carbon monoxide intoxication
Chronic non-healing wounds
Necrotizing soft tissue infections
Clostridial myonecrosis and myositis
Cyanide intoxication
Compartment syndrome or crush injuries
Multiple sclerosis
Intracranial abscess
Thermal burns
Significant anemia
Osteomyelitis
Mucormycosis

from asphyxia as a result of obstruction of the airway compounded by aspiration of blood. Patients may present with severe dyspnea, hemoptysis, aphonia, cyanosis and hypotension. A pneumothorax is often present and a large, persistent air leak notable once a chest tube is inserted. Pneumomediastinum with subcutaneous emphysema will be present if the air leak from the injury does not communicate with the pleural space.

The chest radiograph will be abnormal in 90% of patients with major airway injury, with pneumomediastinum, pneumothorax, or pleural effusion often noted. Also, although uncommon, the presence of a 'dropped lung' sign on X-ray (the apex of the lung is sitting at the level of the hilum, below the bronchial transection) is characteristically seen with mainstem bronchial injury[35]. Atelectasis and pulmonary infiltrates may also appear on X-ray. Flexible bronchoscopy should be performed in all patients with suspected tracheobronchial injury[33,36] to establish the diagnosis, localize the injury and allow for safe endotracheal intubation. Bronchoscopy should be performed in the operating room while maintaining cervical spine precautions. Once the airway is secure and the diagnosis made, consultation with a thoracic surgeon is indicated for repair of the injury. Both blunt and penetrating tracheobronchial trauma is often accompanied by major vascular and esophageal injuries.

Many small tracheobronchial injuries are not diagnosed until after they cause atelectasis and severe pulmonary infections. Delay occurs because the peribronchial tissue may remain intact, allowing for ventilation to continue. Within 2–6 weeks stenosis secondary to the development of granulation tissue occurs, resulting in distal airway collapse with subsequent atelectasis and infection[34,37].

22.9 Blunt aortic injury

Blunt aortic injury (BAI) is the second most common cause of death in blunt trauma patients[38,39]. Only 13–15% of patients with this type of injury reach the hospital with signs of life and those who initially survive have a 30% risk of subsequent rupture and death[38]. Diagnosis of BAI can be made using chest X-ray, aortography (sensitivity 99%, specificity 96%), CT, or transesophageal echocardiography (sensitivity 60–250%, specificity 90%). The 'gold standard' for the diagnosis of an aortic injury is aortography, although CT scanning of the chest is reported to be 100% sensitive, 81–99% specific with a 100% negative predictive value[40,41] (*Figure 22.8*). A widened superior mediastinum is defined as a measured width greater than 8 cm, a mediastinal/chest width ratio of greater than 0.38, or simply the physician's impression or suspicion that the mediastinum is widened, on an erect posterior–anterior view of the chest (*Figure 22.9*). Other chest radiographic findings suggestive for aortic rupture are listed in *Table 22.3*. Once the diagnosis of BAI is made, immediate surgical repair by a cardiovascular surgeon is indicated. Unfortunately, this may not always be possible in patients with multiple trauma who are unstable from intraabdominal injuries or severe head injuries. Additionally, elderly trauma patients with complicated comorbidities that preclude immediate repair are best managed with pharmacological manipulation of their heart rate and blood pressure (see Chapter 9).

Table 22.3 Chest X-ray findings suggestive of aortic injury

Widened mediastinum	Indistinct aortic knob
Depression of left mainstem bronchus	Opacification of aortopulmonary window
Widened paratracheal stripe	Deviation of nasogastric tube to right
Apical capping	First or second rib fracture

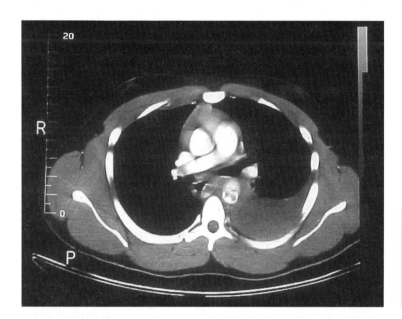

Figure 22.8 Chest CT with intravenous contrast demonstrating active extravasation of contrast from the thoracic aorta with resultant left hemothorax.

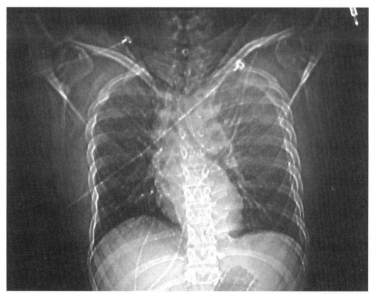

Figure 22.9 Chest X-ray showing widened mediastinum.

In BAI the aortic tear typically occurs distal to the ligamentum arteriosum, and disruption may not always occur through all three layers of the aortic wall. Patients with BAI who survive to reach the hospital often have a subadventitial hematoma or dissection limited to a short segment near the rupture. Traumatic aortic dissection occurs with a frequency between 2 and 12%[42,43] although the true incidence of trauma-related dissection is not known, as aortography can result in false negative results if the false lumen is not opacified. Contrast enhanced chest CT scan and TEE have been used to investigate aortic diseases and both have been shown to be accurate for the diagnosis of dissection[44]. The underlying pathophysiology of aortic dissections involves an intimal tear with formation of a false lumen within the medial layer. The false lumen can extend to the abdominal aorta to occlude visceral or renal branches, resulting in organ infarction[43,45]. Medial aortic dissection seems to occur commonly in patients predisposed to aortic disease (atherosclerosis or hypertension)[43,46,47] although trauma-related dissection may develop without prior aortic disease.

Complications after aortic surgery include paraplegia (5%), renal failure, respiratory complications (pneumonia, empyema), and aortic aneurysm formation from suture line failure. Paraplegia occurs when there is hypoperfusion of the spinal cord resulting from cross-clamping above the artery of Adamkowitz, which supplies the spinal cord but takes off from the aorta at variable levels. Risk factors for the development of paraplegia include intraoperative hypotension and prolonged duration of aortic cross-clamping (>30 min) if using the clamp and sew technique. Cardiopulmonary bypass should be considered if the repair is anticipated to take longer than 30 min.

22.10 Blunt cardiac injury

Blunt cardiac injury is usually the result of a direct precordial blow, and can result in myocardial contusion, cardiac rupture, valvular tears, or coronary thrombosis.

22.10.1 Myocardial contusion

Most patients with myocardial contusions are asymptomatic. Diagnosis is made based on the mechanism of injury (steering wheel damage), bruising and tenderness over the sternum, associated sternal fractures, multiple rib fractures and the presence of cardiogenic shock. There is no highly sensitive or specific test available to make the diagnosis. Cardiac enzyme fractions specific for myocardium (creatinine phosphokinase, lactate dehydrogenase and troponin) are not predictive[48]. Tachyarrythmias are the most common manifestation of cardiac contusions and the admission 12-lead ECG is the most important diagnostic screening tool[49]. Other dysrhythmias include atrial fibrillation or flutter, premature ventricular contractions, ventricular tachycardia or fibrillation. T-wave and ST-segment abnormalities may also be seen and are indicative of a bruised ventricular myocardium. Echocardiogram and radionuclide scans are not effective screening tools. A normal ECG in a hemodynamically stable blunt trauma patient rules out blunt cardiac injury of any clinical significance. Current practice guidelines recommend observation in a telemetry unit to monitor for the development of dysrhythmias or hemodynamic instability, which will require treatment in about 2–5% of patients (see Chapter 11). Delayed complications from myocardial contusions are rare.

22.10.2 Cardiac rupture

This usually occurs at the atrio-caval junction, left atrium, or right ventricular outflow tract[50], often in the setting of acute deceleration, crush injury, or lacerations from chest wall fractures. Patients with blunt cardiac rupture are often dead at the scene or die en route to the hospital. Valvular disruption occurs in 9% of patients with blunt cardiac injury and most often involves the aortic valve[51]. The new onset of a harsh holosystolic murmur implies rupture of a papillary muscle. Subsequent severe left ventricular failure is an indication for early operative repair. Ventricular septal rupture is rare, occurring most often at the muscular portion of the septum near the apex. Coronary vascular thrombosis is rare following blunt thoracic trauma. Its presentation is indistinguishable from atherosclerotic coronary occlusion, but the prognosis is more favorable[52]. Hemodynamic monitoring, fluid managment and inotropic support for blunt cardiac injury follow usual practice as discussed in Chapters 5–8.

References

1. **LoCicero, J. and Mattox, K.L.** (1989) Epidemiology of chest trauma. *Surg. Clin. N. Am.* **59**: 15–19.

2. **Wilson, R.F. and Steiger, Z.** (1999) Thoracic trauma: Chest wall and lung. In: *Trauma: Pitfalls and Practice*, 2nd Edn (ed. R.F. Wilson). Lippincott, Williams & Wilkins, Philadelphia, PA, pp. 314–342.

3. **Richardson, J.D., Miller, F.B., Carrillo, E.H. and Spain**, D.A. (1996) Complex thoracic injuries. *Surg. Clin. N. Am.* **76**(4): 725–748.

4. **Hollinshead, W.H. and Rosse, C.** (eds) (1985) The thorax in general. In: *Textbook of Anatomy*, 4th Edn. Harper & Row, Philadelphia, PA, pp. 465–488.

5. **The American College of Surgeons** (1997) *Advanced Trauma Life Support (ATLS) Manual*, 6th Edn. First Impression, Chicago, IL pp. 21–46.

6. **Chaikhouni, A., Dayas, C.L. Jr, Robinson, J.H., et al.** (1981) Latissimus dorsi free myocutaneous free flap. *J. Trauma* **21**: 398–402.

7. **Landercasper, J. and Cogbill, T.H.** (1985) Long-term follow-up after traumatic asphyxia. *J. Trauma* **25**(9): 838–841.

8. **Jongewaard, W.R., Cogbill, T.H. and Landercasper, J.** (1992) Neurologic consequences of traumatic asphyxia. *J. Trauma* **32**(1): 28–31.

9. **Bulger, E.M., Arneson, M.A., Mock, C.N. and Jurkovich, G.J.** (2000) Rib fractures in the elderly. *J. Trauma* **48**(6): 1040–1046.

10. **Hunt, D.M. and Schwab, F.J.** (1992) Chest trauma. In: *Diagnostic Radiology in Emergency Medicine* (ed. P. Rosen). Mosby Yearbooks, St. Louis, MO, p. 77.

11. **Bassett, J.S., Gibson, R.D. and Wilson, R.F.** (1968) Blunt injuries to the chest. *J. Trauma* **8**(3): 418–429.

12. **Logan, P.M.** (1999) Is there an association between fractures of the cervical spine and first- and second-rib fractures? *Can. Assoc. Radio. J.* **50**(1): 41–43.

13. **Wilson, J.M., Thomas, A.N., Goodman, P.C., et al.** (1978) Severe chest trauma: morbidity implications of first and second rib fractures in 120 patients. *Arch. Surg.* **113**(7): 846–849.

14. **Collins, J.** (2000) Chest wall trauma. *J. Thorac. Imag.* **15**(2): 112–119.

15. **Maloney, J.V., Jr, Schnutzer, K.J. and Raschke, F.** (1961) Paradoxical respiration and 'pendelluft'. *J. Thorac. Cardiovasc. Surg.* **41**: 291.

16. **Restifo, K.M. and Kelen, G.D.** (1994) Case Report: sternal fracture from a seatbelt. *J. Emerg. Med.* **12**: 321–323.

17. **Hamilton, J.R., Dearden, C. and Rutherford, W.H.** (1984) Myocardial contusion associated with fracture of the sternum: important features of the seat belt syndrome. *Injury* **16**(3): 155–156.

18. **Purkiss, S.F. and Graham, T.R.** (1993) Sternal fractures. *Br. J. Hosp. Med.* **50**(2–3): 107–112.

19. **Brookes, J.G., Dunn, R.J. and Rogers, I.R.** (1993) Sternal fractures: A retrospective analysis of 272 cases. *J. Trauma* **35**(1): 46–54.

20. **Roy-Shapiro, A., Levi, I. and Khoda, J.** (1994) Sternal fractures: A red flag or a red herring. *J. Trauma* **37**(1): 59–61.

21. **Henley, M.B., Peter, R.E., Benirschke, S.K., et al.** (1991) External fixation of sternum for thoracic trauma. *J. Ortho. Trauma* **5**(4): 493-497.

22. **Harris, R.D. and Harris, J.H., Jr** (1988) The prevalence and significance of missed scapular fractures in blunt trauma. *Am. J. Radiol.* **151**(4): 747–750.

23. **Fulton, R.L. and Peter, E.T.** (1970) The progressive nature of pulmonary contusion. *Surgery* **67**(3): 499–506.

24. **Trinkle, J.K., Furman, R.W., Hinshaw, M.A., et al.** (1973) Pulmonary contusion. *Ann. Thorac. Surg.* **16**(6): 568–573.

25. **Hoff, S.T., Shotts, S.D., Edd, V.A., et al.** (1994) Outcome of isolated pulmonary contusion in blunt trauma patients. *Am. Surg.* **60**(2): 138–142.

26. **Adoumie, R., Shennib, H., Brown, R., et al.** (1993) Differential lung ventilation. Applications beyond the operating room. *J. Thorac. Cardiovasc. Surg.* **105**(2): 229–233.

27. **Richardson, J.D., Franz, J.L., Grover, F.L., et al.** (1974) Pulmonary contusion and hemorrhage: crystalloid versus colloid replacement. *J. Surg. Res.* **16**(4): 330–336.

28. **Luchette, F.A., Barie, P.S., Oswanski, M.F., et al.** (2000) Practice management guidelines for prophylactic antibiotic use in tube thoracostomy for traumatic hemothorax: The EAST practice management guidelines work group. *J. Trauma* **48**(4): 753–757.

29. **Thomas, A.N.** (1982) Discussion of Graham *et al.* Innominate vascular injury. *J. Trauma* **22**: 655.

30. **O'Brien, J., Cohen, M., Solit, R., et al.** (1994) Thoracoscopic drainage and decortication as definitive treatment for empyema thoracis following penetrating chest injury. *J. Trauma* **36**(4): 536–539.

31. **Nicholas, J.M. and Dulchavsky, S.A.** (1992) Successful use of autologous fibrin gel in traumatic bronchopleural fistula: case report. *J. Trauma* **32**(1): 87–88.

32. **Moylan, J.A., Jr, Witmore, D.W., Mouton, D.E.,** *et al.* (1972) Early diagnosis of inhalation injury using 133-xenon lung scan. *Ann. Surg.* **176**(4): 477–484.

33. **Baumgartner, F., Shepard, B., de Virgilo, C.,** *et al.* (1990) Tracheal and main bronchial disruptions after blunt chest trauma: presentation and management. *Ann. Thorac. Surg.* **50**(1): 569–574.

34. **Deslauriers, J., Beaulieu, M., Archambault, G.** *et al.* (1982) Diagnosis and long term follow-up of major bronchial disruptions due to non-penetrating trauma. *Ann. Thorac. Surg.* **33**(1): 32–39.

35. **Taskinen, S.O., Salo, J.A., Halttunen, P.E.A. and Sovijarvi, A.R.A.** (1989) Tracheobronchial rupture due to blunt chest trauma: a follow-up study. *Ann. Thorac. Surg.* **48**(6): 846–849.

36. **Jones, W.S., Mavroudis, C., Richardson, J.D.,** *et al.* (1984) Management of tracheobronchial disruption resulting from blunt trauma. *Surgery* **95**(3): 319–323.

37. **Roxburgh, J.C.** (1987) Rupture of the tracheobronchial tree. *Thorax* **42**(9): 681–688.

38. **Fabian, T.C., Richardson, J.D., Croce, M.A.,** *et al.* (1997) Prospective study of blunt aortic injury: Multicenter trial of the American Association for the Surgery of Trauma. *J. Trauma* **42**(3): 374–380.

39. **Nagy, K., Fabian, T., Rodman, G., Fulda, G.,** *et al.* (2000) Guidelines for the diagnosis and management of blunt aortic injury: An EAST practice management guidelines work group. *J. Trauma* **48**(6): 1128–1143.

40. **Fabian, T.C., Davis, K.A., Gavant, M.L.,** *et al.* (1998) Prospective study of blunt aortic injury: helical CT is diagnostic and antihypertensive therapy reduces rupture. *Ann. Surg.* **227**(5): 666–676.

41. **Mirvis, S.E., Shanmuganathan, K., Buell, J. and Rodriguez, A.** (1998) Use of spiral computed tomography for the assessment of blunt trauma patients with potential aortic injury. *J. Trauma* **45**(5): 922–930.

42. **Fischer, R.G. and Hadlock, F.** (1981) Laceration of the thoracic aorta and brachiocephalic arteries by blunt trauma: report of 54 cases and review of the literature. *Radiol. Clin. N. Am.* **19**(1): 91–110.

43. **Gates, J.D., Clair, D.G. and Hechtman, D.H.** (1994) Thoracic aortic dissection with renal artery involvement following blunt thoracic trauma: Case report. *J. Trauma* **36**(3): 430–432.

44. **Nienaber, C.A., von Kodolitsch, Y., Nicholas, V.,** *et al.* (1993) The diagnosis of thoracic aortic dissection by noninvasive imaging procedures. *N. Engl. J. Med.* **328**(1): 1–9.

45. **Gammie, J.S., Katz, W.E., Swanson, E.R. and Peitzman, A.B.** (1996) Acute aortic dissection after blunt trauma. *J. Trauma* **40**(1): 126–127.

46. **Perchinsky, M., Gin, K. and Mayo, J.R.** (1998) Trauma-associated dissection of the aorta. *J. Trauma* **45**(3): 626–629.

47. **Faraci, R.M. and Westcott, J.L.** (1976) Dissecting hematoma of the aorta secondary to blunt chest trauma. *Radiology* **123**(3): 569–574.

48. **Fabian, T.C., Cicala, M.R., Croce, M.A.,** *et al.* (1991) A prospective evaluation of myocardial contusion: correlation of significant arrythmia and cardiac output with CPK-MB measurements. *J. Trauma* **31**(5): 653–659.

49. **Feliciano, D.V. and Rozycki, G.S.** (1999) Advances in the diagnosis and treatment of thoracic trauma. *Surg. Clin. N. Am.* **79**(6): 1417–1429.

50. **Williams, J.B., Silver, D.G. and Laws, H.L.** (1981) Successful management of heart rupture from blunt trauma. *J. Trauma* **21**: 534.

51. **Parmley, L.F., Manion, W.C. and Mattingly, T.W.** (1958) Nonpenetrating traumatic injury of the heart. *Circulation* **18**: 371.

52. **Ivatury, R.R.** (1996) Injury to the heart. In: Trauma, 3rd Edn (eds E.E. Moore, K.L. Mattox and D.V. Feliciano DV). Appleton & Lange, Stamford, CT, pp. 409–421.

Chapter 23

Techniques of vascular access for invasive hemodynamic monitoring

William T. McGee, MD, MHA, Jay S. Steingrub, MD, and Thomas L. Higgins, MD

Contents

23.1 **Introduction**

Accessing the circulation is often an initial lifesaving procedure in critically ill patients. Central venous catheterization is the most common invasive procedure performed in hospitalized patients. Although routinely performed safely, significant morbidity and even mortality are reported to complicate central venous cannulation. Physicians performing vascular access procedures require an excellent understanding of relevant anatomy and awareness of potential complications.

23.2 **Intraarterial blood pressure monitoring**

Systemic arterial blood pressure and continuous electrocardiographic (EKG) recording is an essential component of hemodynamic monitoring routinely provided to critically ill patients. Although indirect blood pressure measurements via sphygmomanometry are generally accurate for normotensive or hypertensive individuals, measurements are intermittent, subject to technical error, and tend to underestimate systolic blood pressure in the critically ill, hemodynamically unstable patient. Advantages of indwelling catheters include accuracy, access for blood sampling, and continuous acquisition and display of data. Ongoing surveillance of pressure both permits immediate recognition of hypotension or hypertensive episodes and facilitates titration of pharmacotherapy.

23.2.1 Blood pressure physiology

The pressure in the arterial tree is highest at the aortic valve and falls as a result of the resistance of arterioles, but is also affected by the dynamics of blood flow during each cardiorespiratory cycle. Thus, the arterial waveform and the values of systolic and diastolic pressure may be dissimilar at various locations in the arterial tree or during phases of the cardiorespiratory cycle. Invasive direct measurement of blood pressure best corresponds to actual clinical events and thus best reflects the true 'blood pressure'.

Systolic and diastolic pressures represent estimates of the highs and lows of systemic arterial pressure generated during a cardiac cycle, mean systemic pressure being the average pressure. Pressure transducers convert the pressure-induced movement of a diaphragm to an electrical signal proportional to the inducing pressure. The accuracy of physiological data accumulation is dependent on the system's ability to translate these data without distorting the arterial signal as reflected by a visible waveform.

23.2.2 Site selection for invasive blood pressure measurement

Intraarterial catheters may be inserted in the femoral, radial, axillary or dorsalis pedis artery with no data supporting an optimal site. However, large proximal vessels and larger catheters provide more accurate pressure measurements. Smaller catheter diameter in relation to the vessel diameter minimizes the risk of vessel thrombosis. Ideal arteries are those with rich collateral circulation that will assure distal perfusion in the event of thrombosis. The site should be easily accessible for nursing care and not prone to contamination. The radial arteries are the most frequently cannulated site; success rates are approximately 92%[1,2]. In the presence of circulatory shock, the femoral artery may be most easily cannulated and less prone to thrombosis. Employment of the Seldinger technique, which employs a small needle for vessel cannulation followed by a guidewire over which the catheter is placed, has minimized hemorrhagic complications. Axillary artery cannulation is more difficult and has a greater risk of producing particulate or air embolization when retrograde flow occurs during catheter flushing. Brachial artery catheterization is generally avoided because of the lack of collateral circulation around the vessel and the possibility of median nerve injury. As a result of the distal location of the dorsalis pedis artery, invasive pressure monitoring from this site is more prone to waveform artifact.

23.2.3 Complications

Complications with arterial cannulation are usually related to minor bleeding, resulting in localized hematomas. Although commonly asymptomatic and not clinically significant, arterial thromboses occur in up to 20–48% of the catheterizations of greater than 48 h[1,2]. Most data on arterial thromboses involve radial artery cannulation, with the incidence of thrombosis increasing as the ratio of the catheter diameter to vessel diameter increases. Severe ischemia leading to permanent damage occurs in less than 0.5% of arteries cannulated despite the high prevalence of partial or complete arterial thrombosis, if good collateral flow is available. The Allen test is used clinically to test for collateral flow. The ulnar and radial arteries are simultaneously occluded while the patient's hand is held upright. The patient is then asked to open and close his or her fist until the fingers appear blanched. To check for collateral flow, the ulnar artery is released; evidence of return of circulation should appear promptly. If prolonged beyond 4 s, collateral flow is thought to be insufficient and this site should probably be abandoned in favor of another site. Using a Doppler probe beyond the occlusion of the radial artery to assess the return of a signal when the ulnar artery is released is an alternative method to the visual test. Local neurologic complications of radial and axillary catheterization are rare, but have been attributed to median nerve or brachial plexus compression by hematomas. The incidence of catheter-related sepsis is rare.

23.2.4 Cannulation procedure

The procedure should be explained to the patient, informed consent obtained for non-emergency procedures, and the patient made comfortable with appropriate sedatives and analgesia. An operative field should be large enough so that the sterility of the required catheters and wires can be maintained. Local anesthesia should be obtained through a 25-gauge needle utilizing a 1% lidocaine solution. Infiltration of deeper tissue with local anesthetic is often required for femoral and brachial sites.

23.2.5 Radial artery

The Allen test is performed. The patient's wrist is hyperextended and held in place with an arm board and gauze dressing so that the wrist is exposed. Once the wrist is extended and fixed to the arm board, a wash is performed and a sterile field obtained. The artery is then palpated between the first and second fingers. The entry site is typically 1–1½ cm cephalad from the junction of the arm and the hand. Typically, the best approach is to find the area of maximal arterial pulsation. A 20-gauge or smaller catheter over the needle cannulation is typically used with or without a guidewire. The needle is held at an approximately 30–45° angle above the skin toward the direction of blood flow (i.e. cephalad) aiming directly at the pulsation. Once pulsatile blood flow is noted, the catheter should be gently slipped into the artery with a slight rotatory motion while holding the needle guide perfectly still. If a guidewire is to be used at this point, it should now be inserted through the needle into the vessel and the catheter advanced over it. Occasionally the back wall of the radial artery is penetrated. In this circumstance the pulsatile blood flow will be transient. Simply backing the needle catheter assembly out slowly and assessing for the return of pulsatile blood flow will often locate the vessel in this situation.

The catheter should then be hooked up to the pressure tubing, quickly flushed and then assessed for the adequacy of the arterial tracing. Once confirmed within the artery by visual waveform analysis, the catheter should be secured using tape, a stitch or one of the securing devices without needles such as Stat Lock[3]. If cannulation fails, there may be anatomic or technical problems why this vessel cannot be entered. Radial artery cannulation is associated with a very high success rate, thus we recommend no greater than four separate arterial sticks before abandoning one site and moving to another. Patency of radial artery catheters is enhanced by placing the catheter close to the bend of the wrist[4].

23.2.6 Femoral artery

The femoral artery is palpated just below the inguinal ligament in the groin. It has the advantage of being a fairly large vessel and may be easier to palpate in shock patients. The artery is palpated between the first and second digits attempting to define the medial and lateral extent of the vessel. A fairly steep angle of entry, often between 60 and 90°, must be employed because of the depth of the vessel and the lengths of commonly employed needles. A guidewire is always used as part of this technique and should be inserted through the needle once pulsatile blood return is identified. As with all arterial cannulations, the needle and catheter are advanced toward the blood flow. It is often necessary to drop the insertion angle down more in line with the expected course of the artery to facilitate guidewire entry. Once the guidewire is in place, the needle is removed and then the femoral arterial catheter is placed. Dilation of the skin and muscle is recommended to provide a tract through which the catheter can be easily slid. If the skin entry site is tight, a small stab incision can be made with the Number 11 blade facing away from the wire to allow easier passage of the dilator and catheter.

23.2.7 Dorsalis pedis artery

Assessment of the accuracy of collateral flow should be obtained. Similar to the Allen test, the dorsalis pedis and posterior tibial artery should be simultaneously occluded while assessing blood flow to the great toe. This can be performed by either placing a Doppler along the course of the dorsalis pedis artery distal to the occlusion or using a visual assessment of the great toe while the posterior tibial artery is released. Again, either return of color or prompt return of pulsation would indicate that adequate collateral flow is present. The procedure proceeds similarly to radial artery cannulation. Hyperextension of the foot is sometimes thought to be helpful and typically

a catheter of no greater than 20 gauge should be used.

23.2.8 Axillary artery

Axillary cannulation is rarely used and associated with a higher failure rate. This approach has a more significant potential for cerebral embolization during catheter flushing especially if done on the right side because of the proximity to the central circulation and the carotid artery. For this reason, axillary artery cannulation is almost always done on the left side.

The patient is positioned with their hand under their head to allow maximal exposure of the axilla. The vessel is then palpated and can typically be entered with a catheter over the needle type of device, as the vessel is fairly superficial at this point.

23.2.9 Brachial artery

The brachial artery is uncommonly used, as the collateral circulation around this vessel is often inadequate. The Allen test should be performed before brachial artery cannulation. Because of the close proximity of the radial nerve in this area, arterial bleeding has been associated with a compressive neuropathy of the median nerve in those patients in whom bleeding is a complication of the technique.

23.3 Central venous access

Access to the circulation is required for almost all therapies in hospitalized patients. Besides inability to cannulate the peripheral circulation, there are many other reasons why central venous access may be required. Indications for central venous cannulation are numerous and are listed in *Table 23.1*.

23.3.1 Site selection

Site selection should consider the operator's expertise with any particular technique, and anatomic considerations for a particular patient. Often the subclavian or femoral route is more accessible in an acutely injured patient who may require intubation and also have a

Table 23.1 Indications for central venous cannulation

Diagnostic uses
- Pulmonary artery catheterization (right internal jugular preferred)
- Central venous pressure monitoring
- Endomyocardial biopsies (right internal jugular preferred)
- Pulmonary angiography
- Differentiation of supraventricular from ventricular arrhythmias
- Transvenous hepatic and cardiac biopsy and other rare indications

Therapeutic uses
- Administration of large amounts of fluid, hemodialysis, or total parenteral nutrition
- Access for hemodialysis, hemofiltration or plasmapheresis
- Transvenous pacemaker insertion (right internal jugular preferred)
- Removal of embolized thrombi or catheters
- Aspiration of air from the right atrium during neurosurgical procedures
- Valvuloplasty, angioscopy, and other rare indications

cervical collar in place when first seen. Other anatomic considerations peculiar to individual patients such as a short, thick neck, prior arterial surgery along one of the adjacent arteries, presence of localized skin infection, burns or other unique anatomic variations guide site selection. In patients with chest tubes, it is preferable to use the side where the tube is already in place for subclavian vein cannulations. In patients with a single lung, however, a pneumothorax will not be tolerated, and the side of the solitary lung should be avoided. Femoral venous catheters may pose an independent risk for venous thrombosis, and in those patients already at high risk for this complication this route should be avoided if possible[4,5]. For patients with traumatic brain injury or other causes of increased intracranial pressure, occlusion of the internal jugular vein secondary to thrombosis or hematoma may increase the risk of that approach. In patients with coagulopathy, a compressible vessel is preferred, as bleeding is a common complication of venipuncture and especially inadvertent

arterial puncture. The subclavian vein is not a compressible vein. The relative advantages and disadvantages of internal jugular vein (IJV) versus subclavian vein (SCV) are listed in *Table 23.2*. Although femoral catheters are not truly central venous catheters because they typically do not enter the chest, other than for pressure monitoring, they are used identically to other central venous catheters.

23.3.2 Preparation and equipment

All equipment necessary for this technique should be available at the bedside before a cannulation attempt. This would also include any drugs necessary for sedation, pain control, and local anesthesia, along with cleansing materials for the skin and those materials necessary for the preparation of a sterile field. Patient hair likely to interfere with sterility should be clipped, not shaved, as shaving may increase infection risk. In our practice, cap, mask, gloves and gown are utilized following a thorough washing of the hands.

The surgical site is prepared with antimicrobial solution and gently scrubbed with a circular motion progressing from the center of the site outward. Skin preparation should be performed first so that there is an adequate amount of time (approximately 5 min) for anti-microbial action.

After sterile skin preparation, new gloves should be utilized, and the insertion site draped with sterile towels to prevent any equipment, specifically the catheter or the guidewire, from touching a non-sterile area. A sterile field large enough to accommodate at least twice the length of the guidewire is recommended. The opening in the barrier protection to the skin should be large enough to facilitate cannulation and palpation of landmarks. For cooperative patients, local infiltration of 1% lidocaine often provides adequate analgesia. For patients who are particularly anxious or uncomfortable, systemic therapy with anxiolytics and narcotics may be necessary. Attempting vascular access procedures especially in the chest and neck in an uncooperative or combative patient can result in

Table 23.2 Advantages and disadvantages of neck versus clavicular approaches

	Advantages	Disadvantages
Internal jugular vein	Good landmarks, vein may be visible and palpable Small pneumothorax risk (<0.1%) Compressible bleeding site with good hemostasis after inadvertent arterial puncture Easiest Swan–Ganz and pacemaker passage from right side	Obscured landmarks in obese patients Tracheostomy appliances problematic Dressing hard to secure, possible secretion contamination hazard Relative discomfort in some patients Contraindication with high intracranial pressure
*Subclavian vein**	May be the largest target in vasoconstricted states Fair landmarks, if patient obese, edematous Dressing easily secured Generally comfortable	1–5% pneumothorax risk Avoid with chronic obstructive pulmonary disease, high positive and expiratory pressure, coagulopathies Noncompressible artery if punctured Slightly less ease of passage for Swan–Ganz, pacemaker

*The supraclavicular approach to the subclavian and brachiocephalic veins, as taught and performed by Parsa[6], appears to have comparable success, and lower immediate complication rates, than reported for subclavian and IJV approaches. Reproduced with permission from W.B. Saunders.

inappropriate motion by the patient at critical junctures during the procedure and lead to potentially life-threatening injuries. In select circumstances, intubation and paralysis are required. While the prep solution dries and the local anesthetic takes effect, the operator should remove the catheter from its packaging, flush the port(s) with saline or heparin flush solution, place any necessary end-caps, and lay the prepared catheter on the sterile field where it will be quickly accessible. Using a 25-gauge needle, a skin weal is raised over the anticipated entry site. Following this, a 22-gauge needle is passed through the anesthetized dermis to infiltrate subcutaneous tissue and occasionally bone if contact with the clavicle is expected to be made.

23.3.3 Positioning

Positioning of the patient typically is the final preparation step, as internal jugular and subclavian vein approaches typically involve the head down (Trendelenburg) position. Many patients find this position uncomfortable and it is relatively contraindicated with elevated intracranial pressure as well as associated with increased nosocomial pneumonia risk. For inter-

nal jugular and subclavian vein cannulations, however, the head down (Trendelenburg) position has been shown to significantly increase the diameter of these vessels. A secondary benefit of this position is that not only is the size of the target vessel increased, but also the pressure within the vessel is greater, making the venipuncture simpler. Finally, in spontaneously breathing patients, because of the increased venous pressure, this position significantly reduces the risk of venous air emboli. In general, the more Trendelenburg that the patient can tolerate, the better, as these advantages are enhanced as the venous pressure increases.

For femoral venous approaches the patient should be flat without any bend at the hip with the toes positioned toward the ceiling or allowed to fall slightly to the side. Patient comfort is essential as in complicated cases these positions may have to be maintained for longer than anticipated. Operator comfort when performing this procedure is also important as an awkward or uncomfortable position during the cannulation attempt will result in fatigue and a lower chance of success. Beds that can be placed in full Trendelenburg position and then raised to the appropriate height for the operator are ideal. In the ICU setting, significant attention to positioning of ventilator tubing, IV tubing, and monitors is often necessary.

Patients with difficulty breathing, especially patients with congestive heart failure, may not be able to tolerate even lying flat, let alone head down position. For these patients, attempting to cannulate the vein quickly and then allowing the patient to resume a semi-recumbent position once the risk for air embolization is minimized (i.e. the guidewire is in place), is a possible alternative. Once the guidewire is in place, the rest of the procedure can be performed with the patient in a semi-recumbent position with the head even as high as 45°. Some patients will require intubation and mechanical ventilation before this line placement. We do not recommend attempting this procedure with the head up in a spontaneously breathing patient. In patients with increased intracranial pressure, an attempt can be made with the patient lying flat, but Trendelenburg position is also acceptable as long as the intracranial pressure (ICP) is being monitored. Pre-treatment with pentobarbital, hyperventilation and mannitol can also be employed. The goal should be to have the head down for as short a period of time as possible.

23.3.4 Cannulation procedure

The vessel is entered with either an angiocath or a hollow steel needle. Once the vessel is entered and free flow of venous blood is confirmed, the syringe is gently twisted off the needle or the angiocath advanced into the vessel and the guidewire inserted to approximately half its length. Most guidewires are approximately twice the length of the catheter. For those insertions where there is a potential for the guidewire to enter the heart (internal jugular and subclavian vein approaches) the EKG should be monitored for atrial and ventricular dysrrhythmias. If arrhythmias are encountered, simply withdrawing the wire from the heart, but not out of the vessel, is

usually all that is necessary to terminate the dysrhythmias. Persistent arrhythmias generally respond to a bolus injection (100 mg) of lidocaine (see Chapter 11).

Once the wire is in place, the needle or angiocath is withdrawn. The wire should be held at all times to prevent inadvertent loss within the venous system. Wires do not become pulled into the venous circulation by the flow of blood, but can be inadvertently pushed inward with catheter insertion. Simply clamping the guidewire above the skin frees up the operator's other hand as needed. A Number 11 scalpel blade is be used to cut down along the wire, with the cutting edge of the blade facing away from the wire. The scalpel is then removed, turned 180° and a similar cut is made on the other side of the wire. The depth and width of the cut should be individualized. In thin patients, especially where the vein is visible just below the skin (i.e. some internal jugular vein sites), a very superficial nick of the skin will suffice. In others with lots of muscle mass, fatty tissue or old scarring, deeper cuts will be necessary. In all circumstances, the goal is to open the skin and possibly some of the adjacent subcutaneous tissue and muscle, not the vein itself.

The dilator is now threaded over the wire through the skin and muscle and into the vein. Rarely does more than half the length of the dilator need to go through the skin. Dilators tend to be very stiff and should be advanced only if they move fairly smoothly. Occasionally, the dilator will become stuck on a kink in the wire and will be very difficult to advance. This is remedied by pulling the wire back 1–2 cm, moving the kink back within the dilator, and then proceeding. At no time should the dilator be further advanced if significant resistance is encountered. If the tip of the dilator splays out, it becomes useless and a new dilator will be needed.

Once the dilator is removed, expect fairly significant bleeding through the venipuncture. This is minimized by direct pressure, but more completely by rapid insertion of the central venous catheter. The catheter should have already been prepared by its removal from the package, placement of appropriate caps and flushing of the catheter, typically with a heparinized solution. For a multi-lumen catheter, it should also be noted, ahead of time, which port the wire will exit from so that this cap can be intentionally left off.

The guidewire is now threaded back through the catheter until it can be grabbed at the distal end. Once the guidewire is securely grasped, the catheter is advanced over the wire to the proper position within the vein. When using the femoral approach, the entire catheter should be inserted into the vein. For insertions where the tip of the catheter may potentially enter the heart, i.e. subclavian vein or internal jugular vein sites of entry, the length of catheter to be inserted will vary based on the patient's size. Correct insertion should leave the catheter in the distal superior vena cava, but outside the right atrium. Optimal insertion length for those catheters placed via subclavian or internal jugular veins is 15 cm[7–9]. In shorter patients, especially for right-sided approaches, shorter insertion distances (typically 13 cm) are needed to keep the catheter tip outside of the heart.

The wire is now withdrawn, the catheter is recapped, and all ports are checked for blood return and then flushed. Occasionally, one or more ports will flush easily, but not produce a blood return on aspiration. This can be caused by suction between the catheter port and the vessel wall, and manipulating the catheter within the vein or twisting it often solves the problem.

23.3.5 Post-insertion tasks
Once the catheter has been flushed, it should be secured in place, either with a suture through the appropriate attachment points on the catheter, or using one of the newly available securing devices such as the Stat Lock[3]. Sterile blood cultures may be drawn at this point if desired. It is the operator's responsibility to dispose of all sharp items (needles, scalpels, sutures) and blood-contaminated supplies (dilator, angiocath) in the proper receptacles. A dressing is now applied. Radiographic confirmation of placement and potential complications (i.e. pneumothorax) is not always needed clinically but may be mandated by individual hospital policy.

The catheter tip should be located outside the heart, ideally parallel to the superior vena cava (*Figure 23.1*). A procedure note including the date, time, indication, consent, anesthetic, and particular anatomic or procedural issues should be recorded.

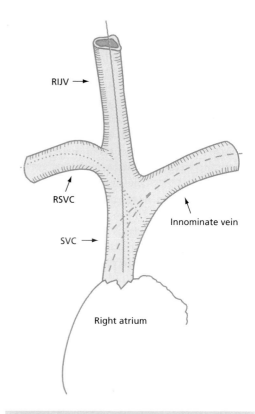

RIJV

RSVC

Innominate vein

SVC

Right atrium

Figure 23.1 Catheter positions relative to the superior vena cava (SVC) based on insertion site and proximity to the right atrium. Catheter angulation relative to the SVC is minimized when the catheter tip is in the distal SVC near the right atrium for all insertion locations other than the right internal jugular vein (RIJV). RIJV insertions tend to be parallel to the vessel wall regardless of location within the SVC.

23.3.6 Precautions

Venous catheterization from any selected site will be unsuccessful up to 35% of the time. We do not recommend more than four needle passes at any selected site. Success is most likely with the first needle pass and diminishes on subsequent attempts, but each pass of the needle carries a risk for puncture of adjacent structures. Thus, the risk–benefit ratio increases with subsequent passes of the needle.

If inadvertent arterial puncture occurs with a finder needle or angiocath, the needle or catheter should be withdrawn as soon as this is recognized and pressure applied to compressible vessel. Direct pressure will be required for longer periods in those patients who do have a coagulopathy. In those patients with coagulopathy in whom this complication is recognized with the catheter already in place, it is probably prudent to correct the coagulopathy before withdrawal of the catheter. Every effort should be made to confirm intravenous and exclude intraarterial placement before using a vessel dilator. If there is any doubt, the pressure in the vessel can be transduced or estimated by the height of blood in attached tubing, or a sample sent for blood gas analysis. Visual inspection of blood pulsatility and color can be unreliable in patients who are hypoxic, in shock, or compromised by tricuspid regurgitation and volume overload.

If the arterial picture is not recognized with the finder needle and the vessel has been dilated (as for triple-lumen or cordis sheath placement) it is best to leave the catheter or dilator in place and obtain an immediate vascular surgery consultation for repair of the vessel.

Besides the hemodynamic clues or obvious external or subcutaneous bleeding, a new pleural effusion in a patient in whom a subclavian vein or low internal jugular venopuncture has been attempted or completed should warrant investigation for hemothorax and evaluation for possible vessel injury.

Never withdraw guidewires against resistance through a needle as the spiral wire may stretch apart or break completely. In those circumstances where the needle is used to guide the wire into the vein, special precautions must be taken to insure the integrity of the wire. If the wire must be withdrawn through the needle and resistance is met, the needle and catheter should be withdrawn simultaneously to prevent shearing of the wire against the needle. Shearing off the wire in an intravascular location is a serious morbid complication. If the wire is withdrawn and intravenous location is reconfirmed, often flipping the wire over from the J end to the straight end will facilitate easier passage.

23.4 Femoral venous cannulation

The femoral venous site typically does not result in central venous cannulation, thus pressure measurements, specifically central venous pressure, cannot be taken. However, for all other reasons for central venous cannulation, the femoral vein is equivalent to other sites. Although some data suggest increased infectious disease risks for this approach, other data do not[10,11]. Thrombotic complications of the deep venous system are probably related to use of femoral venous catheters, especially in a pediatric population[11–13].

Benefits of the femoral approach include accessibility during acute resuscitation, reduced risk of significant mechanical complications, an easily compressible vessel, and, for patients with respiratory failure or increased intracranial pressure, no need to place the patient in Trendelenburg position. Femoral venous cannulation may be the simplest and safest approach for inexperienced operators[13,14].

23.4.1 Anatomy

The femoral pulse is the primary guide for femoral venous cannulation. The vein is located just medial to where the pulse is palpated. The entry site of choice is below the inguinal ligament wherever the pulse is most prominent. Above the inguinal ligament, the vein runs posterior by and becomes the iliac vein. Below the inguinal ligament the vein lies within the femoral sheath just medial to the femoral artery. In pulseless patients, 2 cm below the inguinal ligament and approximately one-third of the way from the pubic tubercle to the anterior–superior iliac spine will serve as a good starting point (*Figure 23.2*).

Once the artery is located by palpation, inserting the needle approximately 1 cm medial to the pulse often results in success. The needle is either inserted in a perpendicular plane or 15–30° off the perpendicular plane with the needle oriented in the direction of blood flow. Negative pressure should be applied to the syringe throughout the entire procedure once the needle has passed through the skin. Evacuating air from the syringe before the procedure will minimize clotting. Although anatomically a superficial structure at this location, 4–6 cm depth of penetration or more is typically required to access the vein. Once a free flow of blood is established, the procedure proceeds as described in Section 23.3.4.

23.4.2 Caveats

Hip flexion has the potential to cause femoral catheter kinking. For sick ICU patients who must be maintained in bed, this is often not an issue. Femoral catheters tend to function even with the head of the bed up to 30 or 45°. If catheter location is inhibiting patients' weaning or rehabilitation progress, a new site should be chosen.

Although a finder needle may be helpful for femoral venous cannulation, those included in most kits may not be long enough to locate the vessel. For the same reason, using a catheter over the needle technique for initial femoral venous access does not provide any advantage and may actually make the procedure more cumbersome.

23.5 Internal jugular vein

The approach from the right internal jugular vein provides the most direct access to the heart, facilitating placement of Swan–Ganz catheters, transvenous pacemakers and

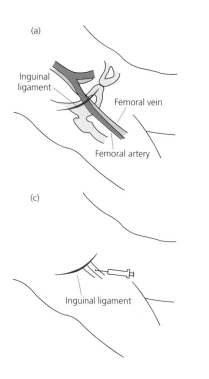
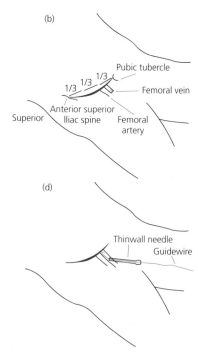

(a)

Inguinal ligament

Femoral vein

Femoral artery

(b)

Pubic tubercle

1/3 1/3 1/3

Femoral vein

Superior

Anterior superior Iliac spine

Femoral artery

(c)

Inguinal ligament

(d)

Thinwall needle

Guidewire

Figure 23.2 Anatomic location of femoral vein below the inguinal ligament.

endomyocardial biopsy. Internal jugular venous cannulation is usually the preferred route for anesthesiologists who are already working at the head of the bed and may have limited access to other anatomic locations. In patients with coagulopathies, the clavicular routes are relatively contraindicated because of inability to compress a bleeding vessel. Finally, because of the extremely low incidence of pleural complications associated with internal jugular venous cannulation, this technique is also preferred in those patients in whom a pneumothorax would not be well tolerated; specifically patients with severe acute or chronic lung disease, or these about to undergo anesthesia and positive pressure ventilation without a chest radiograph to exclude pneumothorax.

23.5.1 Anatomy

The internal jugular vein emerges from the base of the skull through the jugular foramen and enters the carotid sheath anterior and lateral to the internal carotid artery. The cephalad internal jugular vein usually lies medial to the anterior portion of the sternocleidomastoid muscle, runs beneath the triangle formed by the two heads of the sternocleidomastoid in its middle segment, and medial to the anterior portion of the clavicular head of the muscle in the lower segment (*Figure 23.3*). Beneath the clavicle, the right internal jugular vein joins the subclavian vein to form the innominate vein, which continues in a straight path to the superior vena cava. The left internal jugular vein joins the left subclavian vein at almost a right angle. Consequently, any catheter inserted through left-sided approaches must negotiate this turn. The local anatomy is equally important, as complications occur from injury to these structures. The carotid artery usually lies medial to the internal jugular vein throughout its course within the carotid sheath. The artery is usually posterior-medial to and sometimes partially enveloped by the internal jugular vein. Medial and posterior to the internal jugular vein, and the carotid artery, lie the stellate ganglion and the

cervical sympathetic trunk. Deep to this are the roots of the brachial plexus. The phrenic nerve is usually lateral to the vascular bundle, whereas the vagus nerve lies between the internal jugular vein and the carotid artery. Branches of the laryngeal nerves are medial to the vascular bundle. Near the junction of the internal jugular vein and the subclavian vein is the pleural dome. This is usually higher on the left. The thoracic duct lies behind the left internal jugular vein and usually enters the superior margin of the subclavian near the jugular subclavian junction.

23.5.2 Ultrasound and internal jugular venous cannulation

The use of ultrasound has significantly enhanced safety while better defining anatomy of internal jugular venous cannulation[15,16]. Information derived from ultrasound examination gives better appreciation of the following:

- The caliber of the vein usually increases as it progresses toward the clavicle.
- The distance from the skin surface to the vein increases as it approaches the clavicle.

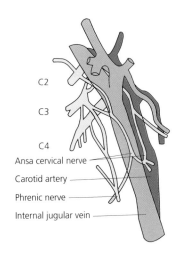

C2
C3
C4
Ansa cervical nerve
Carotid artery
Phrenic nerve
Internal jugular vein

Figure 23.3 Typical anatomy of IJV. The vein lies just lateral to the carotid artery (CA) below the sternocleidomastoid muscle (SCM). Multiple nerves are located in this area.

- Palpation or retraction of the carotid artery during cannulation attempts markedly decreases and occasionally obliterates the ultrasound image of the low-pressure internal jugular vein. Often during veni-puncture, the vein will collapse simply as a result of the pressure exerted by the needle. For this reason, it is important to maintain negative pressure on the syringe as the needle is backed out through the skin, as this is often the time when successful can-nulation is noted. Intravascular volume loading either during or before the pro-cedure may be helpful in increasing the size of the target vessel.

- Occasionally the carotid artery is found posterior to the internal jugular vein, mak-ing it difficult to cannulate with usual familiar landmarks (*Figure 23.4*).

- Placing the patient in the head down Trendelenburg position or using the Valsalva maneuver increases the size of the vessel.

- The internal jugular vein is a superficial structure. The average perpendicular dis-tance from the skin to the vein at the level of the cricoid cartilage is approximately 1.5 cm. For this reason, the needle should

rarely be inserted to beyond 4 cm in most patients (*Figure 23.4*).

- Multiple anatomic variations exist, and for those patients in whom cannulation proceeds with difficulty we recommend early application of ultrasound. Use of ultrasound for cannulation is now recog-nized as an important safety initiative by the Agency for Healthcare Research and Quality (AHRQ).

23.5.3 Cannulation procedure: median approach

Although multiple approaches to the internal jugular vein have been described, our experi-ence has been that knowledge of two approaches (median and anterior) is sufficient.

For the median approach, the two heads of the sternocleidomastoid should be located and followed to their insertions on the clavicle and sternum, respectively. The clavicle forms the base of the sternocleidomastoid triangle. The sternal notch should also be identified as this aids identification of the sternal head of the sternocleidomastoid. The carotid artery should be gently palpated and localized. The angle of the mandible along with the junction between the clavicle and the sternum should also be identified. Identification of the thyroid

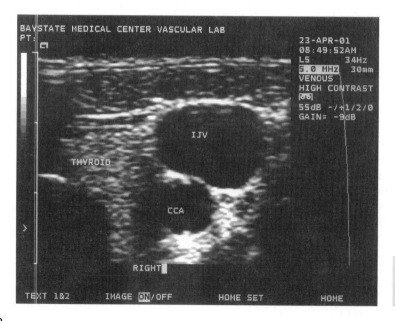

Figure 23.4 Ultrasound image of IJV overlying carotid artery.

cartilage and the cricothyroid membrane may also be useful in difficult cannulations. The more landmarks that can be identified, the easier it will be locate the vessel. However, in many patients the only identifiable landmark will be the carotid pulsation. Even in massively obese patients, the angle of the mandible and medial articulation of the clavicle can be identified. Bisecting a line between these two points will approximate the apex of the sterno-cleidomastoid triangle. This is often found at the level of the cricothyroid membrane. Identifying these additional structures will provide additional assurance that initial site selection is correct.

At a minimum, the carotid artery needs to be identified. Except for urgent or emergent venous access, we use a 22-gauge 2-inch finder needle. The incidence of carotid artery puncture during internal jugular vein cannulation may be as high as 10%[17,18]. If this occurs with a small finder needle, there is typically no adverse consequence and the procedure may still proceed rapidly. If the carotid artery is punctured with either the 18-gauge hollow wall steel needle or the 16-gauge angiocath over 20-gauge needle, a minimum of 5 min of direct pressure over the vessel must be applied.

The needle is placed at the apex of the triangle just lateral to where the carotid pulsation is felt and is advanced in a perpendicular direction with the plane of the needle being midway between the midsternum and ipsilateral nipple (Figure 23.5). Once the vein is found, this needle can be left in place while the catheterizing needle is placed just caudad to it using the same angle of entry and approximate depth. If this proves too cumbersome, the finder needle can be withdrawn, mentally recording the angle and the depth. The cannulating needle is then passed through the identical skin puncture site.

We recommend vessel cannulation using an angiocath rather than a needle, although both are typically provided in most kits. Most kits include a 20-gauge needle with a 16-gauge angiocath over it. Puncturing the carotid artery with a 20-gauge needle is less problem-

atic then when larger cannulating needles are used. The angiocath provides very secure venous access once the vessel is entered, as the entire length of the angiocath can be inserted down the vessel. A problem with this technique is that if the vein is not entered on the first pass of the needle, the angiocath must be held together as it is withdrawn, otherwise the angiocath will separate and potentially make that system non-functional.

A perpendicular approach to the vessel or approximately 30° off the perpendicular with the tip of the needle pointed caudad is the preferred angle to the skin. Once the vessel

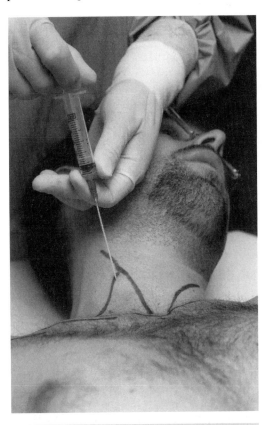

Figure 23.5 Position of cannulating needle for median approach to the IJV. The needle is placed at the apex of the sternocleidomastoid triangle using a steep angle of incidence to the skin (60–90°). It is advanced in a plane midway between the center of the sternum and the ipsilateral nipple. The carotid pulsation should be just medial to the venipuncture.

is entered, the angiocath is further advanced slightly (1–2 mm) while simultaneously placing the syringe more in line with the anatomic direction of the vessel. The syringe is now reaspirated to confirm intravenous location and the angiocath is threaded into the vessel with a twisting motion. Once the angiocath is in place, direct pressure over the internal jugular vein can be applied using three or four fingers to minimize the risk of venous air embolization and back leak. If a hollow steel needle is used, once the vein is accessed the needle should be advanced slightly to assure intravenous location of the entire needle tip. The needle is not advanced further at this point, to prevent laceration of the back wall of the vessel. The guidewire is inserted through the needle hub. Using the plain steel needle requires more attention to detail as slight movements of the needle may inadvertently dislodge the needle tip. The hub of the needle needs to be occluded at all times to prevent air entry. Once the wire is inserted through the needle securely into the vein, further catheterization is similar to the other technique. With the angiocath in place, the wire is threaded through the angiocath, and the angiocath is withdrawn.

If the angiocath becomes unusable and a replacement is to be used, two rules should be followed: assure that the wire will fit through the newly selected angiocath; most guidewires will fit through either a 16- or 18-gauge angiocath. A 1¼ inch angiocath would be the minimum length with 2¼ inch being preferred.

23.5.4 Cannulation procedure: anterior approach
One advantage of the anterior approach is that it can be performed with the patient's head in the midline position. Insertion will be at the level of the cricoid, which is palpated as the first landmark. An imaginary horizontal line is drawn to the anterior border of the sternocleidomastoid. The carotid should be palpable here, and the initial jugular will be just lateral to the carotid. With the needle parallel to the body's long axis and entering at a 30–45° angle to the perpendicular plane, the finder needle is

inserted 1–1.5 cm lateral to the carotid. The internal jugular is usually very superficial, no more than 2–4 cm under the skin except in obese or edematous patients. Once the vessel is identified with the finder needle, the angiocath or larger-bore needle is inserted. As blood is aspirated, the needle or angiocath is aligned more closely to the vessel's direction and free flow assured. The Selinger technique is then used to insert first a guidewire and then the final catheter or introducer. As with the median approach, the carotid artery must be identified and care taken not to exert pressure sufficient to activate carotid reflexes. The risk of carotid puncture using the anterior approach argues for the finder needle technique previously described.

23.6 Subclavian vein cannulation

All approaches to the subclavian vein involve the chest and for this reason the risk of pneumothorax with this approach is significant. Most reports indicate an approximately 5% risk of this complication; however, in experienced hands it is significantly less[19,20]. Although the risk of pneumothorax is greater with this approach, the subclavian approach might be preferable to internal jugular venous cannulation during acute resuscitation when the airway is being secured, with difficult landmarks in the neck, and for patient comfort with long-term cannulations.

23.6.1 Anatomy
The anatomic relationship of the subclavian vein to the subclavian artery and the clavicle along with some of the muscular insertions are shown in *Figure 23.6*. The subclavian vein continues from the axillary vein as it crosses over the first rib then proceeds medially, arching cephalad towards its junction with the internal jugular vein close to the manubrial–clavicular junction. Once joined with the internal jugular vein it forms the brachicephalic vein where it then enters the thorax. As the vein proceeds medially over the first rib and under the clavicle, it is anterior and caudad to the subclavian

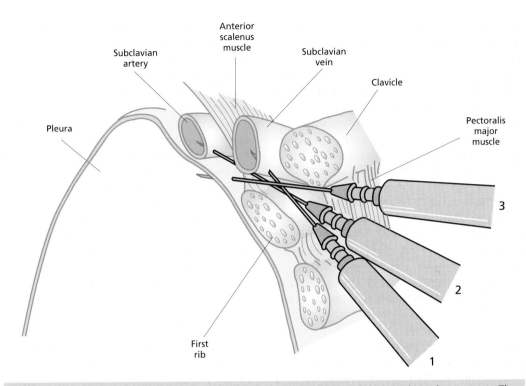

Figure 23.6 Sagittal view of subclavian vein and pertinent superficial and deep perivascular anatomy. The vein is an anterior structure found just underneath the clavicle. Deeper venipuncture attempts are likely to injure either the subclavian artery or pleura.

artery. The vein and artery at this level are separated by the anterior scalenus muscle. As illustrated in *Figure 23.6*, the vein resides just below the clavicle at this point. This is particularly pertinent regarding cannulation of the vein. Approaches just posterior to the clavicle and parallel to it are most likely to result in successful venipuncture. If the position of the needle is moved to form a greater angle relative to the clavicle, the likelihood of subclavian artery or pleural puncture is greater. The vein is covered anteriorly by the pectoralis major muscle, which will always be penetrated first. The medial portions of the vein are completely covered by the clavicle, which will also serve as a guide during cannulation. The pleural dome, which is higher on the left, lies posterior and superior to the subclavian artery. The thoracic duct, which may be a large structure on the left side, crosses the vein just medial to its junction with the internal jugular vein.

Subclavian veins are usually large and often patent as a result of their fibrous attachments. This may be the preferred approach for patients who are hypovolemic or in shock. Multiple approaches to the subclavian vein either above or below the clavicle have been described, but only the two most useful will be presented in detail. All approaches to the subclavian vein are made simpler by placing a small rolled towel between the scapulae to allow the shoulders to fall back. This positioning increases the distance between the first rib and the clavicle.

23.6.2 Supraclavicular approach to the subclavian vein

Supraclavicular approaches to the subclavian vein have primarily been popularized in the emergency room setting especially for hypovolemic patients. This approach to the central circulation provides probably the largest target vessel in the body; the junction of the internal jugular vein (IJV) and subclavian vein. The clavicular notch approach provides easily identifiable landmarks with a very high success rate. As this approach is not terribly different from the medial approach to the internal jugular vein, we find it is easiest with the operator standing at the head of the bed. The base of the triangle formed by the clavicle and the two heads of the sternocleidomastoid muscle is located first. The insertion point for the needle will be just lateral to the mid-point of the base of the triangle, which will also be lateral to where the carotid pulsation is felt. The needle is advanced parallel to the sagittal plane at approximately a 30° angle to place the tip of the needle just under the clavicle (*Figure 23.7*). The vein is typically entered within 4 cm.

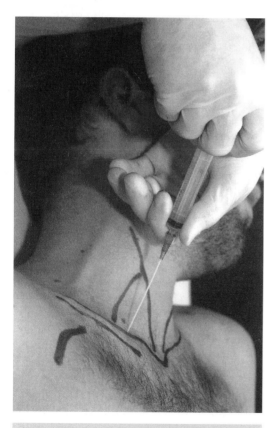

Figure 23.7 Superclavicular approach to subclavian vein (see text).

Picking the needle up towards a more perpendicular location relative to the chest wall is more likely to injure posterior structures. If venipuncture is not accomplished, a slightly more lateral approach may be useful. Essentially, access is at the junction between the internal jugular and subclavian veins. Once blood is aspirated from within the vein, cannulation proceeds as previously described. Because of its similarities to median approaches to the IJV, the use of a finder needle and the angiocath techniques described for the IJV are appropriate in this location. Several variations on this technique exist. Simply moving higher up within the triangle, but using the same needle angles, approximates the low median approach to the internal jugular vein. This is particularly useful in patients who have thick clavicles, which may cause the insertion angle to be greater than desired.

23.6.3 Alternate supraclavicular approach

A second variation on the supraclavicular technique is to place the tip of the cannulating needle just lateral to the clavicular head of the sternocleidomastoid. The tip of the needle is placed at the junction between the clavicle and the clavicular head of the sternocleido-mastoid muscle. The anterior scalene muscle behind which lies the subclavian artery may be appreciated in some patients behind the sternocleidomastoid. The needle is directed somewhat medially to a location below the clavicle above the first rib using a fairly steep approach, approximately 45–60° until blood flow is returned. At that point, the needle is placed more in line with the expected route of the subclavian vein at this location. Again, because the depth of insertion is not expected to be beyond 4 cm in this location, a finder needle and angiocath techniques are appropriate. Although not reported in the literature, because of the initial steeper angle of incidence relative to chest wall, there is some concern for a higher incidence of pneumothorax using these approaches.

23.6.4 Infraclavicular approaches to the subclavian vein

Infraclavicular approaches to the subclavian vein are probably the most common access to this vessel. Positioning a patient for this approach will help facilitate venous access. In addition to placing a roll between the scapulae, another useful technique is to have the arm pulled down under slight traction on the side to be cannulated.

For all infraclavicular approaches, we recommend standing at the side of the bed. The important anatomic landmarks are the clavicle and the suprasternal notch. Multiple initial skin punctures along the clavicle beginning within the distal third and progressing out toward the lateral third have been described. We have had the most success beginning with a point at the mid-clavicle, particularly where the clavicle begins to bend cephalad and the bulk of the insertion of the pectoralis muscle can be felt. These two structures, the clavicle on top and the pectoralis on bottom, form the head of an arrow that aims at the suprasternal notch (*Figure 23.8*). The cannulating needle is grasped such that the tip of the needle is controlled by the index finger. The needle is then inserted directly in line with the arrowhead formed by the clavicle and the major insertion of the pectoralis muscle approximately 1 cm lateral to the clavicle so that it can easily be slipped underneath. The purpose of controlling the tip with the index finger is so that the needle–syringe apparatus can be pressed down toward the patient's bed and the needle advanced under the clavicle with minimal lifting of the syringe. The plane in which the needle travels is as close to parallel to the plane of the floor as possible. If the clavicle is encountered and the hub of the syringe needs to be picked up so that the needle can slide underneath the clavicle, we do not recommend picking the syringe up by any more than 30° off the horizontal plane. Angles above this are much more likely to proceed into deeper structures, such as the subclavian artery and the pleura. It is significantly easier and less risky in

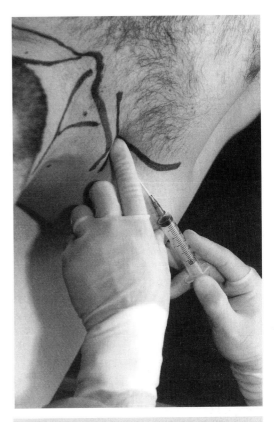

Figure 23.8 Infraclavicular subclavian vein approach. The clavicle on top and the insertion of the pectoralis major on the bottom form the head of an arrow (where the intensivists' index finger is in this figure) that aims at the suprasternal notch. The needle tip is pushed toward the bed and controlled by the index finger to allow the most tangential (close to 0°) insertion possible relative to the chest wall. The needle is advanced toward the suprasternal notch.

these circumstances to choose an insertion point slightly more lateral so that the tip of the needle can be slipped under the clavicle without having to angle the syringe up significantly. The direction of needle travel is now toward the suprasternal notch; constant aspiration on the syringe is maintained as the needle is advanced. In obese patients or those with significant muscle mass, it is not uncommon to have to place the entire length of the needle through the skin, and even encounter dimpling of the skin before the vein is entered.

This provides a particularly challenging situation as the syringe is twisted off the needle, because the pressure from the skin alone may push it out of the vein. It is very important in this circumstance, therefore, to hold the needle in the position in which it is known to be within the vein. The Raulerson syringe, which allows for placement of the guidewire through the hub of the syringe, is particularly useful for infraclavicular subclavian vein approaches when encountering this problem. With this device, once the vein is entered the guidewire can simply be inserted along the hub of the syringe without having to twist the needle off. If in the first pass toward the suprasternal notch the vein is not entered, withdrawing the needle and adjusting the tip slightly more caudad and then reinserting often locates the vessel. If unsuccessful after several passes of the needle (typically no more than four), it is likely that a location more proximal along the clavicle toward the suprasternal notch will be successful compared with a more lateral initial skin puncture.

The clavicle will often be encountered during this approach. As the vein sits just below the clavicle, it is important that the most posterior portion of the clavicle is appreciated and that the needle does not track significantly below this. For this reason, we recommended pushing the needle–syringe assembly down in a plane parallel to the floor utilizing the index finger. Other physicians like to 'march' the needle down the clavicle in small increments until the needle finally slips past. Either approach is fine, as the emphasis should be that the entire assembly of syringe and needle should not be angled to greater than 30° off the plane parallel to the floor.

Orienting the bevel of the needle caudad will safely position the guidewire within the superior vena cava. Because of the typically deeper insertion depth encountered when accessing the subclavian vein, we do not recommend using either a finder needle or an angiocath in this location. Once the vein is entered, central venous cannulation proceeds as previously described.

23.7 Introducer placement

Techniques for placing introducers suitable for the insertion of Swan–Ganz catheters or transvenous pacemakers are different only because of their size. Otherwise, placement of these devices is similar to central venous catheter placement, with a few specific pointers.

23.7.1 Techniques for placing Cordis-type introducers

The introducer should be fully assembled with the dilator in place before venous access. The dilator typically goes through the hemostatic valve and then exits the distal tip of the introducer. It is sometimes easier to first use the dilator by itself to dilate the skin and muscle and then place it through the introducer rather than assembling the whole device initially. A larger skin incision will be necessary than with a central venous catheter. Although more pressure is required to place the introducer through the skin, excessive pressure is not warranted and may damage the introducer. If the introducer is damaged in any way, it should be replaced. Once the introducer assembly is securely placed within the vein, the guidewire and dilator are withdrawn simultaneously. At this point, the stopcock, if utilized, should be open to allow the tubing to fill with blood, and then connected to the desired IV set. These connections should be screwed securely together to prevent inadvertent loss of continuity of the system and the attendant risk of either venous air embolism or bleeding. Intravenous fluids should be continuously run through the introducer to assure patency and the introducer should be securely affixed to the skin. Multiple types of introducers are available depending on the specific requirement. The introducer is typically 1 French greater in diameter than the catheter that will be inserted through it; that is, the common 8½ French introducer will accept a 7 or 7½ French pulmonary artery catheter. The technique for floating a pulmonary artery (Swan–Ganz) catheter is covered in Sections 5.3.3 and 5.3.4.

23.8 **Complications and their prevention**

Complications related to central venous catheterization generally fall into two categories:

- complications occurring during central venous catheter insertion: mechanical complications (*Table 23.3*);
- complications occurring during the indwelling phase of central venous catheterization: septic complications.

23.8.1 Septic complications, catheters and antibiotic coating

Septic complications related to central venous catheterization typically occur after the catheter has been in place for greater than 72 h and are rare before 48 h. Catheter-related blood stream infection occurs in up to 6% of catheterized patients[21-23]. This complication is more likely in patients who are catheterized for longer lengths of time and are more severely ill, with multiple comorbidities and/or therapy with total parenteral nutrition through the central venous catheter. Frequent routine changes of the central venous catheters have not been shown to decrease the incidence of this complication. Antibiotic-impregnated or -coated catheters, on the other hand, have been shown to result in statistically significant decreases in catheter-related blood steam infections, and may be a valuable technique for those patients with expected prolonged duration of catheterization[24-26]. In general, central venous catheters

---

Table 23.3 Major complications of central venous catheterization

	IJV	SCV	Femoral
Arterial puncture	5–10%	1–4%	7%
Pneumothorax	Rare	2–5%	0%
DVT	—	—	Up to 20% esp. pediatrics

	IJV or SCV
Tip malposition within heart	~50% (20 cm CVC) <4% (CVC inserted to 15 cm)

Miscellaneous complications

IJV	SCV
Tracheal puncture	Thoracic duct laceration
Perforation of endotracheal tube cuff	Phrenic nerve paralysis
Horner's syndrome	Brachial plexus palsy
Vocal cord paralysis	
Cerebral vascular accident	

Both

Air embolism
Myocardial injury with tamponade
Hydromediastinum
Catheter embolism
Subcutaneous fluid collection
Fatal exsanguination
Dysrhythmias
Compression of adjacent structures by hematoma
Others

CVC, central venous catheter.

should be removed once they are no longer needed.

23.8.2 Guidewire exchanges

Guidewire exchanges of catheters are reserved for those patients when the risk of venopuncture is thought to be significant (i.e. in patients with severe coagulopathy or serious problems with the alveolar–arterial oxygen gradient who would not tolerate the complications of a pneumothorax). In these circumstances, we recommend that as part of the guidewire exchange procedure, quantitative culture of the catheter tip is obtained. If the culture ultimately grows out greater than 15 colony forming units, the tract through which the catheter was exchanged is considered to be contaminated and central access should then be moved to a new site[22,23]. However, for those catheters with less than 15 colony forming units of growth using this technique, the newly inserted catheter may remain in place and the patient has avoided venipuncture.

For pulmonary artery catheters, there is no consensus on the length of the time that these catheters may remain in place. On the basis of a fairly exhaustive review of current literature, the CDC (Centers for Disease Control) recommends that these catheters be replaced every 5 days[22,23]. It is our experience that the majority of relevant information that can be uncovered with pulmonary artery catheterization has been incorporated into the treatment plan before 5 days, and that pulmonary artery catheterization beyond 5 days is rarely necessary.

23.8.3 Guidewire exchange technique

Sterile guidewire exchanges can be tricky and require a fair amount of expertise. The procedure is as follows:

1. A sterile field is prepared by first scrubbing the skin and then saturating the visible parts of the catheter with an antiseptic solution. The solution should be allowed to soak on the catheter and skin for at least 5 min.

2. The catheter, now disconnected from any IV tubing, is now slowly withdrawn from the skin approximately 4–6 cm. The catheter is now firmly grasped at the skin level or clamped, and cut with sterile scissors approximately 2–3 cm above the skin. This will assure that the part of the catheter being cut was either intravenous or below the dermis. The catheter is cut at a sharp angle to allow easy identification of its internal lumens. The proximal portion of the catheter is discarded and the guidewire is now inserted through the cut portion of the catheter back into the vein. Close attention to detail is important so that the remaining catheter fragment will not be pushed intravenously.

3. Once the guidewire is in place, the catheter can then be withdrawn, leaving the guidewire in an intravenous location. Further catheterization can proceed as previously described.

23.8.4 Catheter malposition

Malposition of central venous catheter tips is the most common complication following central venous catheterization. A review of the practice at five medical centers involving 350 catheterizations showed the incidence of malpositioned tips within the right atrium to be greater than 50%[7]. Using an ECG-guided technique, we were able to eliminate this complication. Simply choosing an insertion length of 15 cm regardless of the site of either internal jugular or subclavian vein catheterization will further reduce the incidence of this complication to less than 5%[8]. Catheter tip position within the right atrium may result in fatal cardiac tamponade typically from the intravenous solution. The Food and Drug Administration (FDA) and manufacturer's guidelines recommend placing the catheter in the superior vena cava above the heart[27,28].

Superior vena caval injuries may also occur especially for those catheters that contact the superior vena cava at high angles of incidence[29,30]. These injuries often require thoracotomy drainage of the pleural space and possibly repair of the blood vessel itself. Placing catheters from the right internal jugular vein virtually eliminates the possibility of this complication. Multiple other malpositioned catheters have been described, although if intravenous these rarely cause significant problems. The primary purpose of the post-procedure chest film is to check for catheter course and tip location.

23.8.5 Dysrhythmias

Dysrhythmias are fairly common during central venous catheterization, especially during pulmonary artery catheter insertion[31–33]. This is thought to be due to mechanical irritation of the right ventricle and rarely causes significant hemodynamic morbidity as it is almost terminated by either advancing the catheter into the pulmonary artery or withdrawing it back to the right atrium. This complication may also occur during guidewire insertion or during placement of the central venous catheter inadvertently within the heart.

23.8.6 Pneumothorax

Pneumothorax is the most significant common complication following clavicular approaches to the central circulation. It is reported to occur up to 5% of the time depending on which series is reviewed[34,35]. Pneumothorax is a rare complication of internal jugular vein cannulation. Of 1338 cases of IV venipuncture reported in large series, the overall pleural complication rate was less than 0.1%[7]. Numerous unique and rare complications have been reported to occur with both internal jugular and subclavian vein catheterizations, usually resulting from laceration of adjacent anatomic structures, vessel dissection or injury caused by vessel dilators or errantly placed catheters.

23.8.7 Ultrasound guidance

Numerous data reported over the past 10 years have shown that ultrasound localization of the internal jugular vein results in faster and safer central venous catheterization[15,36,37]. The primary advantage of the ultrasound technique is real-time visualization of the vessel to be cannulated. Although we do not use this technique in all patients, we strongly recommend it for those patients in whom the catheterization is anticipated to be difficult because of anatomic variations (i.e. obesity, short neck) or the risk of a complication related to inadvertent puncture of adjacent structures are high (i.e. arterial puncture in a patient with serious coagulopathy or pleural injury for patients with large alveolar–arterial oxygen gradients). Early recognition of complications in therapy is mandatory for anyone putting in a central venous catheter. Although not considered the standard of care at this time, ultrasound guidance is now recognized to improve patient safety[38,39]. We have found ultrasound techniques extremely useful, especially as part of our training program in vascular access for housestaff.

References

1. **Bedford, R.F.** (1977) Radial artery function following percutaneous cannulation with 18 and 20 gauge catheters. *Anesthesiology* **47**: 37.

2. **Weiss, B.M. and Gattiker, R.I.** (1986) Complications during and following radial artery cannulation: A prospective study. *Intensive Care Med.* **12**: 424.

3. **Ventec** (2000) Stat lock. Catheter Securement Device. Ventec International, Inc., San Diego, CA.

4. **Kaye, J., Heald, G.R., Morton, J.,** *et al.* (2001) Patency of radial arterial catheters. *Am. J. Crit. Care* **10**: 104–111.

5. **Joynt, G.M., Kew, J., Gomersall, C.D.,** *et al.* (2000) Deep venous thrombosis caused by femoral venous catheter in critically ill adult patients. *Chest* **117**: 178–183.

6. **Parsa, M.H., Taboraf.** (1986) Central Venous Access in critically ill patients in the Emergency Department. Emergency Department management of critical illness. *Emer. Med. Clin. North. Am.* **4**: 709–717.

7. **Durbec, O., Viviand, X., Potie, F.,** *et al.* (1997) Lower extremity deep vein thrombosis: A prospective, randomized, controlled trial in comatose or sedated patients undergoing femoral vein catheterization. *Crit. Care Med.* **25**: 1982–1985.

8. **McGee, W.T. and Moriarty, K.P.** (1996) Accurate placement of central venous catheters

using a 16-cm catheter. *J. Intensive Care Med.* **11:** 19–22.

9. McGee, W.T., Ackerman, B.L., Rouben, L.R., *et al.* (1993) Accurate placement of central venous catheters: A prospective, randomized, multicenter trial. *Crit. Care Med.* **21:** 1118–1123.

10. McGee, W.T. and Martin, R.T. (1999) Safe placement of central venous catheters. *Crit. Care Med.* **27:** A47.

11. Kanter, R.K., Zimmerman, J.J., Strauss, R.H., *et al.* (1986) Central venous catheter insertion by femoral vein: Safety and effectiveness for the pediatric patient. *Pediatrics* **77:** 842–847.

12. Daily, R.H. (1985) Femoral vein cannulation: A review. *J. Emerg. Med.* **2:** 367–372.

13. Newman, B.M., Jewett, T.C., Karp, M.O., *et al.* (1986) Percutaneous central venous catheterization in children. First line choice for venous access. *J. Ped. Surg.* **21:** 685–688.

14. Williams, J.F., Seneff, M., Friedman, B.C., *et al.* (1991) Use of femoral venous catheters in critically ill adults. Prospective study. *Crit. Care Med.* **19:** 550–553.

15. Durbec, O. and Viviand, X. (1997) A prospective evaluation of the use of femoral venous catheters in critically ill adults. *Crit. Care Med.* **25:** 1986–1989.

16. Mallory, D.L., McGee, W.T., Shawker, T.H., *et al.* (1990) Ultrasound guidance improves the success rate of internal jugular vein cannulation: A prospective, randomized trial. *Chest* **98:** 157–160.

17. Mallory, D.L., Shawker, T.H., Evans, G., *et al.* (1990) Effects of clinical maneuvers on sonographically determined internal jugular vein size during venous cannulation. *Crit. Care Med.* **18:** 1269–1273.

18. Brinkman, A.J. and Costley, D.O. (1973) Internal jugular puncture. *JAMA* **223:** 182.

19. Johnson, F.E. (1978) Internal jugular vein catheterization prospective study. *N.Y. State J. Med.* **78:** 2168.

20. Eisenhauer, E.D., Derveloy, R.J. and Hastings, P.R. (1982) Prospective evaluation of central venous pressure (CVP) catheters in a large city–country hospital. *Ann. Surg.* **196:** 560.

21. Sznajder, J.I., Zvebil, F.R., Bitterman, H., *et al.* (1986) Central vein catheterization failure and complication rates by three percutaneous approaches. *Arch. Intern. Med.* **146:** 259.

22. Connors, A.F., Speroff, T., Dawson, N.V., *et al.* (1996) The effectiveness of right heart catheterization in the initial care of critically ill patients. *JAMA* **276:** 889–918.

23. The Hospital Infection Control Practices Advisory Committee (1996) Guideline for prevention of intravascular device-related infections. Part I. Intravascular device-related infections: An overview (Review). *Am. J. Infection Control* **24:** 262–277.

24. **The Hospital Infection Control Practices Advisory Committee** (1996) Guideline for prevention of intravascular device-related infections. Part II. Recommendations for the prevention of nosocomial intravascular device-related infections (Review). *Am. J. Infection Control* **24:** 277–293.

25. Maki, D.G., Stolz, S.M., Wheeler, S., *et al.* (1997) Prevention of central venous catheter-related blood stream infection by use of an anti-septic-impregnated catheter: A randomized, controlled trial. *Ann. Intern. Med.* **127:** 257–266.

26. Marin, M.G., Lee, J.C. and Skurnick, J.H. (2000) Prevention of nosocomial blood stream infections: Effectiveness of antimicrobial-impregnated and heparin-bonded central venous catheters. *Crit. Care Med.* **28:** 3332–3338.

27. Darouiche, R.P., Raad, I.I., Heard, S.O., *et al.* (1999) A comparison of two antimicrobial-impregnated central venous catheters. *N. Engl. J. Med.* **340:** 1–8.

28. **Food and Drug Administration** (1989) Precautions necessary with central venous catheters. FDA Task Force. *FDA Drug Bull.* July: 15–16.

29. **Arrow** (1989) Arrow educational advisory and cautions included as a package insert with all CVC kits. Arrow, Reading, PA.

30. Tocino, I.M. and Watanabe, A. (1986) Impending catheter perforation of superior vena cava: Radiographic recognition. *Am. J. Roentgenol.* **146:** 487–490.

31. Ellis, L.M., Vogel, S.B. and Copeland, E.M. (1989) Central venous catheter vascular erosions. *Ann. Surg.* **209:** 475–478.

32. Sprung, C., Pozen, R., Rozanski, J., *et al.* (1982) Advanced ventricular arrhythmias during bedside pulmonary artery catheterization. *Am. J. Med.* **72:** 203.

33. Iberti, T., Ernest, B., Gruppi, L., *et al.* (1985) Ventricular arrhythmias during pulmonary artery catheterization in the intensive care unit. *Am. J. Med.* **78:** 451.

34. Patel, C., Laboy, V., Venus, B., *et al.* (1986) Acute complications of pulmonary artery catheter insertion in critically ill patients. *Crit. Care Med.* **14:** 195.

35. Feliciano, D.V., Mattox, K.L., Graham, J.M., *et al.* (1979) Major complications of percutaneous subclavian vein catheters. *Am. J. Surg.* **173:** 184.

36. McGee, W.T. and Mallory, D.L. (1988) Cannulation of the internal and external

jugular veins. In: *Problems in Critical Care: Vascular Cannulation, Vol. 2* (eds R.R. Kirby and R.W. Taylor) J.B. Lippincott, Philadelphia, PA, pp. 217–241.

37. **Randolph, A.G., Cook, D.J., Gonzalez, C.A. and Pribble, C.G.** (1996) Ultrasound guidance for placement of central venous catheters: A meta-analysis of the literature. *Crit. Care Med.* **24:** 2053–2058.

38. **Gilbert, T.B., Seneff, M.G. and Becker, R.B.** (1995) Facilitation of internal jugular venous cannulation using an audio-guided Doppler ultrasound vascular access device: Results from a prospective, dual-center, randomized, crossover clinical study. *Crit. Care Med.* **23:** 60–65.

39. **Agency for Healthcare Research and Quality** (2001) Making Health Care Safer—A Critical Analysis of Patient Safety Practices; Summary. Evidence Report/Technology Assessment: Number 43. AHRQ Publications, Rockville, MD.

Index